Complementary and Alternative Therapies in the Aging Population

Complementary and Alternative Therapies in the Aging Population

Edited by
Ronald Ross Watson

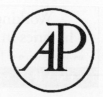

AMSTERDAM • BOSTON • HEIDELBERG • LONDON
NEW YORK • OXFORD • PARIS • SAN DIEGO
SAN FRANCISCO • SINGAPORE • SYDNEY • TOKYO
Academic Press is an imprint of Elsevier

Academic Press is an imprint of Elsevier
525 B Street, Suite 1900, San Diego, CA 92101-4495, USA
30 Corporate Drive, Suite 400, Burlington, MA 01803, USA
32 Jamestown Road, London NW1 7BY, UK
Radarweg 29, PO Box 211, 1000 AE Amsterdam, The Netherlands

Notice
No responsibility is assumed by the publisher for any injury and/or damage to persons
or property as a matter of products liability, negligence or otherwise, or from any use
or operation of any methods, products, instructions or ideas contained in the material
herein. Because of rapid advances in the medical sciences, in particular, independent
verification of diagnoses and drug dosages should be made.

British Library Cataloguing in Publication Data
A catalogue record for this book is available from the British Library

Library of Congress Cataloging-in-Publication Data
A catalog record for this book is available from the Library of Congress

ISBN: 978-0-12-374228-5

For information on all Academic Press publications
visit our web site at books.elsevier.com

Typeset by Charon Tec Ltd., A Macmillan Company.
(www.macmillansolutions.com)

Printed and bound in Great Britain by
CPI Antony Rowe, Chippenham and Eastbourne

Transferred to Digital Printing, 2010

Working together to grow
libraries in developing countries

www.elsevier.com | www.bookaid.org | www.sabre.org

ELSEVIER   BOOK AID
              International   Sabre Foundation

Contents

Chapter 6 *Ginkgo biloba* Extract in Prevention of Age-Associated Diseases in Elderly Population
Yuan Luo and Zhiming Cao

Chapter 9   **Bamboo Extract in the Prevention of Diabetes and Breast Cancer**   159

Jun Panee

Chapter 10   **Cranberry and Other Dietary Supplements for the Treatment of Urinary Tract Infections in Aging Women**   179

Lynn Stothers

Chapter 26   Health Benefits of Traditional
                   Culinary and Medicinal
                   Mediterranean Plants   541
                   *Stephanie C. Degner, Andreas J.
                   Papoutsis and Donato F. Romagnolo*

Chapter 27   Quercetin: A Potential
                   Complementary and Alternative
                   Cancer Therapy   563
                   *Thilakavathy Thangasamy,
                   Sivanandane Sittadjody and Randy Burd*

Preface

Nutrient requirements for optimum health and function of aging physiological systems often are quite distinct from young ones. Recognition and understanding of the special nutrition problems of the aged are being intensively researched and tested, especially due to the increases in the elderly in the general population. In developed countries, economic restrictions and physical inactivity during aging can significantly reduce food intakes, contributing to nutritional stresses and needs. Many disease entities and cancers are found with higher frequency in the aged. Cancer, trauma, or infectious disease can alter intakes and/or requirements for various nutrients. Thus specific foods and nutritional supplementation may be helpful in treatment of aged adults including cancer patients. Many adults and elderly are using foods and nutrients well above the recommended daily allowance, which may not always be needed for optimal health. To some extent, treatment of these conditions with diet or nutritional supplements is a unique problem in the aged. The effects of the aging processes, changes in social status, and financial conditions significantly affect the approaches to treatment and study of nutritional and health problem in the aging adult and the elderly. Increasing numbers of older adults and elderly in the population require detailed study and directed research to understand their health problems, using novel nutraceutical and complementary and alternative medicine (CAM) therapies. Research continues to show that non-nutritional materials in the diet or as supplements can have important health promotion benefits. Those that are antioxidants act, in part, by protecting antioxidant vitamins. However much needs to be learned about benefits and risks of nutriceuticals which have a variety of biological activities in their own right. Therefore botanical extracts and components will be reviewed for their benefits to seniors.

The elderly are frequently using various non-traditional and often unproven CAM therapies, beyond nutritional and nutraceutical supplements. Therefore a variety of physical and psychosocial treatments will be evaluated by experts in CAM research for their benefits/risks and the extent of scientific testing as focused for an aging population.

Diet and nutrition are vital keys to controlling morbidity and mortality from chronic diseases affecting humankind. The multitude of biomolecules in dietary plants, including their purified extracts used as supplements, plays a crucial role in health maintenance. This book brings together experts working on the different aspects of supplementation, foods, and plant extracts, in health promotion and disease prevention. Their expertise and experience provide the most current knowledge to promote future research. Dietary habits need to be altered, for most people. Therefore, the conclusions and recommendations from the various chapters will provide a basis for change as well as application of new extracts and botanicals in health promotion.

Plant extracts are now a multi-billion-dollar business, built upon extremely little research data. For example the US Food and Drug Administration is pushing this industry, with the support of Congress, to base its claims and products on scientific research. While vegetables have traditionally been seen to be good sources of vitamins, the roles of other constituents have only recently become more widely recognized. Most of the expert reviews define and support the actions of bioflavonoids, antioxidants, and similar materials that are part of dietary vegetables, dietary supplements, and nutraceuticals. As non-vitamin minerals with health-promoting activities, nutraceuticals are an increasing body of materials and extracts that may have biological activity. Therefore, their role is a major emphasis, along with discussions of which agents may be the active components.

The goal of this book is to get experts to explore the ways nutraceutical supplements or foods, and herbal medicines prevent disease and promote health. The overall goal is to provide the most current, concise, scientific appraisal of the efficacy of key foods and alternative medicines in dietary plants in preventing and improving the quality of life with special reference to adults and aging adults.

Acknowledgments

The encouragement and research support of Mr. H. B. and Joscyln Wallace through research grants from the Wallace Research Foundation to Ronald Ross Watson was vital to the book's conception and publication. The Wallace Research Foundation has been important in supporting research on nutrition and health promotion in the aged for decades, leading to this book and the previous three editions.

The work of editorial assistant, Bethany L. Stevens, in communicating with authors, working with the manuscripts and the publisher was critical to the successful completion of the book and is much appreciated. Her daily responses to queries and collection of manuscripts and documents were extremely helpful. Support for her work was graciously provided by the National Health Research Institute. This was part of their efforts to educate scientists and the lay public on the health and economic benefits of nutrients in the diet as well as supplements. Finally Nguyen T. Nga of the Arizona Health Sciences library was instrumental in finding the authors and their addresses in the early stages of the book's preparation.

Ronald R. Watson, Ph.D., has edited 65 books, including four on the effects of various dietary nutrients in heart disease. He initiated and directed the Specialized Alcohol Research Center at the University of Arizona College of Medicine for 6 years. The main theme of this National Institute of Alcohol Abuse and Alcoholism Center grant was to understand the role of ethanol-induced immunosuppression with increased oxidation and nutrient loss on disease and disease resistance in animals. For 8 years he directed with Douglas F. Larson several NIH grants studying the effects of retroviral-induced immune dysfunction on cardiac structure and function in a model of AIDS.

Dr. Watson is a member of several national and international societies concerned with nutrition, immunology, and cancer research. He has directed a program studying ways to slow aging using nutritional supplements, funded by the Wallace Genetics Foundation for 30 years. Currently, he is the co-principal investigator on an NIH grant studying the role of immune dysfunction to exacerbate heart disease. He has recently completed studies using complementary and alternative medicines in clinical trials. Dr. Watson and Dr. Larson are co-principal investigators on an NIH grant from the National Center on Complementary and Alternative Medicine to study cytokine dysregulation in cardiac remodeling. Dr. Watson has been funded for a decade to study Pycnogenol, a dietary supplement to reduce diseases of aging, hypertension, osteoarthritis, and diabetes.

Dr. Watson attended the University of Idaho, but graduated from Brigham Young University in Provo, UT, with a degree in chemistry in 1966. He completed his Ph.D. degree in 1971 in biochemistry at Michigan State University. His postdoctoral education was completed at the Harvard School of Public Health in Nutrition and Microbiology, including a 2-year postdoctoral research experience in immunology. He was an Assistant Professor of Immunology and did research at the University of Mississippi Medical Center in Jackson from 1973 to 1974. He was an Assistant Professor of Microbiology and Immunology at the Indiana University Medical School from 1974 to 1978 and an Associate Professor at Purdue University in the Department of Food and Nutrition from 1978 to 1982. In 1982, he joined the faculty at the University of Arizona in the Department of Family and Community Medicine. He is also a professor in the University of Arizona's College of Public Health. He has published 450 research papers and review chapters.

Chapter 1

Botanical and Marine Oils for Treatment of Arthritis

Robert B. Zurier and Ronald G. Rossetti

Department of Medicine, Division of Rheumatology, University of Massachusetts Medical School, Worcester, MA, USA

Keywords: *Fish oil, botanical oil, arthritis, inflammation, fatty acids, prostaglandins*

Abundant experimental evidence supports the view that prostaglandins, thromboxanes, and leukotrienes, collectively termed eicosanoids, participate in development and regulation of immunological and inflammatory responses. Because essential fatty acids are precursors to eicosanoids, and because essential fatty acids are important determinants of cell membrane structure and function, they influence immune responses. Diseases such as rheumatoid arthritis (RA), and systemic lupus erythematosus (SLE), characterized by abnormal immune responses, persistent inflammation, and tissue injury, may therefore be amenable to control by dietary means. Indeed, considerable public interest has been provoked recently by treatment of a variety of disorders, including RA, with plant seed and fish oils. The established and potential uses of unsaturated fatty acids for treatment of inflammatory arthritis and related conditions are examined in this chapter.

Essential fatty acids are "essential" [1] not only because of their physiologic importance, but because they must be derived in either full or partially elaborated form from the diet. Thus, these acids may be classified as vitamins (indeed, they were once called vitamin F). Two groups of fatty acids are essential to the body: the omega-6 (*n*6) series, derived from linoleic acid (18:2 *n*6) and the omega-3 series, derived from α-linolenic acid (18:3 *n*3). In these notations, 18 is the number of carbon atoms in a molecule, the second number is the number of double carbon–carbon bonds (degree of unsaturation), and the number after the "*n*" is the position of the first double bond starting from the methyl (omega) end of the fatty acid chain. The metabolic sequences of the two fatty acid series are shown in Fig. 1.1. Fatty acids provide energy, are an integral part of cell membranes, and are precursors for the eicosanoids. Alteration of the eicosanoid profile by administration of fatty acid precursors other than arachidonic acid is one approach to modulation of host defense.

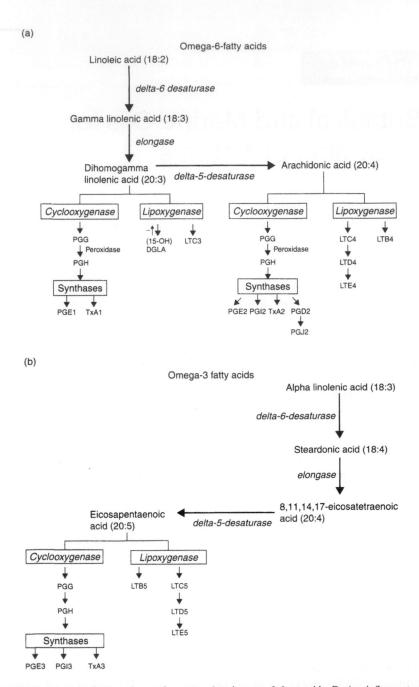

FIGURE 1.1 Metabolic pathways for omega-6 and omega-3 fatty acids. During inflammatory responses, cells are activated to release arachidonic acid or EPA. Activity of the bifunctional enzyme COX oxidizes the precursor fatty acid to PGG and a subsequent peroxidase reaction yields PGH. Then under the influence of terminal synthases, prostaglandins, thromboxanes, and prostacyclins are formed.

Although changes in eicosanoid production due to alteration of fatty acid intake formed the basis of the current hypothesis for antiinflammatory and immunoregulatory effects of this type of treatment, it is likely that the precursor fatty acids themselves influence immune responses. Studies in animals and humans have shown that changes in essential fatty acid intake alter the fatty acid composition of cell membranes [2]. For example, in essential fatty acid deficiency, deprivation of linoleic acid leads to deficiency of arachidonic acid and impairment of prostaglandin synthesis. Essential fatty acid deficiency causes many pathologic changes, but it also reduces the severity of inflammation in experimental animal models. Fasting also has a salutary effect on symptoms of patients with RA [3]. Because neither induction of essential fatty acid deficiency nor fasting are likely to be popular treatments, it follows that it would be more prudent to modify or supplement, rather than delete, lipid intake.

The extraordinary rapidity with which platelets adhere to damaged tissue, aggregate, and release potent biologically active materials, suggests that the platelet is well suited to be a cellular trigger for the inflammatory response [4]. Thus, experiments directed at suppression of thromboxane synthesis, enhancement of prostacyclin production, and inhibition of platelet aggregation, have been conducted in an effort to limit inflammatory responses. Fish oil lipids, rich in eicosapentaenoic acid (EPA; 20:5 n3), inhibit formation of the cyclooxygenase (COX) products thromboxane A_2 (TXA$_2$) and prostaglandin E_2 (PGE$_2$) derived from arachidonic acid. The newly formed thromboxane A_3, has much less ability than TXA$_2$ to constrict blood vessels and aggregate platelets. In addition, production of prostaglandin I_2 (PGI$_2$, prostacyclin) by endothelial cells is not reduced appreciably by increased EPA content, and the physiologic activity of newly synthesized PGI$_3$ is added to that of PGI$_2$ [5]. Moreover, diets enriched in fish oil reduce production of the potent mediator of inflammation leukotriene B_4 (LTB$_4$) via 5-lipoxygenase in stimulated neutrophils and monocytes, and induce the appearance of EPA-derived LTB$_5$, which is far less biologically active than LTB$_4$ [6, 7].

Evidence obtained from experiments *in vitro* and *in vivo* in small animals and in humans suggests that other novel fatty acids may be safe and effective antiinflammatory and immunomodulatory agents. For example, certain botanical lipids, notably those extracted from seeds of the evening primrose and borage plants, contain relatively large amounts of gammalinolenic acid (GLA; 18:3 n6). This fatty acid is converted rapidly to dihomogammalinolenic acid (DGLA; 20:3 n6), the fatty acid precursor of the monoenoic prostaglandins, such as prostaglandin E_1 (PGE$_1$). In humans, the delta-5-desaturase that converts DGLA to arachidonic acid is sluggish. Thus, concentrations of arachidonate do not increase appreciably in patients treated long term with GLA. DGLA competes with arachidonate for oxidative enzymes, thereby reducing synthesis of COX products derived from arachidonate. In addition, DGLA cannot be converted to inflammatory leukotrienes by 5-lipoxygenase. Instead, it is converted to 15-hydroxy-DGLA (Fig. 1.1), which has the additional virtue of suppressing 5-lipoxygenase activity [8].

Enrichment with DGLA of human synovial cells (which line the joint space, and proliferation of which leads to cartilage degradation and bone erosion in patients with RA) in culture leads to a marked reduction of PGE_2 synthesis, a substantial increase in PGE_1 production, and a reduction in interleukin-1β (IL-1β) induced synovial cell proliferation. Addition to cultures of arachidonic acid (which increases PGE_2 substantially) or EPA does not modify synovial cell proliferation. The antiproliferative effect of DGLA is prevented by indomethacin [9]. Although PGE compounds are clearly local mediators of inflammation [10], evidence from both *in vitro* and *in vivo* experiments indicates that they can also suppress diverse effector systems of inflammation [11, 12]. In addition, PGE can both enhance and diminish cellular and humoral immune responses, observations that reinforce a view of these compounds as regulators of cell function. Defective regulation of inflammatory responses, or disordered immune mechanisms, or both, are probably central to the pathologic processes encountered in rheumatic diseases such as RA and SLE. PGE_1, largely by virtue of its ability to influence cellular cyclic nucleotides and signal transduction pathways, appears to be an important regulator of cell function and, therefore, potentially able to influence the function of those cells that participate in tissue injury in these diseases. A regulatory effect of PGE is not without precedent. For example, PGE inhibits the release of noradrenaline from the spleen in response to sympathetic nerve stimulation, and PGE is released from the spleen when it contracts in response to sympathetic nerve stimulation [13]. Thus, by a feedback mechanism, the contracting smooth muscle can reduce the stimulus that is leading to its contraction. PGE release may therefore be a defense mechanism aimed at minimizing potential injury. Certainly PGE compounds serve to protect gastric mucosa and kidney function. Suppression by PGE_1 of leukocyte effector functions and of mediator release suggests that PGE_1 has antiinflammatory effects.

The role of prostaglandins in the inflammatory process is not as well defined as once supposed, because the stable prostaglandins PGE and PGI_2 have antiinflammatory and inflammatory effects [14]. PGJ and lipoxins appear to protect against runaway inflammatory responses. Even LTB4 appears capable of modulating inflammation and immune responses [15]. The observation that PGE_1 inhibits platelet aggregation led to the notion that COX products of arachidonic acid metabolism might have antiinflammatory activity. As it becomes more clear that nonsteroidal antiinflammatory drugs (NSAIDS) have antiinflammatory effects other than interference with COX production and subsequent prostaglandin inhibition [16], the potential protective effects of prostaglandins are being considered.

Other eicosanoids also serve to counter inflammation: PGJ_2, formed from the dehydration of PGD_2, appears to function as a brake on the inflammatory response [17]. Lipoxins are a new class of eicosanoids, which arise from the sequential action of 5- and 15-lipoxygenases. They serve as stop signals in that they prevent leukocyte-mediated tissue injury, thereby facilitating resolution of inflammation [18]. Human endothelial cells treated with aspirin *in vitro* convert EPA to antiinflammatory lipoxins. These novel compounds are also found in inflammatory exudates from animals administered aspirin and fish oil [19].

Thus, it will take exquisitely selective alteration of particular points in the arachidonic acid cascade (as prostaglandin and thromboxane synthases, or eicosanoid receptors) to modify it to the advantage of the host. The selective COX-2 inhibitors were an attempt to do that. It is clear that these agents are equivalent in efficacy to the traditional NSAIDs and that they reduce the more serious gastrointestinal events (ulcer formation, bleeding, and perforation). However, COX-2 is upregulated in stimulated endothelial cells [20]. Thus, selective COX-2 inhibition results in suppression of PGI_2 synthesis by these cells. Because platelets lack COX-2, platelet thromboxane production is spared by selective COX-2 inhibition, and the platelet–blood vessel wall balance mediated between the effects of thromboxane (platelet aggregation, vasoconstriction) and PGI_2 (inhibition of platelet aggregation, vasodilation) is tilted toward promotion of thrombosis. These biochemical truths did indeed translate to the clinical findings that selective COX-2 inhibition is associated with an increased incidence of acute myocardial infarction (coronary artery thrombosis) [21].Thus, botanical and marine oils, which protect the gastric mucosa and counter thrombosis, should find a place in the armamentarium of anti-inflammatory agents.

PGE_1 has remained a bit of an orphan among the eicosanoids, mainly because of a long-held notion that not enough is produced by human cells to be of use, and that its biological effects are no different from those of PGE_2 and PGI_2. Contrary to popular belief, however, PGE_1 is found in physiologically important amounts in humans. Lost in the vast literature on the "arachidonic acid cascade" are the early observations of Bygdeman and Samuelsson [22], who found (using bioassay) the concentration of PGE_1 in human seminal plasma ($16\,\mu g/ml$) to be higher than PGE_2 ($13\,\mu g/ml$), PGE_3 ($3\,\mu g/ml$), $PGF_1\alpha$ ($2\,\mu g/ml$), and $PGF_2\alpha$ ($12\,\mu g/ml$). Furthermore, Karim *et al.* [23] found PGE_1 to be the sole PGE in human thymus. Prostaglandin immunoassays usually do not distinguish between PGE_1 and PGE_2. To identify PGE_1, PGs must first be separated by thin layer or high performance liquid chromatography. When such methods have been used, PGE_1 has been identified consistently in platelets, leukocytes, macrophages, vas deferens, oviducts, uterus, heart, and skin [24]. In addition, concentrations in human tissue of the PGE_1 precursor fatty acid DGLA are not trivial, and are about one-fourth the concentration of arachidonic acid [25]. It is known now that PGE_1, PGE_2, and PGI_2 have separate receptors on cells [26, 27]. Although the biologic activities of corresponding members of the monoenoic (PGE_1) and dienoic (PGE_2) prostaglandins are in many ways qualitatively similar, in other respects, they differ markedly. For example, PGE_1 inhibits aggregation of human platelets *in vitro* whereas PGE_2 does not influence this activity [28]. Also, PGE_1 is more effective than PGE_2 in increasing concentrations of cyclic AMP in human synovial cells in culture, and in suppressing synovial cell proliferation [9]. In addition, PGE_1 relaxes and PGE_2 contracts guinea pig tracheal muscle. More striking are the antagonistic effects of PGE_1 (vasodilation) and PGE_2 (vasoconstriction) on bovine coronary and human chorionic plate arteries [29, 30]. In fact, PGE_1 prevents PGE_2 induced constriction of chorionic plate arteries. Many effects of PGE_1 *in vitro* are seen at concentrations of $10^{-9} - 10^{-13}$ M [31]. Subcutaneous injection of PGE_1 and oral administration of a 15-methylPGE$_1$ analog (at 1/50 the subcutaneous dose) suppress acute and chronic inflammation in a variety of experimental animal models [32].

Much information about the effect of PGE_1 on immune responses derives from studies of immune complex-induced nephritis. A striking protective effect of PGE_1 in murine lupus is associated with increased expression of the characteristically suppressed cell-mediated immune responses [33], reversal of abnormal development of prethymic cells [34], and enhanced functional maturity of thymocytes [35]. PGE_1 treatment does not alter circulating antinuclear antibodies or antibodies to double-stranded DNA in this model; However, PGE_1 treatment can have selective effects on humoral immune responses. An important antigen–antibody system in NZB/NZW F_1 hybrid (lupus) mice includes the major envelope glycoprotein (gp70) of endogenous retroviruses and the corresponding antibody. Large amounts of both are deposited with complement in diseased kidneys and circulate as immune complexes. NZB/NZW mice treated with PGE_1 have far lower levels than untreated controls of circulating gp70 immune complexes [36]. MRL/lpr mice (a lupus model) respond similarly, but BXSB mice maintain high levels of circulating gp70 immune complexes and do not benefit from PGE_1 treatment. PGE_1 treatment does not change antigen formation or quantity; rather, treatment appears to selectively inhibit the humoral response to xenotropic viral gp70. In MRL/lpr mice, PGE_1 suppresses IgG1 antibody and does not affect IgG2 production [36, 37]. IgG2 is the major subclass of anti-DNA antibodies in these animals; hence anti-DNA antibody levels are not influenced, but anti-gp70 levels are reduced by PGE_1 treatment. Further evidence for a regulatory role of PGE on immune responses is furnished by the results of studies that document selective effects of physiologically relevant concentrations of PGE_2 on human B-cell responses. Thus, PGE_2 suppresses DNA and immunoglobulin synthesis, and proliferation of B-cells stimulated by *Staphylococcus aureus*, but has minimal effects on mitogen-stimulated B-cell DNA synthesis [37].

All things considered, it appears that physiologic concentrations of PGE_1 have a range of desirable effects, distinct from other prostaglandins that might be utilized therapeutically. Intravenous infusion can be used for short-term effects, as seen in studies in which intravenous PGE_1 improved renal function in patients with lupus nephritis [38–40]. Intravenous PGE_1 also suppresses human neutrophil activation [40]. When administered by itself in doses approved for human use, the PGE_1 analog misoprostol (given by mouth) does not exhibit immunosuppressive activity [41]. At the upper limit of these doses, misoprostol causes abdominal cramps and diarrhea. In addition, intravenous administration of PGE_1 causes hypotension, flushing tachydysrhythmias, diarrhea, and even shock. It would therefore seem prudent to take a different approach to PGE_1 therapy, first suggested by Willis [2], by providing PGE_1 precursors, such as GLA or DGLA. The extremely short half-lives of natural prostaglandins have a purpose: they allow moment-to-moment regulation of cell function in response to external stimuli and internal messengers. Enrichment of cells with DGLA should enable PGE_1 concentrations to be raised as needed without overriding the physiologic controls that modulate rapid changes in its synthesis and degradation. Hence, both $n6$ and $n3$ eicosanoid precursor lipids have antiinflammatory actions due to their ability to reduce synthesis of oxygenation products of arachidonic acid, which are potent mediators of inflammation.

CLINICAL TRIALS OF GLA THERAPY IN RA PATIENTS

A placebo-controlled study [42] indicated that 20 patients given GLA (360 mg/day) in the form of primrose seed oil for 12 weeks received no benefit from such therapy. It is of interest that although only three patients improved clinically, all but two of the remaining patients were able to complete the study without resorting to other NSAIDS. Thus, although the study was considered to be "negative," the results suggest that GLA might substitute for NSAID treatment. In a double-blind, placebo-controlled study done in Glasgow, Scotland [43], 16 patients received 450 mg/day GLA and 240 mg/day of EPA for 1 year. Patients were kept on their usual doses of NSAIDS, and their physicians were allowed to alter the dose according to clinical responses. Patients did not exhibit changes in objective measures of their disease activity, but over 90% of patients in the treatment group felt subjective improvement in their condition at 12 months, at which time 50% of treated patients had either stopped or reduced substantially the NSAID dose. In a study [44] designed to investigate the effect of GLA on leukocyte function, PGE_2 and LTB_4 production by stimulated leukocytes was reduced markedly, and 6 of 7 RA patients treated 12 weeks with 1.1 g/day GLA in the form of borage seed oil appeared to respond favorably; the study was not placebo-controlled. Unlike the other studies with smaller doses of GLA, RA patients given borage seed oil did exhibit reductions in the duration of painful morning stiffness and the number of tender and swollen joints. Brzeski *et al.* [45] did a 6-month study of 40 patients with RA who had evidence (endoscopic, radiographic, or clinical symptoms) suggestive of upper gastrointestinal lesions, presumably caused by NSAID use. The aim of the study was to determine whether patients given GLA would experience enough improvement in joint symptoms to allow reduction of the NSAID dose. Patients were given either 540 mg GLA/day or 6 g/day of olive oil. Morning stiffness was reduced significantly at both 3 and 6 months in the GLA group, and a reduction in pain and articular index at 6 months was seen in patients given olive oil. However, only 23% of the patients in the GLA group and 18% of patients in the olive oil group were able to reduce the NSAID dose. Although patients in this study had more severe RA than patients in the earlier study [43], none were treated with second line drugs. Beneficial effects of olive oil in RA have been reported [46]. Therefore, olive oil can no longer be considered an inert placebo. Also, individual variations in levels of delta-5-desaturase may alter the response to GLA. It is generally believed that humans have low levels of this enzyme, hence limited conversion of DGLA to arachidonic acid. However, a small but significant increase in serum arachidonate was reported in one group of RA patients who took 1.8 g/day GLA for 3 months [47]. Reduced plasma PGE_2 in these patients was associated with a good therapeutic response to GLA.

GLA treatment of RA was evaluated in a 24-week randomized, double-blind, placebo-controlled (cotton seed oil) trial [48]. Only patients with RA on a stable NSAID and/or low corticosteroid dose (<10 mg/day prednisone or equivalent) that was continued through the study period were allowed to participate. Treatment with GLA (1.4 g/day in borage seed oil) resulted in clinically important reductions in signs and symptoms of disease activity. In contrast, patients given placebo showed no change, or worsening, of disease. GLA reduced the number of tender joints by 36%, tender joint score by 45%, swollen joint count by 28%, and swollen joint score by 41%, whereas the placebo group did not show significant improvement in any measure. Overall clinical responses (more than 25% improvement in four measures) were also significantly better in the treatment group. Platelet counts (increases are associated with inflammation) were reduced significantly in the GLA group, but neither erythrocyte sedimentation rate nor rheumatoid factor changed appreciably in either group. In a larger study [49], 56 patients with active RA were randomized to treatment groups in a 6-month double-blind trial of GLA vs. placebo, followed by a 6-month single-blind trial during which all patients received GLA. Patients were treated with 2.8 g/day of GLA as the free fatty acid or with sunflower seed oil administered in identical capsules. Treatment with GLA for 6 months resulted in statistically significant and clinically relevant reductions in the signs and symptoms of disease activity in patients with RA. Overall meaningful responses were also better in the GLA treatment group (14 of 22 patients vs. 4 of 19 in the placebo group; $p = 0.015$). During the second 6 months, both groups (both on GLA) exhibited improvement in disease activity. Thus, patients taking GLA during the entire study showed progressive improvement during the second 6 months. In this group, 16 of 21 patients showed meaningful improvement at 12 months compared with study entry. The results indicate that GLA at doses used in this study is a well tolerated and effective treatment for active RA. GLA is available as a component of several plant seed oils, and is usually taken in far lower doses than were used in this last trial. It is not approved in the United States for the treatment of any condition, and should not be viewed as therapy for any disease. However, the clinical experience suggests that GLA can be an NSAID substitute. In addition, observations that DGLA suppresses synovial cell proliferation [9], and the results of the study just noted which indicate that RA patients are better after 12 months of GLA treatment than after 6 months, suggest that GLA might function as a so-called DMARD (disease modifying antirheumatic drug). Thus, controlled studies of longer duration on larger numbers of RA patients in which GLA is compared with more established "second line therapy," and which use radiographs to monitor disease progression, are warranted.

Fatty acid analysis of plasma or circulating cells was not used as a measure of compliance in these studies because the amount of GLA or DGLA present after administration of a known amount of GLA varies from person to person, and would not necessarily reflect the number of capsules of GLA ingested. However, it is important to know that plasma and cell concentrations of GLA and/or DGLA during GLA therapy can reach levels equivalent to concentrations of fatty acids which *in vitro* suppress lymphocyte activation and synovial cell proliferation. Plasma levels of GLA and DGLA were increased two- to fourfold in the GLA treated patients to concentrations which exceed those needed to exert effects *in vitro* [49]. Similarly, concentrations of GLA and DGLA in platelets increased as much as eightfold during GLA treatment. Lower doses of GLA used in previous studies (480 to 540 mg/day) were either not effective or reduced pain without effects on physical findings. In controlled clinical trials in which GLA was shown to benefit patients with atopic eczema [50], some patients responded brilliantly, others modestly. Clinical responses seemed to correlate with plasma levels of DGLA. Indeed, in a study in which benefit from GLA was not observed [51], plasma levels of DGLA did not rise. Thus clinical responses to GLA do appear to be dose-dependent.

CLINICAL TRIALS OF FISH OIL IN RA PATIENTS

Each of 12 randomized, placebo-controlled, double-blind trials of fish oil in RA documented clinical improvement, including reduced duration of morning stiffness, reduced number of tender joints, reduced joint pain, reduced time to fatigue, and increased grip strength. Those studies that monitored NSAID use suggest that fish oil treatment has an NSAID-sparing effect (reviewed in [52]). In another study, patients were required to consume less than 10 g/day *n*-6 polyunsaturated fatty acids (PUFAs), considering that a high *n*-6 PUFA intake might reduce the efficacy of fish oil. Patients received 40 mg/kg/day *n*-3 PUFAs (approximately 2–3 g/day) for 15 weeks. Patients in the treatment arm exhibited significant improvements in joint pain and swelling, morning stiffness, and overall health assessment [53]. A combination of EPA and GLA enriched oils exhibits synergy in reduction of synovitis in animal models [54], a result which suggests that a combination of GLA and EPA may be useful therapy for patients with RA. Indeed, treatment of RA patients with black currant seed oil, which contains both the *n*-3 fatty acid α-linolenic acid (which is converted to EPA) and the n-6 GLA suppresses active synovitis in these patients [55].

LIPIDS AND LUPUS

Patients with SLE are uniquely sensitive to suppression of eicosanoid synthesis by the kidneys [56]. Thus, small doses of NSAIDs may impair renal function in patients with lupus nephritis. Antiinflammatory agents which can substitute for NSAIDs would therefore be useful for treatment of SLE patients. Whereas some of the benefits of fish oil in animal models of lupus have been striking [57], results in humans have been modest, but encouraging. Evidence [58] that fish oil administration enhances collagen-induced arthritis in rats and exacerbates vasculitis in autoimmune mice dictates caution in the premature uncontrolled use of fish oil treatments in inflammatory diseases. Nonetheless, clinical studies are warranted. Fish oil treatment of SLE patients for 1 year did not result in clinical benefit, but the frequency of active nephritis may have been reduced in treated patients [59]. In a 34-week placebo (olive oil)-controlled study, administration of 20 g/day of fish oil to SLE patients resulted in improvement of clinical symptoms by patient assessment, but objective data were not reported [60]. As noted above, olive oil is not the best choice for a placebo since it is not inert and may have therapeutic effects [46].

GLA has not been used for the treatment of SLE. However, administration of GLA does delay onset of disease and increase survival time of MRL/lpr mice [61]. Also, GLA enrichment of diet suppresses acute and chronic inflammation as well as joint tissue injury in several experimental animal models [62]. In animals treated with GLA, cells from inflammatory exudates are enriched in GLA and its elongated product, DGLA. Exudate PGE_2 and LTB_4 concentrations are reduced, and leukocyte effector functions (chemotaxis, lysosomal enzyme release) are suppressed. The protective effects of GLA, by virtue of its effects on prostaglandins, may extend to host defense in SLE patients: stimulated peripheral blood monocytes (PBM) from SLE patients with active disease (not on NSAIDs) produce lower quantities of PGE than PBM from patients with mild disease. PBM from two untreated SLE patients with very active disease were low PGE producers until 2 weeks after treatment with high-dose prednisone, at which time lupus activity was diminished and PGE production was equivalent to patients with mild disease [63].

Few adverse effects of marine and botanical lipid administration have been noted: stool softening, belching, and abdominal bloating have been reported. Nonetheless, potential adverse events cannot be dismissed. Experience teaches that the longer a given treatment is used, the greater the incidence of adverse events. Administration of long-chain PUFAs increases the likelihood of lipid peroxidation with its associated toxic effects on cells. It is not known whether increased intake of long-chain unsaturated fatty acids increases the need for antioxidants such as vitamins E and C. Because these novel fatty acids can reduce inflammation and affect immunocytes, the question arises whether they can compromise the immune system. Susceptibility to infection has not been seen but must be considered.

The potential ability of certain fatty acids to regulate cell activation, immune responses, and inflammation is exciting to consider at the clinical, cellular, and molecular levels. A better understanding of how fatty acids modulate function of cells involved in host defense might lead to development of new, benign treatment for diseases characterized by acute and chronic inflammation, and disordered immune responses.

REFERENCES

1. Burr, G. O. & Burr, M. M. (1930). On the nature and role of the fatty acids essential in nutrition. *J Biol Chem* **86**, 587–621.
2. Willis, A. L. (1981). Nutritional and pharmacological factors in eicosanoid biology. *Nutr Rev* **39**, 289–301.
3. Hafstrom, I., Ringertz, B., Gyllenhammar, H., Palmblad, J. & Harms-Ringdatil, M. (1988). Effects of fasting on disease activity, neutrophil function, fatty acid composition and leukotriene biosynthesis in patients with rheumatoid arthritis. *Arthritis Rheum* **31**, 592–595.
4. Mustard, J. F., Packham, M. A. & Kinlough-Rathbone, R. L. (1988). The role of platelets in the early and late stages of atherosclerosis and its clinical applications. *Prog Clin Biol Res* **283**, 639–672.
5. Fisher, S. & Weber, P. C. (1985). Prostaglandin I_3 is formed *in vivo* in man after dietary eicosapentaenoic acid. *Nature* **307**, 165–168.
6. Lee, T. H., Hoover, R. L., Williams, J. D., Sperling, R. I., Revalese, J., Robinson, D. R., Corey, E. J., Lewis, R. A. & Austen, K. F. (1985). Effect of dietary enrichment with eicosapentaenoic and docosahexaenenoic acids on *in vitro* neutrophil and monocytes leukotriene generation and neutrophil function. *New Engl J Med* **312**, 1217–1224.
7. Sperling, R. I., Benincasso, A. I., Knoel, C. T., Larkin, J. K., Austen, K. F. & Robinson, D. R. (1993). Dietary *n*-3 polyunsaturated fatty acids inhibit phosphoinositide formation and chemotaxis in neutrophils. *J Clin Invest* **91**, 651–660.
8. Ziboh, V. A. & Chapkin, R. S. (1987). Biologic significance of polyunsaturated fatty acids in the skin. *Arch Dermatol* **123**, 1686–1690.
9. Baker, D. G., Krakauer, K. A., Tate, G., Laposata, M. & Zurier, R. B. (1989). Suppression of human synovial cell proliferation by dihomo-γ-linoleic acid. *Arthritis Rheum* **32**, 1273–1281.
10. Vane, J. R. (1976). Prostaglandins as mediators of inflammation. *In* Advances in Prostaglandin and Thromboxane Research (B. Samuelsson & R. Paoletti, Eds.), pp. 791–798, Raven Press, New York.
11. Fantone, J. C., Kunkel, S. L. & Zurier, R. B. (1985). Effects of prostaglandins on *in vivo* immune and inflammatory reactions. *In* Prostaglandins and Immunity (J. S. Goodwin, Ed.), pp. 123–146, Marinus Nijhoff, Boston.
12. Endres, S. (1993). Messengers and mediators: Interactions among lipids, eisosanoids, and cytokines. *Am J Clin Nutr* **57**, 7985–8005.

13. Hedqvist, P. (1970). Studies on the effects of prostaglandin E_1 and E_2 on the sympathetic neuromuscular transmission in some animal tissue. *Acta Physiol Scand* **345**(Suppl 79), 1–40.

14. Zurier, R. B. (1993). Prostaglandins, fatty acids, and arthritis. *In* Nutrient Modulation of the Immune Response (S. Cunningham-Rundles, Ed.), pp. 201–209, Marcel Dekker, New York.

15. Haeggstrom, J. Z. & Wetterholm, A. (2002). Enzymes and receptors in the leukotriene cascade. *Cell Mol Life Sci* **59**, 742–753.

16. Abramson, S. B. & Weaver, A. L. (2005). Current state of therapy for pain and inflammation. *Arthritis Res Ther* **7**(Suppl 4), S1–S6.

17. Lawrence, T. & Gilroy, D. W. (2007). Chronic inflammation: A failure of resolution? *Int J Exp Pathol* **88**, 85–94.

18. Serhan, C. N. & Oliw, E. (2001). Unorthodox routes to prostanoid formation: New twists in cycoloxygenase-initiated pathways. *J Clin Investig* **107**, 1481–1489.

19. Serhan, C. N., Cish, C. B. & Brannon, J. (2000). Antimicroinflammatory lipid signals generated from dietary *n*-3 fatty acids via cyclooxygenase-2 and transcellular processing: A novel mechanism for NSAID and *n*-3 PUFA therapeutic actions. *J Physiol Pharmacol* **51**, 643–648.

20. Lipsky, P. E., Brooks, P., Crofford, L. J., DuBois, R., Graham, D., Simon, L. S., vandePutte, l. B. & Abramson, S. B. (2000). Unresolved issues in the role of cyclooxygenase-2 in normal physiologic processes and disease. *Arch Intern Med* **160**, 913–920.

21. Kerr, D. J., Dunn, J. A., Langman, M. J., Smith, J. L., Midgley, R. S., Stanley, A., Stokes, J. C., Julier, P., Iveson, C., Duvvuri, R. & McConkey, C. C. Victor Trial Group (2007). Rofecoxib and cardiovascular adverse events in adjuvant treatment of colorectal cancer. *New Engl J Med* **327**, 360–369.

22. Bygdeman, M. & Samuelsson, B. (1964). Quantitative determination of prostaglandins in human semen. *Clin Chim Acta* **10**, 566–568.

23. Karim, S. M., Sandler, M. & Williams, E. D. (1967). Distribution of prostaglandins in human tissues. *Br J Pharmacol Chemother* **31**, 340–344.

24. Horrobin, D. F. (1988). The roles of essential fatty acids in the development of diabetic neuropathy and other complications of diabetes mellitus. *Prostaglandins, Leukotrienes and Essential Fatty Acids* **31**, 181–197.

25. Holman, R. T., Smythe, L. & Johnson, S. (1979). Effect of sex and age on fatty acid composition of human serum lipids. *Am J Clin Nutr* **32**, 2390–2399.

26. Datta-Roy, A. K., Colman, R. W. & Sinha, A. K. (1983). Prostaglandin E_1 and E_2 receptors of human erythrocyte membranes. *J Cell Biol* **97**, 403–404.

27. Hata, A. N. & Breyer, R. M. (2006). Pharmacology and signaling of prostaglandin receptors: Multiple roles in inflammation and immune modulation. *Pharmacol Ther* **103**, 147–166.

28. Kloeze, J. (1969). Relationship between chemical structure and platelet aggregation activity of prostaglandins. *Biochem Biophys Acta* **187**, 285–292.

29. Suzuki, T., Nakanishi, H. & Nakahata, N. (1982). Antagonism between prostaglandin E_1 and E_2 in bovine coronary arteries. *Fukushima J Med Sci* **29**, 111–117.

30. Kitson, G. E. & Pipkin, F. B. (1981). Effects of interactions of prostaglandins E_1 and E_2 on human chorionic plate arteries. *Am J Obstet Gynecol* **140**, 683–692.

31. Marevich, E. M., Larkin, K. M. & Archakov, A. I. (1985). Influence of cholesterol and prostaglandin E_1 on the molecular organization of phospholipids in the

erythrocyte membrane: A fluorescent polarization study with lipid specific probes. *Biochim Biophys Acta* **815**, 455–460.

32. Tate, G., Mandell, B. F., Schumacher, H. R. & Zurier, R. B. (1988). Suppression of acute inflammation by 15-methylprostaglandin E$_1$. *Lab Investig* **59**, 192–199.

33. Krakauer, K. A., Torrey, S. B. & Zurier, R. B. (1978). Prostaglandin E$_1$ treatment of NZB/W mice. III. Preservation of spleen cell concentration and mitogen induced proliferative responses. *Clin Immunol Immunopathol* **11**, 256–262.

34. Whittum, J., Goldschneider, I., Greiner, D. & Zurier, R. B. (1985). Development abnormalities of terminal deoxynucleotidyl transferase positive bone marrow cells and thymocytes in New Zealand mice: Effects of prostaglandin E$_1$. *J Immunol* **135**, 272–280.

35. Whittum-Hudson, J., Ballow, M. & Zurier, R. B. (1988). Effect of PGE$_1$ treatment on *in vitro* thymocyte function of normal and autoimmune mice. *Immunopharmacology* **166**, 71–78.

36. Izui, S., Kelley, V. E., McConahey, A. & Dixon, F. J. (1981). Selective suppression of retroviral gp70-anti-gp70 immune complex formation by prostaglandin E$_1$ in murine systemic lupus erythematosus. *J Exp Med* **152**, 1645–1658.

37. Thompson, P. A., Jelinek, D. K. & Lipsky, P. E. (1984). Regulation of human B cell proliferation by PGE$_2$. *J Immunol* **133**, 2446–2450.

38. Nagayama, Y., Namura, Y., Tamura, T. & Muso, R. (1988). Beneficial effect of prostaglandin E$_1$ in three cases of lupus nephritis with nephritic syndrome. *Ann Allergy* **61**, 289–295.

39. Yoshikawa, T., Suzuki, H., Kato, H. & Yano, S. (1990). Effects of prostaglandin E$_1$ on collagen diseases with high levels of circulating immune complexes. *J Rheumatol* **17**, 1513–1524.

40. Fantone, J. C., Kunkel, S. L., Ward, P. A. & Zurier, R. B. (1981). Suppression of human polymorphonuclear leucocyte function after intravenous infusion of prostaglandin E$_1$. *Prostag Med* **7**, 195–198.

41. Goodwin, J. S. & Clay, G. A. (1986). Effect of chronic ingestion of a prostaglandin E analogue on immunologic function in healthy elderly subjects. *Int J Immunopharmacol* **8**, 867–875.

42. Mork-Hansen, T., Lerche, A., Kassis, V., Lorenzen, I. & Sondergaard, (1983). Treatment of rheumatoid arthritis with prostaglandin E$_2$, precursors *cis*-linoleic acid and gammalinolenic acid. *Scand J Rheumatol* **12**, 85–88.

43. Belch, J. J. F., Madhok, A. R., O'Dowd, A. & Sturrock, R. D. (1988). Effects of altering dietary essential fatty acids on requirements for nonsteroidal antiinflammatory drugs in patients with rheumatoid arthritis: A double blind controlled study. *Ann Rheum Dis* **47**, 96–104.

44. Pullman-Moar, S. W., Laposata, M., Lem, D., Holman, R. T., Leventhal, L. J., DeMarco, D. & Zurier, R. B. (1980). Alteration of the cellular fatty acid profile and the production of eicosanoids in human monocytes by gammalinoleic acid. *Arthritis Rheum* **33**, 1526–1534.

45. Brezeski, M., Madhok, R. & Capell, H. A. (1991). Evening primrose oil in patients with rheumatoid arthritis and side effects of non-steroidal antiinflammatory drugs. *Br J Rheumatol* **30**, 370–372.

46. Darlington, L. G. & Ramsey, N. W. (1987). Olive oil for rheumatoid patients. *Br J Rheumatol* **26**(Suppl 2), 129–133.

47. Jantti, J., Nikkari, T. & Solakivi, T. (1989). Evening primrose oil in rheumatoid arthritis. Changes in serum lipids and fatty acids. *Ann Rheum Dis* **48**, 124–127.

48. Leventhal, L. J., Boyce, E. G. & Zurier, R. B. (1993). Treatment of rheumatoid arthritis with gammalinolenic acid. *Ann Int Med* **119**, 867–873.

49. Zurier, R. B., Rossetti, R. G., Jacobson, E. W., DeMarco, D. M., Liu, N. Y., Temming, J. E., White, B. M. & Laposata, M. (1996). Gammalinolenic acid, placebo-controlled trial. *Arthritis Rheum* **39**, 1808–1817.

50. Wright, S. & Burton, J. L. (1982). Oral evening primrose improves atopic eczema. *Lancet* **2**, 1120–1122.

51. Bamford, J. T., Gibson, R. W. & Renier, C. M. (1985). Atopic eczema unresponsive to evening primrose oil (linoleic and gammalinolenic acids). *J Acad Dermatol* **13**, 959–965.

52. Calder, P. C. & Zurier, R. B. (2001). Polyunsaturated fatty acids and rheumatoid arthritis. *Curr Opin Clin Nutr Metab Care* **4**, 115–121.

53. Volker, D., Fitzgerald, P., Major, G. & Garg, M. (2000). Efficacy of fish oil concentrate in the treatment of rheumatoid arthritis. *J Rheumatol* **27**, 2343–2346.

54. Tate, G., Mandell, B. F., Karmali, R. A., Laposata, M., Baker, D. G., Schumaker, H. R. & Zurier, R. B. (1988). Suppression of monosodium urate induced inflammation by diets enriched with gamma-linoleic acid and eicosapentaenoic acid. *Arthritis Rheum* **31**, 1543.

55. Leventhal, L. J., Boyce, E. G. & Zurier, R. B. (1994). Treatment of rheumatoid arthritis with black currant seed oil. *Br J Rheumatol* **33**, 847–852.

56. Kimberly, R. P., Gill, J. R., Bowden, R. E., Keiser, H. R. & Plotz, P. H. (1978). Elevated urinary prostaglandins and the effects of aspirin on renal function in lupus erythematosus. *Ann Intern Med* **89**, 336–341.

57. Robinson, D. R., Prickett, J. D., Makoul, G. T., Steinber, A. D. & Colvin, R. B. (1986). Dietary fish oil reduces progression of established renal disease in NZB × NZW F1 mice and delays renal disease in BXSB and MRL/L strains. *Arthritis Rheum* **29**, 539–546.

58. Prickett, J. D., Trentham, D. E. & Robinson, D. R. (1984). Dietary fish oil augments the induction of arthritis in rats immunized with type II collagen. *J Immunol* **132**, 725–729.

59. Moore, G. F., Yarboro, C., Sebring, N., Robinson, D. R. & Steinberg, A. D. (1987). Eicosapentaenoic acid in the treatment of systemic lupus. *Arthritis Rheum* **30**(abstract), 533.

60. Walton, A. J. E., Snaith, M. L., Locniskar, M., Cumberlan, A. G., Morrow, W. J. W. & Isenberg, D. A. (1991). Dietary fish oil and the severity of symptoms in patients with systemic lupus erythematosus. *Ann Rheum Dis* **50**, 463–466.

61. Godfrey, D. C., Stimson, W. H., Watson, J., Belch, J. J. F. & Sturrock, R. D. (1986). The modulation of autoimmunity in the MRL/lpr mouse by dietary fatty acid supplementation. *Prog Lipid Res* **25**, 289–293.

62. Zurier, R. B. (1993). Fatty acids, inflammation, and immune responses. *Prostaglandins, Leukotrienes and Essential Fatty Acids* **48**, 57–62.

63. Freundlich, B., Shoback, B. R. & Zurier, R. B. (1985). Prostaglandin E generation by monocytes from SLE patients. *Arthritis Rheum* **28**(abstract), S48.

Chapter 2

Prolotherapy for Chronic Musculoskeletal Pain[1]

David Rabago

Department of Family Medicine, University of Wisconsin School of Medicine and Public Health, Madison, WI, USA

Abstract

Musculoskeletal pain and resulting disability are among the most common and significant problems facing the elderly today. There is inadequate therapy for several painful chronic musculoskeletal conditions including low back pain, osteoarthritis and several tendinopathies.

Prolotherapy is an injection technique which has been used for musculoskeletal pain for approximately 100 years. While the mechanism of action is not well established, proponents suggest that numerous injections of irritant solutions known as "proliferants" initiate a local healing reaction favoring anabolic processes.

Prolotherapy has been assessed since 1937 in 36 case series and case reports, two non-randomized controlled studies, and seven randomized controlled trials. The case series and reports establish prolotherapy as an ongoing, evolving medical intervention with positive outcomes in patients with difficult musculoskeletal pain conditions. The controlled studies suggest the growing maturity of both the practice and assessment of prolotherapy interventions and suggest efficacy for some indications when evaluated using contemporary "strength of evidence" criteria. The strongest evidence for the efficacy of prolotherapy for any indication comes from one randomized controlled study for severe lateral epicondylosis (tennis elbow), which reported that prolotherapy reduced elbow pain and improved elbow strength compared to control injections. Two case series on Achilles and hip adductor tendinopathies support the use of prolotherapy for these tendinopathies, and suggest that prolotherapy may be effective for painful overuse injury generally. Studies on low back pain and osteoarthritis present more equivocal data for efficacy but clinical recommendations for the use of prolotherapy in patients with cases refractory to standard of care therapies can be made as well.

Keywords: *Prolotherapy, chronic pain, tendinopathy, injection therapy*

---

[1]The tables and parts of the text contain material modified from the paper Rabago, D., Best, T., Beamsly M., *et al.* (2005). A systematic review of prolotherapy for chronic musculoskeletal pain. *Clinical J Sports Med* **15**(5), 376–380.

INTRODUCTION

Prolotherapy is a therapy for chronic musculoskeletal pain in which a small volume of an irritant or sclerosing solution is injected at multiple sites on painful ligament and tendon insertions (entheses [1]), and in adjacent joint spaces. It has been promoted as a treatment for ligament and joint laxity, [2] osteoarthritis and tendinopathies. Injected solutions ("proliferants") are thought to cause local irritation and subsequent inflammation and anabolic healing, resulting in enlargement and strengthening of damaged ligamentous, tendon and intra-articular structures [3, 4]. This is hypothesized to decrease joint laxity and articular dysfunction, improve biomechanics and decrease pain [2, 5]. The three commonly used prolotherapy solutions are reported to act in different ways: hypertonic dextrose by osmotic rupture of local cells, phenol–glycerine–glucose (P2G) by local cellular irritation, and sodium morrhuate by chemotactic attraction of inflammatory mediators [6] and by the sclerosing of pathologic neovascularity associated with tendinopathy [7, 8]. The potential of prolotherapy to stimulate release of growth factors favoring soft tissue healing has been suggested as a possible mechanism [9, 10]. Prolotherapy has been used for approximately 100 years, has been described in the formal medical literature since 1937 and has been evaluated using randomized controlled trial (RCT) methodology since 1987 for low back pain, osteoarthritis and tendinopathy.

While the injection technique is most often called "prolotherapy," it was historically referred to as "sclerotherapy," and more recently as "regenerative injection therapy" or "RIT" [5, 11]. Nomenclature has reflected practitioners' perceptions of the solutions' effect on tissue. Solutions were initially thought to be scar-forming, hence the term sclerotherapy. Later, as new injection agents were used, injected tissue was noted to be larger, or "proliferated" or "regenerated." The most contemporary nomenclature simply names the procedure by the injected solution [12].

Similar to corticosteroid injections, prolotherapy injection is an unregulated procedure without certification by any governing body. It is not formally taught in medical schools or medical residencies. It is however, taught to MD's and other health care providers in semi-formal workshop and continuing medical education (CME) settings by several organizations including medical schools, for example, the annual CME course "The Anatomy, Diagnosis, and Treatment of Chronic Myofascial Pain with Prolotherapy" taught at the University of Wisconsin School of Medicine and Public Health (http://www.cme.wisc.edu/conference.html). It is not approved by the Centers for Medicare and Medicaid Services, formerly the Health Care Financing Administration. Prolotherapy is also not covered by most private health care plans; patients generally pay out-of-pocket.

CURRENT PROLOTHERAPY USE

Prolotherapy is a popular and growing therapy. Exact prevalence is unknown and difficult to estimate; there are no regulatory agencies or umbrella organizations tracking prolotherapy. However, a survey of MD and DO members of two manual medicine associations, the American Association of Orthopaedic Medicine (AAOM) and the American Osteopathic Sclerotherapy Society, about their use of prolotherapy reported that 95 providers had practiced prolotherapy on an estimated 450,000 patients in the United States by 1991 [13]. This likely grossly undercounts the true prevalence of prolotherapy. In this sample, 69% of prolotherapy was done for low back pain, and 20% for cervical and thoracic spine pain. Twenty-six per cent of patients had prolotherapy at one or more peripheral joints. A focused Internet search on "prolotherapy" using the Google™ search engine identified more than 500 sites listing prolotherapy services, training courses, video tapes, books, articles, brochures, references and personal statements [14]. Based on growing membership in organizations that support prolotherapy, and growing attendance in prolotherapy training courses, prolotherapy itself appears to be rapidly growing [15].

While medical practitioners have produced inflammation in order to heal serious traumatic injury since antiquity, the modern use of prolotherapy can be traced to the 1930s [16]. Injection protocols were formalized in the 1950s by George Hackett, a general surgeon in the United States, based on clinical experience over 30 years [2]. Anecdotal reports indicate prolotherapy is used for spinal pain of several etiologies, osteoarthritis, a variety of tendinopathies and other indications; in all over 40 conditions have been identified as appropriate for treatment with prolotherapy by some authors, though the majority have not been subjected to serious assessment in clinical trials [13, 17, 18]. While the rigorous assessment of the clinical and basic science of prolotherapy is in its infancy, a thorough review of the literature reveals: (1) *in vitro* and animal model evidence suggesting biological activity of prolotherapy and (2) considerable clinical evidence of varying methodological strength supporting the safe use of prolotherapy for three major pathologies: low back pain, osteoarthritis and tendinopathy.

IN VITRO AND ANIMAL MODEL EVIDENCE

Three solutions are commonly used in prolotherapy, D-glucose (dextrose), phenol–glucose–glycerin (P2G) and sodium morrhuate [19]. *In vitro* and *in vivo* animal studies have analyzed some aspects of prolotherapy solutions. Increased glucose concentration (D-glucose) causes an increase in cell protein synthesis, [20, 21] DNA synthesis, [20] and cell volume [20]. The effects on cell proliferation are conflicting; some studies report increased proliferation [20] and others report increased apoptosis [21]. Phenol–glucose–glycerin is hypothesized to be a stronger inflammatory stimulator [6]. Phenol has been used in animal models to study acute irritant dermatitis by creating an inflammatory response [22]. However, it has also been shown to be toxic to human colonic epithelial cells [23]. In addition, phenol can temporarily block peripheral nerves in humans [24] and damage the sciatic nerve in rats resulting in partial hind limb paralysis [25]. Sodium morrhuate is an extract of cod liver oil and a sclerosing agent [26]. The hypothesis that prolotherapy causes a selective inflammatory response however, has not been well substantiated experimentally. A recent study compared the inflammatory effect of prolotherapy in a rat model. All three commonly used proliferants were compared to "do-nothing," needle stick and saline injection controls, in healthy rat medial collateral ligaments (MCLs) and assessed using immunohistochemistry techniques for inflammatory mediators [27]. While all prolotherapy groups showed increased inflammation, prolotherapy solutions did not cause an overall inflammatory response that was consistently different from that caused by saline and needle stick controls. Four animal studies have investigated sodium morrhuate as a prolotherapy agent. These studies found an increase in ligament strength, [3, 28] mass, thickness and a trend toward an increase in cell number, glycosaminoglycan content and water content [4] in ligaments injected with sodium morrhuate compared to saline [3, 4] or no injection [28]. Sodium morrhuate injected into healthy rat patellar tendons was recently reported to decrease tendon length and increase in tendon strength compared to the contralateral control (no treatment) 4 weeks after injection [28]. A recent study assessed the effect of dextrose prolotherapy on the physical and mechanical properties of stretch-injured rat MCLs [27]. Rat MCLs injected with dextrose were significantly larger than those injected with saline control solution, those receiving needle stick only and uninjured ligaments. However, changes in biomechanical outcomes (laxity and strength) were not seen [29]. These *in vitro* and *in vivo* reports suggest that sodium morrhuate may produce a biological effect and that a direct effect of inflammation may be less important than initially reported.

CLINICAL TRAIL EVIDENCE

Musculoskeletal pathology, including low back pain, osteoarthritis and tendinopathy are significant causes of pain and disability. They are age-related; given that the US population is aging, the importance of these conditions will increase with time. Prolotherapy has been assessed as a treatment for each of these conditions. Our group recently undertook a comprehensive systematic review of all prolotherapy clinical trial literature involving human subjects [30] (Tables 2.1–2.4).

CASE REPORTS, CASE SERIES AND NON-RANDOMIZED STUDIES (TABLES 2.1 AND 2.2)

The case report and case series provide the earliest and most clinically oriented evidence for prolotherapy. A review of 36 case reports and case series (Table 2.1) shows that 3928 patients from 12 to 88 years old with up to 65 years of pain were evaluated. Report quality varies widely; the internal methodological strength of case studies is consistent with methodology of their publication date.

TABLE 2.1 Description of Case Reports and Case Series

Study author, year	Indication	Subjects	Methods/ Injectant	Outcome measures	Results
Gedney, 1937 [91]	Knee OA[a] pain, knee instability, LBP[b], SI[c] dysfunction	1 F, age 68 years; 1 M, age 45 years	Neo-plasmoid* and MacDonald's Solution* injection	Subjective pain and mobility	Improved mobility, decreased pain
Shuman, 1941 [92]	Recurrent shoulder dislocation	1 F, age 23 years; 3 M, ages 17, 18, 24 years	AC joint capsule injections using one or more of the following: Sodium Linsoleate*, Alparene*, Sylnasol*, Neoplasmoid*	Subjective pain, recurrence of dislocation	No recurrence of dislocation, decreased pain
Bahme, 1945 [93]	SI dysfunction	30 F, 70 M; ages 12–75 years; pain for 0.5–45 years	OM[d] and SI ligament Sylnasol* injections	Subjective pain	50–100% pain relief
Gedney, 1951 [94]	LBP	3 M, ages 19, 32, 34; pain for 0.5–16 years	Sylnasol* injections	Work status, subjective pain	Ability to return to work, decreased pain

continued

TABLE 2.1 (*continued*)

Study author, year	Indication	Subjects	Methods/ Injectant	Outcome measures	Results
Gedney, 1952 [95]	SI dysfunction, LBP	1 F, age 23 years; 1 M, age 30 years; pain for 1 year	SI ligament Sylnasol* injections	Subjective pain	Resolution of pain
Hackett, 1953 [96]	SI dysfunction, LBP	9 M, 8 F; ages 15–52 years; pain for 4 months–20 years	Sylnasol* injections	Subjective pain	Resolution of pain through 2-year follow-up. Occasional exacerbation resolved with re-treatment
Hackett, 1953 [96]	SI dysfunction	119 M, 134 F; ages 15–70; pain for up to 30 years	Not given	Subjective pain	Pain-free for 2–14 years (long-term follow-up questionnaire)
Shuman, 1954 [97]	LBP, knee pain, shoulder separation, other joint pain	93 adults	Not given	Return to work	95% (88) able to return to work, 5% (5) unable to return to work
Hackett, 1954 [98]	SI dysfunction	3 F, ages 40, 56 and 58 years	Not given	Subjective pain	Resolution of pain
Neff, 1960 [99]	LBP, SI dysfunction	3 adults	Sylnasol* injections	Subjective pain	Resolution of pain

Myers, 1961 [100]	LBP	267 adults	Sylnasol/ pontocaine* solution or Zinc/ phenol* solution injections	Subjective pain	Resolution of pain in 82% of subjects
Hackett et al., 1962 [101]	SI dysfunction, other joint pain	1857 subjects (1516: SI dysfunction, 284: other indications); ages 15–88 years; pain/disability for 3 months–65 years	Sylnasol* or P2G[e] injections	Subjective pain	"Satisfactory cure" in 82% (1489) subjects for up to 19 years
Hackett et al., 1962 [101]	Head–neck strain	82 subjects	P2G injections	Subjective pain	"Good to excellent" results in 74 subjects
Kayfetz et al., 1963 [102]	Traumatic (whiplash) or non-traumatic (tension) headache	102 M, 162 F subjects (206 traumatic, 58 non-traumatic headache); pain (average) for 4 years	Sylnasol*, zinc sulfate* or P2G[5] injected during 1–20 sessions	4-point pain scale: from excellent (no pain or symptoms) to poor (no relief of pain or symptoms)	Pain improvement during 6 months–5 years follow-up: excellent: 145; good: 43; fair: 41; poor: 33; Lost to follow-up: 2

continued

TABLE 2.1 (*continued*)

Study author, year	Indication	Subjects	Methods/ Injectant	Outcome measures	Results
Kayfetz, 1963 [103]	Occipito-cervical injury (whiplash)	87 M, 102 F; ages 10–61 years; pain for >1 month in 78%, pain for >1 year in 21% of subjects	Sodium psylliate*, tetradecyl sulfate*, zinc sulfate* injected in 1–20 sessions over 1–6 months	4-item pain scale: from excellent (no pain or symptoms) to poor (no relief of pain or symptoms)	Pain improvement: excellent: 113; good: 15; fair: 34; poor: 27
Peterson, 1963 [104]	LBP	136 adults	P2G injections	Pain improvement (percentage of improvement)	Pain improvement: excellent (>75%): 106; good (50–75%): 114; fair (25–50%): 5; poor (<25%): 11
Barbor, 1964 [105]	LBP	153 adults; pain for 6 months–20 years	P2G injections	Subjective pain relief	Pain relieved to subject's satisfaction: 111; Pain relief failure: 17; Lost to follow-up: 25
Blumenthal, 1974 [106]	Headache	3 adults	P2G injections	Subjective pain	Resolution of pain
Leedy et al., 1976 [107]	LBP	50 adults; ages 25–72 years; pain for 1 month to over 10 years	Not given	Subjective pain at 5-year follow-up	Pain resolution with: 0 exacerbation: 26 1 exacerbation: 18 2 exacerbations: 5 >2 exacerbations: 1

				Subjective pain	Symptom resolution
Leedy, 1977 [108]	Shoulder pain, LBP, costochondritis, epicondylitis	4 M, 4 F	Farnsworth Formula 51* injections	Subjective pain	Symptom resolution
Leedy, 1982 [109]	SI dysfunction	4 M, 18–55 years; 1F, 82 years	Not given	Subjective pain	Symptom relief
Bourdeau, 1988 [110]	LBP	11M, 13 F; ages 19–82 years; pain for 2 months–30 years	12.5% Dextrose injections in 3–10 treatment sessions	4-point pain scale at 5-year follow-up	Excellent (little or no pain for 5 years): 7; Very good (little or no pain for 2–5 years): 10; Good (little or no pain for 1 year): 2; Poor (pain control for less than 6 months): 5
Ongley et al., 1988 [111]	Knee pain, knee laxity	4 subjects	30–40 cc P2G "peppered" into PCL, ACL, LCL, MCL[g] insertions	Laxity measured with "Genucom" knee analysis system; subjective pain and function	Improvement for 90° A–P[h] draw, 90° A–P draw with internal rotation, 30° A–P draw and 80° internal–external rotation ($p < 0.05$); Complete pain resolution: 2; Partial pain improvement: 2; Function improvement: 4
LaCourse et al., 1990 [112]	LBP	8 adults	P2G injections; subjects also received lidocaine and steroid injection, and exercise advice	Pelvic inclination as measured by inclinometer	Decreased pelvic inclination
Dorman et al., 1991 [113]	Low-back, mid-back and neck pain	40 F, 40 M adults	P2G injections; subjects also received lidocaine and steroid injection, and exercise advice	Pain severity, functional capacity, sleep	Decreased pain severity, improved functional status and sleep

continued

TABLE 2.1 (continued)

Study author, year	Indication	Subjects	Methods/ Injectant	Outcome measures	Results
Schwartz et al., 1991 [114]	SI dysfunction	43 adults; ages 20–70 years	Three injections with SM¹ each 2 weeks apart	Pain relief scale at 2-week follow-up	Pain relief: 95%: 20; 75%: 11; 66%: 4; 33%: 1; 0%: 3
Hirschberg et al., 1992 [115]	Iliocostal friction syndrome	6 M, 6 F; ages 38–82 years	12.5–25% Dextrose injections and use of rib compression belt and Hoek corset	Subjective pain	Resolution of pain
Reeves et al., 1994 [116]	Fibromyalgia	31 adults; pain (average) for 7–8 years	12.5% Dextrose injected at 16 fibromyalgia sites an average of 3.5 times	Average pain (0–10 Likert scale); subjective functional status	Average pain improvement of 16%; Improved functional status
Dorman et al., 1995 [117]	LBP	9 adults	Proliferant and protocol not given	Oxygen consumption efficiency while walking	Improved oxygen consumption efficiency while walking
Mathews, 1995 [118]	SI dysfunction	16 subjects	3 series of P2G injections	5-item pain scale	At 4-month follow-up: no pain: 11; slight pain: 1; much better: 1; slightly better: 1; no better: 1; Lost to follow-up: 1
Reeves et al., 1997 [119]	Recurrent knee dislocation	1 F, age 72 years	5% Dextrose injections	Subjective pain; dislocation	Decreased pain Joint relocation

Reeves et al., 2003 [120]	Knee pain, flexion and laxity	16 adults	10% and 25% Dextrose injections	Pain scale; knee laxity	At 3-year follow-up: pain at rest, stair and walk decreased by 35–45%; subjective swelling ($p < 0.05$) and ROM ($p < 0.01$) improved, ligament laxity decreased by 71% ($p < 0.01$).
Hooper et al., 2004 [121]	Cervical, thoracic and lumbar pain	126 F, 51 M subjects; average age 39.5 years; pain for 3 months–27 years (average: 4.8 years)	20% Dextrose injections; weekly set of injections for three sessions with repeated set of three sessions if pain control incomplete	Subjective pain, function and ability to work on three 5-item scales	At mean 9-month follow-up: Pain reduction: 91% of subjects; Function improvement: 84.8% of subjects; Improved ability to work (for those working outside the home): 84% of subjects
Hooper et al. [122]	Cervical pain	1 M subject; neck pain (MVA-related) for 2 years	Intra-articular 20% Dextrose injected under flouroscoopic guidance at zygapophysial joints C2–C6	Neck disability index score (NDI)	NDI score decreased from 24/50 pre-injection to 9/50 at 1 year, and 2/50 at 3 years.
Topol et al., 2005 [65]	Groin pain (osteitis pubis and/or adductor tendinopathy)	24 M rugby and soccer players pain (average) for 15.5 months	12.5% Dextrose injected at the pubis symphysis and ischiopubic ramus at 4-week intervals for 2–6 injection sessions (mean 2.8)	VAS[i], Nirschl Pain Phase Scale	Improvement in both outcome measures ($p < 0.05$); 22/24 subjects plying at full capacity at follow-up (6–32 months)

Continued

TABLE 2.1 (*continued*)

Study author, year	Indication	Subjects	Methods/ Injectant	Outcome measures	Results
Maxwell et al., 2007 [12]	Achilles tendinopathy (insertional and midportion)	11F, 25M adults; ages 23–82 years (mean: 52.6 years); pain for 3–120 months (average: 28.6 months)	25% Dextrose injected into anechoic and hypoechoic areas of the tendon every 6 weeks for mean of 4 sessions (2–11)	100 mm VAS for pain at rest, with activity and during sport; tendon thickness; degree of neovascularity, hypoechogenicity	Sustained at 12-month follow-up: VAS pain at rest: 81% improvement; VAS pain with activity: 84% improvement; VAS pain during sport: 78% improvement; Decrease in tendon thickness, hypoechogenicity and neovascularity.

[a]OA, *osteoarthritis*.
[b]LBP, *low back pain*.
[c]SI, *sacro-iliac*.
[d]OM, *osteopathic manipulation*.
[e]P2G, *phenol–glucose–glycerine*.
[f]SM, *sodium morrhuate*.
[g]PCL, *posterior cruciate ligament*; ACL, *anterior cruciate ligament*; MCL, *medial collateral ligament*; LCL, *lateral collateral ligament*.
[h]A–P, *anterior–posterior*.
[i]VAS, *visual analog scale*.
* No longer used for prolotherapy or no longer available.

TABLE 2.2 Description of Controlled, Non-randomized Prolotherapy Studies

Study author/year	Indication	Subjects	Methods/Injectant	Outcome measures	Results
Naeim et al., 1982 [36]	SI[a] dysfunction	3 M, 13 F; ages 19–80 years	Control: 9 subjects treated with lidocaine injections. Intervention: 7 subjects treated with lidocaine and dextrose injections	2-item scale: "good" subjective improvement, able to conduct daily activities, without pain, no pain medication needed, and negative clinical signs; "poor" results if the above not met	Lidocaine alone: good: 4/9 (44%), poor: 5/9 (56%); Lidocaine and dextrose: good: 6/7 (86%), poor: 1/7 (14%)
Yelland et al., 2000 [31]	LBP[b]	20 M, 13 F; ages 37–63 years; pain for 36–120 months	Control: 13 subjects treated with conservative LBP modalities. Intervention: 20 subjects treated with dextrose injections	VAS[c] on pain intensity; Pain Diagram Disability Score; General Quality of Life score; percentage reaching 50% improvement in pain	Improvement in: VAS leg pain ($p < 0.05$), pain diagram ($p = 0.05$), LBP ($p = 0.07$) and disability scores ($p = 0.08$) compared to controls

[a]SI, sacro-iliac.
[b]LBP, low back pain.
[c]VAS, visual analog scale.

TABLE 2.3 Methods of Randomized Controlled Trials

Feature	Scarpone et al., 2007 [8] (n = 24)	Yelland et al., 2004 [40] (n = 110)	Reeves et al., 2000 [10] (n = 68)	Reeves 2000 [81] (n = 27)	Dechow et al., 1999 [39] (n = 74)	Klein et al., 1993 [38] (n = 79)	Ongley et al., 1987 [37] (n = 81)
Subjects	13 F, 11 M with "tennis elbow;" average age 45.7 years (19–62 years); pain for (average) 1.9 years	63 M, 47 F with LBP[a]; average age 50 years; pain for (average) 14 years	39 M, 29 F with knee OA[b] pain; average age 63 years; pain for minimum of 6 months	11 M, 16 F with finger OA pain; average age 64 years; pain for (average) 4–5 years	36 M, 38 F with LBP; average age 46 years; pain for (average) > 10 years	47 M, 32 F with LBP; average age 44 years; pain for (average) 11 years	38 M, 43 F with LBP; average age 44 years; pain for (average) 10 years
Intervention	Injections at 0, 4 and 8 weeks to supracondylar ridge, lateral epicondyle and annular ligament	On average, 7 bi-weekly injection series to lumbosacral ligaments; 10–30 mL per series	Single 9 mL intra-articular injection to affected knee at 0, 2 and 4 months	Average 6 periarticular injections to DIP, PIP and/or CMC joints at 0, 2 and 4 months	Up to 3 weekly injection series; up to 10 mL per series to lumbosacral ligaments	6 weekly injection series; up to 30 mL per series to lumbosacral ligaments	6 weekly injection series; up to 20 mL per series to lumbosacral ligaments
Proliferant	10.7% Dextrose and 14.7% sodium morrhuate by volume	20% Dextrose and 0.2% lidocaine	10% Dextrose and 0.075% lidocaine in bacteriostatic H_2O	10% Dextrose and 0.075% lidocaine in bacteriostatic H_2O	P2G[c]	P2G[c]	P2G[c]
Placebo	Saline	Saline	H_2O/Lidocaine	H_2O/Lidocaine	Saline/Lidocaine	Saline/Lidocaine	Saline/Lidocaine
Ancillary treatment	None	Subjects stratified in 2 × 2 fashion to receive dextrose or saline injections	Injections at 6, 8 and 10 months; unblinded follow-up	Injections at 6, 8, 10, and 12 months, and as needed;	None	Initial spinal manipulation for all subjects,	Intervention group: initially 60 mL lidocaine injection and forceful spinal manipulation, followed by triamcinolone/ lidocaine injection. Control

		with either flexion/extension exercises or normal activity; all subjects received daily oral vitamin C, zinc and manganese supplements		unblinded follow-up		followed by steroid injection at tender points; all subjects advised to do back exercises	group: initially 10 mL lidocaine injection, followed by non-forceful spinal manipulation; both groups encouraged to do routine activity and 150 flexion exercises daily
Follow-up	8, 16, 52 weeks	2.5, 4, 6, 12, 24 months	6, 12 months	6, 12 months	1, 3, 6 months	6 months	1, 3, 6 months
Outcomes	VAS[d] overall elbow pain; Eccentric Strength, Jamar Grip Strength; continuity of improvement at 52 weeks	Percentage of subjects achieving 50% pain or disability reduction; prior week pain VAS[d]; medication use; pain diagram; physical and mental health	Multiple VAS[d] assessments for knee pain, swelling, stability; leg buckling frequency; knee laxity arthrometry; joint space X-ray	Pain scores at rest, with movement, grip and flexion; average pain score; ROM[e] goniometry; joint space X-ray	Percentage of subjects achieving 50% pain reduction; McGill Pain Questionnaire; pain drawing; Somatic Perception Questionnaire; Depression Scale; Oswestry Disability Scale; objective assessment of ROM[e]	Percentage of subjects achieving 50% pain reduction; VAS[d] pain intensity; Roland-Morris Disability Scale; pain grid; ROM[e] by Triaxial dynamometer	Percentage of subjects achieving 50% pain reduction; VAS[d] pain intensity; Roland-Morris Disability Scale; clinical signs (ROM[e], tenderness)

[a]LBP, low back pain.
[b]OA, osteoarthritis (by X-ray and clinical criteria).
[c]P2G, phenol–glucose–glycerine.
[d]VAS, visual analog scale.
[e]ROM, range of motion.

TABLE 2.4 Results of Randomized Controlled Trials

Study	Scarpone et al., 2007 [8]	Yelland, 2004 [40]	Reeves and Hassanein, 2000 [10] (Knee)	Reeves and Hassanein, 2000 [10] (Finger)	Dechow et al., 1999 [39]	Klein et al., 1993 [38]	Ongley et al., 1987 [37]
Jadad score (x/5)	5	5	4	5	5	5	4
Delphi score (x/9)	8	9	7	9	8	7	7
Findings	Statistically and clinically significant improvements on pain ($p < 0.001$) and isometric strength ($p < 0.01$) testing compared to control injections, and grip strength compared to baseline	No significant improvement in primary or secondary outcome scores compared to controls. In all 4 groups, 36–46% of subjects achieved 50%	Reported improved pain, swelling, buckling and knee flexion compared to controls ($p < 0.05$). Improved lateral (increased) patellofemoral cartilage thickness ($p < 0.05$) compared to controls. Significant 6- and	Improvement in pain with finger movement compared to controls ($p < 0.05$). Improved flexion range compared to controls ($p < 0.01$). Non-significant ($p = 0.096$)	No significant improvement between groups in primary or secondary outcome scores. Small trends toward improvement in both control	77% of intervention subjects achieved >50% pain reduction vs. 53% in control group ($p < 0.05$). Intervention subjects improved in pain grid scores ($p < 0.05$) and showed a trend toward improvement	88% of intervention subjects achieved >50% pain reduction vs. 39% in control group ($p < 0.05$). Intervention subjects improved their mean pain ($p < 0.001$) and disability ($p < 0.001$) scores. No significant scores.

$(p < 0.01)$. Clinical improvement maintained at 52 weeks. Control subjects did not improve at 52 weeks.	pain reduction and 34–42% achieved 50% disability reduction.	12-month improvement in all assessments for knee pain, swelling and buckling compared to baseline. Decreased laxity $(p < 0.05)$, increased flexion $(p < 0.01)$ in uncontrolled follow-up compared to baseline.	improvement in multiple pain scores compared to controls. Improved joint space narrowing compared to controls at 1 year $(p < 0.01)$.	and intervention groups on McGill, pain drawing, somatic and ROM[b] scores. No change in depression or disability scores.	in pain $(p = 0.056)$ and disability $(p = 0.068)$ scores. Both intervention and control subjects improved compared to baseline on VAS[a], pain grid and disability scores $(p < 0.001)$.	difference between intervention and control groups in clinical signs.
Limitations	Small size, lack of consistent long-term follow-up	Lack of non-injection control group	Lack of non-injection control group; difficult to interpret the results of comparison between the groups	Lack of non-injection control group	Lack of non-injection control group; data presented graphically, no numerical data for any outcomes; unclear blinding of allocation and prolotherapist	Lack of non-injection control group; experimental group had statistically worse baseline pain	Lack of non-injection control group; different ancillary interventions for intervention and control groups making these groups non-comparable

[a] VAS, visual analog scale.

[b] ROM, range of motion.

The older case studies report materials and methods that have changed over time; solutions such as sylnasol and zinc sulfate are no longer used, while contemporary solutions are seen starting with P2G in the 1960s, dextrose in the 1980s and sodium morrhuate in the early 1990s. The case reports and case series highlight the fact that prolotherapy has over time been used and studied for a growing set of clinical indications. Case series have also been used as pilot studies to develop new assessment techniques that attempt to elucidate pathophysiology of the condition in question [12] and test methods for later use in more robust randomized studies [31]. The focus on "real-life" trial methods has been termed "pragmatic" [32]. Studies using pragmatic methods have the advantage of assessing effectiveness under conditions that patients encounter, thereby avoiding confounders associated with highly standardized trial settings. The case studies report consistently positive patient outcomes and the general satisfaction of physicians using prolotherapy for patients with often long-standing, debilitating pain. Pragmatic aspects of these studies include the ability of the prolotherapist to select the patient and individually tailor the injection protocol. More focused controlled studies have been termed "fastidious" and allow for improved hypothesis testing through the use of randomization, control groups and subject and investigator blinding. Seven RCTs have been conducted to date assessing prolotherapy for low back pain, osteoarthritis and tendinopathy. Evidence from the RCTs is the basis on which clinical recommendations in this chapter are made.

CASE SERIES AND NON-RANDOMIZED PROLOTHERAPY STUDIES FOR LOW BACK PAIN

Approximately 80% of Americans experience low back pain during their lifetime. An estimated 15–20% develop protracted pain, and approximately 2–8% have chronic pain. Every year, 3–4% of the population is temporarily disabled, and 1% of the working-age population is disabled totally and permanently because of low back pain. Low back pain is second only to the common cold as a cause of lost work time; it is the fifth most frequent cause for hospitalization and the third most common reason to undergo a surgical procedure. Productivity losses from chronic low back pain approach $28 billion annually in the United States [33]. Medication in the form of analgesics, antidepressants and non-steroidal anti-inflammatory drugs (NSAIDS) are likely to be beneficial. Exercise, intensive multidisciplinary treatment programs, acupuncture, back schools behavioral therapy and spinal manipulation are all beneficial or likely to be beneficial. Local injections are of unknown effectiveness [34].

Most of the case reports and case series involving prolotherapy concern low back pain or sacro-iliac dysfunction (2691/3741, 72%). Collectively, these studies describe subjective positive outcomes with minimum adverse effects. The most dramatic study is the career-long 21-year series by Hackett who reported an overall 82% "cure" rate for a variety of indications in 1857 patients [35]. Two non-randomized, controlled low back pain studies compared the treatment effects of prolotherapy with dextrose and lidocaine to either lidocaine alone [36] or conservative low back pain modalities [31] (Table 2.2). Naim *et al.* [36] reported a higher positive response rate in the treatment arm compared to controls, though the differences were not reported as significant. Yelland *et al.* [31] comparing subjects receiving prolotherapy to those receiving conservative low back pain therapy, reported significant improvement in leg pain score and pain diagram scores; disability and back pain scores trended toward significance.

CLINICAL TRIALS ASSESSING PROLOTHERAPY FOR LOW BACK PAIN (TABLES 2.3 AND 2.4)

Most existing RCTs for prolotherapy also concern low back pain. Four trials report on prolotherapy for musculoskeletal low back pain three used P2G as the injectant [37–39] and the fourth used Dextrose [40]. Each used a protocol involving injections to the ligamentous insertions of the L4-S1 spinous processes, sacrum and ilium. While outcome measures varied, a common measure was the number of participants showing a >50% improvement in pain/disability scores at 6 months.

Two studies reported positive findings compared to control injections. Ongley *et al.* [37] and Klein *et al.* [38] compared the treatment effects of prolotherapy in conjunction with injected steroids, spinal manipulation and exercise. In the Ongley study [37] 88% of subjects in the experimental group reported 50% pain reduction compared to 39% in the control group ($p < 0.03$). Significant ($p < 0.001$) improvement of experimental compared to control subjects was reported for low back pain, disability and pain grid scores. Klein *et al.* [38] compared two groups with more similar treatment protocols. Significant differences were reported between groups; 77% of experimental subjects improved 50% or more on pain score or disability, compared to 53% in the control group ($p = 0.04$). Pain grid scores were also significantly better in the experimental group ($p = 0.03$), although pain ($p = 0.06$) and disability ($p = 0.07$) scores individually trended toward significance compared to the control group. Both groups utilized steroid injections and spinal manipulation prior to prolotherapy. In the Ongley study, the intervention and control groups varied markedly on the make-up of initial injections and type of spinal manipulation associated with the injections.

Dechow *et al.* [39] and Yelland *et al.* [40] reported negative outcomes compared to control injections. Dechow *et al.* [39] refined protocol complexity in their study. All subjects underwent three injection sets without spinal manipulation or physical therapy. While both groups improved on a pain questionnaire, pain grid and somatic perception score, these were not significantly different within or between groups; improvement by 6 months for both groups was smaller than that of the other RCTs.

The largest and most methodologically rigorous prolotherapy study to date is by Yelland *et al.* [40]. One hundred and ten subjects with an average of 14 years of low back pain were randomized to one of four intervention regimens: dextrose and physical therapy, dextrose and "normal activity," saline injections and physical therapy, and saline injections with "normal activity." The investigators used a non-standard injection protocol that has generated editorial controversy [41, 42]. By 12 months, subjects in all groups had improved pain scores (26–44%) and disability scores (30–44%); there was no significant difference between groups. Fifty-five percent of subjects reported that their improvement had been worth the effort of the trial for both pain and disability. The percentage of subjects who reached 50% pain reduction varied between 36% and 46% in each of the four groups, though again the differences between groups were not significant.

Because the active and control groups receive very different treatment protocols, it is impossible to attribute effects to prolotherapy or any specific intervention. However, all four low back pain RCTs report improvements for pain and disability in all treatment groups. In particular, Yelland et al. [40] reported clinical improvement in excess of minimal clinical important difference, [43–45] and in excess of subjects' own perception of the minimum improvement necessary for prolotherapy to be worthwhile (25% for pain and 35% for disability) [31, 40].

CLINICAL TRIALS ASSESSING PROLOTHERAPY FOR TENDINOPATHIES

The strongest data that prolotherapy is an effective treatment for any musculoskeletal condition compared to control injections is for chronic painful overuse tendon disease. These conditions were formerly called "tendonitis" and are now more correctly termed "tendinosis" or "tendinopathy." Patients with a variety of tendinopathies commonly present to family practitioners and various medical specialists [46, 47]. They are discussed as a group because the current understanding of over-use tendinopathies identifies them as sharing underlying non-inflammatory pathology, that of repetitive motion/overuse injury and resulting painful degenerative tissue. Light microscopy of biopsies in patients undergoing surgery for tendon pain reveals collagen separation [48] and thin, frayed and fragile tendon fibrils, separated from each other lengthwise and disrupted in cross section. There is an apparent increase in tenocytes with myofibroblastic differentiation (tendon repair cells) with increased proteoglycan ground substance and neovascularization. Classic inflammatory cells are usually absent [48]. This aspect of tendinosis was first described 25 years ago, [49]; experts have advocated a change in nomenclature [50] but the misnomer continues [51].

Prolotherapy has been assessed as a treatment for three tendon disorders: lateral epicondylosis (LE) ("tennis elbow"), hip adductor and Achilles tendinopathies (Tables 2.1, 2.3 and 2.4). LE ("tennis elbow") is an important condition of the upper extremity with an incidence of 4–7/1000 patients per year in primary care settings [52–54]. Its greatest impact is on workers with repetitive and high load upper extremity tasks and on athletes. The most common cause of LE may be low-load, high-repetition activities such as keyboarding, though formal data is lacking [55]. Cost and time away from job or activity are significant [56, 57]. While many non-surgical therapies have been tested for LE refractory to conservative measures, none have shown to be uniformly effective in the long term [58–60]. Scarpone *et al.* conducted an RCT to determine whether prolotherapy improves elbow pain, grip strength and extension strength in patients with LE. Twenty adults with at least 6 months of LE refractory to rest, NSAIDS and corticosteroid injections were randomized to prolotherapy with dextrose and sodium morrhuate or 0.9% saline. Three injections were made at the supracondylar ridge, lateral epicondyl and annular ligament. Pain scores were improved at 8 weeks compared to controls and dramatically improved by 16 weeks ($p < 0.001$). Prolotherapy subjects also reported improvement extension strength compared to controls ($p < 0.01$) and grip strength compared to baseline ($p < 0.05$). Clinical improvement in prolotherapy subjects was maintained at 52 weeks.

Chronic Achilles tendinopathy is a common overuse injury that is seen not only in athletes but also in the general population. This condition is painful and a cause of considerable distress and disability [61]. Maxwell *et al.* conducted a well-designed case series to assess whether intratendinous 25% dextrose injected in hypoechoic regions of the Achilles tendon under ultrasound guidance at intervals of 6 weeks would decrease pain. Interestingly, they also assessed the thickness of the tendon and the degree of hypoechogenicity and neovascularity, ultrasound findings recently reported to be associated with tendinopathy [62, 63]. They reported that pain decreased by 88%, 84% and 78% on visual analog scales during rest, activity or sport respectively. Tendon thickness decreased significantly; the overall grade of tendon pathology, hypoechoic and anechoic regions tendons and neovascularity were all improved in some subjects but not in others. Therefore the relationship between these characteristics, prolotherapy and clinical improvement remains unclear.

Groin pain is a common problem among those who engage in kicking sports [64]. Topol *et al.* conducted a case series assessing prolotherapy for chronic groin pain, a condition involving pain and tenderness at both tendon and ligament insertions [65]. Male athletes with an average of 15.5 months of groin pain were injected with 12.5% dextrose at the thigh adductor origins, supra-pubic abdominal insertions and symphysis pubis at 4-week intervals until pain resolved or subjects had no improvement for two consecutive sessions. Subjects reported dramatic improvements on a VAS Pain Scale and on the Nirschl Pain Phase Scale; 20 of 24 subjects had no pain and 22 of 24 were unrestricted with sports after therapy.

CLINICAL TRIALS ASSESSING PROLOTHERAPY FOR OSTEOARTHRITIS

Prolotherapy has been assessed as a treatment for knee and finger osteoarthritis (Tables 2.3 and 2.4) [66] and is the subject of ongoing NIH assessment [67].

Arthritis is a leading cause of disability in the world and in the United States where it affects 43 million persons [68–70]. Osteoarthritis is the most common form of arthritis, and the most common joint disorder [71]. In the United States, knee osteoarthritis is present and symptomatic in up to 6% of the population over 30, [71] and has an incidence of 360,000 new, symptomatic cases per year [72]. Incidence increases up to 10-fold from ages 30 to 65 and more thereafter [73]. Osteoarthritis results in a high burden of disease and economic impact through high prevalence, time off work and frequent utilization of health care resources [68, 74]. Osteoarthritis is also associated with significant disability, the main source of which is pain in performance of activities of daily living [38, 75, 76]. The disability impact of knee osteoarthritis is similar to that of cardiovascular disease and has an impact that may equal that of any other medical condition in the elderly [77].

Allopathic and complementary and alternative medicine (CAM) treatment recommendations aimed at correcting modifiable risk factors, symptom control and disease modification have been published [78, 79]. Non-pharmacologic measures include patient education and social support, weight loss, physical and occupational therapy, aerobic exercise and a variety of assist and brace devices. Pharmacologic management includes acetaminophen, NSAIDS, cyclooxygenase 2-specific inhibitors, steroid injections, tramadol, opioids, topical capsacin and methysalicylate. While they may help some patients, none have proven to provide definitive pain or disease modification for patients with knee osteoarthritis. The Agency for Research Health and Quality (AHRC) has recently evaluated glucosamine, chondroitin viscosupplementation and arthroscopic debridement [80]. These too have not shown to be effective compared to placebo. The high burden of knee osteoarthritis and the absence of cure continue to stimulate intense search for new agents to modify disease and control symptoms.

Reeves *et al.* have assessed prolotherapy as a treatment for knee and finger osteoarthritis [10, 81]. Subjects with finger or knee pain and radiological evidence of osteoarthritis underwent three sessions of prolotherapy with 10% dextrose and lidocaine, or lidocaine and bacteriostatic water. In the finger osteoarthritis trial, intervention subjects improved in "pain with movement" ($p = 0.027$) and "flexion range" ($p = 0.003$) compared to controls, while pain at rest and with grip showed non-significant improvement. In the knee osteoarthritis trial, subjects in both groups reported significant improvement in multiple pain scores, swelling, number of buckling episodes and flexion range of motion compared to baseline.

Both osteoarthritis studies had 6-month open-label follow-up. Surprising and potentially important 12-month findings on plain X-ray included decreased joint space narrowing and improved osteophyte grade in the finger study, and increased patellofemoral cartilage thickness in the knee study. Whether or not subjects had concomitant meniscal pathology in the knee study was not reported or included in entry criteria. Furthermore, the ability of plain X-ray to quantify patellofemoral cartilage thickness is questionable, limiting the impact of the authors' conclusions.

ADVERSE EFFECTS OF PROLOTHERAPY

Injection of ligaments and joints with irritant solutions raises safety concerns, especially when performed for perispinal or rib indications. Historically, a small number of significant complications have been reported in perispinal prolotherapy for back or neck pain using very concentrated prolotherapy solutions, including five cases of neurologic impairment from spinal cord irritation [82–84] and one death in 1959 following prolotherapy with zinc sulfate for low back pain [82]. Neither zinc sulfate nor concentrated prolotherapy solutions are currently in general use. In a retrospective survey of 95 doctors using prolotherapy, there were 29 reports of pneumothoraces after prolotherapy for back and neck pain, two of which required hospitalization for a chest tube. Fourteen cases of allergic reactions were reported, none classified as serious [13]. A more recent survey of practicing prolotherapists yielded similar results for spinal prolotherapy [19]. Spinal headache, pneumothoraces, nerve damage and non-severe spinal cord insult and disk injury were reported. The authors concluded these events were no more common in prolotherapy than for other spinal injection procedures. Prolotherapy has much less risk when used on peripheral joint indications. Minor side effects have been reported in two trials of dextrose prolotherapy for knee and finger osteoarthritis [10, 81] and in one trial for LE, [8] including temporary discomfort and stiffness, a flare in pain requiring steroid injection and, in the fingers, a transient restriction of venous return due to pressure effects.

PROLOTHERAPY RESEARCH

Prolotherapy research methods are evolving amidst significant debate; [41, 42, 85–87] existing studies are far from definitive. Several research methods require refinement. First, the RCT control therapies in studies using control injections may have affected outcomes. No RCT contained a control arm without injections. In both the control and intervention groups, the effect of needle-to-bone contact, pressure–volume relationships at the bone–ligament junction, and especially the irritant effects of blood [88, 89] may have induced similar effects irrespective of the injectant. The similarity of control and intervention therapies could account for the fact that clinically relevant improvements were not different across groups. The independent effect of control injections in prolotherapy has not been adequately assessed in basic science studies or clinical trials. This seems to be far more a factor in the low back pain studies than the osteoarthritis and tendinopathy studies.

Second, RCT results to date may not reflect ideal subject selection. Prolotherapy is an operator-dependent procedure in which injection protocols are in part exam-dependent. Experienced prolotherapists decide who should be treated based on both diagnosis and exam findings. The Dechow study reported the smallest improvement in subject outcomes but also noted that the prolotherapist considered a subset of subjects inappropriate for prolotherapy, even though they met the study's entry criteria [39]. The entry criteria of all RCTs evaluated were diagnosis-driven; none reported that exam findings by the prolotherapist could exclude a subject. Results may therefore be skewed away from a positive effect, should one exist.

CLINICAL RECOMMENDATIONS

Present data suggest that prolotherapy is likely an effective therapy for painful overuse tendinopathy. Specifically, the Scarpone study reports significant reduction in pain and improved isometric strength scores in subjects with refractory LE treated with prolotherapy using dextrose and sodium morrhuate compared to control injections. It provides level 1B evidence (high-quality RCT in a setting of less than two consistent RCTs evaluating patient oriented evidence) [90] that prolotherapy is an effective therapy for LE. It is supported by the Maxwell and Topol studies, which report very strong case series results for Achilles and hip adductor respectively. These studies provide level 2B evidence that prolotherapy is effective for Achilles and adductor tendinopathies compared to a patient's baseline condition [90]. Given that the underlying mechanism of injury and pathophysiologic effect is similar for tendinopathies, prolotherapy is a reasonable option for both of these conditions as well. RCTs for all three tendinopathies and for other tendinopathies are indicated.

Recommendations are more difficult to make for osteoarthritis and low back pain, both of which are associated with more complex anatomy and less clear pathophysiology than seen in tendinopathies. Side effect and potential adverse events of prolotherapy are likely to be more serious when performed for spinal or intra-articular indications and must be weighed against the potential for improvement. Existing studies provide level 2B evidence that prolotherapy is effective for low back pain compared to a patient's baseline condition (studies with inconsistent findings [90]). Given that subjects with refractory, disabling low back pain significantly improved compared to their own baseline status in the Yelland study, patients may reasonably try prolotherapy when performed by an experienced operator. Existing studies provide level 2B evidence that prolotherapy is effective for osteoarthritis compared to control injections (lower quality clinical trial [90]). Based on evidence from the two Reeves RCTs, patients may reasonably try prolotherapy for significant osteoarthritic knee or finger pain.

REFERENCES

1.   McGonagle, D., Marzo-Ortega, H., Benjamin, M. & Emery, P. (2003). Report on the second international enthesitis workshop. *Arthritis Rheum* **48**, 896–905.
2.   Hackett, G. S., Hemwall, G. A. & Montgomery, G. A. (1993). *Ligament and Tendon Relaxation Treated by Prolotherapy*, Gustav A, Hemwall, Oak Park.
3.   Liu, Y. K., Tipton, C. M., Matthes, R. D., Bedford, T. G., Maynard, J. A. & Walmer, H. C. (1983). An *in-situ* study of the influence of a sclerosing solution in rabbit medial collateral ligaments and its junction strength. *Connect Tissue Res* **11**, 95–102.

4. Maynard, J. A., Pedrini, V. A., Pedrini-Mille, A., Romanus, B. & Ohlerking, F. (1985). Morphological and biochemical effects of sodium morrhuate on tendons. *J Orthop Res* **3**, 236–248.

5. Linetsky, F. S., FRafael, M. & Saberski, L. (2002). Pain management with regenerative injection therapy (RIT). *In* Pain Management (R. S. Weiner, Ed.), pp. 381–402, CRC Press, Boca Raton.

6. Banks, A. (1991). A rationale for prolotherapy. *J Orthop Med* **13**, 54–59.

7. Hoksrud, A., Ohberg, L., Alfredson, H. & Bahr, R. (2006). Ultrasound-guided sclerosis of neovessels in painful chronic patellar tendinopathy. *Am J Sports Med* **34**, 1738–1746.

8. Scarpone, M., Rabago, D., Zgierska, A., Arbogest, J. & Snell, E. D. (2007). The efficacy of prolotherapy for lateral epicondylosis: A pilot study. *Clin J Sports Med*, In Review.

9. Kim, S. R., Stitik, T. P. & Foye, P. M. (2004). Critical review of prolotherapy for osteoarthritis low back pain and other musculoskeletal conditions: A physiatric perspective. *J Phys Med Rehabil* **83**, 379–389.

10. Reeves, K. D. & Hassanein, K. (2000). Randomized prospective double-blind placebo-controlled study of dextrose prolotherapy for knee osteoarthritis with or without ACL laxity. *Alternative Ther Health Med* **6**, 68–80.

11. Linetsky, F. S., Botwin, K., Gorfin, L. & Jay, G. W. (2001). Regeneration injection therapy (RIT): Effectiveness and Appropriate Usage. Florida Academy of Pain Medicine http://www.gracermedicalgroup.com/resources/articles/rf_file_0025.pdf

12. Maxwell, N. J., Ryan, M. B., Taunton, J. E., Gillies, J. H. & Wong, A. D. (2007). Sonographically guided intratendinous injection of hyperosmolar dextrose to treat chronic tendinosis of the Achilles tendon: A pilot study. *Am J Roentgenol* **189**, W215–W220.

13. Dorman, T. A. (1993). Prolotherapy: A survey. *J Orthop Med* **15**, 49–50.

14. Google (2003)

15. Fleck, M. (2002). Director American Association of Orthopaedic Medicine.

16. Schultz, L. (1937). A treatment for subluxation of the temporomandibular joint. *J Am Med Assoc* **109**, 1032–1035.

17. Schnirring, L. (2000). Are your patients asking about prolotherapy? *Physician and Sportsmedicine* **28**, 15–17.

18. Matthews, J. H. (1999). Nonsurgical treatment of pain in lumbar spinal stenosis: Letter to the editor. *Am Fam Physician* **59**, 280–284.

19. Dagenais, S., Ogunseitan, O., Haldeman, S., Wooley, J. R. & Newcomb, R. L. (2006). Side effects and adverse events related to intraligamentous injection of sclerosing solutions (prolotherapy) for back and neck pain: A survey of practitioners. *Arch Phys Med Rehabil* **87**, 909–913.

20. Natarajan, R., Gonzalez, N., Xu, L. & Nadler, J. L. (1992). Vascular smooth muscle cells exhibit increased growth in response to elevated glucose. *Biochem Biophys Res Commun* **187**, 552–560.

21. McGinn, S., Poronnik, P. & King, M. (2003). High glucose and endothelial cell growth: Novel effects independent of autocine TGF-beta 1 and hyperosmolaraity. *Am J Cell Physiol* **284**, C1374–C1386.

22. Kondo, S., Beissert, S. & Wang, B. (1996). Hyporesponsiveness in contact hypersensitivity and irritant contact dermatitis in CD4 gene targeted mouse. *J Invest Dermatol* **106**.

23. Pedersen, G., Brynskov, J. & Saermark, T. (2002). Phenol toxicity and congugation in human colonic epithelial cells. *Scand J Gastroenterol* **37**, 74–79.

24. Gunduz, S., Kalyon, T. A. & Dursun, H. (1992). Peripheral nerve block with phenol to treat spasticity in spinal cord injured patients. *Paraplegia* **30**, 808–811.

25. Westerlund, T., Vuorinen, V., Kirvela, O. & Roytta, M. (1999). The endoneurial response to neurolytic agents is highly dependent on the mode of application. *Reg Anesth Pain Med* **24**, 294–302.

26. de lorimer, A. A. (1995). Sclerotherapy for venous malformations. *J Pediatr Surg* **30**, 1729–1734.

27. Jensen, K., Rabago, D., Best, T. M., Patterson, J. J. & Vanderby, R. (2007). Early inflammatory response of knee ligaments to prolotherapy in a rat model. *J Ortho Res*, In Press.

28. Aneja, A., Spero, G., Weinhold, P. *et al.* (2005). Suture plication thermal shrinkage and sclerosing agents. *Am J Sports Med* **33**, 1729–1734.

29. Jensen, K. T., Rabago, D., Best, T. M., Patterson, J. J. & Vanderby, R. (2007). Longer term response of knee ligaments to prolotherapy in a rat injury model. *Am J Sports Med*, Comment: In Review.

30. Rabago, D., Best, T., Beamsly, M. & Patterson, J. (2005). A systematic review of prolotherapy for chronic musculoskeletal pain. *Clin J Sports Med* **15**, 376–380.

31. Yelland, M., Yeo, M. & Schluter, P. (2000). Prolotherapy injections for chronic low back pain: Results of a pilot comparative study. *Aust Musculoskel Med* **5**, 20–30.

32. Ernst, E., Pittler, M. H., Stevinson, C. & White, A. (2001). *Randomised clinical trials: Pragmatic or fastidious? Focus on alternative and complementary therapies* **63**, 179–180.

33. Wheeler, A. H. (2007). Pathophysiology of Chronic Back Pain. http://www.emedicine.com/neuro/topic516.htm

34. van Tulder, M. & Koes, B. (2006). Low back pain (chronic). BMJ Clin Evid http://clinicalevidence.bmj.com/ceweb/conditions/msd/1116/1116.jsp

35. Hackett, G. S. & Huang, T. C. (1961). Prolotherapy for Sciatica from weak pelvic ligaments and bone dystrophy. *Clin Med* **8**, 2301–2316.

36. Naeim, F., Froetscher, L. & Hirschberg, G. G. (1982). Treatment of the chronic iliolumbar syndrome by infiltration of the iliolumbar ligament. *West J Med* **136**, 372–374.

37. Ongley, M. J., Klein, R. G., Dorman, T. A., Eek, B. C. & Hubert, L. J. (1987). A new approach to the treatment of chronic low back pain. *Lancet* **2**, 143–146.

38. Klein, R. G., Eek, B. C., DeLong, W. B. & Mooney, V. (1993). A randomized double-blind trial of dextrose–glycerine–phenol injections for chronic low back pain. *J Spinal Disord* **6**, 23–33.

39. Dechow, E., Davies, R. K., Carr, A. J. & Thompson, P. W. (1999). A randomized double-blind placebo-controlled trial of sclerosing injections in patients with chronic low back pain. *Rheumatology* **38**, 1255–1259.

40. Yelland, M., Glasziou, P., Bogduk, N., Schluter, P. & McKernon, M. (2004). Prolotherapy injections saline injections and exercises for chronic low back pain: A randomized trial. *Spine* **29**, 9–16.

41. Reeves, K. D., Klein, R. G. & DeLong, W. B. (2004). Letter to the editor. *Spine* **29**, 1839–1840.

42. Linetsky, F. S., Saberski, L. & Dubin, J. A. (2004). Letter to the editor. *Spine* **29**, 1840–1841.
43. Bellamy, N., Carr, A., Dougados, M., Shea, B. & Wells, G. (2001). Towards a definition of "difference" in osteoarthritis. *J Rheumatol* **28**, 427–430.
44. Redelmeier, D. A., Guyatt, G. H. & Goldstein, R. S. (1996). Assessing the minimal important difference in symptoms: A comparison of two techniques. *J Clin Epidemiol* **49**, 1215–1219.
45. Wells, G. A., Tugwell, P., Kraag, G. R., Baker, P. R., Groh, J. & Redelmeier, D. A. (1993). Minimum important difference between patients with rheumatoid arthritis: The patient's perspective. *J Rheumatol* **20**, 557–560.
46. Bongers, P. M. (2001). The cost of shoulder pain at work. Variation in work tasks and good job opportunities are essential for prevention. *BMJ* **322**, 64–65.
47. Wilson, J. J. & Best, T. M. (2005). Common overuse tendon problems: A review and recommendations for treatment. *Am Fam Physician* **72**, 811–818.
48. Khan, K. M., Cook, J. L., Bonar, F., Harcourt, P. & Astrom, M. (1999). Histopathology of tendinopathies. Update and implications for clinical management. *Sports Med* **27**, 393–408.
49. Puddu, G., Ippolito, E. & Postacchini, F. A. (1976). Classification of Achilles tendon disease. *Am J Sports Med* **4**, 145–150.
50. Khan, K. M., Cook, J. L., Kannus, P., Maffuli, N. & Bonar, S. F. (2002). Time to abandon the "tendinitis" myth. *BMJ* **324**, 626–627.
51. Johnson, G. W., Cadwallader, K., Scheffel, S. B. & Epperly, T. D. (2007). Treatment of lateral epicondylitis. *Am Fam Physician* **76**, 843–848, 849–850, 853.
52. Verhar, J. (1994). Tennis elbow: Anatomical epidemiological and therapeutic aspects. *Int Orthop* **18**, 263–267.
53. Hamilton, P. (1986). The prevalence of humeral epicondylitis: A survey in general practice. *J Roy Coll Gen Pract* **36**, 464–465.
54. Kivi, P. (1983). The etiology and conservative treatment of lateral epicondylitis. *Scand J Rehabil Med* **15**, 37–41.
55. Gabel, G. T. (1999). Acute and chronic tendinopathies at the elbow. *Curr Opin Rheumatol* **11**, 138–148.
56. Ono, Y., Nakamura, R., Shimaoka, M., Hattori, Y. & Ichihara, G. (1998). Epicondylitis among cooks in nursery schools. *Occup Environ Med* **55**, 172–179.
57. Ritz, B. R. (1995). Humeral epicondylitis among gas and waterworks employees. *Scand J Work Environ Health* **21**, 478–486.
58. Buchbinder, R., Green, S., White, M., et al. (2002) Shock wave therapy for lateral elbow pain. *Cochrane Database of Systematic Reviews* **1** (Art. No.: CD003524. DOI: 10.1002/14651858.CD003524.pub2).
59. Smidt, N., van der Windt, D. A., Assendelft, W. J., Deville, W. L., Korthals-deBos, I. B. & Bouter, L. M. (2002). Corticosteroid injections physiotherapy or a wait-and-see policy for lateral epicondylitis: A randomised controlled trial. *Lancet* **359**, 657–662.
60. Struijs, P. A., Smidt, N., Arola, H., Dijk, C. N.v., Buchbinder, R. & Assendelft, W. J. (2005). Orthotic devices for the treatment of tennis elbow. *The Cochrane Collaboration* **3**.
61. Kvist, M. (1994). Achilles tendon injuries in athletes. *Sports Med* **18**, 173–2001.
62. Zeisig, E., Ohberg, L. & Alfredson, H. (2006). Extensor origin vascularity related to pain in patients with tennis elbow. *Knee Surg Sports Traumatol Arthrosc* **14**, 659–663.

63. Alfredson, H. & Ohberg, L. (2005). Sclerosing injections to areas of neovascularization reduce pain in chronic Achilles tendinopathy: A double-blind randomised trial. *Knee Surg Sports Traumatol Arthrosc* **13**, 338–344.

64. Holmich, P., Uhrskou, P. & Ulnits, L. (1999). Effectiveness of active physical training as treatment of long-standing adductor-related groin pain in athletes: A randomized controlled trial. *Lancet* **353**, 439–443.

65. Topol, G. A., Reeves, K. D. & Hassanein, K. M. (2005). Efficacy of dextrose prolotherapy in elite male kicking-sport athletes with groin pain. *Arch Phys Rehabil* **86**, 697–702.

66. Reeves, K. D. (2000). Randomized prospective double-blind placebo-controlled study of dextrose prolotherapy for knee osteoarthritis with or without ACL laxity. *Alternative Ther* **6**, 68–80.

67. Rabago, D. (In Progress). The Efficacy of Prolotherapy in Osteoarthritic Knee Pain. NIH-NCCAM Grant, 1K23 AT001879-01.

68. Reginster, J. Y. (2002). The prevalence and burden of arthritis. *Rheumatology* **41**, 3–6.

69. CDC (1998) Prevalence and impact of chronic joint symptoms – seven states (1996). *MMWR* **47**, 345–351.

70. CDC (1994) Prevalence of disabilities and associated health conditions – United States (1991–1992). *MMWR* **43**, 730–739.

71. Felson, D. T. & Zhang, Y. (1998). An update on the epidemiology of knee and hip osteoarthritis with a view to prevention. *Arthritis Rheum* **41**, 1343–1355.

72. Wilson, M. G., Michet, C. J., Ilstrup, D. M. & Melton, L. J. (1990). Ideopathic symptomatic osteoarthritis of the hip and knee: A population-based incidence study. *Mayo Clic Proc* **65**, 1214–1221.

73. Oliveria, S. A., Felson, D. T., Klein, R. A., Reed, J. I. & Walker, A. M. (1996). Estrogen replacement therapy and the development of osteoarthritis. *Epidemiology* **7**, 415–419.

74. Levy, E., Ferme, A., Perocheau, D. *et al.* (1993). Socioeconomic costs of osteoarthritis in France. *Rev Rhum* **60**, 63S–67S.

75. Callahan, L. F., Brooks, R. H., Summey, J. A. & Pincus, T. (1987). Quantitative pain assessment for routine care of rheumatoid arthritis patients using a pain scale based on activities of daily living and a visual analog pain scale. *Arthritis Rheum* **30**, 630–636.

76. Bellamy, N., Buchanan, W. W., Goldsmith, C. H., Campbell, J. & Stitt, L. W. (1988). Validation study of WOMAC: A health status instrument for measuring clinically important patient relevant outcomes in antirheumatic drug therapy in patients with osteoarthritis of the knee. *J Rheumatol* **15**, 1833–1840.

77. Guccione, A. A., Felson, D. T., Anderson, J. J., Anthony, J. M., Zhang, Y., Wilson, P. W., Kelly-Hayes, M., Wolf, P. A., Kreger, B. E. & Kannel, W. B. (1994). The effects of specific medical conditions on the functional limitations of elders in the Framingham study. *Am J Publ Health* **84**, 351–358.

78. Felson, D. T., Lawrence, R. C., Hochberg, M. C. *et al.* (2000). Osteoarthritis: New insights part 2: Treatment approaches. *Ann Intern Med* **133**, 726–737.

79. American College of Rheumatology Subcommittee on Osteoarthritis Guidelines (2000). Recommendations for the medical management of osteoarthritis of the hip and knee. *Arthritis Rheum* **43**, 1905–1915.

80. Samson, D. J., Grant, M. D., Ratko, T. A., Bonnell, C. J., Ziegler, K. M. & Aronson, N. (2007). Treatment of primary and secondary osteoarthritis of the knee. *Agency for Healthcare Research and Quality: Evidence Report/Technology Assessment* **151**.

81. Reeves, K. D. & Hassanein, K. (2000). Randomized prospective placebo-controlled double-blind study of dextrose prolotherapy for osteoarthritic thumb and finger (DIP PIP and Trapeziometacarpal) joints: Evidence of clinical efficacy. *J Altern Complem Med* **6**, 311–320.

82. Schneider, R. C., Williams, J. J. & Liss, L. (1959). Fatality after injection of sclerosing agent to precipitate fibro-osseous proliferation. *J Am Med Assoc* **170**, 1768–1772.

83. Keplinger, J. E. & Bucy, P. C. (1960). Paraplegia from treatment with sclerosing agents – report of a case. *J Am Med Assoc* **173**, 1333–1336.

84. Hunt, W. E. & Baird, W. C. (1961). Complications following injection of sclerosing agent to precipitate fibro-osseous proliferation. *J Neurosurg* **18**, 461–465.

85. Loeser, J. D. (2004). Point of view. *Spine* **29**, 16.

86. Kidd, R. (2004). Letter to the editor. *Spine* **29**, 1841–1842.

87. Yelland, M. (2004). Letter to the editor. *Spine* **29**, 1842–1843.

88. Taylor, M. A., Norman, T. L., Clovis, N. B. *et al.* (2002). The response of rabbit patellar tendons after autologous blood injection. *Med Sci Sports Exerc* **34**, 70–73.

89. Edwards, S. G. & Calandruccio, J. H. (2003). Autologous blood injections for refractory lateral epicondylitis. *J Hand Surgery Am* **28**, 272–278.

90. Ebell, M. H., Siwek, J., Weiss, B. D., Woolf, S. H., Susman, J., Ewigman, B. & Bowman, M. (2004). Strength of recommendation taxonomy (SORT): A patient-centered approach to grading evidence in the medical literature. *Am Fam Physician* **69**, 548–556.

91. Gedney, E. (1937). Special technic hypermobile joint: A preliminary report. *Osteopath Profession* **4**, 30–31.

92. Shuman, D. (1941). Luxation recurring in the shoulder. *Osteopath Profession* **8**, 11–14.

93. Bahme, B. B. (1945). Observations on the treatment of hypermotile joints by injection. *J Am Osteopath Assoc* **45**, 101–109.

94. Gedney, E. H. (1951). Disk syndrome: New approach in the treatment of symptomatic intervertebral disk. *Osteopath Profession* **18**, 11–14.

95. Gedney, E. H. (1952). Technique for sclerotherapy in the management of hypermobile sacroiliac. *Osteopath Profession* **16–19**, 37–38.

96. Hackett, G. S. (1953). Joint stabilization through induced ligament sclerosis. *Ohio State Med J* **49**, 877–884.

97. Shuman, D. (1954). Sclerotherapy: Statisitics on its effectiveness of unstable joint conditions. *Osteopath Profession* **11–15**, 37–38.

98. Hackett, G. S. (1954). Shearing injury to the sacroiliam joint. *J Int Coll Surg* **XXII**, 631–642.

99. Neff, F. (1960). Low back pain and disability. *West Med* **1**, 12–14, 27–33.

100. Myers, A. (1961). Prolotherapy treatment of low back pain and sciatica. *Bull Hosp Joint Dis* **22**, 48–55.

101. Hackett, G. S. & Huang, T. C. (1962). Prolotherapy for headache. *Headache* **2**, 20–28.

102. Kayfetz, D. O., Blumenthal, L. S., Hackett, G. S., Hemwall, G. A. & Neff, F. E. (1963). Whiplash injury and other ligamentous headache – Its managment with prolotherapy. *Headache*, 21–28.
103. Kayfetz, D. O. (1963). Occipito-cervical (Whiplash) injuries treated by prolotherapy. *Medical Trial Tech Quarter* **3**, 9–29.
104. Peterson, T. H. (1963). Injection treatment for back pain. *Am J Orthoped*, 320–321.
105. Barbor, R. (1964). A Treatment for Chronic Low Back Pain. *Proceedings of IV International Congress of Physical Medicine*, Paris, 661–664.
106. Blumenthal, L. (1974). Injury to the cervical spine as a cause of headache. *Postgrad Med* **53**, 147–152.
107. Leedy, R. & Kulik, A. L. (1976). Analysis of 50 low back cases 6 years after treatment by joint ligament sclerotherapy (prolotherapy). *Osteopath Med* **6**, 15–22.
108. Leedy, R. F. (1977). Applications of sclerotherapy to specific problems. *Osteopath Med*, 79–97.
109. Leedy, R. (1982). The challenge of a new skill. *New Jersey Assoc Osteopat Phys Surg J* **81**, 9–13.
110. Bourdeau, Y. (1988). Five-year follow-up on sclerotherapy/prolotherapy for low back pain. *Manual Med* **3**, 155–157.
111. Ongley, M. J., Dorman, T. A., Eck, B. C., Lundgren, D. & Klein, R. G. (1988). Ligament instability of knees: A new approach to treatment. *Manual Med* **3**, 152–154.
112. LaCourse, M., Moore, K., David, K., Fune, M. & Dorman, T. A. (1990). A report on the asymmetry of iliac inclinations. *J Orthop Med* **12**, 69–72.
113. Dorman, T. A. (1991). Treatment for spinal pain arising in ligaments using prolotherapy: A retrospective study. *J Orthop Med* **13**, 13–19.
114. Schwartz, R. G. & Sagedy, N. (1991). Prolotherapy: A literature review and retrospective study. *J Neurol Orth Med S* **12**, 220–223.
115. Hirschberg, G. G., Williams, K. A. & Byrd, J. B. (1992). Diagnosis and treatment of ileocostal friction syndromes. *West J Med* **14**, 35–39.
116. Reeves, K. D. (1994). Treatment of consecutive severe fibromyalgia patients with prolotherapy. *J Orthop Med* **16**, 84–89.
117. Dorman, T. A., Cohen, R. E., Dasig, D., Jeng, S., Fischer, N. & deJong, A. (1995). Energy efficiency during human walking before and after prolotherapy. *J Orthop Med* **17**, 24–26.
118. Matthews, J. S. N., Altman, D. G., Campbell, M. J. & Royston, P. (1990). Analysis of serial measurements in medical research. *BMJ* **300**, 230–235.
119. Reeves, K. D. & Harris, A. I. (1997). Recurrent dislocation of total knee prostheses in a large patient: Case report of dextrose proliferant use. *Arch Phys Med Rehabil* **78**, 1039.
120. Reeves, K. D. & Hassanein, K. M. (2003). Long-term effects of dextrose prolotherapy for anterior cruciate ligament therapy. *Alternative Ther Health Med* **9**, 58–62.
121. Hooper, R. A. & Ding, M. (2004). Retrospective case series on patients with chronic spinal pain treated with dextrose prolotherapy. *J Alternative Compl Med* **10**, 670–674.
122. Hooper, R. A., Sherman, S. T. & Frizzell, J. B. (2005). Case report of whiplash related chronic neck pain treated with intraarticular prolotherapy. *Journal of Whiplash and Related Disorders* **2**, 23–27.

Chapter 3

Soy and Cognition in the Aging Population

Lauren L. Drogos[1], Stacie Geller[3] and Pauline M. Maki[1,2]

[1]Department of Psychology, University of Illinois, Chicago, IL, USA
[2]Department of Psychiatry, University of Illinois, Chicago, IL, USA
[3]Department of Obstetrics and Gynecology, University of Illinois, Chicago, IL, USA

Abstract

Phytoestrogens are naturally occurring estrogen compounds found in plants. One of the most abundant and readily available sources of these compounds is soy products. Concerns about the risks of hormone therapy to women's health led to an increase in the use of soy and soy supplements for menopausal symptoms and general health. There is evidence that estrogen might benefit memory and other cognitive abilities in younger postmenopausal women, suggesting that soy might act in a similar manner to enhance cognition. Animal studies support the view that soy isoflavones can benefit memory and other cognitive abilities. Similarly, small clinical trials provide evidence that soy can positively impact cognition in premenopausal and postmenopausal women under age 65. Larger studies in older postmenopausal women show no cognitive benefits with soy, suggesting that any benefits might be limited to younger postmenopausal women. Animal studies indicate that the effects of soy may be sex-specific, benefitting females but not males, though this has not been tested extensively in humans. Additional studies are needed to investigate the possible influence of age and sex in modulating the cognitive effects of soy.

Keywords: *Phytoestrogens, soy and soy isoflavones, aging, women health*

INTRODUCTION

The use of botanicals and their derivatives as supplements for both mental and physical health can be traced back many centuries. Traditional Chinese medicine stressed the ability of certain herbs, plants and foods to act as preventative or curative medical treatments. In modern medical practice, the idea of complementary alternative medicine has grown in popularity, and there is a related need for systematic investigations into the putative benefits of these compounds. Herbal medicines are widely marketed as cognitive enhancers,

45

despite the lack of strong evidence for benefits. In the Study of Women's Health Across the Nation, a large epidemiological study of midlife women in the United States, 17% of women used soy supplements [1]. With many women now using botanical supplements as "safe" alternatives to hormone therapy for relieving menopausal symptoms and improving memory, there is increased interest in research aimed at determining the effectiveness and safety of these various compounds. This chapter reviews the evidence pertaining to soy isoflavones, one of the main nutraceuticals used for sustaining cognitive function, particularly in women.

USE OF SOY AND SOY ISOFLAVONES

Interest in soy isoflavones as a possible treatment for menopausal symptoms is based on anecdotal evidence from cultures where soy consumption is high [2] and evidence of estrogenic properties conducive to cognitive enhancement [3]. The frequency of menopausal symptoms and the prevalence of estrogen-related diseases, such as breast cancer and osteoporosis, vary in low soy consuming countries, like the United States, compared with high soy consuming countries like Japan [2]. This variation is frequently used as evidence of the significance of estrogenic action of soy-containing foods and supplements for women's health.

Soybeans and soybean-based foods such as tofu and tempeh are one of the richest plant sources for one type of bioactive antioxidants known as isoflavones. Isoflavones act as both antioxidants and phytoestrogens. Phytoestrogens are plant-derived compounds that resemble steroid hormones in both structure and function. Isoflavones from soy can be ingested either from whole food sources such as tofu or through a supplement in powder or pill form. There is evidence of differential absorption and bioavailability (i.e., the degree which the compounds are available for use within the body) depending on the administration medium for the isoflavones (e.g., food type and supplement type) [4]. The bioavailability of these compounds is highly dependent on how they are metabolized within the digestive tract. The most common side effects of soy isoflavones supplements are gastrointestinal and musculoskeletal symptoms [5]. Soy supplements in particular are commonly used by midlife women.

ESTROGEN, SOY AND BRAIN FUNCTION

Soy isoflavones are broken down into three bioactive compounds: daidzein, genistein and glycitein. All metabolites can bind to both types of estrogen receptors (ERs) (i.e., ERα and ERβ), however the estrogenic properties of isoflavone metabolites are primarily limited to the compound's effect on the estrogen receptor beta (ERβ) [6]. Genistein has a higher affinity for ERβ that is similar to endogenous circulating 17β-estradiol, whereas it has a very low affinity to ER-alpha (ERα) [7]. Genistein binds at ERβ at an affinity that is approximately 20 times less than [6] 17β-estradiol (E$_2$). Genistein at concentrations of 10–100 nM can induce protein synthesis within the cell similar to that seen with E_2 [7]. Daidzein is metabolized within the gut, by particular intestinal flora, to produce the bioactive compound equol. Equol has very strong estrogenic qualities which are much higher than its precursor daidzein. Also, unlike the other metabolites of soy isoflavones, equol has potent binding capabilities at both ER, although still stronger at ERβ [8]. Despite the promising endocrine profile of equol, only about 30% of the population is able to produce equol from daidzein. It has been suggested that this subpopulation of equol producers benefit the most from soy isoflavone treatment [9].

Investigations into soy and brain regions critical for cognitive function demonstrate that isoflavones, like estrogens, can exert significant effects within the central nervous system, acting directly on cell functioning and subsequent behavior [10]. Estrogens and estrogen-like compounds such as isoflavones exert their effects on the brain and cognition through ERs. They are highly expressed throughout the brain, and are known to have a large influence on cognition through receptors in two main areas within the brain: the hippocampus and the prefrontal cortex [11, 12]. Estrogen therapy is associated with enhanced activity in the hippocampus and prefrontal cortex as postmenopausal women age [13, 14]. Conversely, suppressing ovarian hormones pharmacologically leads to decreased brain activation in the prefrontal cortex and anterior cingulate gyrus during verbal memory tasks in women [15]. Behavioral and structural studies have revealed that the prefrontal cortex is sensitive to the effects of soy isoflavones [15–21].

As with estrogen, treatment with soy isoflavones or their metabolites can lead to increases in spine density in the hippocampus and prefrontal cortex in female rats [20]. This change in brain function was associated with improvement on a test of spatial memory; female rats receiving soy treatment also performed better on a task of spatial memory compared to the rats receiving placebo treatment [20] (see Fig. 3.1). Female rats fed soy diets or soy supplements exhibited less anxiety-related behavior in a well-validated behavioral maze task compared to control-fed counterparts [18, 21]. These parallel mechanisms of action for estrogen and soy isoflavones raise the possibility that both compounds would have similar effects on cognitive function in women. However, compared to humans, rats can readily produce equol when digesting soy isoflavones. Therefore, they may have a higher response to isoflavone treatment due to increased exposure to equol, the strongest estrogenic metabolite of soy.

COGNITIVE-ENHANCING EFFECTS OF ESTROGEN

Throughout the course of menopause, circulating levels of estrogens decrease dramatically [22]. Across this hormonal transition, women also report changes in cognition, most often citing memory as a problem [23]. The decrease in circulating hormones has been implicated as a possible cause of changes in cognition, in particular memory [24]. Acute withdrawal from estrogen, via surgical

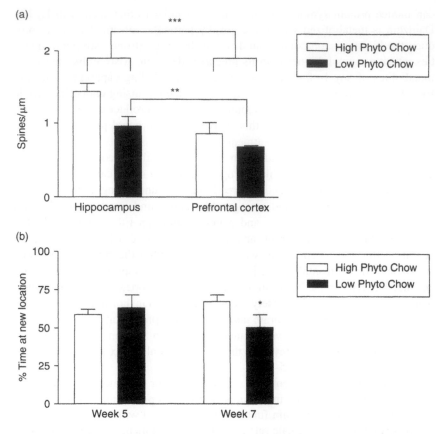

FIGURE 3.1 High soy diets increase dendritic spine density in the hippocampus and prefrontal cortex of rats and improve memory for spatial location. *Note*: Surgically menopausal adult female rats fed high phytoestrogen diet show enhanced spine density in brain regions subserving memory (a) and enhanced memory for the placement of objects (b) compared with controls fed low phytoestrogen diets for 7–9 weeks. ***p < .001 for higher spine density in hippocampus versus prefrontal cortex; **p < .01 for greater spine density with high versus low phytoestrogen diet; *p < .05 for enhanced memory for object placement with high versus low phytoestrogen diet. From Ref. [20].

removal of the ovaries in women in their 40s also leads to declines in verbal memory, but these declines can be prevented by estrogen treatment [25]. A similar pattern of reversible declines in verbal memory is evident following pharmacological suppression of estrogen [26]. Evidence from randomized clinical trials of estrogen in young women indicates cognitive benefit, particularly to verbal memory [27]. A smaller, but growing literature indicates that estrogens also have effects on cognitive functions mediated by the frontal lobes [27].

Despite the promising effects of estrogen treatment in premenopausal and young women, there is no evidence of cognitive benefit following initiation of estrogen treatment in women over the age of 65 [28]. These results suggest that the brain may not be responding in the same manner to estrogen in early postmenopausal women, compared to late postmenopausal women. A prominent theory suggests there is a critical period or window early in the menopause within which estrogen confers cognitive benefits and that beyond this period of efficacy treatment with estrogen is not helpful in ameliorating cognitive deficits, and may in fact increase the risk for dementia [29, 30]. The critical period may also apply to soy, as noted below.

COGNITIVE-ENHANCING EFFECTS OF SOY IN WOMEN

There is evidence that soy isoflavones improve cognitive functioning in healthy young adults. The beneficial effects of soy have been observed on cognitive tests that rely heavily on both the hippocampus and the prefrontal cortex. Studies investigating the effects of soy isoflavones in healthy young adults have shown improvements in cognition, primarily in memory and mental flexibility [17, 31]. One trial investigated the effects of a 10 week low (0.5 mg total isoflavones/day) or high (100 mg total isoflavones/day) soy diet in young healthy volunteers (male = 15; female = 12) [32]. Improvements in cognition were only seen in the high soy diet intervention group, with improvements on both verbal and figural memory, and also executive functioning. Another study investigated the effects of acute, moderate intake of soy isoflavones, between 1080 and 3780 mg per week in 16 healthy young female volunteers. After the soy treatment, there was an increase in mental rotation ability and spatial visualization [31]. Together these studies suggest that phytoestrogens have the ability to improve cognition in healthy young adults.

However, there has been limited investigation into the use of soy isofla vones as a treatment for cognitive changes seen across the menopause and with aging. Seven randomized, double-blind, placebo-controlled clinical trials have examined the effect of dietary or supplemental soy isoflavones on cognition in postmenopausal women. These trials show inconsistent evidence, with some trials showing a benefit of soy treatment, and some showing a detriment or no effect in response to soy treatment. However, as with estrogen, a clearer picture evolves when considering studies involving early postmenopausal women and those involving late postmenopausal women separately. Such an analysis suggests that phytoestrogens may be effective cognitive enhancers in women who are early postmenopausal, but not those who are late postmenopausal.

The first clinical trial to examine the effect of soy isoflavone treatment on cognitive functioning in both early and late post menopausal women investigated the effects of 110 mg of isoflavones per day on verbal memory, verbal fluency, attention and vasomotor tracking ability. Fifty-three women between the ages of 55 and 74 completed the 6-month intervention [19]. When comparing the placebo and the soy groups, there was a significant overall effect of treatment on category fluency performance such that women who were receiving the soy treatment were able to produce more exemplars of a category (e.g., saying all the animals that come to mind) than women who were receiving the placebo treatment. The results became much more interesting when age was taken into consideration and the data was split into two age groups: young (50–59 years) and older (60–74 years). The young group of participants experienced more benefit from the phytoestrogen treatment than the older group. The young women showed improvements on verbal memory, category fluency and attention. The group of older women who were treated with soy improved in category fluency performance, however decreased in verbal memory performance [19]. This study concluded that the effects of soy isoflavones may be differential, depending on menopausal stage.

A second study of soy isoflavones investigated the effects of a 3-month intervention in 33 early postmenopausal women (age range: 50–65) using 60 mg of soy isoflavones per day [33]. Women receiving the soy intervention showed greater improvements compared to the placebo group on measures of executive function, verbal memory and figural memory. Soy intervention did not have significant effects on factors such as anxiety, depression or menopausal symptoms. This led to the conclusion that soy was not indirectly enhancing memory and executive functions, at least through the physiological and psychological constructs that were measured.

In a larger follow-up study, 50 postmenopausal women (age range: 51–66 years) completed a 6-week intervention of 60 mg isoflavones per day [17]. After treatment, women receiving the soy supplement performed better than the placebo group on measures of non-verbal short-term memory, planning ability and mental flexibility (see Fig. 3.2). Although a later study by this same group replicated the effects on mental flexibility and planning, they did not replicate the effects on memory [33]. This study concluded that soy supplements have beneficial effects on executive function (i.e., mental flexibility and planning ability), but that there may not be a robust effect of soy treatment on memory ability in postmenopausal women.

The effects of soy isoflavones in early postmenopausal women was explored in a study using a crossover design [34]. Women (age range: 46–65 years) were randomized to receive 60 mg isoflavones per day for 6 months or placebo, followed by a 1 month washout period. After this washout period, each woman received whichever treatment (soy or placebo) that she had not previously been given. Cognitive testing was completed following each treatment period. Women performed better on a working memory task when they were receiving the soy isoflavones compared to when they were receiving placebo. During the soy treatment, women also reported significantly reduced depression and fatigue. However, there was no decrease in the amount of self-reported anxiety.

A study conducted in early postmenopausal women used two methods of administration of soy isoflavones, dietary and supplement. Seventy-eight women (mean age: 50 years) were randomized to one of the three treatment conditions for 16 weeks: cow's milk and placebo supplement, soy milk (72 mg

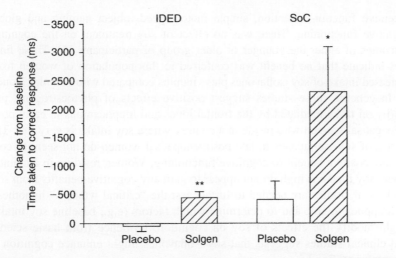

FIGURE 3.2 Soy supplements improve performance on executive function tasks in postmenopausal women. *Note*: In a clinical trial, postmenopausal women (mean age 50–65) randomized to receive 60 mg total isoflavones per day from a soy isoflavone supplement (Solgen) showed significant improvements on two executive function tests, the IDED (Intradimensional/Extradimensional Shift; a test of mental flexibility) and the SoC (Stockings of Cambridge; a test of planning ability), compared with women randomized to receive placebo. **p < .01 for enhanced performance with soy supplementation. *p < .05 for enhanced performance with soy supplementation. From Ref. [33].

isoflavones/day) and placebo supplement, or cow's milk and soy isoflavone supplement (70 mg isoflavones/day) [35]. Both before and after the soy intervention, women completed a psychological test battery which included tests of attention, executive function, working memory and delayed memory (i.e., visual and verbal). There were no significant improvements on any cognitive measure after treatment [35]. In fact, the group randomized to receive soy milk showed a decrease in performance in a measure of working memory.

The largest study to date in postmenopausal women followed 202 late postmenopausal women (mean age: 67) treated for 1 year with 99 mg isoflavones per day or placebo. Memory, verbal fluency and attention were the main cognitive outcomes tested in this study. However, after a year of treatment there were no significant differences between soy and placebo treatment on any cognitive outcome [9].

Soy isoflavone supplementation has also been studied in postmenopausal women residing in a high soy consuming culture. A large sample of 191 women (age range: 55–76) living in Hong Kong and surrounding areas were randomized to receive either 80 mg of soy isoflavones per day or placebo for 6 months. In addition to study treatment, all subjects were given a vitamin supplement containing calcium, zinc, magnesium and vitamin D. Subjects were split into two age groups: younger than 65 and older than 65 years of age. The cognitive battery included tests of verbal and figural memory, working memory, verbal fluency, executive function, attention, simple motor speed, object naming and global cognitive functioning. There was no effect of soy treatment on the cognitive outcomes in either the younger or older group of participants [5]. These findings indicate that no benefit was conferred to this population of women from increased intake of soy isoflavones plus vitamins compared with vitamins alone.

In general, these studies suggest positive effects of phytoestrogens, primarily on tasks mediated by the frontal lobes and hippocampus in early postmenopausal women who reside in a country where soy intake is very low. The effects of soy isoflavones in late postmenopausal women do not seem to confer any positive benefit to cognitive functioning. Women residing in a country where soy intake is high do not appear to gain any cognitive benefits from soy. Additional studies are needed to further test the "critical window" hypothesis as it applies to soy, and to determine which factors (e.g., baseline soy intake) might modify the effects of soy on cognition. Evidence from basic science and clinical studies suggests that soy isoflavones might enhance cognition in women under age 65.

EVIDENCE THAT MALES MAY NOT BENEFIT FROM SOY

There is some evidence from animal studies that soy treatment may confer potential cognitive risks to male animals and humans. For example, a study in adult male and female rats investigated the effects of both acute and lifelong administration of a phytoestrogen-rich diet on spatial memory measured by a radial arm maze [36]. Females fed a lifelong phytoestrogen-rich diet learned more quickly than females fed a phytoestrogen-free diet, whereas for males the effect was the opposite. Furthermore, female rats that were switched to a phytoestrogen-free diet performed worse on the memory portion of the task compared to females who continued on the high isoflavone diet, while the opposite effect was seen in the male rats. Similarly, another animal study investigated the effects of a high and low soy diet on spatial memory in aged male rats [37]. Male rats that were fed a low soy diet had better memory than the male rats that were fed a high soy diet. Rats fed a control, isoflavone-free diet performed similarly to the rats that were fed a high soy diet. Together these two studies suggest that high doses of soy may be detrimental to cognitive functioning in males, however low doses of soy may still be able to enhance cognition.

Evidence from an observational (i.e., not randomized) study suggested that intake of high amounts of soy products can also be harmful to aging adult men [38]. This study involved a cohort of 948 Japanese-American men living on the Oahu Island of Hawaii. High tofu consumption during middle age was associated with higher incidence of cognitive impairment, low brain weight and enlargement of the ventricles within the brain [38]. The study had several noted limitations, including reliance on self-reports of tofu intake that were not reliable over time. To date, no randomized clinical trials have been published on the effects of soy on cognition in aging adult men. However, one randomized clinical trial has investigated the effect of acute soy supplementation on cognition in young adult males. A 10-week treatment of 100 mg of soy per day increased cognitive function (i.e., verbal and figural memory and executive function) compared to placebo in healthy college aged men (and women) [32]. These results contradict the animal studies and suggest that high soy intake could have positive effects in healthy young men. However, these results may not generalize to an aging population due to changes in metabolism, disease and general physiological changes with aging.

GENERAL SUMMARY

As the population of older adults steadily increases, interest in botanical compounds as memory enhancers will continue to grow. There are not yet enough conclusive findings to draw any meaningful conclusions about the effects of soy on cognition in aging men, though early studies suggest a need for further investigation to ensure that soy does not impair cognition in men. Overall, soy isoflavones taken in a supplement form or incorporated into the diet appear to confer cognitive benefit in young women and early postmenopausal women. However, there is not enough evidence to support the use of phytoestrogens as cognition enhancers in late menopausal women. Further studies are needed to better understand the effects of soy on cognitive function.

REFERENCES

1. Gold, E. B., Bair, Y., Zhang, G., Utts, J., Greendale, G. A., Upchurch, D., Chyu, L., Sternfeld, B. & Adler, S. (2007). Cross-sectional analysis of specific complementary and alternative medicine (CAM) use by racial/ethnic group and menopausal status: The Study of Women's Health Across the Nation (SWAN). *Menopause* **14**, 612–623.
2. Grodstein, F., Mayeux, R. & Stampfer, M. J. (2000). Tofu and cognitive function: Food for thought. *J Am Coll Nutr* **19**, 207–209.
3. Pan, Y., Anthony, M. & Clarkson, T. B. (1999). Effect of estradiol and soy phytoestrogens on choline acetyltransferase and nerve growth factor mRNAs in the frontal cortex and hippocampus of female rats. *Proc Soc Exp Biol Med* **221**, 118–125.
4. de Pascual-Teresa, S., Hallund, J., Talbot, D., Schroot, J., Williams, C. M., Bugel, S. & Cassidy, A. (2006). Absorption of isoflavones in humans: Effects of food matrix and processing. *J Nutr Biochem* **17**, 257–264.
5. Ho, S. C., Chan, A. S., Ho, Y. P., So, E. K., Sham, A., Zee, B. & Woo, J. L. (2007). Effects of soy isoflavone supplementation on cognitive function in Chinese postmenopausal women: A double-blind, randomized, controlled trial. *Menopause* **14**, 489–499.
6. Kuiper, G. G., Lemmen, J. G., Carlsson, B., Corton, J. C., Safe, S. H., van der Saag, P. T., van der Burg, B. & Gustafsson, J. A. (1998). Interaction of estrogenic chemicals and phytoestrogens with estrogen receptor beta. *Endocrinology* **139**, 4252–4263.

7. Kim, H., Xia, H., Li, L. & Gewin, J. (2000). Attenuation of neurodegeneration-relevant modifications of brain proteins by dietary soy. *Biofactors* **12**, 243–250.

8. Axelson, M., Kirk, D. N., Farrant, R. D., Cooley, G., Lawson, A. M. & Setchell, K. D. (1982). The identification of the weak oestrogen equol [7-hydroxy-3-(4'-hydroxyphenyl)chroman] in human urine. *Biochem J* **201**, 353–357.

9. Kreijkamp-Kaspers, S., Kok, L., Grobbee, D. E., de Haan, E. H., Aleman, A., Lampe, J. W. & van der Schouw, Y. T. (2004). Effect of soy protein containing isoflavones on cognitive function, bone mineral density, and plasma lipids in postmenopausal women: A randomized controlled trial. *JAMA* **292**, 65–74.

10. Cameron, H. A. & McKay, R. D. (2001). Adult neurogenesis produces a large pool of new granule cells in the dentate gyrus. *J Comp Neurol* **435**, 406–417.

11. Maki, P. M. & Resnick, S. M. (2001). Effects of estrogen on patterns of brain activity at rest and during cognitive activity: A review of neuroimaging studies. *Neuroimage* **14**, 789–801.

12. Woolley, C. S. & McEwen, B. S. (1993). Roles of estradiol and progesterone in regulation of hippocampal dendritic spine density during the estrous cycle in the rat. *J Comp Neurol* **336**, 293–306.

13. Maki, P. M. & Resnick, S. M. (2000). Longitudinal effects of estrogen replacement therapy on PET cerebral blood flow and cognition. *Neurobiol Aging* **21**, 373–383.

14. Joffe, H., Hall, J. E., Gruber, S., Sarmiento, I. A., Cohen, L. S., Yurgelun-Todd, D. & Martin, K. A. (2006). Estrogen therapy selectively enhances prefrontal cognitive processes: A randomized, double-blind, placebo-controlled study with functional magnetic resonance imaging in perimenopausal and recently postmenopausal women. *Menopause* **13**, 411–422.

15. Craig, M. C., Fletcher, P. C., Daly, E. M., Rymer, J., Cutter, W. J., Brammer, M., Giampietro, V., Wickham, H., Maki, P. M. & Murphy, D. G. (2007). Gonadotropin hormone releasing hormone agonists alter prefrontal function during verbal encoding in young women. *Psychoneuroendocrinology* **32**, 1116–1127.

16. Duffy, R., Wiseman, H. & File, S. E. (2003). Improved cognitive function in postmenopausal women after 12 weeks of consumption of a soya extract containing isoflavones. *Pharmacol Biochem Behav* **75**, 721–729.

17. File, S. E., Hartley, D. E., Elsabagh, S., Duffy, R. & Wiseman, H. (2005). Cognitive improvement after 6 weeks of soy supplements in postmenopausal women is limited to frontal lobe function. *Menopause* **12**, 193–201.

18. Kessler, R. C., Berglund, P., Demler, O., Jin, R., Merikangas, K. R. & Walters, E. E. (2005). Lifetime prevalence and age-of-onset distributions of DSM-IV disorders in the National Comorbidity Survey Replication. *Arch Gen Psychiatr* **62**, 593–602.

19. Kritz-Silverstein, D., Von Muhlen, D., Barrett-Connor, E. & Bressel, M. A. (2003). Isoflavones and cognitive function in older women: the Soy and Postmenopausal Health In Aging (SOPHIA) Study. *Menopause* **10**, 196–202.

20. Luine, V., Attalla, S., Mohan, G., Costa, A. & Frankfurt, M. (2006). Dietary phytoestrogens enhance spatial memory and spine density in the hippocampus and prefrontal cortex of ovariectomized rats. *Brain Res* **1126**, 183–187.

21. Patisaul, H. B., Blum, A., Luskin, J. R. & Wilson, M. E. (2005). Dietary soy supplements produce opposite effects on anxiety in intact male and female rats in the elevated plus-maze. *Behav Neurosci* **119**, 587–594.
22. Burger, H. G., Dudley, E. C., Hopper, J. L., Shelley, J. M., Green, A., Smith, A., Dennerstein, L. & Morse, C. (1995). The endocrinology of the menopausal transition: A cross-sectional study of a population-based sample. *J Clin Endocrinol Metabol* **80**, 3537–3545.
23. Woods, N. F., Mitchell, E. S. & Adams, C. (2000). Memory functioning among midlife women: Observations from the Seattle Midlife Women's Health Study. *Menopause* **7**, 257–265.
24. Maki, P. & Hogervorst, E. (2003). The menopause and HRT. HRT and cognitive decline. *Best Pract Res Clin Endocrinol Metabol* **17**, 105–122.
25. Sherwin, B. B. (1988). Estrogen and/or androgen replacement therapy and cognitive functioning in surgically menopausal women. *Psychoneuroendocrinology* **13**, 345–357.
26. Sherwin, B. B. & Tulandi, T. (1996). "Add-back" estrogen reverses cognitive deficits induced by a gonadotropin-releasing hormone agonist in women with leiomyomata uteri. *J Clin Endocrinol Metabol* **81**, 2545–2549.
27. Maki, P. M. (2005). Estrogen effects on the hippocampus and frontal lobes. *Int J Fertil Womens Med* **50**, 67–71.
28. Maki, P. M. (2005). A systematic review of clinical trials of hormone therapy on cognitive function: Effects of age at initiation and progestin use. *Ann NY Acad Sci* **1052**, 182–197.
29. Resnick, S. M. & Henderson, V. W. (2002). Hormone therapy and risk of Alzheimer disease: A critical time. *JAMA* **288**.
30. Maki, P. M. (2006). Hormone therapy and cognitive function: Is there a critical period for benefit? *Neuroscience* **138**, 1027–1030.
31. Celec, P., Ostatnikova, D., Caganova, M., Zuchova, S., Hodosy, J., Putz, Z., Bernadic, M. & Kudela, M. (2005). Endocrine and cognitive effects of short-time soybean consumption in women. *Gynecol Obstet Investig* **59**, 62–66.
32. File, S. E., Jarrett, N., Fluck, E., Duffy, R., Casey, K. & Wiseman, H. (2001). Eating soya improves human memory. *Psychopharmacology* **157**, 430–436.
33. Duffy, R., Wiseman, H. & File, S. E. (2003). Improved cognitive function in postmenopausal women after 12 weeks of consumption of a soya extract containing isoflavones. *Pharmacol Biochem Behav* **75**, 721–729.
34. Casini, M. L., Marelli, G., Papaleo, E., Ferrari, A., D'Ambrosio, F. & Unfer, V. (2006). Psychological assessment of the effects of treatment with phytoestrogens on postmenopausal women: A randomized, double-blind, crossover, placebo-controlled study. *Fertil Steril* **85**, 972–978.
35. Fournier, L. R., Ryan Borchers, T. A., Robison, L. M., Wiediger, M., Park, J. S., Chew, B. P., McGuire, M. K., Sclar, D. A., Skaer, T. L. & Beerman, K. A. (2007). The effects of soy milk and isoflavone supplements on cognitive performance in healthy, postmenopausal women. *J Nutr Health Aging* **11**, 155–164.
36. Lund, T. D., West, T. W., Tian, L. Y., Bu, L. H., Simmons, D. L., Setchell, K. D., Adlercreutz, H. & Lephart, E. D. (2001). Visual spatial memory is enhanced in female rats (but inhibited in males) by dietary soy phytoestrogens. *BMC Neurosci* **2**, 20.

37. Lee, Y. B., Lee, H. J., Won, M. H., Hwang, I. K., Kang, T. C., Lee, J. Y., Nam, S. Y., Kim, K. S., Kim, E., Cheon, S. H. & Sohn, H. S. (2004). Soy isoflavones improve spatial delayed matching-to-place performance and reduce cholinergic neuron loss in elderly male rats. *J Nutr* **134**, 1827–1831.

38. White, L. R., Petrovitch, H., Ross, G. W., Masaki, K., Hardman, J., Nelson, J., Davis, D. & Markesbery, W. (2000). Brain aging and midlife tofu consumption. *J Am Coll Nutr* **19**, 242–255.

Chapter 4

Valerian and Other CAM Botanicals in Treatment of Sleep Disturbances

Diana M. Taibi and Carol A. Landis

Department of Biobehavioral Nursing and Health Systems, School of Nursing, University of Washington, Seattle, WA, USA

Keywords: *Sleep disorders, insomnia, valerian, hops, lemon balm, lavender, passion flower, kava, chamomile, melatonin, L-tryptophan, 5–hydroxytryptophan*

Sleep disturbances are one of the most prevalent health problems in older adults. As many as 50% of older adults report problems sleeping including difficulty falling asleep, awakening frequently or for long periods of time during the night, or awakening early in the morning without being able to return to sleep [1]. Older adults often use prescription hypnotics, sedating antidepressants, or over-the-counter (OTC) sedating medications (e.g., antihistamines, anticholinergics) as sleep aids [2, 3]. Many of these drugs further disrupt sleep and have adverse side effects including daytime sleepiness, drug tolerance, memory impairments, dry mouth, constipation, urinary retention, and rebound sleep disturbance on withdrawal of the medication [4–6]. Many adults have turned to herbal products as a "natural" alternative for treating their sleep disturbances [7]. National surveys in the United States show that over 50% of middle-aged to older adults use daily dietary supplements, particularly herbal sleep aids, and use of these agents is estimated to increase over the next few decades [8–10].

The purpose of this chapter is to provide an overview of botanical products commonly used for sleep disturbance and evidence on the effectiveness and safety of these products in older adults. The chapter focuses primarily on valerian, which is a commonly used herbal sedative and has been the most extensively studied [11]. We briefly review other herbal sleep aids, including hops, lemon balm, lavender, passion flower, kava, and chamomile as well as selected non-botanical substances including melatonin, L-tryptophan, and 5-hydroxytryptophan. This chapter begins with a discussion of changes in sleep associated with aging and common types of sleep disturbances in older adults before addressing botanicals and other supplements that are commonly used as sleep aids.

SLEEP AND AGING

Changes in sleep associated with increasing age begin in midlife and are sustained throughout old age. Sleep becomes lighter with less slow wave or deep sleep, more light and transitional stages of sleep, longer sleep latency (time between going to bed and falling asleep), shorter total sleep time, and steady decline in sleep efficiency (the percentage of time in bed spent asleep) from midlife throughout old age [12]. Because of the shift towards lighter and less consolidated sleep, older adults are more easily awakened and have an increased number of nighttime awakenings [13]. Many older adults with disturbed sleep spend more time in bed trying to sleep, which only intensifies poor sleep efficiency. Although these age-related changes are fairly universal and increase susceptibility for insomnia, only about half of older adults complain of insomnia symptoms. Many adjust their expectations about sleep, attributing problems to "getting older," rather than considering changes in sleep as symptoms of a sleep disorder.

Insomnia

Broadly defined, insomnia is a sleep-wake disorder often associated with an inadequate amount of sleep and with both nighttime sleep disturbance symptoms and daytime consequences [14]. Insomnia nighttime symptoms include difficulty falling asleep (long sleep latency), frequent awakenings (fragmented sleep), prolonged awakenings (wake after sleep onset), or awakening too early and not being able to fall back to sleep (early morning awakening). Awakening feeling unrefreshed (also called non-restorative sleep) is considered a nighttime symptom of insomnia. The most common daytime consequences of insomnia include fatigue, mood disturbance (anxiety and depression), decreased motivation, impaired memory and work productivity, and reduced quality of life [15–17]. Insomnia occurs when an individual has an adequate amount of time for sleep. This differentiates it from insufficient sleep syndrome, which also is associated with an inadequate amount of sleep, but occurs because an individual restricts the time available for sleep [18].

Primary insomnia occurs in the absence of a contributing medical or psychiatric condition [19]. In healthy older individuals, certain behavioral patterns, in addition to the natural tendency toward lighter sleep, increase the risk of primary insomnia. For instance, many older adults have reduced physical activity and reduced exposure to natural light, both of which are factors that affect sleep intensity and duration [13]. Retired individuals with excess free time may spend long periods of time in bed due to boredom, resulting in sleep that is fragmented rather than consolidated, which is considered more restful sleep and of higher quality. Treatment of these problems may require addressing the specific contributing factor (e.g., going for daily walks for exercise and daylight exposure), providing education about typical changes in sleep with age, and cognitive-behavioral approaches for managing insomnia complaints.

Co-morbid insomnia occurs concurrent with medical or psychiatric disorders and is the most common type of insomnia, especially in older adults [6, 17, 20]. Medical and psychiatric conditions associated with co-morbid insomnia include arthritis, heart disease, pulmonary disease, depression, and nocturia [21]. Many medications individuals take to treat these conditions may also disrupt sleep, for example, bronchodilators, decongestants, steroids, beta blockers, antidepressants. Furthermore, risk of anxiety and depression increases with age, and both of these conditions exacerbate and are exacerbated by insomnia [13]. Finally, many women experience vasomotor symptoms during and after the menopause transition that, in some cases, persist into old age. Vasomotor symptoms, commonly called "night sweats" have been associated with frequent awakenings and arousals (sleep disruption just below the threshold of awakening) throughout the night, and these disruptions may result in a pattern of insomnia [22–24]. Relieving these symptoms with low dose hormone replacement therapy or antidepressant medications may help to alleviate insomnia [23], but it often persists and specific treatment is required.

Cognitive and behavioral therapies (CBT) for insomnia are efficacious and recommended as first-line treatment for insomnia [6, 25]. These therapies aim to change insomnia-promoting or "sleep effort" behaviors (e.g., spending excessive amounts of time in bed, getting inadequate daylight exposure) and negative cognitions (e.g., rumination and worry about not being able to sleep during nocturnal awakenings). Although most CBT research has been done in primary insomnia, it also has been shown to improve sleep in older adults with chronic illness and co-morbid insomnia [26]. CBT has long lasting effects on sleep because an individual's beliefs and behaviors about sleep have been altered. Hypnotic medications are best reserved for temporary episodes of insomnia because they are effective only when they are taken. Despite the benefits of CBT, this type of therapy is not widely available in clinical practice and many older adults commonly rely on chronic use of sedating medications. Benzodiazepines (e.g., lorazepam, temazepam) have been prescribed for many years as sleep aids and have numerous well-known side effects, including daytime sleepiness, drug tolerance, memory impairments, dry mouth, constipation, and rebound sleep disturbance on withdrawal of the medication [4, 5]. The newer non-benzodiazepine hypnotics (e.g., zolpidem, zaleplon, eszopiclone) have shorter half-lives and fewer side effects than benzodiazepines [27], but compared to CBT, the long term efficacy of these agents has not been established, especially in older adults. Typically, randomized controlled trials of hypnotic medications are conducted for 2–4 weeks duration. Only one drug, eszopiclone, has been evaluated for 6 months of consistent nightly use [28]. Tricyclic antidepressants and antihistamines are also used as sleep aids because of their sedative effects. However, both classes of medications are associated with adverse effects including urinary retention, confusion, and daytime sleepiness that are problematic for older adults.

Advanced Sleep Phase Disorder (ASPD)

Another common age-related change is advanced sleep phase, in which the physiological circadian timing of sleep is advanced, such that sleepiness occurs earlier in the evening than desired (e.g., 8 p.m.) and morning awakening also occurs earlier than desired (e.g., 4 a.m.) [14]. This condition is not considered a disorder unless it is disruptive to an individual's total sleep time and quality of life [13]. For instance, an individual may oppose the urge to sleep early in the evening and maintain a later bedtime, yet still awaken in the early morning, resulting in reduced total sleep time and exacerbation of daytime sleepiness [13]. Bright light exposure in the late afternoon or early evening, either by spending time outdoors or using a therapeutic light box, is an effective treatment because it shifts the circadian timing of sleep onset and offset to a later time in the evening and morning, respectively [13, 29].

Periodic Limb Movements in Sleep (PLMS) and Restless Legs Syndrome (RLS)

The prevalence of periodic limb movements in sleep (PLMS) and of restless legs syndrome (RLS) is increased in older adults [30]. PLMS are characterized by periodic, repetitive jerking of the limbs, most commonly the legs, during sleep. RLS is the urge to move limbs, usually the legs, when at rest which is accompanied by unpleasant sensations, such as "creeping" or "pulling" [31]. Most individuals with RLS also have PLMS, but PLMS frequently occur without RLS [13, 30]. The prevalence of PLMS is over 45% in older adults and they occur commonly in persons with obstructive sleep apnea [30]. The prevalence of RLS is 20% in the adult population [30, 32]. Insomnia complaints are common both in PLMS and RLS, as these conditions commonly cause difficulty falling asleep and numerous awakenings [30, 33]. Although the causes of PLMS and RLS are unknown, the conditions are associated with iron deficiency, and iron supplementation relieves symptoms in some individuals [32]. Dopamine central nervous system (CNS) mechanisms are believed to be involved in the pathophysiology of PLMS and RLS based on observations that dopaminergic drugs such as pramipexole and ropinirole relieve symptoms [31].

Sleep Disordered Breathing

Sleep disordered breathing (SDB) involves complete (apnea) and partial (hypopnea) collapse of the airway during sleep, resulting in loud snoring, many brief arousals, and intermittent hypoxic episodes. SDB is often first recognized by a patient's bed partner because of loud snoring or witnessing actual apneic events. Increasing age and obesity are common risk factors for SDB [34, 35]. SDB severity ranges from mild (5–15 events/hour) to severe (>30 events/hour) [36], and disease severity has been linked with increased risk of hypertension, cardiovascular disease, nocturia, cognitive impairment, sleepiness-related motor vehicle accidents, and mortality [34]. SDB is associated with excessive daytime sleepiness and fatigue because of frequent disruptions of sleep and hypercapnea from hypoventilation. SDB is diagnosed by overnight polysomnography (PSG), a test in which brain activity, muscle tone, eye movements, respiratory effort, and hemoglobin oxygen saturation are monitored. Treatment for SDB is the use of continuous positive airway pressure (CPAP), which maintains positive pressure in the airway via a face mask to prevent airway collapse [36].

Consequences of Sleep Disturbances in Older Adults

Sleep disturbance is a significant health risk for older adults. Serious daytime impairment with excessive sleepiness and reduced quality of life may result from all the sleep disruptions discussed above. Older adults with disturbed sleep are at increased risk for medical-related morbidity and mortality as well as psychosocial consequences including depression, fatigue, poor daytime functioning, and poor quality of life [13]. Insomnia in older adults is associated with the risk of injury from motor vehicle accidents and falls [13]. Older adults may have more than one sleep disturbance, complicating diagnosis and treatment.

HERBS USED AS SLEEP AIDS (COMMISSION E RECOMMENDED)

Numerous herbs are used for their purportedly sedating qualities. Many of these herbs are recommended by the German Commission E, known internationally for a comprehensive series of monographs on medicinal herbs [37]. Herbs recommended for the general indication of sleep disturbance due to restlessness or anxiety include valerian, hops, lemon balm, and lavender. Other herbs are used as sedatives, but are not specifically recommended for sleep by the Commission E. These include passion flower, kava, and chamomile.

Valerian

Valerian is among the top-selling herbs in the United States and has long been used as a remedy for sleep disorders and anxiety [38]. It has been recommended as potentially useful for older adults with sleep difficulties [39]. Valerian is typically used as a sedative for insomnia symptoms but is not commonly used for other sleep disorders, although one study has evaluated its use to reduce sleep-related movements in patients with Parkinson's disease [40] and one study is currently investigating valerian for RLS [41].

Valerian is produced from the root of various plants in the *Valeriana* species, including *Valeriana officinalis* (the species most commonly used in commercial products in the United States), *Valeriana wallichii* (Indian valerian), and *Valeriana edulis* (Mexican valerian). Valerian contains a variety of chemical compounds including valerenic acid, valepotriates, amino acids, and lignans that may act synergistically to exert sedative effects [42]. The diluent used for the extraction process (water alone vs. a water–alcohol mixture) affects the constituents present in the final product [43], potentially resulting in varying physiological effects. The herbal product is made from the dried whole root or dried root extract and administered medicinally in a capsule or tablet, as a tincture, or made into tea. To demonstrate product quality, commercially formulated valerian capsules, tablets, or tinctures are commonly standardized on 0.08% valerenic acid, a pharmacologically active marker compound.

Based on *in vitro* and animal studies, valerian affects gamma-aminobutyric acid (GABA) [44, 45], adenosine [46–48], and serotonin [49] neurotransmitter mechanisms involved in sleep regulation. Several components of valerian, specifically valerenic acids and amino acids, have affinity for GABA receptors, which are involved in the promotion and maintenance of sleep. Valerian constituents also have been shown to promote release and inhibit reuptake of synaptic GABA [44, 45, 50]. Valerian constituents have affinity for adenosine receptors [46–48] that exert inhibitory effects in the CNS and are thought to induce sleepiness as time awake increases [51]. Adenosine also is involved in the regulation of both rapid-eye-movement (REM) sleep and non-REM sleep stages. Although valerian has been shown to affect specific components of sleep regulation mechanisms, little is known about how the herb gains access to the CNS or what component of herb has active sedation properties. Numerous animal studies have shown general sedative effects of valerian and its constituents [52].

Few studies have specifically investigated the effects of valerian on sleep in older adults. One double-blind, placebo-controlled randomized crossover clinical trial (RCCT) of older adults with mild sleep complaints tested an ethanolic extract of valerian root *V. officinalis* (a 300 or 600 mg dose), the type of valerian product similar to those most commonly used in the United States and found no significant differences between valerian and placebo on PSG or self-reported sleep outcomes [53]. This study may be criticized because valerian was administered for only one night, and because it is commonly recommended that valerian requires at least 2 weeks of use to achieve effectiveness. However, two double-blind, placebo-controlled randomized clinical trials (RCTs) and one RCCT of the same valerian product (LI 156, or Sedonium®) in younger adults for 14–28 nights also showed no significant differences between valerian and placebo in self-rated or PSG sleep outcomes [54–56]. Other studies in older adults tested different types of valerian preparations: aqueous extracts (extracted with water alone) or preparations high in valepotriate content. One double-blind, placebo-controlled RCT tested the effects of an aqueous valerian extract given three times daily for 8 days to 14 older women with insomnia and found no significant differences between the valerian and placebo on self-report or PSG sleep outcomes [57]. A double-blind, placebo-controlled RCT tested an aqueous extract of valerian given three times daily for 30 days to German elder home residents with behavioral disturbance and sleep problems. A greater proportion of those given valerian than those given placebo had reduced sleep disturbance ratings but the significance of this finding was not reported [58]. A non-randomized, double-blind, placebo-controlled clinical trial of elder home residents with sleep disturbance tested 14 days of a high-valepotriate valerian preparation and found that a significantly greater proportion of individuals given valerian than placebo reported reduced sleep latency and improved sleep maintenance [59]. The type of valerian preparation used in this study is not available in the United States because of cytotoxic effects of valepotriates.

Although two studies showed positive effects of valerian in older adults [58, 59], the studies were not rigorously designed, and findings were based on self-reported and less validated outcomes compared to more recent trials. Two of the trials that measured both self-report and PSG sleep outcomes found no significant effects of valerian on sleep [53, 57], consistent with the larger body of literature on valerian. A recent comprehensive systematic review of valerian examined 37 clinical trials of valerian and found that the overall evidence on valerian failed to show efficacy for sleep disturbances [11]. Most of the studies were small and underpowered to find significant changes. However, several recent studies with adequate power and rigorous designs have shown no significant effects of valerian on sleep disturbance [54, 60–63], which corroborates the null findings from the broader body of research literature on valerian.

Although valerian is not effective for improving sleep, it is among one of the safest herbs. Several large post-marketing studies have been done on valerian preparations and preparations of valerian in combination with hops, lemon balm, and/or passion flower. The majority of patients (70–90%) in these studies rated the tolerability of the preparations as good or very good, and side effects were rare and mild. Side effects reported with valerian are usually mild and include gastrointestinal effects (e.g., nausea, diarrhea) or cognitive/nervous system effects (dizziness, morning "hangover," drowsiness) [53–55, 59, 60, 64–66]. One case report associated valerian with paradoxical stimulation [37].

Valerian has only tenuously been linked to cases of transient hepatic dysfunction [67, 68]. In these cases, contribution of other ingested substances, particularly the herbs mistletoe and skullcap, could not be ruled out. In several cases of intentional overdose, effects were serious, but non-life threatening (tremor, stupor, elevated liver function tests) and resolved over several days to weeks [69–72]. Of particular concern are the valepotriate constituents of valerian. Metabolites of these constituents produced in the stomach and bowel (baldrinals) have been shown to have mutagenic properties. It is suspected that the GI tract and liver are at greatest risk of potential adverse effects of bald-rinals [52]. Although toxicity has not been shown in humans, adverse effects would likely be cumulative from long-term use. Therefore, experts generally recommend avoiding preparations containing high levels of valepotriates. Valepotriate content is minimal in the *V. officinalis* species, but high levels occur in *V. edulis* and *V. wallichii* [73].

Hops

Hops (*Humulus lupulus*) is plant from which the strobiles (female flower) are used for a variety of purposes including as a sleep aid. Hops is rarely available in single-herb preparations and is usually combined with valerian, lemon balm, passion flower, skullcap, and/or kava. The main constituents of hops are the bitter acids, lupulone, and humulone [73, 74]. Constituents of hops extract have been shown to bind to melatonin and serotonin receptors, although it remains unknown whether this binding produces receptor agonist or antagonist effects [75]. Hops has been shown in animal studies to exert sedative effects, primarily through the alpha-bitter acid constituents [74, 76].

No studies have specifically tested hops in older adults with sleep disturbance. The product most commonly tested is the valerian–hops combination, ZE 91019 (Alluna®). Two 4-week placebo-controlled, double-blind RCTs of this product showed no significant differences from placebo on self-report or PSG sleep outcomes in persons with insomnia [61, 77]. A double-blind RCT comparing 2 weeks of valerian–hops to the benzodiazepine, bromazepam, in persons with insomnia showed significant improvement on a sleep quality scale over time and no significant difference between the two treatments [78]. Although this study showed equivalence between valerian–hops and a benzodiazepine, the magnitude of change was small and there was no placebo group. Finally, a recent placebo-controlled, double-blind RCT comparing a valerian–hops combination (ZE 91019) to valerian alone (ZE 911, the same valerian in the ZE 91019 combination) for 4 weeks showed significant reduction of self-reported sleep latency with valerian–hops but not valerian compared to placebo [79]. Neither treatment significantly affected total sleep or wake times. Overall, evidence from combination preparations suggests that hops may have some sedative properties, at least in combination with valerian, but improvements in sleep tended to be non-significant when compared to placebo and in some studies placebo effects could not be ruled out. In summary, the findings in one study showed that valerian–hops was associated with a large reduction in sleep latency [79], but overall evidence does not currently support the efficacy of hops (used in combination with valerian) as a sleep aid.

Potential side effects from hops are mostly from anecdotal evidence and include upset stomach, topical or respiratory allergy, nervousness, or depression [78, 80]. Hops has also been reported to have estrogenic effects and should be avoided for history of estrogen receptor-positive breast cancer [80].

Lemon Balm

Lemon balm (*Melissa officinalis*) leaves are used as a tea, tincture, or formulated as pills for multiple uses, including as a sedative. As with hops, lemon balm is commonly combined with other sedative herbs. Lemon balm contains numerous physiologically active constituents including volatile oils that could contribute to the herb's purported sedative effects [81]. One study showed moderate affinity of lemon balm extract for the $GABA_A$-benzodiazepine receptor site [82].

Little evidence exists about the sedative effects of lemon balm in older adults. Lemon balm has dose-dependent sedative effects in mice [83], and several studies investigated lemon balm in combination with valerian in humans, although no studies specifically tested lemon balm alone or in combination with another herb in older adults. In one double-blind, placebo-controlled RCT of a valerian–lemon balm combination in healthy adults, there was no significant difference from placebo in sleep quality ratings after 30 days of treatment [84]. In a placebo-controlled, double-blind RCT of healthy adults, one night of a valerian–lemon balm combination did not improve PSG-measured sleep efficiency, sleep latency, or wake after sleep onset compared to a placebo [85]. A 14-day placebo-controlled, double-blind RCT of valerian–lemon balm given twice a day to adults with insomnia showed significant improvement in self-reported sleep quality and sleep latency compared to the placebo [86]. Finally, in a placebo-controlled, double-blind RCCT of adults with sleep disturbance, a significantly greater proportion of participants reported that their sleep quality was "perfect" after a single dose of a valerian–hops–lemon balm combination compared to hops–lemon balm alone [87], suggesting that valerian was the active component rather than the other two herbs. The overall evidence for lemon balm is mixed and is insufficient to recommend therapeutic use of the herb for insomnia.

Potential side effects are mostly from anecdotal evidence and include hypersensitivity, contact dermatitis, headache, nausea, and palpitations. Caution is advisable in persons with glaucoma as lemon balm has been anecdotally reported to increase intraocular pressure [88].

Lavender

Lavender is a family of highly fragrant garden plants that have a wide range of traditional uses. For sedative effects, lavender oil, produced mainly from flowering part of the plant, is either inhaled (e.g., aromatherapy) or applied topically in massage oil. One of the main constituents of lavender oil, linalyl acetate, was detectable in blood samples after both massage and inhalation of lavender vapor [89]. The effects of lavender on reduction of stress and sleep disturbance are believed to be related both to the aroma being considered pleasant and to CNS activity of absorbed oil. The main sedative components of lavender are linalool and linalyl acetate, which may affect CNS GABA mechanisms [89].

Few studies have investigated the effects of lavender (topical or aromatherapy) on sleep, and participants in these trials cannot be blinded to treatment allocation due to the recognizable aroma of the active treatment. One RCCT comparing the aroma of lavender, sweet orange, and tea tree, to no aroma in older adults with dementia reported no effects on behavioral disturbances [90], but no controlled trials have tested lavender for sleep disturbance in older adults. A RCCT compared 1 week of the aroma of lavender to 1 week of sweet almond oil for mild insomnia [91]. Self-reported sleep quality with the lavender did not differ significantly from the comparison, but the study was confounded by poor compliance in using the noisy aromatherapy device. In another RCCT, diffused lavender significantly increased deep sleep stages (Stages 3 and 4) compared to distilled water, but the change was small (1.2%) [92]. One other RCT compared massage (30 minute massage weekly), massage with lavender oil (30 minutes weekly), and no treatment in hospice cancer patients [93], and reported significant improvement in self-reported sleep quality in the lavender massage group (but not the massage alone group) compared to no treatment. In summary, the few studies available provide only tenuous evidence of the sedative effects of lavender, and more rigorous studies are needed before any conclusions about efficacy may be reached.

Lavender is a mild and safe herb, although mild allergic reactions have been reported with direct contact from lavender pillows and topical applications (e.g., lavender-containing lotion) [94]. Small amounts of lavender may safely be ingested (e.g., lavender teas), but large amounts have been associated with acute toxicity in animals (ataxia, depression, tremors, hypothermia) and pure lavender oils should not be ingested. Lavender may interact with antiseizure medications and should be avoided in persons with epilepsy [94].

OTHER HERBS USED AS SLEEP AIDS

Passion Flower

Passion flower (*Passiflora incarnata*) is recommended by the German Commission E for nervous restlessness, but not specifically for sleep [37]. It is commonly used in sedative herb combinations and is rarely used alone. Biologically active constituents include flavonoids (e.g., apigenin, quercetin) and alkaloids, among numerous other constituents [52, 95]. Little evidence exists about the sedative effects or safety of the herb and no controlled trials have been conducted on the effects of passion flower on sleep in older adults. Animal studies have shown sedative effects [74, 95–97] that are blocked by a benzodiazepine receptor antagonist [98]. Equivalent sedating effects of passion flower extracts and benzodiazepines have been shown in two human studies of anxiety [99–101]. One open-labeled study of a valerian–hops–passion flower combination reported improvement in self-reported sleep latency and overall sleep quality in a general adult population. In this study, over 90% of the 190 participants rated the tolerability of the product "good" or "very good" and no side effects occurred [102]. Reported potential side effects of passion flower include cardiac dysrhythmia, headache, allergic reactions, and asthma. Overdoses may cause CNS depression, nausea, and vomiting [95, 101, 103].

Kava

Kava is an herbal product extracted from the rhizome (underground stem) of the *Piper methysticum* plant [52]. Kava has been used for centuries as an intoxicating ceremonial drink in South Pacific islands, where many people currently frequent "kava bars" for recreational consumption of kava drinks. The German Commission E recommends kava for anxiety and restlessness but not specifically for sleep problems [37]. Two meta-analyses support the effectiveness of kava for anxiety reduction, although the magnitude of effect was small [104, 105]. Active constituents of kava are the kavalactones (also called kavapyrones). Kava products are generally standardized to contain 70% kavalactones [106]. Evidence suggests that kava may have a general inhibitory effect on the limbic system and may also exert sedative effects at the GABA receptors [52, 107].

Few studies have investigated the effects of kava on sleep, none of which specifically tested kava in older adults. One double-blind, placebo-controlled RCT compared the effects of 4 weeks of daily kava extract, valerian, and placebo on anxiety and insomnia ratings in persons with both anxiety and insomnia [60]. Neither kava nor valerian differed significantly from placebo; in fact, the magnitude of improvement was greatest with placebo. Another double-blind, placebo-controlled RCT tested kava extract for sleep disturbance associated with anxiety disorders [108]. Sleep quality ratings improved in both groups but were significantly more improved with kava than placebo. Finally, a one-group open-label trial tested 6 weeks of kava extract to improve stress-induced insomnia [109]. Participants had significant reductions in stress ratings and insomnia severity scores after 6 weeks of kava compared to baseline, but a placebo effect cannot be excluded. Overall, evidence suggests that kava may provide mild reduction of anxiety, but research on efficacy for anxiety-related insomnia is scant and mixed. Because kava is not a sedative, it may not be useful as a sleep aid except in cases associated with anxiety.

Few side effects have been reported with kava and include gastrointestinal complaints, headache, restlessness, drowsiness, tremor, tiredness [104, 107]. The hepatotoxicity profile of kava has been highly controversial in recent years. Several case reports of severe liver dysfunction, some resulting in liver transplantation or death, were reported in kava users, resulting in a ban of kava products in the European Union and Canada and issuance of a consumer advisory in the United States [107]. However, the causal link between kava and these occurrences is speculative, and other factors (e.g., concurrent use of potentially hepatotoxic medications) may have been involved. Several large studies with over 1500 participants each monitored the safety of daily kava use over 4–7 weeks, none of which had any occurrence of hepatotoxicity [110]. At present, caution is especially advisable in individuals with current or past liver dysfunction and in older adults who often have reduced hepatic capacity to metabolize pharmaceuticals. Older adults may require conservative doses of kava, but no dose-response studies exist on which the balance of efficacy and safety can be based.

Chamomile

Tea made from chamomile (*Matricaria recutita*) is widely consumed as a calming agent to aid in relaxation and sleep onset. The German Commission E has approved use of chamomile externally for skin inflammation and consumption for gastrointestinal discomfort but does not specifically mention sedative uses [37]. Apigenin, along with other flavonoid constituents, is considered the primary agent responsible for sedative properties in chamomile [111]. Apigenin has been shown to bind to the benzodiazepine receptor [112], but it remains unclear whether this is the sedative mechanism of chamomile [113]. Although sedative effects and sleep promotion have been demonstrated in animals [111, 114], no controlled studies have investigated the effects of chamomile as a sedative or sleep aid in humans. Chamomile is generally safe, with few reported side effects. Because chamomile is in the Compositae family, individuals allergic to asters, ragweed, or related plants may have cross-sensitivity to chamomile [115]. Allergic reactions are uncommon [115], and severe allergic reactions have only been reported in cases of excessive exposure (chamomile-containing enemas) [116]. Additionally, chamomile contains naturally occurring anti-platelet substances (coumarins) and should be avoided by individuals with coagulopathies and those taking warfarin [111]. This interaction is hypothetical, and no other herb–drug interactions with chamomile have been reported.

NON-BOTANICAL SUPPLEMENTS

Melatonin

Melatonin is a naturally occurring neurohormone that is often taken medicinally as a sleep aid. Because melatonin is regulated as a supplement, it is often considered a CAM product. Endogenous melatonin secretion is suppressed by light exposure and rises during darkness [117]. Exposure of retinal cells to light and to dark "signals" controls the timing of melatonin secretion by the pineal gland [117]. Melatonin secretion exerts chronobiologic effects, altering the circadian timing of core body temperature and other rhythms such as sleep and wake. The rise of melatonin in the evening is associated with a decline in body temperature, which has been linked to increased sleepiness and to sleep onset [118]. Melatonin also directly affects CNS mechanisms involved in sleep timing, particularly in the thalamus [119]. Although some age-related changes in the timing and the amount of melatonin secreted have been observed, the relevance of these changes to sleep disturbance in older adults remains unclear [120]. While some evidence has shown nocturnal melatonin plasma concentration to peak earlier in the night and to reach a lower amplitude in older adults compared to younger adults, other studies have shown no differences [117, 119, 120]. Additionally, age-related changes may differ by gender in that older men, but not older women, have shown a lower plasma concentration of melatonin during sleep [120].

A recent meta-analysis published by the US Agency for Healthcare Research and Quality (AHRQ) concluded that research evidence supports use of exogenous melatonin as a "phase re-setter" for circadian sleep disorders rather than as a general hypnotic [121]. Melatonin has been shown effective in altering circadian sleep timing, and the American Academy of Sleep Medicine (AASM) recently published recommendations supporting the use of melatonin for both advanced sleep phase disorder (ASPD) and delayed sleep phase disorder (DSPD) [122]. Melatonin supplementation for ASPD is administered in the morning to exert phase delay in sleep onset the next evening [123]. Administration of melatonin in the evening advances sleep onset, which is useful for DSPD but could exacerbate ASPD [119]. ASPD is the most common type of circadian rhythm sleep disorder in older adults. Because ASPD requires careful evaluation, persons with ASPD should seek the care of a health care provider with experience in chronobiologic disorders if they are interested in using melatonin. Furthermore, evening light therapy is very effective for delaying sleep onset and improving sleep in ASPD and is recommended in the AASM practice guidelines [122, 123]. In summary, melatonin is recommended for ASPD, but this recommendation is based solely on theoretical effects and a favorable safety profile, and no current research evidence exists.

According to the AHRQ meta-analysis, current evidence does not support the clinical effectiveness of melatonin to treat primary or secondary insomnia [121]. However, melatonin is potentially useful for older adults with melatonin deficiency [119]. Placebo-controlled RCTs of melatonin in older adults with low nocturnal melatonin levels showed improvement in sleep maintenance on PSG and actigraphy compared to placebo [124–126]. Thus, melatonin may be potentially effective for individuals with a deficiency, but it is not effective for treating insomnia.

Although short-term melatonin has a high safety profile, it has immunostimulatory effects, and the safety of melatonin for long-term use and for use in persons with autoimmune disease is not known [117]. Side effects of melatonin are dose-dependent and include nausea, dizziness, drowsiness, fatigue, headache, confusion, agitation, depression, alteration of other hormones, nightmares, and cardiovascular effects [121, 127]. Several drug interactions have been shown: melatonin metabolism is reduced (resulting in increased levels) by several antidepressant, sedative, and antipsychotic medications. Melatonin levels are reduced by fluoxetine, and melatonin is an antagonist of calcium channel blocking antihypertensives. Melatonin may exacerbate depression and may variably affect seizure disorders. Finally, melatonin is metabolized by the liver and levels may be affected by altered hepatic function [127].

L-tryptophan and 5-HTP

L-tryptophan is an essential amino acid that may be taken as a supplement or consumed in dietary protein both from animal and plant sources. L-tryptophan and its metabolite 5-hydroxytryptophan (5-HTP), the immediate precursor of serotonin, have been used for improving sleep because serotonin is known to have multiple functions in the regulation of wake and sleep states [128]. Because serotonin is a precursor of melatonin, sleep promotion through L-tryptophan administration may also result from increased melatonin levels. Whereas the conversion of L-tryptophan to serotonin is limited by the availability of the metabolizing enzyme tryptophan hydroxylase and protein transporters that are shared with other amino acids, 5-HTP conversion is not limited by these factors and may be more efficiently converted to serotonin [129], although more research is needed on the clinical effects of this difference.

Early studies on L-tryptophan generally used small samples and produced mixed results. Some research showed that L-tryptophan or 5-HTP supplementation reduced sleep latency [129]. Additionally, some evidence suggests that consumption on foods rich in L-tryptophan along with carbohydrates (which promotes L-tryptophan uptake) also reduces sleep latency [130], and CBT strategies include a bedtime snack with foods high in this amino acid. After the occurrence of a 1989 epidemic of the life-threatening condition eosinophilia-myalgia syndrome (EMS) associated with L-tryptophan, research on L-tryptophan for sleep ceased, and only recently have investigators begun to study its effects on sleep. One double-blind, placebo controlled RCT showed improvement in self-reported total sleep time, sleep efficiency, total wake time, and sleep quality with both pharmaceutical grade L-tryptophan and specifically formulated L-tryptophan/carbohydrate food bars [131]. Another study showed that REM sleep suppression caused by use of a serotonin-reuptake inhibiting antidepressant was reversed by concurrent L-tryptophan supplementation [132]. At present, insufficient evidence exists to determine the clinical efficacy of L-tryptophan and 5-HTP for sleep disturbance.

Safety concerns regarding L-tryptophan were raised in 1989 following an epidemic of EMS that resulted in at least 37 reported deaths [133]. In most cases, EMS was linked to a contaminated product from Japan, but individual susceptibility could not be excluded as a contributing factor. The US Food and Drug Administration (FDA) issued an advisory and banned the sale of most tryptophan products. Only recently has marketing of L-tryptophan been allowed in the United States again, but an advisory remains in effect and restrictions remain on imported L-tryptophan products [133]. Other than the rare but serious risk of EMS, L-tryptophan and 5-HTP supplements have few reported side effects and are not associated with residual sedation. Nausea is a common side effect of L-tryptophan doses above 5 mg [103].Although some evidence suggests that concurrent use of serotonin precursors (L-tryptophan or 5-HTP) with antidepressants may be beneficial, such use should be avoided until more is known about potential product interactions due to risk of serotonin syndrome, a dangerous condition associated with hyperthermia, hyperreflexia, and risk of death.

GENERAL SAFETY CONSIDERATIONS FOR OLDER ADULTS

In addition to the specific side effects and safety issues discussed above, some general safety concerns apply to all purportedly sedative products, with some specific cautions applied to older adults. First, because hepatic and renal clearance may be reduced [134], active constituents of botanical supplements may have prolonged half-lives in older adults, and doses may need to be reduced accordingly. Because no rigorous dose-response studies have investigated botanical sedatives, there is no evidence on which to base such adjustment.

Given that polypharmacy is common in older adults, drug–herb interactions are of particular concern. Sedating herbs may cause risk of additive sedation in older adults taking the benzodiazepine receptor medications (e.g., Ambien® or Lunesta®) or medications for which sedation is a major side effect (e.g., opioids, first generation antihistamines). In animal models, valerian [135], hops [74, 76], and lemon balm [83] have been shown to increase barbiturate-induced sleep time. Given this evidence, concurrent use of these herbs with sedating medications should be avoided, especially in older adults in whom sedative effects are unpredictable.

Altered drug metabolism is another potential drug–herb interaction that could pose the risk of serious harm to older adults. Various herbs may inhibit or induce enzymes that metabolize drugs during the first pass through the small intestine and liver following ingestion and initial absorption. Inhibition of these enzymes (cytochrome P450 isoenzymes) reduces drug metabolism and may cause risk of increased drug levels and toxicity; induction of the enzymes increases drug metabolism and may reduce or abolish the therapeutic actions of the affected drugs. Although *in vitro* studies suggest that caution is warranted, the effects suggested in these studies do not always occur *in vivo* in humans. An example of this is valerian, which was shown *in vitro* to have mild to moderate inhibitory effects on P450 enzymes [136–138], but had no effects on the levels of medications metabolized by these enzymes when tested in humans [139, 140]. Other botanicals shown *in vitro* to inhibit drug-metabolizing enzymes include kava [140, 141], chamomile [142, 143], and hops [144]. Until safety *in vivo* is demonstrated, caution is warranted when using these herbs with other medications metabolized by affected enzymes.

SUMMARY AND CONCLUSIONS

Sleep disturbance is common in older adults and may pose health risks and reduce quality of life. Particular sleep disturbances that become more common with increasing age include co-morbid insomnia, advanced sleep phase disorder, sleep apnea, periodic limb movements in sleep, and restless legs syndrome. Non-pharmaceutical products commonly used for sedative effects include the botanicals valerian, hops, lemon balm, lavender, passion flower, kava, and chamomile as well as non-botanical products melatonin, L-tryptophan, and 5-HTP. Although valerian is widely used and accepted as a sedative, numerous studies have failed to show sleep-promoting effects of valerian that are superior to placebo. Evidence suggests that kava may be helpful as a sleep aid for anxiety disorders, but more research is needed and caution is strongly recommended in persons at risk for liver problems. Melatonin has shown efficacy as chronobiologic agent but is not recommended for the treatment of insomnia. Insufficient evidence currently exists to determine the sedative efficacy of hops, lavender, chamomile, passion flower, L-tryptophan, and 5-HTP.

Side effects of most of the botanicals and supplements reviewed are generally mild at recommended doses. Two notable exceptions are kava, which was associated with idiosyncratic cases of hepatotoxicity, and L-tryptophan (likely from a contaminated source) which was associated with EMS. Valerian, hops, lemon balm, and passion flower have been shown to have good safety and tolerability in several large open-labeled trials (144–3447 participants) [102, 145–147].

Overall, insufficient evidence supports the efficacy of botanicals for the treatment of sleep disturbances in older adults. Most appear unlikely to cause harm should individuals elect to use these products, but such use should always be discussed with a health care provider, especially for evaluation of potential drug–herb interactions.

REFERENCES

1. Foley, D. J., Monjan, A. A., Brown, S. L., Simonsick, E. M., Wallace, R. B. & Blazer, D. G. (1995). Sleep complaints among elderly persons: An epidemiologic study of three communities. *Sleep* **18**, 425–432.
2. Basu, R., Dodge, H., Stoehr, G. P. & Ganguli, M. (2003). Sedative-hypnotic use of diphenhydramine in a rural, older adult, community-based cohort: Effects on cognition. *Am J Geriatr Psychiatry* **11**, 205–213.
3. Aparasu, R. R., Mort, J. R. & Brandt, H. (2003). Psychotropic prescription use by community-dwelling elderly in the United States. *J Am Geriatr Soc* **51**, 671–677.
4. Glass, J. R., Sproule, B. A., Herrmann, N., Streiner, D. & Busto, U. E. (2003). Acute pharmacological effects of temazepam, diphenhydramine, and valerian in healthy elderly subjects. *J Clin Psychopharmacol* **23**, 260–268.
5. Wagner, J., Wagner, M. L. & Hening, W. A. (1998). Beyond benzodiazepines: Alternative pharmacologic agents for the treatment of insomnia. *Ann Pharmacother* **32**, 680–691.

6. State-of-the-Science Panel (2005). National Institutes of Health State of the Science Conference statement on Manifestations and Management of Chronic Insomnia in Adults, June 13–15, 2005. *Sleep* **28**, 1049–1057.

7. Pearson, N. J., Johnson, L. L. & Nahin, R. L. (2006). Insomnia, trouble sleeping, and complementary and alternative medicine: Analysis of the 2002 National Health Interview Survey data. *Arch Intern Med* **166**, 1775–1782.

8. Eisenberg, D. M., Kessler, R. C., Van Rompay, M. I., Kaptchuk, T. J., Wilkey, S. A., Appel, S. & Davis, R. B. (2001). Perceptions about complementary therapies relative to conventional therapies among adults who use both: Results from a national survey. *Ann Intern Med* **135**, 344–351.

9. Kessler, R. C., Davis, R. B., Foster, D. F., Van Rompay, M. I., Walters, E. E., Wilkey, S. A., Kaptchuk, T. J. & Eisenberg, D. M. (2001). Long-term trends in the use of complementary and alternative medical therapies in the United States. *Ann Intern Med* **135**, 262–268.

10. Ni, H., Simile, C. & Hardy, A. M. (2002). Utilization of complementary and alternative medicine by United States adults: Results from the 1999 National Health Interview Survey. *Med Care* **40**, 353–358.

11. Taibi, D. M., Landis, C. A., Petry, H. & Vitiello, M. V. (2007). A systematic review of valerian as a sleep aid: Safe but not effective. *Sleep Med Rev* **11**, 209–230.

12. Ohayon, M. M., Carskadon, M. A., Guilleminault, C. & Vitiello, M. V. (2004). Meta-analysis of quantitative sleep parameters from childhood to old age in healthy individuals: Developing normative sleep values across the human lifespan. *Sleep* **27**, 1255–1273.

13. Ancoli-Israel, S. & Cooke, J. R. (2005). Prevalence and comorbidity of insomnia and effect on functioning in elderly populations. *J Am Geriatr Soc* **53**, S264–S271.

14. American Academy of Sleep Medicine (2001). *The International Classification of Sleep Disorders, Revised*, American Academy of Sleep Medicine, Westchester, IL.

15. Sateia, M. J. & Nowell, P. D. (2004). Insomnia. *Lancet* **364**, 1959–1973.

16. Zammit, G. K., Weiner, J., Damato, N., Sillup, G. P. & McMillan, C. A. (1999). Quality of life in people with insomnia. *Sleep* **22**, S379–S385.

17. Stewart, R., Besset, A., Bebbington, P., Brugha, T., Lindesay, J., Jenkins, R., Singleton, N. & Meltzer, H. (2006). Insomnia comorbidity and impact and hypnotic use by age group in a national survey population aged 16 to 74 years. *Sleep* **29**, 1391–1397.

18. Buysse, D. J., Ancoli-Israel, S., Edinger, J. D., Lichstein, K. L. & Morin, C. M. (2006). Recommendations for a standard research assessment of insomnia. *Sleep* **29**, 1155–1173.

19. Edinger, J. D., Bonnet, M. H., Bootzin, R. R., Doghramji, K., Dorsey, C. M., Espie, C. A., Jamieson, A. O., McCall, W. V., Morin, C. M. & Stepanski, E. J. (2004). Derivation of research diagnostic criteria for insomnia: Report of an American Academy of Sleep Medicine Work Group. *Sleep* **27**, 1567–1596.

20. Taylor, D. J., Mallory, L. J., Lichstein, K. L., Durrence, H. H., Riedel, B. W. & Bush, A. J. (2007). Comorbidity of chronic insomnia with medical problems. *Sleep* **30**, 213–218.

21. Foley, D., Ancoli-Israel, S., Britz, P. & Walsh, J. (2004). Sleep disturbances and chronic disease in older adults: Results of the 2003 National Sleep Foundation Sleep in America Survey. *J Psychosom Res* **56**, 497–502.

22. Krystal, A. D., Edinger, J., Wohlgemuth, W. & Marsh, G. R. (1998). Sleep in perimenopausal and post-menopausal women. *Sleep Med Rev* **2**, 243–253.

23. Landis, C. A. & Moe, K. E. (2004). Sleep and menopause. *Nurs Clin North Am* **39**, 97–115.

24. Woods, N. F. & Mitchell, E. S. (2005). Symptoms during the perimenopause: Prevalence, severity, trajectory, and significance in women's lives. *Am J Med* **118**, 14–24.

25. McCall, W. V. (2005). Diagnosis and management of insomnia in older people. *J Am Geriatr Soc* **53**, S272–S277.

26. Rybarczyk, B., Stepanski, E., Fogg, L., Lopez, M., Barry, P. & Davis, A. (2005). A placebo-controlled test of cognitive-behavioral therapy for comorbid insomnia in older adults. *J Consult Clin Psychol* **73**, 1164–1174.

27. Allain, H., Bentue-Ferrer, D., Polard, E., Akwa, Y. & Patat, A. (2005). Postural instability and consequent falls and hip fractures associated with use of hypnotics in the elderly: A comparative review. *Drugs Aging* **22**, 749–765.

28. Krystal, A. D., Walsh, J. K., Laska, E., Caron, J., Amato, D. A., Wessel, T. C. & Roth, T. (2003). Sustained efficacy of eszopiclone over 6 months of nightly treatment: Results of a randomized, double-blind, placebo-controlled study in adults with chronic insomnia. *Sleep* **26**, 793–799.

29. Shaw, D., Leon, C., Kolev, S. & Murray, V. (1997). Traditional remedies and food supplements. A 5-year toxicological study (1991–1995). *Drug Saf* **17**, 342–356.

30. Hornyak, M., Feige, B., Riemann, D. & Voderholzer, U. (2006). Periodic leg movements in sleep and periodic limb movement disorder: Prevalence, clinical significance and treatment. *Sleep Med Rev* **10**, 169–177.

31. Trenkwalder, C., Kohnen, R., Allen, R. P., Benes, H., Ferini-Strambi, L., Garcia-Borreguero, D., Hadjigeorgiou, G. M., Happe, S., Hogl, B., Hornyak, M., Klein, C., Nass, A., Montagna, P., Oertel, W. H., O'Keeffe, S., Paulus, W., Poewe, W., Provini, F., Pramstaller, P. P., Sieminski, M., Sonka, K., Stiasny-Kolster, K., de Weerd, A., Wetter, T. C., Winkelmann, J. & Zucconi, M. (2007). Clinical trials in restless legs syndrome – Recommendations of the European RLS Study Group (EURLSSG). *Mov Disord*, (http://www3.interscience.wiley.com/)

32. Allen, R. P. (2007). Controversies and challenges in defining the etiology and pathophysiology of restless legs syndrome. *Am J Med* **120**, S13–S21.

33. Cuellar, N. G., Strumpf, N. E. & Ratcliffe, S. J. (2007). Symptoms of restless legs syndrome in older adults: Outcomes on sleep quality, sleepiness, fatigue, depression, and quality of life. *J Am Geriatr Soc* **55**, 1387–1392.

34. Launois, S. H., Pepin, J. L. & Levy, P. (2007). Sleep apnea in the elderly: A specific entity? *Sleep Med Rev* **11**, 87–97.

35. Young, T., Peppard, P. E. & Taheri, S. (2005). Excess weight and sleep-disordered breathing. *J Appl Physiol* **99**, 1592–1599.

36. Kushida, C. A., Littner, M. R., Hirshkowitz, M., Morgenthaler, T. I., Alessi, C. A., Bailey, D., Boehlecke, B., Brown, T. M., Coleman, J., Jr., Friedman, L., Kapen, S., Kapur, V. K., Kramer, M., Lee-Chiong, T., Owens, J., Pancer, J. P., Swick, T. J. & Wise, M. S. (2006). Practice parameters for the use of continuous and bilevel

positive airway pressure devices to treat adult patients with sleep-related breathing disorders. *Sleep* **29**, 375–380.

37. Blumenthal, M. (1998). *The Complete German Commission E Monographs: Therapeutic Guide to Herbal Medicines*, American Botanical Council, Integrative Medicine Communications, Boston, MA.

38. National Center for Complementary and Alternative Medicine (2007). *Valerian.* Bethesda, MD: NCCAM, National Institutes of Health, Herbs at a glance, (http://www.nccam.nih.gov/health/valerian/)

39. Cuellar, N. G., Rogers, A. E. & Hisghman, V. (2007). Evidenced based research of complementary and alternative medicine (CAM) for sleep in the community dwelling older adult. *Geriatr Nurs* **28**, 46–52.

40. Bliwise, D., Saunders, D., Wood-Siverio, C., Greer, S., Pour Ansari, F., Rye, D., Hitchcock, S. & Decker, M. (2007). Double-blind, placebo (PLO)-controlled, polysomnographic randomized clinical trial (RCT) of valerian (VAL) for sleep in Parkinson's disease (PD). *Sleep* **30**, A41.

41. Cuellar, N. (2007). *The use of valerian on sleep in persons with restless legs syndrome*, National Institutes of Health, Bethesda, MD, (http://www.crisp.cit.nih.gov/)

42. Houghton, P. J. (1999). The scientific basis for the reputed activity of Valerian. *J Pharm Pharmacol* **51**, 505–512.

43. Upton, R. (1999). Valerian root: *Valeriana officinalis*, analytical quality control, and therapeutic monograph. *American Herbal Pharmacopoeia and Therapeutic Compendium* (http://www.herbal-ahp.org/documents/sample/valerian.pdf).

44. Ortiz, J. G., Rassi, N., Maldonado, P. M., Gonzalez-Cabrera, S. & Ramos, I. (2006). Commercial valerian interactions with [3 H]Flunitrazepam and [3 H]MK-801 binding to rat synaptic membranes. *Phytother Res* **20**, 794–798.

45. Yuan, C. S., Mehendale, S., Xiao, Y., Aung, H. H., Xie, J. T. & Ang-Lee, M. K. (2004). The gamma-aminobutyric acidergic effects of valerian and valerenic acid on rat brainstem neuronal activity. *Anesth Analg* **98**, 353–358.

46. Schumacher, B., Scholle, S., Holzl, J., Khudeir, N., Hess, S. & Muller, C. E. (2002). Lignans isolated from valerian: Identification and characterization of a new olivil derivative with partial agonistic activity at A(1) adenosine receptors. *J Nat Prod* **65**, 1479–1485.

47. Lacher, S. K., Mayer, R., Sichardt, K., Nieber, K. & Muller, C. E. (2007). Interaction of valerian extracts of different polarity with adenosine receptors: Identification of isovaltrate as an inverse agonist at A1 receptors. *Biochem Pharmacol* **73**, 248–258.

48. Muller, C. E., Schumacher, B., Brattstrom, A., Abourashed, E. A. & Koetter, U. (2002). Interactions of valerian extracts and a fixed valerian-hop extract combination with adenosine receptors. *Life Sci* **71**, 1939–1949.

49. Dietz, B. M., Mahady, G. B., Pauli, G. F. & Farnsworth, N. R. (2005). Valerian extract and valerenic acid are partial agonists of the 5-HT5a receptor *in vitro*. *Brain Res Mol Brain Res* **138**, 191–197.

50. Khom, S., Baburin, I., Timin, E., Hohaus, A., Trauner, G., Kopp, B. & Hering, S. (2007). Valerenic acid potentiates and inhibits GABA(A) receptors: Molecular mechanism and subunit specificity. *Neuropharmacology* **53**, 178–187.

51. Porkka-Heiskanen, T., Alanko, L., Kalinchuk, A. & Stenberg, D. (2002). Adenosine and sleep. *Sleep Med Rev* **6**, 321–332.

52. Schulz, V., Hansel, R. & Tyler, V. E. (2001). *Rational Phytotherapy*, 4th ed., Springer-Verlag, Berlin.

53. Diaper, A. & Hindmarch, I. (2004). A double-blind, placebo-controlled investigation of the effects of two doses of a valerian preparation on the sleep, cognitive and psychomotor function of sleep-disturbed older adults. *Phytother Res* **18**, 831–836.

54. Vorbach, E. U., Gortelmeyer, R. & Bruning, J. (1996). Therapie von Insomnien: Wirksamkeit und Veträglichkeit eines Baldrianpräparats. *Psychopharmakotherapie* **3**, 109–115.

55. Donath, F., Quispe, S., Diefenbach, K., Maurer, A., Fietze, I. & Roots, I. (2000). Critical evaluation of the effect of valerian extract on sleep structure and sleep quality. *Pharmacopsychiatry* **33**, 47–53.

56. Kuhlmann, J., Berger, W., Podzuweit, H. & Schmidt, U. (1999). The influence of valerian treatment on "reaction time, alertness and concentration" in volunteers. *Pharmacopsychiatry* **32**, 235–241.

57. Schulz, H., Stolz, C. & Muller, J. (1994). The effect of valerian extract on sleep polygraphy in poor sleepers: A pilot study. *Pharmacopsychiatry* **27**, 147–151.

58. Jansen, W. (1977). Double blind trial of a mixture of valerian extract with valepotriates. *Therapiewoche* **27**, 2779–2786.

59. Kamm Kohl, A. V., Jansen, W. & Brockmann, P. (1984). Moderne Baldriantherapie gegen nervöse Störungen im Senium. *Med Welt* **35**, 1450–1454.

60. Jacobs, B. P., Bent, S., Tice, J. A., Blackwell, T. & Cummings, S. R. (2005). An internet-based randomized, placebo-controlled trial of kava and valerian for anxiety and insomnia. *Medicine* **84**, 197–207.

61. Morin, C. M., Koetter, U., Bastien, C., Ware, J. C. & Wooten, V. (2005). Valerian–hops combination and diphenhydramine for treating insomnia: A randomized placebo-controlled clinical trial. *Sleep* **28**, 1465–1471.

62. Coxeter, P. D., Schluter, P. J., Eastwood, H. L., Nikles, C. J. & Glasziou, P. P. (2003). Valerian does not appear to reduce symptoms for patients with chronic insomnia in general practice using a series of randomised n-of-1 trials. *Complement Ther Med* **11**, 215–222.

63. Brattstrom, A. (2007). Scientific evidence for a fixed extract combination (Ze 91019) from valerian and hops traditionally used as a sleep-inducing aid. *Wien Med Wochenschr* **157**, 367–370.

64. Ziegler, G., Ploch, M., Miettinen-Baumann, A. & Collet, W. (2002). Efficacy and tolerability of valerian extract LI 156 compared with oxazepam in the treatment of non-organic insomnia: A randomized, double-blind, comparative clinical study. *Eur J Med Res* **7**, 480–486.

65. Leathwood, P. D., Chauffard, F., Heck, E. & Munoz-Box, R. (1982). Aqueous extract of valerian root (*Valeriana officinalis* L.) improves sleep quality in man. *Pharmacol Biochem Behav* **17**, 65–71.

66. Leathwood, P. D. & Chauffard, F. (1985). Aqueous extract of valerian reduces latency to fall asleep in man. *Planta Med* **51**, 144–148.

67. Caldwell, S. H., Feeley, J. W., Wieboldt, T. F., Featherston, P. L. & Dickson, R. C. (1994). Acute hepatitis with use of over-the-counter herbal remedies. *Va Med Q* **121**, 31–33.

68. MacGregor, F. B., Abernethy, V. E., Dahabra, S., Cobden, I. & Hayes, P. C. (1989). Hepatotoxicity of herbal remedies. *BMJ* **299**, 1156–1157.

69. Chan, T. Y. (1998). An assessment of the delayed effects associated with valerian overdose. *Int J Clin Pharmacol Ther* **36**, 569.
70. Chan, T. Y., Tang, C. H. & Critchley, J. A. (1995). Poisoning due to an over-the-counter hypnotic, Sleep-Qik (hyoscine, cyproheptadine, valerian). *Postgrad Med J* **71**, 227–228.
71. Willey, L. B., Mady, S. P., Cobaugh, D. J. & Wax, P. M. (1995). Valerian overdose: A case report. *Vet Hum Toxicol* **37**, 364–365.
72. Mullins, M. E. & Horowitz, B. Z. (1998). The case of the salad shooters: Intravenous injection of wild lettuce extract. *Vet Hum Toxicol* **40**, 290–291.
73. Bos, R., Woerdenbag, H. J., DeSmet, P. A. G. M. & Scheffer, J. J. (1997). Valeriana species. In *Adverse Effects of Herbal Drugs* (P. A. G. M. DeSmet, K. Keller, R. Hansel & R. F. Chandler, Eds.), Vol. 3, pp. 165–180, Springer-Verlag, Berlin.
74. Zanoli, P., Avallone, R. & Baraldi, M. (2000). Behavioral characterisation of the flavonoids apigenin and chrysin. *Fitoterapia* **71**, S117–S123.
75. Abourashed, E. A., Koetter, U. & Brattstrom, A. (2004). *In vitro* binding experiments with a valerian, hops and their fixed combination extract (Ze91019) to selected central nervous system receptors. *Phytomedicine* **11**, 633–638.
76. Schiller, H., Forster, A., Vonhoff, C., Hegger, M., Biller, A. & Winterhoff, H. (2006). Sedating effects of *Humulus lupulus* L. extracts. *Phytomedicine* **13**, 535–541.
77. Rodenbeck, A., Simen, S., Cohrs, S., Jordan, W., Kinkelbur, J., Staedt, J. & Hajak, G. (1998). Veranderte Schafstadienstruktur als Hinweis auf die GABAerge Wirking eines Baldrian-Hopfen-Präparates bei Patienten mit psychophysiologischer Insomnie. *Somnologie* **2**, 26–31.
78. Schmitz, M. & Jackel, M. (1998). Vergleichsstudie zur Untersuchung der Lebensqualität von Patienten mit exogenen Schlafstörungen (vorübergehenden Ein- und Durchschlafstörungen) unter Therapie mit einem Hopfen-Baldrian-Präparat und einem Benzodiazepin-Präparat. *Wien Med Wochenschr* **148**, 291–298.
79. Koetter, U., Schrader, E., Kaufeler, R. & Brattstrom, A. (2007). A randomized, double blind, placebo-controlled, prospective clinical study to demonstrate clinical efficacy of a fixed valerian hops extract combination (Ze 91019) in patients suffering from non-organic sleep disorder. *Phytother Res* **21**, 847–851.
80. AltMedDex® System, Vol. 2007. Thomson Healthcare, Greenwood Village, CO.
81. Gardiner, P. (2000). *Lemon balm (Melissa officinalis)*, Longwood Herbal Task Force, (http://www.mcp.edu/herbal)
82. Salah, S. M. & Jager, A. K. (2005). Screening of traditionally used Lebanese herbs for neurological activities. *J Ethnopharmacol* **97**, 145–149.
83. Soulimani, R., Fleurentin, J., Mortier, F., Misslin, R., Derrieu, G. & Pelt, J. M. (1991). Neurotropic action of the hydroalcoholic extract of *Melissa officinalis* in the mouse. *Planta Med* **57**, 105–109.
84. Cerny, A. & Schmid, K. (1999). Tolerability and efficacy of valerian/lemon balm in healthy volunteers (a double-blind, placebo-controlled, multicentre study). *Fitoterapia* **70**, 221–228.
85. Dressing, H., Riemann, D., Low, H., Schredl, M., Reh, C., Laux, P. & Muller, W. E. (1992). Baldrian-Melisse-Kombinationen versus Benzodiadepin. Bei schlafstörungen gleichwertig? *Therapiewoche* **42**, 726–736.

86. Dressing, H., Kohler, S. & Muller, W. E. (1996). Verbessering der Schlafqualität mit einem hochdosierten Baldrian-Melisse-Präparat: eine plazebokontrollierte doppelblinde. *Psychopharmakotherapie* **3**, 123–130.
87. Lindahl, O. & Lindwall, L. (1989). Double blind study of a valerian preparation. *Pharmacol Biochem Behav* **32**, 1065–1066.
88. Ulbricht, C., Brendler, T., Gruenwald, J., Kligler, B., Keifer, D., Abrams, T. R., Woods, J., Boon, H., Kirkwood, C. D., Hackman, D. A., Basch, E. & Lafferty, H. J. (2005). Lemon balm (*Melissa officinalis* L.): An evidence-based systematic review by the Natural Standard Research Collaboration. *J Herb Pharmacother* **5**, 71–114.
89. Cavanagh, H. M. & Wilkinson, J. M. (2002). Biological activities of lavender essential oil. *Phytother Res* **16**, 301–308.
90. Gray, S. G. & Clair, A. A. (2002). Influence of aromatherapy on medication administration to residential-care residents with dementia and behavioral challenges. *Am J Alzheimers Dis Other Demen* **17**, 169–174.
91. Lewith, G. T., Godfrey, A. D. & Prescott, P. (2005). A single-blinded, randomized pilot study evaluating the aroma of *Lavandula augustifolia* as a treatment for mild insomnia. *J Altern Complement Med* **11**, 631–637.
92. Goel, N., Kim, H. & Lao, R. P. (2005). An olfactory stimulus modifies nighttime sleep in young men and women. *Chronobiol Int* **22**, 889–904.
93. Soden, K., Vincent, K., Craske, S., Lucas, C. & Ashley, S. (2004). A randomized controlled trial of aromatherapy massage in a hospice setting. *Palliat Med* **18**, 87–92.
94. Chu, C. J. & Kemper, K. J. (2001). *Lavender (Lavandula spp.)*, Longwood Herbal Task Force, (http://www.mcp.edu/herbal).
95. Dhawan, K., Dhawan, S. & Sharma, A. (2004). Passiflora: A review update. *J Ethnopharmacol* **94**, 1–23.
96. de Castro, P. C., Hoshino, A., da Silva, J. C. & Mendes, F. R. (2007). Possible anxiolytic effect of two extracts of *Passiflora quadrangularis* L. in experimental models. *Phytother Res* **21**, 481–484.
97. Capasso, A. & Sorrentino, L. (2005). Pharmacological studies on the sedative and hypnotic effect of Kava kava and Passiflora extracts combination. *Phytomedicine* **12**, 39–45.
98. Lolli, L. F., Sato, C. M., Romanini, C. V., Villas-Boas Lde, B., Santos, C. A. & de Oliveira, R. M. (2007). Possible involvement of GABA A-benzodiazepine receptor in the anxiolytic-like effect induced by *Passiflora actinia* extracts in mice. *J Ethnopharmacol* **111**, 308–314.
99. Mori, A., Hasegawa, K., Murasaki, M., Yamauchi, T. *et al.* (2000). Clinical evaluation of Passiflamin (passiflora extract) on neurosis: Multicenter double blind study in comparison with mexazolam. *Clinical Evaluation* **21**, 383–440.
100. Akhondzadeh, S., Naghavi, H. R., Vazirian, M., Shayeganpour, A., Rashidi, H. & Khani, M. (2001). Passionflower in the treatment of generalized anxiety: A pilot double-blind randomized controlled trial with oxazepam. *J Clin Pharm Ther* **26**, 363–367.
101. Miyasaka, L. S., Atallah, A. N. & Soares, B. G. (2007). Passiflora for anxiety disorder. *Cochrane Database Syst Rev*, CD004518.
102. Staiger, C. & Wegener, T. (2006). Pflanzliche Dreierkombination bei Schlafstörungen und Unruhezuständen: eine Anwendungsbeobachtung. *Z Phytother* **27**, 12–15.
103. POISINDEX® System, Vol. 2007. Thomson Healthcare, Greenwood Village, CO.

104. Pittler, M. H. & Ernst, E. (2000). Efficacy of kava extract for treating anxiety: Systematic review and meta-analysis. *J Clin Psychopharmacol* **20**, 84–89.

105. Witte, S., Loew, D. & Gaus, W. (2005). Meta-analysis of the efficacy of the acetonic kava-kava extract WS 1490 in patients with non-psychotic anxiety disorders. *Phytother Res* **19**, 183–188.

106. Gyllenhaal, C., Merritt, S. L., Peterson, S. D., Block, K. I. & Gochenour, T. (2000). Efficacy and safety of herbal stimulants and sedatives in sleep disorders. *Sleep Med Rev* **4**, 229–251.

107. Clouatre, D. L. (2004). Kava kava: Examining new reports of toxicity. *Toxicol Lett* **150**, 85–96.

108. Lehrl, S. (2004). Clinical efficacy of kava extract WS 1490 in sleep disturbances associated with anxiety disorders. Results of a multicenter, randomized, placebo-controlled, double-blind clinical trial. *J Affect Disord* **78**, 101–110.

109. Wheatley, D. (2001). Kava and valerian in the treatment of stress-induced insomnia. *Phytother Res* **15**, 549–551.

110. Pittler, M. H. & Ernst, E. (2003). Kava extract for treating anxiety. *Cochrane Database Syst Rev*, CD003383.

111. McKay, D. L. & Blumberg, J. B. (2006). A review of the bioactivity and potential health benefits of chamomile tea (*Matricaria recutita* L.). *Phytother Res* **20**, 519–530.

112. Mills, S. & Bone, K. (2000). German chamomile. *Principles and Practice of Phytotherapy*, Churchill Livingstone, New York.

113. Avallone, R., Zanoli, P., Puia, G., Kleinschnitz, M., Schreier, P. & Baraldi, M. (2000). Pharmacological profile of apigenin, a flavonoid isolated from *Matricaria chamomilla*. *Biochem Pharmacol* **59**, 1387–1394.

114. Shinomiya, K., Inoue, T., Utsu, Y., Tokunaga, S., Masuoka, T., Ohmori, A. & Kamei, C. (2005). Hypnotic activities of chamomile and passiflora extracts in sleep-disturbed rats. *Biol Pharm Bull* **28**, 808–810.

115. Gardiner, P. (1999). *Chamomile (Matricaria recutita, Anthemis nobilis)*, Longwood Herbal Task Force, (http://www.mcp.edu/herbal)

116. Reider, N., Sepp, N., Fritsch, P., Weinlich, G. & Jensen-Jarolim, E. (2000). Anaphylaxis to camomile: Clinical features and allergen cross-reactivity. *Clin Exp Allergy* **30**, 1436–1443.

117. Reiter, R. J. (2003). Melatonin: Clinical relevance. *Best Pract Res Clin Endocrinol Metab* **17**, 273–285.

118. Krauchi, K., Cajochen, C., Werth, E. & Wirz-Justice, A. (2000). Functional link between distal vasodilation and sleep-onset latency. *Am J Physiol Regul Integr Comp Physiol* **278**, R741–R748.

119. Pandi-Perumal, S. R., Zisapel, N., Srinivasan, V. & Cardinali, D. P. (2005). Melatonin and sleep in aging population. *Exp Gerontol* **40**, 911–925.

120. Zeitzer, J. M., Duffy, J. F., Lockley, S. W., Dijk, D. J. & Czeisler, C. A. (2007). Plasma melatonin rhythms in young and older humans during sleep, sleep deprivation, and wake. *Sleep* **30**, 1437–1443.

121. Buscemi, N., Vandermeer, B., Pandya, R., Hooton, N., Tjosvold, L., Hartling, L., Baker, G., Vohra, S. & Klassen, T. (2004). Melatonin for treatment of sleep disorders. *Evidence Report Technology Assessment No. 108*. AHRQ Publication No. 05-E002-2. Rockville, MD.

122. Morgenthaler, T. I., Lee-Chiong, T., Alessi, C., Friedman, L., Aurora, N., Boehlecke, B., Brown, T., Chesson, A. & Kapur, V. (2007). Practice parameters

for the clinical evaluation and treatment of circadian rhythm disorders: An American Academy of Sleep Medicine Report. *Sleep* **30**, 1445–1459.

123. Sack, R. L., Auckley, D., Auger, R., Carsakdon, M. A., Wright, K. P., Vitiello, M. V. & Zhdanova, I. V. (2007). Circadian rhythm sleep disorders: Part II, advanced sleep phase disorder, delayed sleep phase disorder, free-running disorder, and irregular sleep-wake rhythm. *Sleep* **30**, 1484–1501.

124. Haimov, I., Lavie, P., Laudon, M., Herer, P., Vigder, C. & Zisapel, N. (1995). Melatonin replacement therapy of elderly insomniacs. *Sleep* **18**, 598–603.

125. Zhdanova, I. V., Wurtman, R. J., Regan, M. M., Taylor, J. A., Shi, J. P. & Leclair, O. U. (2001). Melatonin treatment for age-related insomnia. *J Clin Endocrinol Metab* **86**, 4727–4730.

126. Garfinkel, D., Laudon, M. & Zisapel, N. (1997). Improvement of sleep quality by controlled-release melatonin in benzodiazepine-treated elderly insomniacs. *Arch Gerontol Geriatr* **24**, 223–231.

127. Committee on the Framework for Evaluating the Safety of Dietary Supplements (2004). *Prototype monograph on melatonin*, Institute of Medicine and National Research Council, Washington, D.C., (http://www.iom.edu/?id=31934).

128. Ursin, R. (2002). Serotonin and sleep. *Sleep Med Rev* **6**, 55–69.

129. Birdsall, T. C. (1998). 5-Hydroxytryptophan: A clinically-effective serotonin precursor. *Altern Med Rev* **3**, 271–280.

130. Anonymous (2006). L-Tryptophan. Monograph. *Altern Med Rev* **11**, 52–56.

131. Hudson, C., Hudson, S. P., Hecht, T. & MacKenzie, J. (2005). Protein source tryptophan versus pharmaceutical grade tryptophan as an efficacious treatment for chronic insomnia. *Nutr Neurosci* **8**, 121–127.

132. Levitan, R. D., Shen, J. H., Jindal, R., Driver, H. S., Kennedy, S. H. & Shapiro, C. M. (2000). Preliminary randomized double-blind placebo-controlled trial of tryptophan combined with fluoxetine to treat major depressive disorder: Antidepressant and hypnotic effects. *J Psychiatry Neurosci* **25**, 337–346.

133. U.S. Food and Drug Administration (2001). *Information paper on L-tryptophan and 5-hydroxytryptophan*, FDA Center for Food Safety and Applied Nutrition, Washington, D.C., (http://www.cfsan.fda.gov)

134. Dorne, J. L. (2007). Human variability in hepatic and renal elimination: Implications for risk assessment. *J Appl Toxicol* **27**, 411–420.

135. Leuschner, J., Muller, J. & Rudmann, M. (1993). Characterisation of the central nervous depressant activity of a commercially available valerian root extract. *Arzneimittelforschung* **43**, 638–641.

136. Lefebvre, T., Foster, B. C., Drouin, C. E., Krantis, A., Livesey, J. F. & Jordan, S. A. (2004). *In vitro* activity of commercial valerian root extracts against human cytochrome P450 3A4. *J Pharm Pharm Sci* **7**, 265–273.

137. Budzinski, J. W., Foster, B. C., Vandenhoek, S. & Arnason, J. T. (2000). An *in vitro* evaluation of human cytochrome P450 3A4 inhibition by selected commercial herbal extracts and tinctures. *Phytomedicine* **7**, 273–282.

138. Strandell, J., Neil, A. & Carlin, G. (2004). An approach to the *in vitro* evaluation of potential for cytochrome P450 enzyme inhibition from herbals and other natural remedies. *Phytomedicine* **11**, 98–104.

139. Donovan, J. L., DeVane, C. L., Chavin, K. D., Wang, J. S., Gibson, B. B., Gefroh, H. A. & Markowitz, J. S. (2004). Multiple night-time doses of valerian

(*Valeriana officinalis*) had minimal effects on CYP3A4 activity and no effect on CYP2D6 activity in healthy volunteers. *Drug Metab Dispos* **32**, 1333–1336.

140. Gurley, B. J., Gardner, S. F., Hubbard, M. A., Williams, D. K., Gentry, W. B., Khan, I. A. & Shah, A. (2005). *In vivo* effects of goldenseal, kava kava, black cohosh, and valerian on human cytochrome P450 1A2, 2D6, 2E1, and 3A4/5 phenotypes. *Clin Pharm Ther* **77**, 415–426.

141. Cote, C. S., Kor, C., Cohen, J. & Auclair, K. (2004). Composition and biological activity of traditional and commercial kava extracts. *Biochem Biophys Res Commun* **322**, 147–152.

142. Ganzera, M., Schneider, P. & Stuppner, H. (2006). Inhibitory effects of the essential oil of chamomile (*Matricaria recutita* L.) and its major constituents on human cytochrome P450 enzymes. *Life Sci* **78**, 856–861.

143. Maliakal, P. P. & Wanwimolruk, S. (2001). Effect of herbal teas on hepatic drug metabolizing enzymes in rats. *J Pharm Pharmacol* **53**, 1323–1329.

144. Henderson, M. C., Miranda, C. L., Stevens, J. F., Deinzer, M. L. & Buhler, D. R. (2000). *In vitro* inhibition of human P450 enzymes by prenylated flavonoids from hops. *Humulus lupulus. Xenobiotica,* **30**, 235–251.

145. Volk, S., Friede, M., Hasenfuss, I. & Wüstenberg, P. (1999). Phytosedativum gegen nervöse Unruhezustände und Einschlafstörungen: Wirksamkeit und Veträglichkeit eines pflanzlichen Kombinations-präparates aus Baldrianwurzeln, Hofenzapfen und Melissenblättern. *Z Phytother* **20**, 337–344.

146. Notter, D., Brattström, A. & Ullrich, N. (2004). Therapie von Schlafstörungen. *Dtsch Apoth Ztg* **144**, 147–148.

147. Kubisch, U., Ullrich, N. & Muller, C. E. (2004). Therapie von Schlarstörungen mit einem Baldrian-Hopfen-Extrakt. *Schweiz Zschr Ganzheits Medizin* **16**, 348–354.

Chapter 5

Botanicals and Nutrition in the Treatment of Epilepsy

Siegward-M. Elsas

Department of Neurology, Oregon Center for Complementary and Alternative, Medicine in Neurological Disorders, Oregon Health and Science University, Portland, OR

Abstract

Among natural treatments for epilepsy, the strongest data exists to support the use of the ketogenic diet for children. More recently, a modified Atkins diet which is more easily applied, also seems to be promising. Natural progesterone has been shown to exert powerful anticonvulsant effects for women with epilepsy. Limited evidence exists to consider the use of melatonin as an adjunct to anticonvulsant treatment.

In contrast, clinical data on botanical treatments and other nutritional supplements for seizures is scarce. Interactions of botanicals with anticonvulsant medications need to be considered to ensure safety of their use (Samuels, N., Finkelstein, Y., Singer, S. & Oberbaum, M. (2008). Herbal medicine and epilepsy: Proconvulsive effects and interactions with antiepileptic drugs. *Epilepsia* 49(3), 373–380). Most clinical studies on botanicals were performed in China but did not meet the rigorous standards of clinical studies as performed in western countries. Nevertheless, their results draw attention to potentially efficacious anticonvulsant botanicals. Botanicals of Western origin, that seem promising for further studies, may be Passiflora and Viscum. GABA could be of potential use as a supplement if its blood–brain barrier penetration could be improved. Clinical studies of botanicals and nutritional supplements are needed to clarify their safety and therapeutic potential for epilepsy.

Keywords: *Seizure, CAM, herbs, diet, supplement, hormonal therapy*

INTRODUCTION

Epilepsy is a disabling neurological disorder with a prevalence of about 0.5% in the general population [1]. Epilepsy can cause a severe impact on quality of life [2], a high risk for injury or mortality and patients often carry a social stigma. The incidence follows a bimodal distribution with peaks in early childhood and in old age [1, 3]. Epileptic seizures fall into two large groups: primary generalized epilepsy (which includes absence, myoclonic seizures and primary generalized tonic-clonic seizures), and partial epilepsy (which includes simple or complex partial and secondarily generalized tonic-clonic seizures). While primary generalized epilepsies are mostly due to genetic changes, partial epilepsies may be due to multiple etiologies (genetic, head injuries, stroke, brain tumors, and others) [4].

Conventional treatment options for partial epilepsy include classic and newer antiepileptic drugs, the ketogenic diet, vagal nerve stimulation, and resective surgery. Since approximately 25% of epilepsy patients remain insufficiently controlled by current conventional approaches [5], interest in alternative treatments is high. In addition, many epilepsy patients may try to pursue alternative treatment options to avoid the well-known cognitive side effects of most anticonvulsant medications [6, 7], which include sedation, psychomotor slowing, and dyscoordination.

Up to 44% of epilepsy patients use CAM (complementary and alternative medicine) therapies [8–10]. Most commonly used are prayer (44%), stress management (22%), and botanicals (12%) [8]. Of the methods used, stress management (in 68%), yoga (in 57%), and botanicals (in 55%) were reported by patients to be most helpful [8]. Recent reviews of CAM treatments for epilepsy [10, 11] conclude that while there are few studies, the most promising treatments include botanicals [12] and strategies using behavioral therapy [13], biofeedback [14, 15] or other methods of self-control in mind–body medicine.

The number of botanicals, which have been used for epilepsy in various settings, is large. In most cases, efficacy is unknown or not documented. While many botanicals may have anticonvulsant potential, some may have proconvulsant effects as well (see below). In addition, the use of botanicals may affect the level of anticonvulsant medications, with the potential of either lowering seizure threshold or causing undesired anticonvulsant side effects.

The majority of the available scientific literature covers testing of herbs in animal models of epilepsy. Potential anticonvulsant or proconvulsant effects of herbal medicines were reviewed by Tyagi and Delanty [16]. A recent review by Nsour *et al.* [12] lists over 150 botanicals traditionally used for the treatment of epilepsy which have shown some promise in *in vivo* or *in vitro* studies. In contrast, the same review lists only four clinical studies, which have some methodological problems. Clinical studies are clearly needed to evaluate the efficacy of promising botanicals in clinical use.

In the following, a limited number of the most commonly used or studied herbs and some, which are of interest due to controversy, will be discussed in the context of the alternative medical systems in which they are used.

WESTERN HERBAL MEDICINE

Ginkgo biloba

Ginkgo biloba is most commonly used botanical in the general population [17] as well as in the elderly [18]. While Ginkgo extracts are primarily used to prevent cognitive impairment, they are also recommended by some for the treatment of epilepsy due to its tonic and possible antioxidant effects, for example [19]. In contrast, there is some evidence to suggest proconvulsant effects of Ginkgo. A recent report describes two patients with epilepsy well-controlled by valproate who developed frequent generalized seizures about 2 weeks after beginning regular use of ginkgo biloba extracts for cognitive impairment [20]. Ingestion so large quantities of ginkgo seeds during a food shortage was associated with seizures [21]. The FDA has received seven reports of seizure as an adverse reaction to ginkgo [22]. Despite this potential concern, ginkgo remains the most commonly used botanical even in the elderly with a diagnosis of epilepsy [18]. More detailed information from clinical studies is needed to solve this controversy.

Marijuana

Cannabis sativa is occasionally recommended for the treatment of epilepsy, for example [19]. Gowers reports about its use in the 19th century and prescribed it himself sometimes [23]. The recent conflicting evidence regarding marijuana and epilepsy has been reviewed by Gordon and Devinsky [24]. They report that animal studies show both anticonvulsant and proconvulsant effects of the primary psychoactive constituent delta-9-tetrahydrocannabinol (THC), and mild anticonvulsant effects of cannabidiol, the primary nonpsychoactive constituent. Clinical data is inconclusive about the overall usefulness of marijuana for the treatment of epilepsy.

Passionflower

The medicinal use of *Passiflora incarnata* originated with native Americans [25], and its most popular uses are for insomnia [26], anxiety [27], and epilepsy [25]. While its active ingredients have not yet been conclusively defined [27], available data suggests flavonoids as most likely active ingredients [28–30]. Studies in animal models show efficacy of *Passiflora* extracts and flavonoid fractions against pentylenetetrazole-induced seizures [29, 31], which can be inhibited by the benzodiazepine antagonist Ro 15-1788 [32]. Purified flavonoids have been shown to have anxiolytic properties in mice similar to benzodiazepines [33, 34].

   Passionflower extract is a popular botanical currently sold over the counter in many different preparations in many countries. In light of the common use, very few reports on undesirable effects have been reported. One patient with hypersensitivity developed cutaneous vasculitis and urticaria following ingestion of tablets including passionflower extract [35]. One patient developed nausea, vomiting, prolonged QT-interval in the EKG and reversible nonsustained ventricular arrythmias after ingestion of a total of 3.5 grams of *Passiflora incarnata* extract [36]. A clinical pilot trial has been published, which shows similar efficacy of

Passiflora incarnata extract with oxazepam for treatment of anxiety [37]. While this trial did not include a placebo, a trial of 182 patients with anxiety found a reduced Ham-A score in 43% of patients treated with a combination botanical extract which included *Passiflora* compared to 25% in the placebo group ($p = 0.012$) [38].

TRADITIONAL CHINESE MEDICINE (TCM)

Piper nigrum/Antiepilepsirine

Among other herbs, pepper is used in traditional Chinese medicine to treat epilepsy. Antiepilepsirine (AES) is an isolation of a piperine derivative which has been identified as a probable active ingredient which is commercially available in China. AES was evaluated in a 6-month double-blind cross-over clinical trial as adjunctive treatment to conventional anticonvulsants in 34 children [39]. During AES treatment, 18 of 34 had a response (seizure freedom or a reduction in seizure frequency of at least 50%) compared to 11 of 34 during treatment with placebo.

Prescriptions in Chinese medicine are commonly a mixture of many ingredients. One example is "Zhenxianling" [40], which consists of herbal tablets including valerian, antelope's horn powder, human placenta, and seven other ingredients, and also of a plaster placed on the umbilicus, which included semen strychni, semen hyoscyami and *Cynanchum otophyllum*, and five other ingredients. This prescription was used on 239 patients with 95.4% having a reduction in seizure frequency by at least 50%. Regarding the interpretation of such results I was cautioned by a western practitioner of TCM that physicians in Chinese hospitals are under significant pressure to produce positive research results.

Another herbal treatment for epilepsy in Chinese medicine is "Qingyangshen" prepared from the root of *Cynanchum otophyllum*. Kuang *et al.* [41] reports on the effects of "Qingyangshen" as an adjunctive treatment in 32 patients with grand mal seizures which were refractory to conventional treatment. Twenty-eight of the 32 patients showed at least 50% reduction in seizure frequency within 1 month of treatment. After 2–9 months, 9 patients became seizure free.

Similar observations in large groups of patients are described for other TCM formulas such as "Wuhuzhuifeng San" [42] or "Wuchong San" [43], which are all described to have similar efficacy when compared to control groups treated with conventional anticonvulsants such as phenytoin, carbamazepine, or valproate. Additional, uncontrolled studies are described in a review of TCM for epilepsy [44].

In summary, it appears there may be promise in some botanicals used in TCM formulas, but much research is needed to clarify which ingredients are essential, effective, and safe for clinical use.

AYURVEDIC MEDICINE

Ayurvedic medicines often contain a mixture of many different herbs, often composed on the basis of individual constitutional problems of the patient. Among other herbal preparations, such as "Ashwagandha" (*Withania somnifera*), "Brahmi ghrita" is recommended for epilepsy [45]. "Brahmi" is the Indian name for *Herpestis monniera* (also named *Bacopa monniera*), an herb which is otherwise commonly recommended for cognitive impairment. "Ghrita" describes the form of preparation which in this case is a paste used as a supplement to food and includes *Acorus calamus*, pachak root and the root of *Canscora decussata* in addition to *Herpestis monniera* [45]. Unfortunately, information on the efficacy of Brahmi ghrita for epilepsy is not available.

Since some ayurvedic preparations include heavy metals [46], safety is an important issue with ayurvedic medicines [47]. Ayurvedic preparations should be used with extreme caution and only when all ingredients of a preparation are clearly known.

ANTHROPOSOPHIC MEDICINE AND HOMEOPATHY

Viscum

Botanical extracts from *Viscum album* (Mistletoe) have traditionally been used in Europe for the treatment of epilepsy and other conditions. In a mouse experiment, a mistletoe extract was protective against pentylenetetrazole and bicuculline induced seizures [48]. Madeleyn [49] reports six cases of infantile spasms, one 9-year-old child and two adult patients with epilepsy, which became seizure free on *Viscum album* treatment. In addition to oral preparations, sterile injectable preparations are available from several companies in Europe and the US, since mistletoe is widely used as an adjunctive treatment for cancer.

In classic homeopathy there are no remedies for generic conditions. Instead, remedies are identified for the individual patient on the basis of similarity of symptoms or even the personality which matches the profile of remedies [50]. There are, however, some homeopathic remedies whose profile includes symptoms such as convulsions, which are typically associated with epilepsy. Most of these remedies are also commonly used for epilepsy in the context of anthroposophic medicine. In the following, only a few examples will be mentioned.

Belladonna and Hyoscyamus

These plants from the family Solanaceae contain the anticholinergic alkaloids atropine and scopolamine which in toxic doses can produce symptoms reminiscent of epileptic seizures. The same plants given in high dilutions are used in homeopathy to treat epileptic patients. Madeleyn [49] describes five children with epilepsy which, in combination with other anthroposophic remedies, became seizure free with homeopathic dilutions of Belladonna or Hyoscyamus.

Bufo Rana

A preparation made from the poison glands of toads is also used in homeopathy for the treatment of epileptic patients. Soldner and Stellmann [51] describe a 3-year-old boy with Lennox-Gastaut syndrome who became seizure free after treatment with a homeopathic dilution (C200) of Bufo Rana.

Arnica

Preparations from this plant of the composite family have been used to treat epilepsy either in homeopathic dilution or in the form of a bath. Charette [50] describes a 30-year-old patient with posttraumatic epilepsy who became seizure free after homeopathic treatment with Arnica (C6). Madeleyn [49] describes a 7-year-old child with Lennox-Gastaut syndrome who became seizure free after using baths with arnica extract 3 times a week.

NUTRITIONAL APPROACHES TO EPILEPSY

Ketogenic Diet

The high fat, low carbohydrate ketogenic diet [52] is used in many epilepsy centers as an adjunct to medical treatment for children with medically refractory seizures. This diet was designed in the 1920s to mimic the effects of starvation, which can have dramatic and long-lasting effects on seizure control. It is not known how the diet works, but it is assumed that ketones, which are produced in metabolism in the absence of carbohydrates, have anticonvulsant effects [53]. High fat foods such as mayonnaise, butter, and cream make up 80–90% of the diet, which requires supplementation with vitamins and minerals. Even small amounts of carbohydrates can reverse the ketotic state and reduce seizure control. Pursuing this diet takes an enormous commitment, and supervision by an experienced physician including the monitoring of metabolic parameters in blood. Serious adverse events can occur, including death from pancreatitis [54]. Success rates in seizure control in children vary somewhat between centers; about 25% of study participants in a multicenter trial had a reduction in seizures by 50% or more [55]. A small study of the ketogenic diet for seizure control in adults found a 54% responder rate [56].

Modified Atkins Diet

More recently, the potential usefulness a less strict diet, such as a modified Atkins diet, for seizure control has been evaluated in several small studies in children [57] and adults [58, 59]. Compared to the ketogenic diet, this modified Atkins diet is more feasible since it does not require a fasting period or hospital admission, and has no restriction on protein consumption. Carbohydrates are limited to 15 g/day, high fat foods are encouraged, and urine ketones are monitored. A prospective study in 30 adults showed a 47% responder rate after 1 and 3 months, and 33% responders after 6 months [58].

In addition to whole diets, certain nutritional supplements are sometimes recommended for epilepsy [60], some of which will be briefly discussed below.

GABA

The amino acid GABA (gamma aminobutyric acid) serves as the main inhibitory neurotransmitter in the brain, and its presence is essential to maintain the balance between neuronal excitation and inhibition, which controls the threshold for epileptic seizures. Naturally, GABA metabolism has been a target for anticonvulsant drug design. Benzodiazepines potentiate effects of intrinsic synaptic GABA. Vigabatrin blocks the enzyme GABA transaminase, which inactivates GABA; Tiagabine blocks reuptake of GABA, both actions are designed to elevate GABA levels in the brain [61]. It would seem a natural choice to use GABA as a nutritional supplement, as commonly done in naturopathic practice. However, GABA does not reliably pass the blood–brain barrier, so that increased dietary levels of GABA will not penetrate into the brain consistently enough to have an effect on seizure control [62]. To improve on this, the anticonvulsant drug Gabapentin was designed as a GABA molecule with an added aromatic ring to facilitate the penetration of the blood–brain barrier; however the actual mechanism of action of Gabapentin appears to be more complex than that of a GABA agonist [63].

Progesterone

The anticonvulsive properties of progesterone [64] were discovered as a result of the observation that over one third of women with epilepsy have increased seizure activity during certain times of their menstrual cycle (during ovulation or premenstrual), a phenomenon termed "catamenial epilepsy" [65]. Estradiol, in contrast, has proconvulsive effects [66]. Catamenial epilepsy responds only to natural progesterone (available as Prometrium®), not synthetic progestins such as those included in hormone replacement therapy [67]. This may be due to the fact that only natural progesterone is metabolized to allopregnanolone, whose anticonvulsant effects are more potent than barbiturates [68]. The net result of hormone replacement therapy using synthetic progestins likely has proconvulsant effects, since the proconvulsant effects of estrogen are unopposed by the anticonvulsant effects of natural progesterone. This can be corrected by adding natural progesterone (e.g., Prometrium®). Several open label studies of natural progesterone have shown that about 75% of women with intractable catamenial partial onset epilepsy experienced a reduction in seizures by more than 50% [69, 70]. An NIH-funded multicenter, double-blind controlled trial of progesterone for women with epilepsy began in 2000.

Melatonin

Melatonin, a hormone produced by the pineal gland, helps regulate the sleep/wake cycle and is commonly taken as a supplement for insomnia. Adequate sleep is essential for good seizure control, so a relationship of melatonin to seizure control seems logical. In a study of patients with intractable temporal lobe epilepsy, melatonin levels before seizures were found to be lower than normal individuals, and increased after seizures, which could be interpreted as a compensatory release of an endogenous anticonvulsant [71]. Melatonin might have some anticonvulsant activity as suggested by a study in mice, which appeared to be protected from kainate induced seizures when preinjected with melatonin [72]. Several studies in children with medically refractory epilepsy suggest that melatonin supplementation improved seizure control, with worsening of seizures when melatonin was discontinued and improvement on resuming melatonin [73–75]. In contrast to these findings, it is possible that nocturnal seizures could be exacerbated by increased melatonin [76]. More research is needed to clarify the effect of the circadian changes of melatonin on seizures. Since melatonin is not known to cause significant side effects or to interfere with anticonvulsant levels [77], it may be a useful adjunct to anticonvulsant therapy of seizures.

Taurine

Taurine, a conditionally essential amino acid, has inhibitory effects in the central nervous system, and evidence of decreased taurine levels in epileptic patients have been used to advocate its use as adjunctive treatment for seizures [78]. Two small, uncontrolled studies suggested a mild anticonvulsant effect of taurine [79, 80]. However, results have been variable, and the use of taurine in the treatment of epilepsy remains controversial. For some patients, high doses of taurine can lead to peptic ulcers [81].

Pyridoxine

Pyridoxine (Vitamin B_6) is necessary for the synthesis of the inhibitory neurotransmitter GABA and is effective when seizures are due to pyridoxine deficiency [82]. There is no evidence that pyridoxine is useful in the treatment of other forms of epilepsy. High doses of pyridoxine can be dehydrating and can cause gait problems and reversible distal numbness [81].

Magnesium

Decreased levels of magnesium can predispose to epileptic seizures, and obstetricians commonly use intravenous magnesium to control seizures in eclampsia [83]. However, there is no evidence of a beneficial effect of oral magnesium supplementation in epilepsy outside these indications. High doses of oral magnesium can occasionally cause diarrhea [81].

Zinc

Zinc has been found to be synaptically released and to act as a neuromodulator in the hippocampus [84], a region of the cerebral cortex commonly implicated in partial epilepsy. While synaptic zinc release may increase in the course of epilepsy [85], it is not clear whether the complex actions of zinc result in protection from or in enhancement of seizures [86]. In either case there is no evidence so far to suggest a role of zinc supplements in the treatment of epilepsy.

ACKNOWLEDGMENTS

This study was supported by NIH NCCAM grant AT01993-01 to S.M.E. The author wishes to thank Garrett White and Gaddiel Navarro for assistance with this review.

REFERENCES

1. Hauser, W. A. (1997). Incidence and prevalence. *In* Epilepsy: A Comprehensive Textbook (J. J. Engel & T. A. Pedley, Eds.), pp. 47–57, Lippincott-Raven, Philadelphia.
2. Birbeck, G. L., Hays, R. D. & Cui, X. (2002). Seizure reduction and quality of life improvements in people with epilepsy. *Epilepsia* **43**(5), 535–538.
3. Olafsson, E., Hauser, W. A., Ludvigsson, P. & Gudmundsson, G. (1996). Incidence of epilepsy in rural Iceland: A population-based study. *Epilepsia* **37**(10), 951–955.
4. Wolf, P. (1994). *Epileptic Seizures and Syndromes*, J Libbey, London.
5. Aicardi, J. & Shorvon, S. D. (1997). Intractable epilepsy. *In* Epilepsy: A Comprehensive Textbook (J. J. Engel & T. A. Pedley, Eds.), pp. 1325–1331, Lippincott-Raven, Philadelphia.
6. Meador, K. J., Loring, D. W., Moore, E. E., Thompson, W. O., Nichols, M. E., Oberzan, R. E., Durkin, M. W., Gallagher, B. B. & King, D. W. (1995). Comparative cognitive effects of phenobarbital, phenytoin, and valproate in healthy adults. *Neurology* **45**(8), 1494–1499.

7. Salinsky, M. C., Oken, B. S. & Binder, L. M. (1996). Assessment of drowsiness in epilepsy patients receiving chronic antiepileptic drug therapy. *Epilepsia* **37**(2), 181–187.
8. Sirven, J. I., Drazkowski, M. D., Zimmerman, R. S., Bortz, J. J. et al. (2003). Complementary/alternative medicine for epilepsy in Arizona. *Neurology* **61**, 576–577.
9. Ryan, M. & Johnson, M. S. (2002). Use of alternative medications in patients with neurologic disorders. *Ann Pharmacother* **36**(10), 1540–1545.
10. Sonnen, A. E. (1997). Alternative and Folk remedies. *In* Epilepsy: A Comprehensive Textbook (J. J. Engel & T. A. Pedley, Eds.), pp. 1365–1378, Lippincott-Raven, Philadelphia.
11. Elsas, S. M. (2003). Epilepsy. *In* Complementary Therapies in Neurology: An Evidence-based Approach (B. S. Oken, Ed.), pp. 265–277, Parthenon, London.
12. Nsour, W. M., Lau, C. B. & Wong, I. C. (2000). Review on phytotherapy in epilepsy. *Seizure* **9**(2), 96–107.
13. Wolf, P. (1997). Behavioral Therapy. *In* Epilepsy: A Comprehensive Textbook (J. J. Engel & T. A. Pedley, Eds.), pp. 1359–1364, Lippincott-Raven, Philadelphia.
14. Kotchoubey, B., Strehl, U., Uhlmann, C., Holzapfel, S., König, M., Fröscher, W., Blankenhorn, V. & Birbaumer, N. (2001). Modification of slow cortical potentials in patients with refractory epilepsy: a controlled outcome study. *Epilepsia* **42**(3), 406–416.
15. Sterman, M. B. (2000). Basic concepts and clinical findings in the treatment of seizure disorders with EEG operant conditioning. *Clin Electroencephal* **31**(1), 45–55.
16. Tyagi, A. & Delanty, N. (2003). Herbal remedies, dietary supplements, and seizures. *Epilepsia* **44**(2), 228–235.
17. Mar, C. & Bent, S. (1999). An evidence-based review of the 10 most commonly used herbs. *Western J Med* **171**, 168–171.
18. Harms, S., Garrard, J., Schwinghammer, P., Eberly, L., Chang, Y. & Leppik, I. (2006). *Ginkgo biloba* use in nursing home elderly with epilepsy or seizure disorder. *Epilepisa* **47**(2), 323–329.
19. Murphy, P. A. (2002). *Treating Epilepsy Naturally*, McGraw-Hill, New York.
20. Granger, A. S. (2001). Ginkgo biloba precipitating epileptic seizures. *Age and Ageing* **30**(6), 523–525.
21. Kajiyama, Y., Fujii, K., Takeuchi, H. et al. (2002). Ginkgo seed poisoning. *Pediatrics* **109**, 325–327.
22. Gregory, P. (2001). Seizure associated with *Ginkgo biloba*. *Ann Intern Med* **134**, 344.
23. Gowers, W. R. (1861). *Epilepsy and Other Chronic Convulsive Disorders*, Churchill, London.
24. Gordon, E. & Devinsky, O. (2001). Alcohol and marijuana: Effects on epilepsy and use by patients with epilepsy. *Epilepsia* **42**(10), 1266–1272.
25. Spinella, M. (2001). Herbal medicines and epilepsy: The potential for benefit and adverse effects. *Epilepsy and Behavior* **2**, 524–532.
26. Krenn, L. (2002). *Passiflora incarnata* L. – a reliable herbal sedative. *Wien Med Wochenschr* **152**(15–16), 404–406.

27. Carlini, E. A. (2003). Plants and the central nervous system. *Pharmacol Biochem Behav* **75**, 501–512.
28. Dhawan, K., Kumar, S. & Sharma, A. (2001). Anti-anxiety studies on extracts of *Passiflora incarnata* L. *J Ethnopharmacol* **78**, 165–170.
29. Speroni, E. & Minghetti, A. (1988). Neuropharmacological activity of extracts from *Passiflora incarnate*. *Planta Med* **54**, 488–491.
30. Dhawan, K., Dhawan, S. & Chhabra, S. (2003). Attenuation of benzodiazepine dependence in mice by a tri-substituted benzoflavone moiety of *Passiflora incarnata* Linneaus: A non-habit forming anxiolytic. *J Pharm Pharmaceut Sci* **6**(2), 215–222.
31. Speroni, E. & Billi, R. (1996). Sedative effects of crude extract of *Passiflora incarnata* after oral administration. *Phytother Res* **10**, S92–S94.
32. Medina, J. H., Paladini, A. C., Wolfman, C. et al. (1990). Chrysin (5,7-di-OH-flavone), a naturally-occurring ligand for benzodiazepine receptors, with anticonvulsant properties. *Biochem Pharmacol* **40**(10), 2227–2231.
33. Wolfman, C., Viola, H., Paladini, A. C. et al. (1994). Possible anxiolytic effects of chrysin, a central benzodiazepine receptor ligand isolated from *Passiflora coerulea*. *Pharmacol Biochem Behav* **47**, 1–4.
34. Zanoli, P., Avallone, R. & Baraldi, M. (2000). Behavioral characterisation of the flavonoids apigenin and chrysin. *Fitoterapia* **71**(S1), S117–S123.
35. Smith, G., Chalmers, T. & Nuki, G. (1993). Vasculitis associated with herbal preparation containing *Passiflora* extract. *Br J Rheumatol* **32**, 87–88.
36. Fisher, A., Purcell, P. & Le Couteur, D. (2000). Toxicity of *Passiflora incarnata* L. *Clin Toxicol* **38**(1), 63–66.
37. Akhondzadeh, S., Naghavi, H. R. & Vazirian, M. (2001). Passionflower in the treatment of generalized anxiety: A pilot double-blind randomized controlled trial with oxazepam. *J Clin Pharm Therapeut* **26**, 363–367.
38. Bourin, M., Bougerol, T., Guitton, B. & Broutin, E. (1997). A combination of plant extracts in the treatment of outpatients with adjustment disorder with anxious mood: Controlled study versus placebo. *Fundam Clin Pharmacol* **11**(2), 127–132.
39. Wang, L., Zhao, D., Zhang, Z., Zuo, C., Zhang, Y., Pei, Y. Q. & Lo, Y. Q. (1999). Trial of antiepilepsirine (AES) in children with epilepsy. *Brain & Development* **21**(1), 36–40.
40. Wang, T. (1996). Effects of Chinese medicine zhenxianling in 239 cases of epilepsy. *Journal of Traditional Chinese Medicine* **16**(2), 94–97.
41. Kuang, P. G., Wu, Y. X., Meng, F. J., Kuang, P. Z., Shao, D. S. & Mu, Q. Z. (1981). Treatment of grand mal seizures with "Qingyangshen" (root of *Cynanchum otophyllum*) and observations on experimental animals. *Journal of Traditional Chinese Medicine* **1**(1), 19–24.
42. Li, Y. (1997). A report on 153 cases on epilepsy treated by modified Wuhuzhuifeng San. *TCM Forum* **4**, 26.
43. Vesta, K. & Medina, P. (2003). Valproic acid-induced neutropenia. *AnnPharmacother* **37**, 819–821.

44. Wang, S. & Li, Y. (2005). Traditional Chinese Medicine. *In* Complementary and Alternative Therapies for Epilepsy (O. Devinsky, S. Schachter & S. Pacia, Eds.), pp. 177–182, Demos, New York.

45. Nadkarni, K. M. (1976). *Indian Materia Medica*, Popular Prakashan, Bombay.

46. Parab, S., Kulkarni, R. & Thatte, U. (2003). Heavy metals in "herbal" medicines. *Indian J Gastroenterol* **22**(3), 111–112.

47. Gogtay, N. J., Bhatt, H. A., Dalvi, S. S. & Kshirsagar, N. A. (2002). The use and safety of non-allopathic Indian medicines. *Drug Safety* **25**(14), 1005–1019.

48. Amabeoku, G. J., Leng, M. J. & Syce, J. A. (1998). Antimicrobial and anticonvulsant activities of *Viscum capense*. *J Ethnopharmacol* **61**(3), 237–241.

49. Madeleyn, R. (1998). Aspects of epilepsy and methods of its treatment in pediatrics. *J Anthroposophical Medicine* **15**(1), 8–26.

50. Charette, G. (1958). *Homöopathische Arzneimittellehre für die Praxis*, Hippocrates, Stuttgart.

51. Soldner, G. & Stellmann, H. M. (2001). *Individuelle Pädiatrie*, Wissenschaftliche Verlagsgesellschaft, Stuttgart.

52. Freeman, J. M., Kelly, M. & Freeman, J. B. (2000). *The Ketogenic Diet: A Treatment for Epilepsy*, Demos Medical Publishing, New York.

53. Likhodii, S. S. & Burnham, W. M. (2002). Ketogenic diet: Does acetone stop seizures? *Med Sci Mon* **8**(8), 19–24.

54. Stewart, W. A., Gordon, K. & Camfield, P. (2001). Acute pancreatitis causing death in a child on the ketogenic diet. *J Child Neurol* **16**, 682.

55. Coppola, G., Veggiotti, P., Cusmai, R., Bertoli, S., Cardinali, S., Dionisi-Vici, C., Elia, C., Lispi, M., Sarnelli, M., Tagliabue, C., Toraldo, A. & Pascotto, A. (2002). The ketogenic diet in children, adolescents and young adults with refractory epilepsy: An Italian multicentric experience. *Epilepsy Res* **48**, 221–227.

56. Sirven, J., Whedon, B., Caplan, D., Liporace, J., Glosser, D., O'Dwyer, J. & Sperling., M. (1999). The ketogenic diet for intractable epilepsy in adults: Preliminary results. *Epilepsia* **40**, 1721–1726.

57. Kossoff, E., Turner, Z., Bluml, R., Pyzik, P. & Vining., E. (2007). A randomized, crossover comparison of daily carbohydrate limits using the modified Atkins diet. *Epilepsy and Behavior* **10**, 432–436.

58. Kossoff, E., Rowley, H., Sinha, S. & Vining, E. (2008). A prospective study of the modified Atkins diet for intractable epilepsy in adults. *Epilepsia* **49**(2), 316–319.

59. Kossoff, E., Krauss, G., McGrogan, J. & Freeman, J. (2003). Efficacy of the Atkins diet as therapy for intractable epilepsy. *Neurology* **61**, 1789–1791.

60. Rudderham, M., Laff, R. & Devinsky, O. (2003). Nutrition and Epilepsy. *In* Complementary and Alternative Therapies for Epilepsy (O. Devinsky, S. Schachter & S. Pacia, Eds.), pp. 191–203, Demos, New York.

61. Czuczwar, S. J. & Patsalos, P. N. (2001). The new generation of GABA enhancers. Potential in the treatment of epilepsy. *CNS Drugs* **15**(5), 339–350.

62. Shyamaladevi, N., Jayakumar, A. R., Sujatha, R., Paul, P. & Subramanian, E. H. (2002). Evidence that nitric oxide production increases gamma-amino butyric acid permeability of blood–brain barrier. *Brain Res Bullet* **57**(2), 231–236.

63. Treiman, D. M. (2001). GABAergic mechanisms in epilepsy. *Epilepsia* **42**(supplementary 3), 8–12.

64. Bäckström, T., Zetterlund, B., Blom, S. & Romano, M. (1984). Effects of intravenous progesterone infusions on the epileptic discharge frequency in women with partial epilepsy. *Acta Neurol Scand* **69**, 240–248.

65. Herzog, A. G., Klein, P. & Ransil, B. J. (1997). Three patterns of catamenial epilepsy. *Epilepsia* **38**(10), 1082–1088.

66. Hardy, R. W. (1970). Unit activity in premarin-induced cortical epileptogenic foci. *Epilepsia* **11**, 179–186.

67. Jacobs, A. R. (2005). Hormonal therapy. *In* Complementary and Alternative Therapies for Epilepsy (O. Devinsky, S. Schachter & S. Pacia, Eds.), pp. 225–230, Demos, New York.

68. Smith, S. S., Gong, Q. H., Hsu, F., Markowitz, R. S., French-Mullen, J. M. H. & Li, X. (1998). GABA (A) receptor alpha 4 subunit suppression prevents withdrawal properties of an endogenous steroid. *Nature* **392**(6679), 926–930.

69. Herzog, A. G. (1995). Progesterone therapy in women with comlpex partial and secondary generalized seizures. *Neurology* **45**(9), 1660–1662.

70. Herzog, A. G. (1986). Intermittent progesterone therapy and frequency of complex partial seizures in women with menstrual disorders. *Neurology*, 1607–1610.

71. Bazil, C. W., Short, D., Crispin, D. & Zheng, W. (2000). Patients with intractable epilepsy have low melatonin, which increases following seizures. *Neurology* **55**, 1716–1748.

72. Mohanan, P. V. & Yamamoto, H. A. (2002). Preventive effect of melatonin against brain mitochondrial DNA damage, lipid peroxidation and seizures induced by kainic acid. *Toxicology Lett* **129**(1–2), 99–105.

73. Peled, N., Shorer, Z., Peled, E. & Pillar, G. (2001). Melatonin effect on seizures in children with severe neurologic deficit disorders. *Epilepsia* **42**(9), 1208–1210.

74. Fauteck, J., Schmidt, H., Lerchl, A., Kurlemann, G. & Wittkowski, W. (1999). Melatonin in epilepsy: First results of replacement therapy and first clinical results. *Biological Signals and Receptors* **8**(1–2), 105–110.

75. Carballo, Molina-A., Hoyos, Muñoz-A., Reiter, R. et al. (1997). Utility of high doses of melatonin as adjunctive anticonvulsant therapy in a child with severe myoclonic epilepsy: Two years experience. *J Pineal Res* **23**(2), 97–105.

76. Sandyk, R., Tsagas, N. & Anninos, P. A. (1992). Melatonin as a proconvulsive hormone in humans. *Int J Neurosci* **63**(1–2), 125–135.

77. Siddiqui, M. A. A., Nazmi, A. S., Karim, S., Khan, R., Pillai, K. K. & Pal, S. N. (2001). Effect of melatonin and valproate in epilepsy and depression. *Indian J Pharmacol* **33**, 378–381.

78. Oja, S. S. & Kontro, P. (1983). Free amino acids in epilepsy: Possible role of taurine. *Acta Neurol Scand (Suppl)* **93**.

79. Fukuyama, Y. & Ochiai, Y. (1982). Therapeutic trial by taurine for intractable childhood epilepsies. *Brain & Development* **4**(1), 63–69.

80. König, P., Kriechbaum, vonG., Presslich, O., Schubert, H., Schuster, P. & Sieghart, W. (1977). Orally-administered tauringe in therapy-resistant epilepsy. *Wien Klin Wochenschr* **89**(4), 111–113.

81. Richard, A. & Reiter, J. (1995). *Epilepsy: A new approach*, Walker and Co., New York.

82. Swaiman, K. F. & Milstein, J. M. (1970). Pyridoxine dependency and penicillamine. *Neurology* **20**(1), 78–81.
83. Group, E.T.C. (1995). Which anticonvulsant for women with eclampsia? Evidence from the collaborative Eclampsia trial. *Lancet* **345**(8963), 1455–1463.
84. Harrison, N. L. & Gibbons, S. J. (1994). Zn2+: An endogenous modulator of ligand- and voltage-gated ion channels. *Neuropharmacol* **33**(8), 935–952.
85. Takeda, A., Hanajima, T., Ijiro, H., Ishige, A., Iizuka, S., Okada, S. & Oku., N. (1999). Release of zinc from the brain of El (epilepsy) mice during seizure induction. *Brain Res* **828**(1–2), 174–178.
86. Elsas, S. M., Hazany, S. & Mody, I. (2003). Zinc delays the development of seizures in a kinding model of epilepsy. *Neurology* **60**(S1), A72.

Chapter 6

Ginkgo biloba Extract in Prevention of Age-Associated Diseases in Elderly Population

Yuan Luo[1,2] and Zhiming Cao[1]

[1]Department of Pharmaceutical Sciences, School of Pharmacy, University of Maryland, Baltimore, MD, USA

[2]Center for Integrative Medicine, School of Medicine, University of Maryland, Baltimore, MD, USA

Abstract

The standard *Gingko biloba* leaf extract EGb 761 has been given routinely as prescript drug in many countries, and as dietary supplement in US, for Alzheimer's dementia. Numerous clinical data has demonstrated possible improvement of dementia by EGb 761 in Alzheimer patients. Two large-scale Alzheimer's disease prevention trials by EGb 761 in normal aging population are ongoing and expected to finish by 2010. EGb 761 protects brain from damage in experimental animals and neuronal cells. Polypotent and multitarget actions (antioxidative, platelet activating factor (PAF) receptor antagonist, inhibiting amyloid oligomerization) of EGb 761 may underlie its clinical efficacy. EGb 761 exhibits good side effect profile in clinical studies. It may cause potential bleeding when used with other anticoagulant drugs. Product quality of EGb 761 should be taken into consideration when used as a dietary supplement.

Keywords: *Ginkgo biloba, Alzheimers, sarcopenia, neurodegenerative diseases*

INTRODUCTION

Age-associated diseases such as Alzheimer's disease (AD) are threatening elderly population worldwide. Current available therapeutic treatment for AD exhibits only symptomatic modification of the disease and improves cognitive functions only in some patients. An ancient tree *Ginkgo biloba* leaf extract offers beneficial effect to Alzheimer dementia at a similar degree as the current front-runner medication. Experimental evidence provides possible mechanism of action for its beneficial effects in human. Current prevention trails may offer evidence-based therapy for protecting elderly population against dementia. Prospective and limitation, safety and quality issues of this extract are also discussed.

AGE-DEPENDENT DEGENERATIVE DISEASES IN ELDERLY

In broad terms, an age-dependent degenerative disease is widely used to describe a condition in which the function or structure of affected tissues or organs experience progressively deterioration over time, such as cardiovascular diseases, nervous system dysfunction, immune system decline and skeleton muscle degeneration.

Neurodegenerative disease associated with aging is a disorder resulting from the gradual and progressive loss of neuronal cells, leading to nervous system dysfunction. The disorder is often associated with the deterioration of certain nerve cells in the central or peripheral nervous system; the changes in these cells cause them to function abnormally and eventually dead.

Amongst a variety of neurodegenerative diseases, Alzheimer's disease (AD) is the most prevalent and devastating disorder in the growing population of the elderly. It is estimated that there were 4.5 million Americans diagnosed with AD in 2000, with an annual estimated cost of $100 billion. It is predicted that the number will continue climb and reach 13.2 million by 2050 in US population [1]. Globally, approximately 24 million people worldwide are living with AD today. Clinical signs of Alzheimer's disease are characterized by progressive memory loss and cognitive deterioration usually with an onset after 65 years old. AD is the most common cause of dementia and accounts for about 70% patients with dementia in the elderly. Extracellular senile plaques and intracellular neurofibrillary tangles in the brains of AD patients have been identified as pathological hallmarks of AD.

Parkinson's disease (PD) is also one of the most common age-related neurodegenerative diseases. As opposed to cognitive deficits in AD, PD is a movement disorder resulting from selective loss of dopaminergic neurons in the brain. Although PD and AD largely differ from their clinical symptoms and course of disease, both disorders are basically provoked by progressive loss of neurons in different neuronal system, which eventually cause neural system function abnormally.

In contrast to neurodegenerative diseases, sarcopenia, an age-related progressive loss of skeletal muscle mass and strength in senescence, is a degenerative disorder that accompanies a natural aging process. Although sarcopenia is not directly lethal to affected individuals, the severity of sarcopenia could prevent older people from living independently and impose a remarkably adverse impact on the quality of life of the geriatric population.

Owing to the rapidly growing number of elderly people and increased life expectancy in past decades, neurodegenerative dementias, neurodegenerative movement disorders and other degenerative diseases, such as sarcopenia, have been recognized as marked problems in the developed world because of its health care concerns as well as socioeconomic implications. Unfortunately, in spite of great progress made in understanding the pathogenesis of those diseases, there is no cure for those disorders, only symptomatic treatments are available. Moreover, diagnosis of AD can only be made psychologically by variety of cognitive tests or neuropathologically from postmortem brain by examining the amyloid plaques and tangles.

CURRENT THERAPEUTIC APPLICATIONS FOR AD

Cholinesterase inhibitors are the earliest developed and still the first line prescript drug available in US for patients with mild to moderate AD. By inhibiting the hydrolysis of neurotransmitter acetylcholine in the synaptic cleft and prolonging the levels of acetylcholine, these drugs restore the neurotransmitter in the lost neurons in the brain of AD patients. Tacrine was the first cholinesterase inhibitor approved by US Food and Drug Administration (FDA) for symptomatic treatment of AD but was problematic due to hepatotoxicity. Therefore, three new compounds, donepezil, galantamine and ricastigmine, with similar efficacy but improved safety profiles replaced it.

Recently, an *N*-methyl-*D*-aspartate (NMDA) receptor antagonist, memantine, was approved for the symptomatic treatment of moderate to severe AD. By noncompetitively inhibiting NMDA receptor, memantine counteract on "excitotoxic" glutamate, the major excitatory neurotransmitter in the brain. It turns out that memantine is well tolerated and its efficacy is comparable to the cholinesterase inhibitors. Nevertheless, its potential side effects on overall cognitive function are questioned.

Much effort has been focused on development of disease-modifying medications. Guided by the "amyloid cascade hypothesis" [2], inhibition of γ-secretase or β-secretase, or enhancement of α-secratase, would decrease amyloid beta (Aβ) peptide production. Several of these compounds are currently undergoing clinical trials by Wyeth and other pharmaceutical companies [3]. Along the same line, one interesting approach initiated by Schenk and colleagues [4] is the active and passive immunotherapy to lower brain Aβ levels and improved memory [5]. The subsequent problem with micro hemorrhage could be potentially overcome by deglycosylation of the antibody structure [6].

Anti-inflammatory medication for AD was originated from epidemiological evidence, which suggests that use of nonsteroidal anti-inflammatory (NSAID) medication earlier in life may reduce the risk of developing AD [7]. However, clinical trials for this practice are not conclusive. Similarly, clinical data for antioxidant therapy such as vitamin E, vitamin C and selegiline, was discouraging. Trials of antioxidant vitamin "cocktails" as possible prevention strategies have been proposed [8]. *Ginkgo biloba* leaf extract was classified as an antioxidant for treatment of AD, though it has multiple properties [9]. Some of them have disease-modification potential. Prospective clinical trials of EGb 761 to delay the onset of AD in older people without dementia are currently being conducted in United States [10] and Europe [11].

GINKGO BILOBA EXTRACT EGB 761

The *Ginkgo biloba* tree is a tall and ancient tree with remarkable long life span of more than 4000 years due, in part, to high tolerance to pollution and resistance to infections. The tree is described as a "living fossil" without close living relatives. The medical use of fan-shaped Ginkgo leaves can be traced back to approximately 5000 years to origins of traditional Chinese medicine and modern Chinese pharmacopoeia introduced leaves as treatment for dysfunctions of heart and lung and as a promoter of longevity. In 1965, Dr. Willmar Schwabe, a German physician-pharmacist introduced the extract of *Ginkgo biloba* leaves into medical practice, and first registered EGb 761 as a medication by Dr. W. Schwabe company. Since then, EGb 761 (trade names Tebonin®, Tanakan®, Rokan®) is a well-defined and patented product developed and commercialized by IPSEN in France and Dr. Willmar Schwabe Pharmaceuticals in Germany in the early 1970s. Standardized extracts of the *Ginkgo biloba* leaves are presently widely prescribed in Europe as a treatment for "cerebral insufficiency," which is a general term used for nonspecific age-related deterioration of mental functions, including AD [12, 13]. In the United States, EGb 761 has been a top-sell dietary supplement that is used for enhancement of blood circulation and memory. EGb 761 consists of 24% flavonol glycosides and 6% terpenoid lactones. The flavonoid fraction is primarily composed of quercetin, kaempferol and isorhamnetin. The terpene lactones are represented by the ginkgolides A, B, C, J and M, as well as bilobalide.

During the past decades, a wealth of accumulating evidence *in vivo* or *in vitro* studies indicated that EGb 761 or its single component exhibits a wide range of biomedical and pharmacological effects on various model systems. Substantial experimental evidence has shown EGb 761 to be a multifunctional antioxidant and potent free radical scavenger that can effectively protect organisms against oxidative stress, which may, at least in part, contribute to its therapeutic potential on many disorders or diseases. Other major activities of EGb 761 include: inhibition of membrane lipid peroxidation [14] cognition enhancement particularly in aging rats and alleviating stress in the experimental animals [15, 16], anti-PAF activity contributing to improvements in cerebral insufficiency [17] enhancing neuronal plasticity [18] anti-inflammatory effects [19], stimulation of choline uptake in the hippocampus, inhibition of Aβ aggregation, and anti-apoptotic activities in neuronal cells [20–22].

It is still not determined which component, alone or in combination, in EGb 761 is responsible for the proposed health-enhancing properties, but it has been suggested that many of effects of EGb 761 are so called "polyvalent" actions. That is the therapeutic activity of EGb 761 is the net effect of interactions between various biological activities of the principle substances in the extract, acting at different levels of the body. This multi-faceted mode of action by EGb 761 is opposed to pharmacologically manufactured or synthetic drugs, which provide a single target for a single receptor as its mechanism of action. Since the etiology of neurodegenerative diseases is often multifactorial, the multiplicity of neuroprotective effects by EGb 761 strongly implicates therapeutic potentials in patients with AD and other age-related neurodegenerative disorders.

EGB 761 EXTENDS LIFE SPAN, DELAYS SACROPENIA AND Aβ-INDUCED TOXICITY IN EXPERIMENTAL ANIMALS

In the past years, we have used the model organism *Caenorhabditis elegans* to evaluate pharmacological effects of EGb 761 on aging. We demonstrated that treatment of the worms with EGb 761 extended their median life span by 8% (Fig. 6.1B). Amongst several purified components of EGb 761, the flavonoid fraction showed the most dramatic effect: it extended the median life span by 25%. Furthermore, EGb 761 increased the worm's resistance to acute oxidative stress by 33% (Fig. 6.1A). It appears that oxidative stress, a major determinant of life span, as well as other types of stress, can be successfully counteracted by the *Ginkgo biloba* extract EGb 761. These results suggest that EGb 761 extends the life span by increasing resistance to oxidative stress via augmenting natural antioxidant defenses [23].

Life span enhancing by EGb 761 lead us to hypothesize that age-associated tissue degeneration can be modulated by EGb 761. Age-related muscle deterioration not only occurs in the skeletal muscle of human and other mammalian species, but also in invertebrates. It has been demonstrated that sarcopenia accompanies the age-dependent functional decline in the nematode, similar to those longer-lived vertebrates. When examined the major cellular changes of a number of important cell types in aging worms, it was revealed that the nervous system in senescent nematodes stays largely intact, although the muscles experience a gradual and progressive deterioration, that is, sarcopenia [24]. Using a combination of

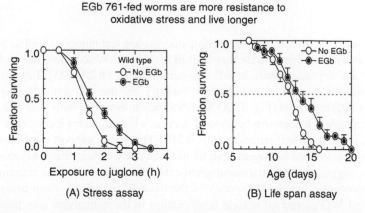

FIGURE 6.1 Effects of EGb 761 on stress response (A) and life span (B) of *C. elegans*. (A) Survival curve of *C. elegans* pre-exposed to oxidative stress (40 µM juglone in food for 24 hours) with (filled circles) or without (open circles) EGb 761 treatment. Total number of worms in each group was 48 and 42, respectively. (B) Life span of adult worms, which were fed with *E. coli* OP50 supplemented with either 100µg/ml EGb 761 (filled circles) or control vehicles (open circles). Data was obtained from three independent experimented each contains 100 worms [23].

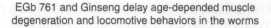

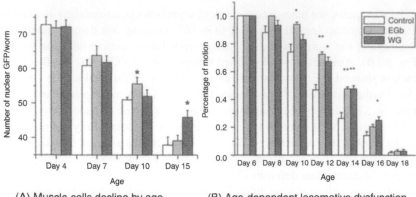

(A) Muscle cells decline by age　　　(B) Age-dependent locomotive dysfunction

FIGURE 6.2　Age-associated decline of *C. elegans* body wall muscle (A) or locomotive behavior (B). (A) Fluorescent images were captured in live worms under the microscope and the number of GFP labeled nuclei of body wall muscle in the worms treated with either vehicle (clear bars), or EGb 761 (filled bars), or WG (dashed bars). The decline of GFP signals in control worms over time was faster than that of drug-treated animals. EGb treated day 10 animals retain significantly more GFP labeled nuclei of muscle cells than other animals. The delay of the muscle cell deterioration in worms fed with WG is significantly different from the control animals at day 15. (B) Age-related locomotive behavioral decline and the effects of the treatment. The worms at indicated ages were untreated (open column), fed with EGb 761 (filled column) or WG (dashed column). The locomotor decline was significantly delayed by both EGb 761 and WG in the worms at 12, 14 and 16 days, compared with the age-matched worms without treatment [25]. *$p < 0.05$, **$p < 0.01$.

fluorescent and transmission electronic microscope techniques as well as behavioral assays, we demonstrate that both EGb 761 and Wisconsin Ginseng (WG) delay age-dependent muscle cell degeneration (Fig. 6.2A) [25]. Interestingly, the reduced decline of muscle cell integrity by the two extracts displayed an age different onset (Fig. 6.2A), which seems to correlate with their effects on age-dependent locomotive behavioral decline which includes locomotion, body bend, and pharyngeal pumping (Fig. 6.2B). These data support our hypothesis that age-associated sarcopenia can be modulated by certain life span-extending drugs, suggesting that pharmacological extension of life span is a consequence of maintaining functional capacity of the tissue. The insights from using EGb 761 and WG extract on muscle deterioration in the nematodes may provide a basis for developing pharmacological interventions for human sarcopenia [25].

EGb 761 has being viewed as an antioxidant, which may underlie its life span extension and sarcopenia alleviation properties. However, others and we described a specific inhibitory effect of EGb 761 on Aβ [24, 26]. In a follow up study, we use the transgenic *C. elegans* model [27] that exhibits several

EGb 761 inhibits Aβ aggregation and deposits

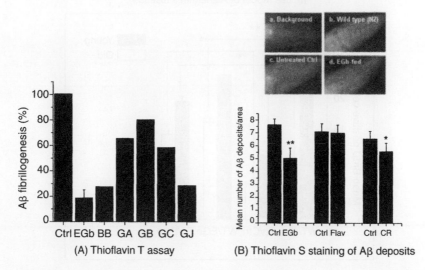

(A) Thioflavin T assay

(B) Thioflavin S staining of Aβ deposits

FIGURE 6.3   EGb 761 inhibits Aβ aggregation *in vitro* (A) and in transgenic *C. elegans* express-ing Aβ (B). (A) Thioflavin T fluorescence assay. Aβ was incubated in the absence (Ctrl) or pres-ence of EGb 761 (EGb) or bilobalide (BB), ginkgolides A, B, C and J (GA, GB, GC and GJ, respectively). (B) Aβ deposits in transgenic *C. elegans* CL2006 fed with or without drugs. Inset: Representative images of background fluorescence in a *C. elegans* without staining (a), with thio-flavin S staining in the wild type (b), or in the transgenic strain CL2006 fed with (d) or with-out EGb 761 (c). The numbers of deposits (arrowheads) were scored in the worm head, which is separated from the body by pharyngeal bulb (arrows). Graph: Quantitative analysis of β amyloid deposits in the transgenic *C. elegans* CL2006 fed with different chemicals for 48 hours (EGb 761, the flavonoid fraction of EGb 761 Congo Red) [22, 30]. *$p = 0.025$ and **$p = 0.002$.

pathological behaviors to associate Aβ species with Aβ-induced abnormal behaviors in the organism. We reported that EGb 761 and one of its compo-nents, ginkgolide A, alleviated Aβ-induced pathological behaviors, including paralysis, and reduced chemotaxis behavior and 5-hydroxytryptamine (5-HT) hypersensitivity in a transgenic *C. elegans*. We also showed that EGb 761 inhib-ited Aβ oligomerization and Aβ deposits in the worms (Fig. 6.3B). Moreover, we revealed that reducing oxidative stress is not the mechanism by which EGb 761 and ginkgolide A suppress Aβ-induced paralysis since the antioxidant L-ascorbic acid reduced intracellular levels of hydrogen peroxide to the same extent as EGb 761, but was not nearly as effective in suppressing paralysis in the transgenic *C. elegans*. This study further supports multi-potent function as mechanism of EGb 761 protection. It is likely that the pharmacological efficacy manifested in the transgenic worms share the similar mechanisms with the cog-nitive impairment in mammals.

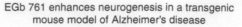

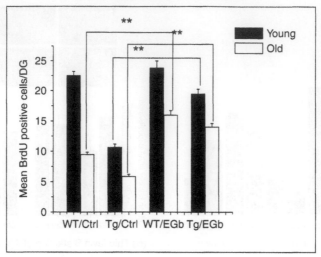

FIGURE 6.4 EGb 761 enhances cell proliferation in the hippocampus of transgenic (TgAPP/PS1) mice. BrdU positive cells in the Dentate Gyrus (DG) of young and old, WT and Tg mice maintained on a dietary regiment supplemented with or without 100 mg/kg of EGb 761 for 1 month and intraperitonially injected with BrdU (75 mg/kg/daily) for 7 consecutive days were quantified. BrdU positive cells were counted in both DG of one brain section taken out of every consecutive seven, and were expressed as the Mean ± SEM of total number of BrdU positive cells/DG of 3–4 WT or Tg mice per treatment category. **$p < 0.01$ indicates the most striking differences (three way ANOVA) [32].

Considering the beneficial effects of EGb 761 on cognitive impairment in AD patients [28] and AD mice [29], and its ability to inhibit Aβ oligomerization *in vitro* [26, 22] and in the worm model [30], we further examined the neurogenic potential of EGb 761 in the hippocampus of a mouse model of AD (TgAPP/PS1) [31]. EGb 761 significantly increases cell proliferation in the hippocampus of the TgAPP/PS1 mice (Fig. 6.4) [32]. Administration of EGb 761 reduces Aβ oligomers and restores CREB phosphorylation in the hippocampus of these mice. These findings suggest that (1) enhanced neurogenesis by EGb 761 may be mediated by activation of CREB, (2) stimulation of neurogenesis by EGb 761 may contribute to its beneficial effects in AD patients and cognitive functions in the mouse model of AD and (3) EGb 761 has therapeutic potential for the prevention and treatment of AD. Neurodegenerative disorder seen in AD is believed to start with synaptic dysfunction and subsequent loss of neuronal cells [33]. Evidence of

TABLE 6.1 The Transcriptional Effects of *Ginkgo biloba* on the hippocampus and cortex (Genes Whose Expression Changed Threefold or More

Probe set	Gene/description	Fold change
Hippocampus		
Pre-albumin		
D00073	Transthyretin	16
Cortex		
Growth factors/Neuromodulators		
X02891	Growth hormone	11.1
X04418	Prolactin	11
Transcription factors		
Y07688	NfiX1 protein	7.3
U02098	Purinergic region binding protein α	5.1
Ion channels		
AF029347	Chloride channel protein 3	4.5
AF029347	Chloride channel protein 3	6.2
AF077739	Calcium channel	3.8
L32372	GluRB (AMPA-2)	3.9
Signal transduction		
X95518	Neuronal tyrosine/threonine phosphatase	7.3
Cytoskeletal		
M18775	Microtubule-associated τ	3.1
M18775	Microtubule-associated τ	4.4

Source: Ref. [38]

neurogenesis in the adult rodent's brain [34, 35] raised the hope that the replacement of lost neurons could represent a therapeutic approach for the management of AD [36]. Given the deleterious impact of the association between aging and Aβ, the role of newly generated neurons in hippocampal-dependent learning and memory [37], the neurogenic enhancing property of EGb 761 succeed this top selling dietary supplement as a therapeutic candidate in the management of Alzheimer's dementia [32].

Advance in molecular biology offers new tools to reveal overall gene transcription changes using DNA microarrays analysis. The transcriptional effects of EGb 761 in the cortex and hippocampus of mice showed a more than threefold change in several neuromodulatory genes. All of which were associated with brain function and were up-regulated (Table 6.1) [38] demonstrating that EGb 761 have neuromodulatory effects *in vivo* and the validity of genome-wide expression monitoring to investigate the biological actions of complex extracts.

CLINICAL EVIDENCE SUPPORTING EFFICACY OF EGB 761 IN AD DEMENTIA

Available data from human studies has confirmed the clinical efficacy of EGb 761 in patients with multi-infarct dementia or primary degenerative dementia of Alzheimer's type or mixed types of dementia [39]. As early as in 1992, Kleijnen and Knipschild systematically reviewed eight well-conducted clinical trials conclude that *Ginkgo biloba* extracts reduce the symptoms of dementia and cerebral insufficiency to an extent that was clinically relevant [40]. The first randomized, double-blind, placebo-controlled, multicenter-involved clinical trial, lasted 52 weeks, of EGb 761 treatment for multi-infarct dementia or dementia of the Alzheimer type was conducted in New York Institute for Medical Research by Le Bars and colleagues [28]. A serial of standardized neuropsychological measures including Alzheimer's disease assessment scale-cognitive subscale (ADAS-Cog), Geriatric Evaluation by Relative's Rating Instrument (GERRI), and Clinical Global Impression of Change (CGIC) was employed for assessment of efficacy of 52 weeks of treatment with EGb 120 mg/day. Consistent with previous studies, they made a conclusion that a treatment effect of EGb showed clinically significant benefits with respect to cognitive performance (ADAS-Cog) and social functioning (GERRI) in patients with mild to moderate Alzheimer's dementia. No change occurred by CGIC evaluation. Total 309 mild to severe demented outpatients (>45 year old) were divided into two groups, EGb group (120 mg/d) had ADAS-Cog score 1.4 points better than the placebo group ($p = 0.04$); 27% patients treated with EGb achieved 4 point improvement on ADAS-Cog, compared with 14% taking placebo ($p = 0.005$). No significant differences were observed in number of patients reporting adverse events or incidence between EGb and placebo treated group. The authors concluded that EGb was safe and capable of stabilizing and improving the cognitive performance and social function of demented patients for 6 months to 1 year. Specifically, EGb 761 was more effective than placebo in AD patients treated for 12–24 weeks, at 120–240 mg/day [13, 41, 42].

In 1998, Oken *et al.* [12] preformed a meta-analysis of 50 clinical studies using EGb 761 for treatment of dementia and cognitive function associated with AD. There were total of 212 subjects in each of placebo or drug treatment group among four randomized, double-blind, placebo-controlled studies. Patients diagnosed with AD received 120–240 mg *Ginkgo biloba* extract with the duration of 3–6 months, ADAS-Cog was used as the primary efficacy assessment of cognitive function. It was concluded that there was a modest but statistically significant effect that translated into 3% improvement on the ADAS-Cog, and no significant adverse effect observed in the drug treatment group [12]. A later systematical review of nine studies of ginkgo extract by Pittler and Ernst [43] reported similar findings that *Ginkgo biloba* extracts showed a safe and positive effect for treatment of dementia symptoms beyond placebo. Standard extract EGb 761 was used in the most studies aforementioned.

Regarding clinical study of EGb 761 in dementia of normal aging, the data is controversial [44]. A study by Mix and David Crews reported that EGb 761 was also more effective than placebo in cognitively intact 60-year-old adult ($n = 131$) treated with 180 mg/day EGb 761 for 6 weeks, in certain neuropsychological/memory process [45]. A case study shown that no significant association of AD onset with EGb 761 for 2 years in 345 women over 75 year old, followed up for 7 years [46]. However, a 6 week randomized controlled trial, included >60-year-old male and female healthy volunteers administrated EGb 40 mg 3 times/day ($n = 115$), placebo ($n = 115$) showed that no effect of EGb 761 administration compared with placebo in healthy volunteers [47].

A more recent meta-analysis [39] of 33 randomized trials, involving 3106 participants further demonstrated that there are benefits associated with Ginkgo for AD compared with placebo in AD patients' cognition, activity of daily living (ADL), and mood and emotion. They concluded that *Ginkgo biloba* appears to be safe in use with no excess side effects compared with placebo. Overall there is promising evidence of improvement in AD patient's cognition and function associated with ginkgo. Nevertheless, the authors emphasized a need for modern, larger trials [39]. Obviously there are some limitations of studies used in meta-analyses, such as: (a) non standardized diagnostic practices; (b) relatively short duration of many studies; (c) inconsistent potency/ dosing across the studies; (d) standardization of test products not clear; (e) use of inexperienced investigators; (f) some studies not placebo-controlled, and (g) blinding may have been inadequate (i.e., failure to adequately mask the taste and color of EGb 761).

EGB COMPARED WITH THE FIRST LINE DRUG FOR AD (ARICEPT)

EGb 761 has been used as a prescribed medicine in Europe for symptomatic treatment for age-related cerebral insufficiency and cognitive impairments associated with a range of neurological disorders. A review further addressing an issue regarding the efficacy of EGb 761 compared with other prescribed drugs such as the first line drug donepezil (Aricept) approved by the US Food and Drug Administration (FDA) for symptomatic treatment of mild to moderate Alzheimer's dementia. The review concluded that second-generation cholinesterase inhibitors and Ginkgo special extract EGb 761 were equally effective in treating mild to moderate Alzheimer's dementia.

An Italian group performed a 24-week randomized, double-blind, placebo-controlled study to directly compare the therapeutic efficacy of

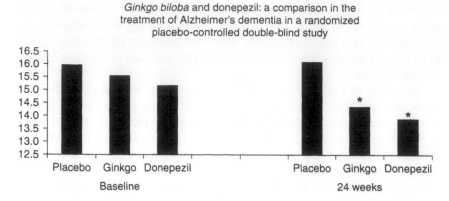

FIGURE 6.5   The *in vivo* neuromodulatory effects by *Ginkgo biloba* extract administration of experimental mice using DNA microarray assay for profiles of transcription changes [48]. *$p = 0.01$.

EGb 761 (160 mg daily dose) and donepezil (5 mg daily dose) in patients suffering from mild to moderate degenerative dementia of Alzheimer type [48].
The degree of severity of dementia was assessed by the Syndrome Kurz test
(SKT) and the Mini-Mental State Examination (MMSE). The changes in
patients' condition were examined by Clinical Global Impression (CGI) score.
As a result, they demonstrated that there were significant clinical improvements in cognitive functions observed in patients of tested medication groups
regarding three measures aforementioned (Fig. 6.5). There was no evidence
of relevant differences in the efficacy of EGb 761 and donepezil in treatment
of mild to moderate Alzheimer's dementia (Fig. 6.5). In addition, EGb 761
showed a good tolerability and side effect profile in comparison of adverse
events (diarrhea, nausea, vomiting and restlessness) occurred in donepezil
group. Their findings provide solid evidence to support beneficial effects of
EGb 761 on slowing down Alzheimer's degenerative progression and stabilizing cognitive decline comparable with clinical efficacy of second-generation
cholinesterase inhibitors.

"AN OZ PREVENTION IS WORTH A POND OF CURE": THE ONGOING PREVENTION TRIAL FOR EGB 761 ON DEMENTIA

Given that Alzheimer's disease being leading causes of morbidity and mortality in industrialized countries as a result of increased life expectancy and the
lack of the curative therapy for treatment of AD, finding strategies to prevent
or delay the onset of AD become one of the important challenges [1]. It was
predicted that delaying the onset of AD by 5 years would reduce the number
of incidence of the AD by half in the next decade.

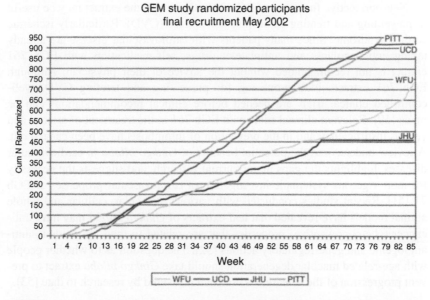

FIGURE 6.6 Rate of successful randomization of GEM Study participants by site over 21 months of recruitment (September 2000 through June 2002) [49].

Considering the importance of AD prevention, two phase III clinical trials, GEM (Ginkgo evaluation of memory) in United States and GuidAge in France, focus on evaluation of its efficacy of prevention of AD in subjects over 70 year old. Both trials included randomized more than 3000 individuals. GEM was designed as a 7 years, with 8.5 years of participant follow up, randomized, double-blind, placebo-controlled trail of *Ginkgo biloba*, administrated in a dose of 120 mg twice daily, in prevention of dementia in normal elderly or those with mild cognitive impairment [10]. From September 2000 through June 2002, GEM study successfully recruited 3072 participants age 75 years and older at four US sites (Fig. 6.6) [49]. Primary outcome is the incidence of all-cause dementia. Secondary outcome includes the rate of cognitive and functional decline, the incidence of cardiovascular and cerebrovascular events and mortality. The assessments are repeated every 6-month and side effects and adverse events are tracked [10]. Similarly, the GuidAge study is a 5-year double-blind, randomized trial conducted in France to evaluate the efficacy of 240 mg daily of EGb 761 in the prevention of AD. The study have enrolled elderly individuals with spontaneous memory complaint and the primary outcomes is the incidence of AD during a 5-year follow up period. This study is the largest clinical trials carried out in Europe on the prevention of AD. The anticipated final results would be available in 2010 [11].

Neuroprotective functions of EGb 761suggest that the extract may be useful in preventing and treating cardiovascular disease (CVD). Particularly ischemic cardiac syndrome. Since many patients with cardiovascular disease are already taking anticoagulants and antiplatelet drugs, self-medication with EGb 761 extract is not recommended without the advice of their physician. Although EGb 761 extracts look promising for preventing and treating CVD, well-controlled clinical trials are needed before clinical recommendations can be made [50]. Relevant clinical trials with EGb 761 in the treatment of arterial and venous insufficiency and in the prevention of thrombosis have been carried out. A review underscored the potential benefits of *Ginkgo biloba* in cardiovascular diseases, highlights the gaps in our current research, and suggests the necessity for more rigorous systematic investigation of cardiovascular properties of EGb 71 [51]. Recent studies conducted with various molecular, cellular and whole animal models have revealed that leaf extracts of *Ginkgo biloba* may have anti-cancer (chemopreventive) properties that are related to their antioxidant, anti-angiogenic and gene-regulatory actions [52]. The question as to whether people with age-related macular degeneration should take *Ginkgo biloba* extract to prevent progression of the disease has not been answered by research to date [53].

SIDE EFFECTS AND QUALITY ISSUE OF EGB 761

As summarized in Table 6.2, common side effects including headache, nausea, gastrointestinal upset, diarrhea, dizziness or allergic skin reaction, in EGb 761

TABLE 6.2 Side Effects and Caution

Adverse effect	Drugs	References
Headache, nausea, gastrointestinal upset, diarrhea, dizziness, or allergic skin reaction.	No significant difference from placebo	
Could increase bleeding risk, for people who take anticoagulant drugs, have bleeding disorders, during surgery or dental procedure or (discontinue 36 h prior to). Alone no inhibit of blood coagulation, or platelet aggregation.	With Aspirinspontaneous hyphema With Warfarin – intracerebral hemorrhage	[55] [56] [54]
Reduce effectiveness of anticonvulsant for seizer. Uncooked ginkgo seeds contain ginkotoxin, which can cause seizers.	With Carbamazapine or valproic acid – seizer	[57] National Center for Complementary and Alternative Medicine (NCCAM), http://nccam.nih.gov

treated group are not different compare with that in placebo group. It should be noted that EGb 761 could increase bleeding risk [54], for people who take anti-coagulant drugs, have bleeding disorders, or during surgery or dental procedure (discontinue 36 hours prior to surgery are recommended by the physicians). For example, when taken with Aspirin, spontaneous hyphema could occur [55], when used with Warfarin, intracerebral hemorrhage could happen [56]. Interestingly, EGb 761 was found to reduce effectiveness of anticonvulsant for seizer [57]. Seizer could also be caused by non-cooked ginkgo seeds containing ginkotoxin.

As with any natural products, standardization and quality concerns could impact on all studies. The problems of complex herbals could adversely affect assay sensitivity of any clinical trial. Furthermore, standardization of herb against one active marker group may not necessarily assure standardization of the activity of the extract. In general, phytochemical composition can vary depending on variability in the raw material from which the extract is obtained, for example harvesting period, drying process, storage conditions and method of extraction, for example solvent composition, ratio of raw material to extraction fluid, etc. Based on a survey of 27 US brands (tabs and caps) of EGb 761 tested for content [58]: flavone glycosides varied from 24% to 36%; terpene lactones ranged from 4% to 11%; Ginkgolic acid ranged from ∼500 ppm to 90,000 ppm (should not exceed 5 ppm). Of 14 produces tested for dissolution: 10 exhibited >75% dissolution of glycosides and lactones in 30 minutes; 2 exhibited about 55–70%; 1 about 10% dissolution in 30 minutes. The authors warned that many of the investigated products can not be considered to be pharmaceutically equivalent to the patented original product by Schwabe [58].

ACKNOWLEDGMENT

Studies in this laboratory have been supported by NIH grant R01AT001928-03A1 (YL) from the National Center for Complementary and Alternative Medicine, and by IPSEN, Paris, France.

REFERENCES

1. Brookmeyer, R., Gray, S. & Kawas, C. (1998). Projections of Alzheimer's disease in the United States and the public health impact of delaying disease onset. *Am J Public Health* **88**(9), 1337–1342.
2. Hardy, J. & Selkoe, D. J. (2002). The amyloid hypothesis of Alzheimer's disease: Progress and problems on the road to therapeutics. *Science* **297**(5580), 353–356.
3. Jacobsen, J. S., Reinhart, P. & Pangalos, M. N. (2005). Current concepts in therapeutic strategies targeting cognitive decline and disease modification in Alzheimer's disease. *NeuroRx* **2**(4), 612–626.
4. Schenk, D., Barbour, R., Dunn, W., Gordon, G., Grajeda, H., Guido, T., Hu, K., Huang, J., Johnson-Wood, K., Khan, K., Kholodenko, D., Lee, M., Liao, Z., Lieberburg, I., Motter, R., Mutter, L., Soriano, F., Shopp, G., Vasquez, N., Vandevert, C., Walker, S., Wogulis, M., Yednock, T., Games, D. &

Seubert, P. (1999). Immunization with amyloid-beta attenuates Alzheimer-disease-like pathology in the PDAPP mouse. *Nature* **400**(6740), 173–177.

5. Morgan, D., Diamond, D. M., Gottschall, P. E., Ugen, K. E., Dickey, C., Hardy, J., Duff, K., Jantzen, P., DiCarlo, G., Wilcock, D., Connor, K., Hatcher, J., Hope, C., Gordon, M. & Arendash, G. W. (2000). A beta peptide vaccination prevents memory loss in an animal model of Alzheimer's disease. *Nature* **408**(6815), 982–985.

6. Carty, N. C., Wilcock, D. M., Rosenthal, A., Grimm, J., Pons, J., Ronan, V., Gottschall, P. E., Gordon, M. N. & Morgan, D. (2006). Intracranial administration of deglycosylated C-terminal-specific anti-Abeta antibody efficiently clears amyloid plaques without activating microglia in amyloid-depositing transgenic mice. *J Neuroinflammation* **3**, 11.

7. Moore, A. H. & O'Banion, M. K. (2002). Neuroinflammation and anti-inflammatory therapy for Alzheimer's disease. *Adv Drug Deliv Rev* **54**(12), 1627–1656.

8. Tariot, P. N. & Federoff, H. J. (2003). Current treatment for Alzheimer disease and future prospects. *Alzheimer Dis Assoc Disord* **17**(Suppl 4), S105–S113.

9. Smith, J. V. & Luo, Y. (2004). Studies on molecular mechanisms of *Ginkgo biloba* extract. *Appl Microbiol Biotechnol* **64**(4), 465–472.

10. DeKosky, S. T., Fitzpatrick, A., Ives, D. G., Saxton, J., Williamson, J., Lopez, O. L., Burke, G., Fried, L., Kuller, L. H., Robbins, J., Tracy, R., Woolard, N., Dunn, L., Kronmal, R., Nahin, R. & Furberg, C. (2006). The Ginkgo Evaluation of Memory (GEM) study: Design and baseline data of a randomized trial of *Ginkgo biloba* extract in prevention of dementia. *Contemp Clin Trials* **27**(3), 238–253.

11. Vellas, B., Andrieu, S., Ousset, P. J., Ouzid, M. & Mathiex-Fortunet, H. (2006). The GuidAge study: Methodological issues. A 5-year double-blind randomized trial of the efficacy of EGb 761 for prevention of Alzheimer disease in patients over 70 with a memory complaint. *Neurology* **67**(9 Suppl 3), S6–S11.

12. Oken, B. S., Storzbach, D. M. & Kaye, J. A. (1998). The efficacy of *Ginkgo biloba* on cognitive function in Alzheimer disease. *Arch Neurol* **55**(11), 1409–1415.

13. Maurer, K., Ihl, R., Dierks, T. & Frolich, L. (1997). Clinical efficacy of *Ginkgo biloba* special extract EGb 761 in dementia of the Alzheimer type. *J Psychiatr Res* **31**(6), 645–655.

14. DeFeudis, F. V. & Drieu, K. (2000). *Ginkgo biloba* extract (EGb 761) and CNS functions: Basic studies and clinical applications. *Curr Drug Targets* **1**(1), 25–58.

15. Winter, E. (1991). Effects of an extract of *Ginkgo biloba* on learning and memory in mice. *Pharmacol Biochem Behav* **38**(1), 109–114.

16. Winter, J. C. (1998). The effects of an extract of *Ginkgo biloba*, EGb 761, on cognitive behavior and longevity in the rat. *Physiol Behav* **63**(3), 425–433.

17. Smith, P. F., Maclennan, K. & Darlington, C. L. (1996). The neuroprotective properties of the *Ginkgo biloba* leaf: A review of the possible relationship to platelet-activating factor (PAF). *J Ethnopharmacol* **50**(3), 131–139.

18. Gohil, K. & Packer, L. (2002). Global gene expression analysis identifies cell and tissue specific actions of *Ginkgo biloba* extract, EGb 761. *Cell Mol Biol (Noisy-le-grand)* **48**(6), 625–631.

19. Oberpichler, H., Sauer, D., Rossberg, C., Mennel, H. D. & Krieglstein, J. (1990). PAF antagonist ginkgolide B reduces postischemic neuronal damage in rat brain hippocampus. *J Cereb Blood Flow Metab* **10**(1), 133–135.

20. Bastianetto, S., Ramassamy, C., Dore, S., Christen, Y., Poirier, J. & Quirion, R. (2000). The *Ginkgo biloba* extract (EGb 761) protects hippocampal neurons against cell death induced by beta-amyloid. *Eur J Neurosci* **12**(6), 1882–1890.

21. Yao, Z., Drieu, K. & Papadopoulos, V. (2001). The *Ginkgo biloba* extract EGb 761 rescues the PC12 neuronal cells from beta-amyloid-induced cell death by inhibiting the formation of beta-amyloid-derived diffusible neurotoxic ligands. *Brain Res* **889**(1–2), 181–190.

22. Luo, Y., Smith, J. V., Paramasivam, V., Burdick, A., Curry, K. J., Buford, J. P., Khan, I., Netzer, W. J., Xu, H. & Butko, P. (2002). Inhibition of amyloid-beta aggregation and caspase-3 activation by the *Ginkgo biloba* extract EGb 761. *Proc Natl Acad Sci U S A* **99**(19), 12197–12202.

23. Wu, Z., Smith, J. V., Paramasivam, V., Butko, P., Khan, I., Cypser, J. R. & Luo, Y. (2002). *Ginkgo biloba* extract EGb 761 increases stress resistance and extends life span of *Caenorhabditis elegans. Cell Mol Biol (Noisy-le-grand)* **48**(6), 725–731.

24. Herndon, L. A., Schmeissner, P. J., Dudaronek, J. M., Brown, P. A., Listner, K. M., Sakano, Y., Paupard, M. C., Hall, D. H. & Driscoll, M. (2002). Stochastic and genetic factors influence tissue-specific decline in ageing *C. elegans. Nature* **419**(6909), 808–814.

25. Cao, Z., Wu, Y., Curry, K., Wu, Z., Christen, Y. & Luo, Y. (2007). *Ginkgo biloba* extract EGb 761 and Wisconsin ginseng delay sarcopenia in *C. elegans. J. Gerontology* **62**, 1337–45.

26. Chromy, B. A., Nowak, R. J., Lambert, M. P., Viola, K. L., Chang, L., Velasco, P. T., Jones, B. W., Fernandez, S. J., Lacor, P. N., Horowitz, P., Finch, C. E., Krafft, G. A. & Klein, W. L. (2003). Self-assembly of Abeta(1–42) into globular neurotoxins. *Biochemistry* **42**(44), 12749–12760.

27. Link, C. D. (1995). Expression of human beta-amyloid peptide in transgenic *Caenorhabditis elegans. Proc Natl Acad Sci U S A* **92**(20), 9368–9372.

28. Le Bars, P. L., Katz, M. M., Berman, N., Itil, T. M., Freedman, A. M. & Schatzberg, A. F. (1997). A placebo-controlled, double-blind, randomized trial of an extract of *Ginkgo biloba* for dementia. North American EGb Study Group. *JAMA* **278**(16), 1327–1332.

29. Stackman, R. W., Eckenstein, F., Frei, B., Kulhanek, D., Nowlin, J. & Quinn, J. F. (2003). Prevention of age-related spatial memory deficits in a transgenic mouse model of Alzheimer's disease by chronic *Ginkgo biloba* treatment. *Exp Neurol* **184**(1), 510–520.

30. Wu, Y., Wu, Z., Butko, P., Christen, Y., Lambert, M. P., Klein, W. L., Link, C. D. & Luo, Y. (2006). Amyloid-beta-induced pathological behaviors are suppressed by *Ginkgo biloba* extract EGb 761 and ginkgolides in transgenic *Caenorhabditis elegans. J Neurosci* **26**(50), 13102–13113.

31. Price, D. L. & Sisodia, S. S. (1998). Mutant genes in familial Alzheimer's disease and transgenic models. *Ann Rev Neurosci* **21**, 479–505.

32. Tchantchou, F., Xu, Y., Wu, Y., Christen, Y. & Luo, Y. (2007). EGb 761 enhances adult hippocampal neurogenesis and phosphorylation of CREB in transgenic mouse model of Alzheimer's disease. *Faseb J* **21**, 2400–2408.

33. Lacor, P. N., Buniel, M. C., Chang, L., Fernandez, S. J., Gong, Y., Viola, K. L., Lambert, M. P., Velasco, P. T., Bigio, E. H., Finch, C. E., Krafft, G. A. & Klein, W. L. (2004). Synaptic targeting by Alzheimer's-related amyloid beta oligomers. *J Neurosci* **24**(45), 10191–10200.

34. Altman, J. & Das, G. D. (1965). Autoradiographic and histological evidence of postnatal hippocampal neurogenesis in rats. *J Comp Neurol* **124**(3), 319–335.

35. Gould, E., Tanapat, P., Hastings, N. B. & Shors, T. J. (1999). Neurogenesis in adulthood: A possible role in learning. *Trends Cogn Sci* **3**(5), 186–192.

36. Brinton, R. D. & Wang, J. M. (2006). Therapeutic potential of neurogenesis for prevention and recovery from Alzheimer's disease: Allopregnanolone as a proof of concept neurogenic agent. *Curr Alzheimer Res* **3**(3), 185–190.

37. Shors, T. J., Miesegaes, G., Beylin, A., Zhao, M., Rydel, T. & Gould, E. (2001). Neurogenesis in the adult is involved in the formation of trace memories. *Nature* **410**(6826), 372–376.

38. Watanabe, C. M., Wolffram, S., Ader, P., Rimbach, G., Packer, L., Maguire, J. J., Schultz, P. G. & Gohil, K. (2001). The *in vivo* neuromodulatory effects of the herbal medicine *Ginkgo biloba*. *Proc Natl Acad Sci U S A* **98**(12), 6577–6580.

39. Birks, J., Grimley, E. V. & Van Dongen, M. (2002). *Ginkgo biloba* for cognitive impairment and dementia. *Cochrane Database Syst Rev* (4), CD003120.

40. Kleijnen, J. & Knipschild, P. (1992). *Ginkgo biloba* for cerebral insufficiency. *Br J Clin Pharmacol* **34**(4), 352–358.

41. Le Bars, P. L. (2003). Magnitude of effect and special approach to *Ginkgo biloba* extract EGb 761 in cognitive disorders. *Pharmacopsychiatry* **36**(Suppl 1), S44–S49.

42. Hopfenmuller, W. (1994). [Evidence for a therapeutic effect of *Ginkgo biloba* special extract. Meta-analysis of 11 clinical studies in patients with cerebrovascular insufficiency in old age]. *Arzneimittelforschung* **44**(9), 1005–1013.

43. Pittler, M. H. & Ernst, E. (2000). *Ginkgo biloba* extract for the treatment of intermittent claudication: A meta-analysis of randomized trials. *Am J Med* **108**(4), 276–281.

44. Canter, P. H. & Ernst, E. (2007). *Ginkgo biloba* is not a smart drug: An updated systematic review of randomised clinical trials testing the nootropic effects of *G. biloba* extracts in healthy people. *Hum Psychopharmacol* **22**(5), 265–278.

45. Mix, J. A. & David Crews, W., Jr (2002). A double-blind, placebo-controlled, randomized trial of *Ginkgo biloba* extract EGb 761(R) in a sample of cognitively intact older adults: Neuropsychological findings. *Hum Psychopharmacol* **17**(6), 267–277.

46. Andrieu, S., Gillette, S., Amouyal, K., Nourhashemi, F., Reynish, E., Ousset, P. J., Albarede, J. L., Vellas, B. & Grandjean, H. (2003). Association of Alzheimer's disease onset with *Ginkgo biloba* and other symptomatic cognitive treatments in a population of women aged 75 years and older from the EPIDOS study. *J Gerontol A Biol Sci Med Sci* **58**(4), 372–377.

47. Solomon, P. R., Adams, F., Silver, A., Zimmer, J. & DeVeaux, R. (2002). Ginkgo for memory enhancement: A randomized controlled trial. *JAMA* **288**(7), 835–840.

48. Mazza, M., Capuano, A., Bria, P. & Mazza, S. (2006). *Ginkgo biloba* and donepezil: A comparison in the treatment of Alzheimer's dementia in a randomized placebo-controlled double-blind study. *Eur J Neurol* **13**(9), 981–985.

49. Fitzpatrick, A. L., Fried, L. P., Williamson, J., Crowley, P., Posey, D., Kwong, L., Bonk, J., Moyer, R., Chabot, J., Kidoguchi, L., Furberg, C. D. & DeKosky, S. T. (2006). Recruitment of the elderly into a pharmacologic prevention trial: The Ginkgo Evaluation of Memory Study experience. *Contemp Clin Trials* **27**(6), 541–553.

50. Mahady, G. B. (2002). *Ginkgo biloba* for the prevention and treatment of cardiovascular disease: A review of the literature. *J Cardiovasc Nurs* **16**(4), 21–32.
51. Zhou, W., Chai, H., Lin, P. H., Lumsden, A. B., Yao, Q. & Chen, C. (2004). Clinical use and molecular mechanisms of action of extract of *Ginkgo biloba* leaves in cardiovascular diseases. *Cardiovasc Drug Rev* **22**(4), 309–319.
52. DeFeudis, F. V., Papadopoulos, V. & Drieu, K. (2003). *Ginkgo biloba* extracts and cancer: A research area in its infancy. *Fundam Clin Pharmacol* **17**(4), 405–417.
53. Evans, J. R. (2000). *Ginkgo biloba* extract for age-related macular degeneration. *Cochrane Database Syst Rev2*, CD001775.
54. Kohler, S., Funk, P. & Kieser, M. (2004). Influence of a 7-day treatment with *Ginkgo biloba* special extract EGb 761 on bleeding time and coagulation: A randomized, placebo-controlled, double-blind study in healthy volunteers. *Blood Coagul Fibrinolysis* **15**(4), 303–309.
55. Rosenblatt, M. & Mindel, J. (1997). Spontaneous hyphema associated with ingestion of *Ginkgo biloba* extract. *N Engl J Med* **336**(15), 1108.
56. Matthews, M. K., Jr (1998). Association of *Ginkgo biloba* with intracerebral hemorrhage. *Neurology* **50**(6), 1933–1934.
57. Kupiec, T. & Raj, V. (2005). Fatal seizures due to potential herb–drug interactions with *Ginkgo biloba*. *J Anal Toxicol* **29**(7), 755–758.
58. Kressmann, S., Muller, W. E. & Blume, H. H. (2002). Pharmaceutical quality of different *Ginkgo biloba* brands. *J Pharm Pharmacol* **54**(5), 661–669.

Chapter 7

Policosanol to Manage Dyslipidemia in Older Adults

Barbara Swanson and Joyce Keithley

Rush University College of Nursing, Chicago, IL, USA

Abstract

Policosanol (*Saccharum officinarum*) is a dietary supplement that is widely used in Latin America to normalize dyslipidemic profiles, as well as to reduce hypertriglyceridemia. Consisting of fatty alcohols derived from plant waxes, policosanol has shown comparable efficacy and better safety than statins for raising HDL and lowering LDL cholesterol levels. However, nearly all published trials of policosanol have been conducted by a single group of investigators in Cuba, and more recent studies outside of Cuba haven't replicated these findings. This chapter presents current information on the pharmacological properties of policosanol and reviews recent studies with a focus on those that target elderly populations. Additional studies are needed in elderly populations to further describe its efficacy, especially when directly compared with statins, and to characterize its mechanism of action and potential pleiotropic effects.

Keywords: *Policosanol, dietary supplements, plant waxes, cholesterol, triglycerides, older adults*

Policosanol is an over-the-counter dietary supplement that consists of fatty alcohols derived from plant wax, generally sugar cane (*Saccharum officinarum*). Widely used in Latin American countries to promote cardiovascular health, policosanol is a natural remedy that has been shown in several Cuban studies to be efficacious for normalizing dyslipidemic lipoprotein profiles, as well as for reducing hypertriglyceridemia. However, more recent studies from the United States, Europe, South Africa, and Canada have failed to replicate these findings, raising questions about the role of policosanol in the management of dyslipidemia.

PHARMACOLOGICAL PROFILE

Chemistry

Policosanol is also known as 32–C, dotriacontanol, heptacosanol, hexacosanol, nonacosanol, octacosanol, tetracosanol, tetratriacontanol, triacontanol.

It is composed of aliphatic primary alcohols that are isolated from purified sugar cane wax by hydrolytic cleavage. Its chemical formula is $CH_3\text{-}(CH_2)_n\text{-}CH_2OH$ with a chain length varying from 24 to 34 carbon atoms [1]. Most policosanol preparations contain aliphatic alcohols in the following proportions: 66–67% octacosanol, 12–14% triacosanol, 7–8% hexacosanol, and 11–15% other carbon alcohols [2].

Policosanol has been shown to melt without decomposition and to remain stable at temperatures up to 185°C [3]. It has low solubility in water. At temperatures of 25°C and 40°C, solubility has been reported to be 1.7×10^{-15} mg/ml and 2.5×10^{-15} mg/ml [3].

Mechanism of Action

The primary effect of policosanol is to reduce low-density lipoprotein (LDL) cholesterol concentration, although it has also been shown to raise high-density lipoprotein (HDL) cholesterol [4] and lower triglycerides (TG) [4–7]. Significant effects have been observed after 6–8 weeks of treatment [8–9]. Although the mechanism of action remains uncertain, policosanol is hypothesized to exert its lipid-altering effects via two mechanisms. First, a growing body of *in vitro* and animal studies suggest that policosanol inhibits cholesterol synthesis prior to the formation of mevalonate [10], thus suggesting a modulatory effect on 3-hydroxy-3-methylglutaryl-coenzyme A (HMG-CoA) reductase, the target for statin drugs (Fig. 7.1). Recent data suggest that policosanol inhibits *de novo* synthesis of HMG-CoA reductase and/or stimulates its degradation [11]. Other data suggest that policosanol upregulates hepatic

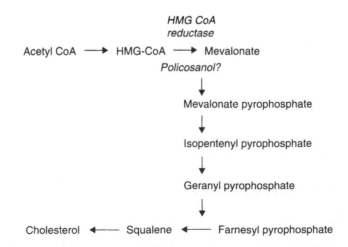

FIGURE 7.1   Cholesterol biosynthesis pathway.

AMP-kinase phosphorylation, an action known to suppress HMG-CoA activity [12]. Second, policosanol has been shown to increase receptor-mediated uptake of LDL in the liver [13]. A third mechanism, inhibition of bile acid absorption, has been reported, but additional data are needed to substantiate this finding [14]. Other effects of policosanol that are relevant to reducing atherogenic risk include inhibition of platelet aggregation, blocking the effects of cholesterol on smooth muscle proliferation, inhibition of foam cell formation, and prevention of LDL peroxidation [10, 15–17], although conflicting data exist on policosanol's antioxidant effects [14].

It is not clear if policosanol-induced inhibition of cholesterol synthesis is due to a single constituent or is the result of the interaction or synergy among multiple constituents. A study of cholesterol synthesis *in vitro* found that triacontanol, a minor component in most policosanol preparations, decreased HMG-CoA reductase activity in rat hepatoma cells, but not in microsomal fractions from Harlan Sprague–Dawley rats [12]. This suggests that triacontanol may be transformed to an active metabolite that inhibits cholesterol synthesis or, alternatively, it may act via intracellular pathways.

Pharmacokinetics

To date, there are no validated methods to measure plasma concentrations of long-chain alcohols or their metabolites in humans following therapeutic doses, thus restricting investigation of the pharmacokinetic properties of policosanol [1]. Studies of pharmacokinetics in animal models have involved measurement of total radioactivity following administration of radiolabeled octacosanol, rather than the parent drug, limiting the conclusions that can be drawn. Although the findings must be viewed cautiously, rat studies have found that the bioavailability of oral octacosanol ranges from 5% to 12% and that its half-life is 1–2 hours [18]. Orally administered octacosanol distributes to the tissues, with accumulations of greater than 1% of the administered dose in the liver and brown and white adipose tissues, and less than 0.4% in the spleen, kidney, heart, lung, brain, and muscle [13]. *In vitro*, octacosanol is metabolized to octacosanoic acid; *in vivo*, oral octacosanol is associated with the formation of shortened saturated and unsaturated fatty acids. This suggests that octacosanol and fatty acids are metabolized via shared pathways [19].

Toxicity

At doses that are between 100 and 3500 times greater than the recommended dosage, there have been no reports of policosanol-related toxicity in any published animal or human trials [1, 20]. A review of four clinical trials of policosanol in healthy volunteers and persons with dyslipidemia (total $N = 308$ persons treated with policosanol for between 8 weeks and 14 months) revealed the following adverse events: (a) significant, but mild, decrease in serum liver transaminase levels that remained within normal limits and one case of abdominal pain with nausea [4], (b) significant decrease in serum creatinine levels, although no values were outside the normal range [21], (c) transient dizziness, nausea, and diarrhea in two participants [4], and (d) somnolence ($n = 1$) and headache ($n = 1$) [14]. A large surveillance study followed 27,879 policosanol-treated patients for an average of 2.7 years and found that only 86 (0.31%) patients reported adverse effects. The most commonly occurring adverse effects included weight loss (0.08%), polyuria (0.07%), insomnia (0.05%), and polyphagia (0.05%) [22].

There have been no reports of carcinogenicity associated with policosanol supplementation. In one study, mice who were administered excessive doses of policosanol (50–500 mg/kg) for 18 months did not show increased neoplastic disease compared with control mice [23]. This finding corroborated earlier animal studies that found no evidence of policosanol-related toxicities, including neoplasms, in doses of up to 500 mg/kg administered over a period of 12–24 months [24–26].

Several studies have shown that policosanol supplementation reduces platelet aggregation [5, 21, 27]. Although this could provide protection against thrombotic events, it could also be associated with bleeding tendencies. To date, no published clinical trials have reported the occurrence of bleeding or hemorrhagic events during policosanol supplementation.

There has been one published report on the perinatal and postnatal effects of policosanol in an animal model. In that study, pregnant Sprague-Dawley rats were administered policosanol at doses of up to 500 mg/kg/day from day 15 of pregnancy to day 21 post-parturition. No toxic effects were observed in the dams during pregnancy, while the pups showed no adverse effects related to postnatal growth, behaviors, or reproductive ability [28].

Drug Interactions

In clinical trials, policosanol has been concomitantly administered with a number of medications, including, but not limited to, calcium channel blockers, angiotensin-converting enzyme inhibitors, diuretics, antidepressants, oral hypoglycemics, and nonsteroidal anti-inflammatory drugs. There have been no reports of any adverse drug interactions with policosanol [1]. In one randomized controlled trial (RCT), two of three policosanol-treated participants (2 mg/day for 14 months) who concomitantly received beta-adrenoceptor antagonists showed an increase in TG and no change in total cholesterol [29]. Beta-adrenoceptor antagonists are known to increase TG and very low-density lipoprotein (VLDL) cholesterol, and to decrease HDL cholesterol [30, 31]. Suprapharmacological doses of policosanol have been shown to significantly increase propanolol-induced hypotension in spontaneously hypertensive rats, while having no effect on blood pressure when concomitantly administered with nifidepine [32].

REVIEW OF STUDIES

Overview of Older Studies/Systematic Reviews

To our knowledge, two systematic reviews have evaluated the safety and efficacy of policosanol as a lipid-lowering agent. The first of these reviews [1] considered randomized double-blind placebo-controlled or randomized double-blind comparative trials in healthy volunteers, patients with hypercholesterolemia, and special populations, such as elderly patients and postmenopausal women. All 21 included studies reported significant changes in total cholesterol at doses of 10–20 mg/day, and 20 of the 21 studies reported significant changes in LDL cholesterol. Neither TG nor HDL cholesterol were significantly altered in the majority of studies. Most studies were done in the Caribbean using policosanol derived from Cuban sugar cane. The reviewers concluded that policosanol was well-tolerated and safe in reducing total and LDL cholesterol and that additional studies need to be conducted in other countries and research centers.

The second systematic review compared the safety and efficacy of plant sterols and stanols (e.g., fortified margarines) to policosanol for reducing LDL cholesterol [33]. Fifty-two randomized double-blind placebo-controlled studies (23 plant sterol and stanol; 29 policosanol) met all inclusion criteria. Similar to the first review, a variety of patient populations were studied, including patients with normal and elevated cholesterol levels, as well as patients with type 2 diabetes mellitus, post-myocardial infarction, and other disorders. In the 52 included studies, plant sterols and stanols and policosanol were significantly more effective than placebo ($p < 0.0001$) in reducing LDL cholesterol. Although none of the studies directly compared plant sterols and stanols to policosanol, policosanol was associated with greater reductions in LDL cholesterol than plant sterols and stanols ($p < 0.0001$). Among the authors' conclusions were that all three products – plant sterols and stanols and policosanol – were well-tolerated and safe, and that policosanol was more effective in reducing LDL cholesterol than plant sterols and stanols.

Review of Recent Studies: 2004–2007

Since the publication of the systematic reviews, 12 additional studies of policosanol for dyslipidemia have been published and are summarized in Table 7.1 [34–45]. Consistent with the findings reported in the systematic reviews, six studies showed that daily supplementation with policosanol produced significant reductions in some or all of the lipid parameters. Three of the six positive studies were conducted by the prominent Cuban research team; and three were conducted by researchers in Croatia, the United States, and Italy. With the exception of one retrospective, comparative study, all studies employed randomized, prospective, clinical trial designs. Study sample sizes ranged from 21 to 100 adults with hypercholesterolemia; and policosanol dosages ranged

TABLE 7.1 Recent Studies of Policosanol for Dyslipidemia: 2004–2007

Reference	Design	N	Dose/(Product source)	Duration	Results
Lin et al. (2004) (Netherlands) [34]	Randomized, double-blind, parallel placebo-controlled	58 adults with normal or mildly elevated cholesterol levels	20 mg wheat germ policosanol administered via chocolate pellets (Garuda Intl., Inc., USA, California; composition similar to sugar cane-derived policosanol)	4 weeks	No change in LDL, TC, HDL, TG No short-term adverse effects
Castano et al. (2005) (Cuba) [35]	Randomized, double-blind, comparative	90 patients with type II hypercholesterolemia	3 groups: 2 omega-3 fatty acids + placebo; 2 omega-3 fatty acids + 5 mg policosanol; 2 omega-3 fatty acids + 10 mg policosanol (Dalmar Labs, Havana, Cuba)	8 weeks	Decreased LDL, TC, TG, and increased HDL in both policosanol groups Only TG reduced in omega-3 fatty acids + placebo group Well-tolerated
Castano et al. (2005) (Cuba) [36]	Randomized, double-blind, comparative	100 patients with type II hypercholesterolemia	D-003, 5 or 10 mg, or policosanol, 5 or 10 mg (Dalmar Labs, Havana, Cuba; D-003 = mixture of high molecular weight aliphatic acids purified from sugar cane wax)	8 weeks	Decreased LDL, TC, and increased HDL in both groups at both dosages; with greater changes in both D-003 groups No change in TG Both agents well-tolerated

Study	Design	Subjects	Intervention	Duration	Results
Reiner et al. (2005) (Croatia) [37]	Randomized, double-blind, placebo-controlled, crossover	67 patients with moderate hypercholesterolemia	Policosanol 10 mg (rice-derived policosanol)	8 weeks	Significant decrease in TC and increase in apoprotein A I No change in LDL, HDL, TG, homocysteine, CRP No adverse effects
Wright et al. (2005) (USA, Kentucky) [38]	Retrospective, comparative	21 adults with elevated cholesterol levels: 15 treated with policosanol and 6 treated with policosanol and statin therapy	Policosanol 10 mg/coenzyme Q 15 mg combination twice/day, or above + statin (product source not stated)	156 ± 63 days	Decreased LDL, $p < 0.001$ and TC, $p < 0.001$ in both groups No change in HDL, TG
Berthold et al. (2006) (Germany) [39]	Multi-center, randomized double-blind, placebo-controlled	143 patients with hypercholesterolemia or combined hyperlipidemia	5 groups: 10, 20, 40, or 80 mg policosanol, or placebo (Dalmar Labs, Havana, Cuba)	12 weeks	No change in LDL, TC, HDL, TG, VLDL, lipoprotein a, LDL:HDL, TC:HDL All dosages well-tolerated
Castano et al. (2006) (Cuba) [40]	Randomized, double-blind, comparative	54 outpatients with atherosclerotic risk factors	1 omega-3 fatty acids + 10 mg policosanol, or 1 omega-3 fatty acids + placebo (Dalmar Labs, Havana, Cuba)	21 days	17% decrease in LDL, 10% decrease in TC, 18% increase in HDL No change in TG Policosanol + omega-3 fatty acids more effective in inhibiting platelet aggregation than omega-3 fatty acids alone

(Continued)

TABLE 7.1 (*Continued*)

Reference	Design	N	Dose/(Product source)	Duration	Results
Cubeddu *et al.* (2006) (USA, Florida) [41]	Randomized, double-blind, double dummy, placebo-controlled	99 patients with LDL levels 140–189 mg/dL	Four groups: policosanol 20 mg, atorvastatin 10 mg, combination therapy, placebo (Cholesstor, Pharmed Group, USA, Florida)	12 weeks	No change in LDL, TC, HDL, TG, either alone or as combination therapy Well-tolerated
Dulin *et al.* (2006) (USA, North Carolina) [42]	Randomized, double-blind, placebo-controlled	40 adults with mild hypercholesterolemia	Policosanol 20 mg per day (Garuda Intl., Inc., USA, California)	8 weeks	No change in LDL, TC, HDL, TG, C-reactive protein, NMRS-determined profiles
Greyling *et al.* (2006) (South Africa) [43]	Randomized, double-blind, placebo-controlled, cross-over	35 patients with hypercholesterolemia or familial hypercholesterolemia	Policosanol 20 mg per day (Garuda Intl., Inc., USA, California)	12 weeks	No change in LDL, TC, HDL, TG
Kassis and Jones (2006) (Canada) [44]	Randomized, double-blind, placebo-controlled, cross-over	21 hypercholesterolemic males and post-menopausal females	Policosanol 10 mg incorporated in margarine (Dalmar Labs, Havana, Cuba)	4 weeks	No change in LDL, TC, HDL, TG
Cicero *et al.* (2007) (Italy) [45]	Randomized, single-blind, parallel groups	40 patients with moderate dyslipidemias	Berberine (plant alkaloid) or combination of berberine, policosanol, red yeast extract, folic acid, astasanthin	4 weeks	Decreased TC, LDL, TG, ApoB in both groups; increased HDL in both groups No adverse events in either group

Abbreviations: HDL, *HDL-cholesterol*; LDL, *LDL-cholesterol*; TC, *total cholesterol*; TG, *triglycerides*; VLDL, *VLDL-cholesterol*; CRP, *C-reactive protein*; NMRS, *nuclear magnetic resonance spectroscopy* from 5 to 10 mg, either alone or in combination with other agents, such as omega-3 fatty acids, coenzyme Q, or berberine. Policosanol source was sugar cane-derived in three studies, rice-derived in one study, and not identified in two studies. Study duration ranged from 4 weeks to 6 months. The majority of studies reported significant decreases in LDL-cholesterol, total cholesterol, and TG, and significant increases in HDL-cholesterol. Also similar to the systematic reviews, policosanol was well-tolerated and associated with no adverse effects in any of studies.

The other six studies reported results that were in marked contrast to the studies included in the systematic reviews. All six studies were double-blind, randomized, placebo-controlled clinical trials conducted with adults (N range, 40–143) who had normal or mild hypercholesterolemia or dyslipidemia. Policosanol dosages ranged from 10 to 80 mg daily, either alone or in combination with other agents, primarily sugar-cane derived and from Dalmar Labs, Havana, Cuba or Garuda International, Inc., California. Study duration ranged from 4 to 12 weeks, and policosanol was well-tolerated. The majority of these studies found no change in any of the lipid parameters, including LDL-cholesterol, HDL-cholesterol, total cholesterol, and TG.

The divergence of these findings raises several questions: First, do differences in dietary patterns across countries affect policosanol bioavailability and subsequent efficacy? It has been shown, for example, that oleyl alcohol, a component of fish oil, inhibits absorption of long-chain alcohols in the rat gut [46]. Second, what is the variability in the composition of the policosanol products provided by Dalmar Laboratories, Havana, Cuba and Garuda International, Inc., California? It is well-established that plant-based supplements can vary from lot to lot and crop to crop. Third, do other differences in the composition of policosanol account for the disparate findings, such as the presence of other ingredients, or the use of other preparation or delivery techniques, such as chocolate pellets or margarine? Fourth, do genetic or other differences in the samples account for the discrepant findings? Or, fifth, do study duration, sample sizes, heterogeneous samples, or other limitations account for the variable findings?

Studies of Older Adults

Eight clinical trials and one surveillance study focusing on the aging population (>60 years) and including 3763 participants are summarized in Table 7.2 [47–55]. In dosages ranging from 5 to 20 mg, policosanol was administered, either alone ($n = 8$ studies) or in combination with a beta-blocker ($n = 1$ study). Policosanol was compared against placebo, simvastatin, pravastatin, or atorvastatin. The studies encompassed a mix of small sample sizes and large multi-center samples and ranged in length from 8 weeks to 12 months. With the exception of one study conducted by researchers in Argentina, all studies were conducted by a Cuban research team. Policosanol was more effective

TABLE 7.2 Policosanol and Aging Studies

Reference	Design	N	Dose	Duration	Results
Castano et al. (1995) [47]	Multi-center, randomized, double-blind, placebo-controlled	62 patients (60–75 years) with hypercholesterolemia	Policosanol, 10 mg	12 months	Decreased LDL, TC, LDL:HDL, TC:HDL, $p < 0.00001$ HDL increased 8% No change in TG Mild/transient adverse effects
Ortensi et al. (1997) (Argentina) [48]	Randomized, double-blind, parallel-group, comparative	53 patients (60–77 years) with primary hypercholesterolemia	Policosanol or Simvastatin, 10 mg	8 weeks	Both drugs significantly/similarly decreased LDL, TC, TG, TC:HDL, LDL:HDL No change in HDL No serious adverse events
Castano et al. (1999) [49]	Randomized, double-blind	68 patients (60–80 years) with hypercholesterolemia	Policosanol, or Pravastatin, 10 mg	8 weeks	Policosanol decreased LDL, TC, LDL:HDL, TC:HDL, $p < 0.00001$ Pravastatin decreased LDL, TC, LDL:HDL, TC:HDL, $p < 0.00001$ Policosanol increased HDL, $p < 0.001$ and decreased TG, $p < 0.01$ Policosanol decreased platelet aggregation, $p < 0.05$ and endothelemia levels, $p < 0.001$ Both agents well-tolerated

Reference	Study design	Patient population	Treatment	Duration	Results
Castano et al. (2001) [50]	Multi-center, randomized, placebo-controlled	179 patients (60–78 years) with type II hypercholesterolemia and >1 concomitant atherosclerotic risk factor	Policosanol, 5 mg for 12 weeks; then 10 mg for 12 weeks	24 weeks	Both doses decreased LDL, TC, $p < 0.001$; and LDL:HDL, TC:HDL, $p < 0.01$ Both doses increased HDL, $p < 0.01$ and improved cardiovascular capacity, $p = 0.01$ No change in TG No serious adverse events, $p < 0.01$
Mas et al. (2001) [51]	Multi-centered, randomized, placebo-controlled	280 patients ($\geq$60 years) with type II hypercholesterolemia and CHD	Policosanol 5 mg for 6 months; increased to 10 mg if pre-defined cholesterol goals not reached by 6 months	12 months	Decreased LDL, TC, TC:HDL, LDL:HDL, $p < 0.00001$ Decreased TG, $p < 0.001$ Increased HDL, $p < 0.001$ Decreased cardiac and vascular events and hospitalizations, $p < 0.001$ Well-tolerated
Castano et al. (2002) [52]	Multi-center, randomized, double-blind, placebo-controlled, parallel groups	589 patients ($\geq$60 years) with hypertension and type II hypercholesterolemia	Policosanol 5 mg for 6 months; increased to 10 mg if pre-defined cholesterol goals not reached by 6 months	12 months	Decreased LDL, TC, TG, TC:HDL, LDL:HDL, $p < 0.00001$ Increased HDL, $p < 0.0001$ Decreased vascular and all-cause serious adverse events, $p < 0.05$, and total adverse events, $p < 0.01$

(Continued)

TABLE 7.2 (*Continued*)

Reference	Design	N	Dose	Duration	Results
Castano et al. (2003) [53]	Randomized, single-blind, parallel group	75 older patients (60–80 years) with type II hypercholesterolemia	Policosanol or Atorvastatin, 10 mg	8 weeks	Both agents decreased TC, LDL:HDL, TC:HDL, $p < 0.0001$, and TG, $p < 0.001$. Atorvastatin more effectively decreased LDL and TC. Policosanol increased HDL, $p < 0.05$. Nine adverse events with Atorvasatin; none with policosanol
Castano et al. (2004) [54]	Randomized, placebo-controlled	205 patients ($\geq$60 years) with hypercholesterolemia	Policosanol 5 mg plus beta-blocker, or placebo	3 years	Decreased LDL, TC, TG, $p < 0.00001$. Increased HDL, $p < 0.00001$. Decreased BP in policosanol/beta-blocker group. Fewer adverse events in policosanol/beta-blocker group (3.1%) vs. placebo group (14.0%)
Fernandez et al. (2004) [55]	Multi-site surveillance for tolerability	2252 patients ($\geq$60 years) with high coronary risk	Policosanol 5, 10, and 20 mg	Variable: 6–36 months	Serious adverse events: 1.4%. Hospitalization: 0.6%. Mild to moderate adverse events: 2.7%

Abbreviations: HDL, HDL-*cholesterol*; LDL, LDL-*cholesterol*; TC, *total cholesterol*; TG, *triglycerides*; CHD, *coronary heart disease* than placebo in improving lipid parameters. Comparisons between policosanol and the three different statin agents suggested that policosanol was equivalent ($n = 2$) or superior ($n = 1$) in efficacy. With the exception of atorvastatin, policosanol and the other agents were associated with only mild or transient side effects. Because of the preponderance of studies conducted in one country with one type of policosanol, study findings may not be generalizable to other settings and populations and may be unique to the people of Cuba.

IMPLICATIONS FOR OLDER ADULTS

Although statins remain the cornerstone therapy for dyslipidemia, their high cost may preclude their use by persons on Medicare. For those individuals, policosanol may represent a cost-effective alternative. In November 2005, the average Medicare drug plan cost for a 1-month supply of simvastatin (Zocor®) was $132 [56]. In contrast, a 1-month supply of policosanol costs $12.00. Another consideration is older adult polypharmacy. With the exception of pravastatin and rosuvastatin, all statins are extensively biotransformed by the cytochrome P450 system and hence their plasma concentrations may be altered when P450 inducers or inhibitors are concomitantly administered. Competitive CYP inhibitors can increase statin plasma concentrations to potentially toxic levels, resulting in myopathy and rhabdomyolysis. CYP inhibitors that are commonly administered to the elderly include calcium channel blockers, warfarin, and sildenafil [57]. Digoxin can also increase the area under the curve (AUC) for statins through its effects on the P glycoprotein, a physiological drug transporter [58]. Given the interactions between statins and drugs commonly prescribed for older adults, policosanol may be a safer lipid-lowering alterative. Additional pharmacokinetic studies are needed to identify the effects of policosanol on CYP P450 isoforms and drug transporters.

Statins are characterized by cardioprotective pleiotropic actions that are independent of their lipid lowering effects. These pleiotropic actions include improved endothelial cell dysfunction, increased myocardial perfusion, increased bioavailability of nitric oxide, antioxidant and anti-inflammatory effects, and stabilization of plaque formation [59]. Additionally, statins have extrahepatic effects that may be beneficial to older adults. In the central nervous system, statins have been associated with reduced rates of Alzheimer's disease and other dementias, an effect not seen with non-statin lipid lowering therapies [60, 61]. One study found that persons receiving long-term statin therapy had lower depression and anxiety levels compared with statin-naïve persons [62]. However, the mechanisms underlying potential psychotropic effects of statins remain unknown. It is not known if policosanol shares these beneficial pleiotropic effects and additional studies are needed to characterize its pharmacodynamic spectrum.

Despite the widespread use of statins, it is unclear if they are associated with an increased or decreased risk of cancer. A recent meta-analysis of

23 statin treatment arms that encompassed 309,506 person-years of follow-up found an inverse relationship between achieved LDL-cholesterol levels and incidence of cancer [63]. However, other studies have either failed to find an association between statin use and cancer [64], or have concluded that statins reduce cancer risk [65]. While animal studies suggest no increased cancer risk with short-term suprapharmacological doses of policosanol, studies of long-term use in humans are needed.

CONCLUSIONS

There are conflicting findings on the efficacy of policosanol to normalize dyslipidemic profiles. The majority of studies that support policosanol's lipid-lowering properties have been conducted by the same team of Cuban researchers. Given the possibly unique properties of Cuban sugar cane or differences in sample/population characteristics, these findings must be viewed cautiously. Several recent studies conducted outside the Caribbean have failed to replicate the Cuban findings. However, direct comparisons of clinical trial findings have been limited by differences in regional dietary patterns and unknown variability in the composition of the policosanol products that were tested.

There is little disagreement that policosanol is safe, even when administered in amounts that exceed recommended doses. To date, there have been no published reports of serious toxic effects related to policosanol. This is significant because Americans' use of policosanol likely increased following the 2005 release of One-A-Day Cholesterol Plus®, a multivitamin that contains 10 mg of policosanol.

It remains unclear whether policosanol is an effective alternative to conventional lipid lowering therapies. Additional studies are needed to further describe its efficacy, especially when directly compared with statins, and to further characterize its mechanism of action and potential pleiotropic effects. Moreover, clinical trials in elderly populations are needed to determine the safety and efficacy of policosanol within the context of polypharmacy and age-related reductions in drug biotransformation and elimination.

REFERENCES

1. Gouni-Berthold, I. & Berthold, H. K. (2002). Policosanol: Clinical pharmacology and therapeutic significance of a new lipid-lowering agent. *Am Heart J* **143**, 356–365.
2. Natural Medicines Comprehensive Database, online version (2007).
3. Uribarri, E., Laguna, A., Sierra, R. & Ricardo, Y. (2002). Physico-mechanical characterization of policosanol, a novel hypocholesterolemic drug. *Drug Dev Ind Pharm* **28**, 89–93.
4. Mas, R., Castano, G., Illnait, J., Fernandez, L., Fernandez, J., Aleman, C., Pontigas, V. & Lescay, M. (1999). Effects of policosanol in patients with type II hypercholesterolemia and additional coronary risk factors. *Clin Pharmacol Ther* **65**, 439–447.

5. Castano, G., Mas, R., Arruzazabala, M. L., Noa, M., Illnait, J., Fernandez, J. C., Molina, V. & Menendez, A. (1999). Effects of policosanol and pravastatin on lipid profile, platelet aggregation, and endothelemia in older hypercholesterolemic patients. *Int J Clin Pharmacol Res* **19**, 105–116.

6. Castano, G., Mas, R., Fernandez, J. C., Lopez, L. E. & Fernandez, L. (1999). A long-term, open-label study of the efficacy and tolerability of policosanol in patients with high global coronary risk. *Curr Ther Res* **60**, 379–391.

7. Castano, G., Mas, R., Fernandez, J. C., Fernandez, L., Illnait, J. & Lopez, E. (2002). Effects of policosanol on older patients with hypertension and type II hypercholesterolemia. *Drugs R D* **3**, 159–172.

8. Illnait, J., Castano, G., Mas, R. & Fernandez, J. C. (1997). A comparative study on the efficacy and tolerability of policosanol and simvastatin for treating type II hypercholesterolemia [Abstract]. *Can J Cardiol* **13**(Suppl B), 342B.

9. Pons, P., Illnait, J., Mas, R., Rodriquez, M., Aleman, C., Fernandez, J. C., Fernandez, L. & Martin, M. (1997). A comparative study of policosanol versus probucol in patients with hypercholesterolemia. *Curr Ther Res* **58**, 26–35.

10. Menendez, R., Fernandez, S. I., Del Rio, A., Gonzalez, R. M., Fraga, V., Amor, A. M. & Mas, R. M. (1994). Policosanol inhibits cholesterol biosynthesis and enhances low density lipoprotein processing in cultured human fibroblasts. *Biol Res* **27**, 199–203.

11. Menendez, R., Amor, A. M., Rodeiro, I., Gonzalez, R. M., Gonzalez, P. C., Alfonso, J. L. & Mas, R. (2001). Policosanol modulates HMG-CoA reductase activity in cultured fibroblasts. *Arch Med Res* **32**, 8–12.

12. Singh, D. K., Li, L. & Porter, T. D. (2006). Policosanol inhibits cholesterol synthesis in hepatoma cells by activation of AMP-kinase. *J Pharmacol Exp Ther* **318**, 1020–1026.

13. Kabir, Y. & Kimura, S. (1993). Biodistribution and metabolism of orally administered octacosanol in rats. *Ann Nutr Metab* **37**, 33–38.

14. Ng, C., Leung, K. Y., Huang, Y. & Chen, Z. Y. (2005). Policosanol has no antioxidant activity in human low-density lipoprotein but increases excretion of bile acids in hamsters. *J Agric Food Chem* **53**, 6289–6298.

15. Menendez, R., Mas, R., Amor, A. M., Gonzalez, R. M., Fernandez, J. C., Rodeiro, I., Zayas, M. & Jimenez, S. (2000). Effects of policosanol treatment on the susceptibility of low density lipoprotein (LDL) isolated from healthy volunteers to oxidative modification in vitro. *Br J Clin Pharmacol* **50**, 255–262.

16. Noa, M., Mas, R. & Mesa, R. (1998). Effect of policosanol on intimal thickening in rabbit cuffed carotid artery. *Int J Cardiol* **67**, 124–132.

17. Noa, M., de la Rosa, M. C. & Mas, R. (1996). Effect of policosanol on foam-cell formation in carrageenan-induced granulomas in rats. *J Pharm Pharmacol* **48**, 306–309.

18. Kabir, Y. & Kimura, S. (1993). Biodistribution and metabolism of orally administered octacosanol in rats. *Ann Nutr Metab* **37**, 33–38.

19. Menendez, R., Maarrero, D., Mas, R., Fernandez, I., Gonzalez, L. & Gonzalez, R. M. (2005). *In vitro* and *in vivo* study of octacosanol metabolism. *Arch Med Res* **36**, 113–119.

20. Janikula, M. (2002). Policosanol: A new treatment for cardiovascular disease. *Altern Med Rev* **7**, 203–217.

21. Alcocer, L., Fernandez, L., Campos, E. & Mas, R. (1999). A comparative study of policosanol versus acipimox in patients with type II hypercholesterolemia. *Int J Tissue React* **21**, 85–92.

22. Fernandez, L., Mas, R., Illnait, J. & Fernandez, J. C. (1998). Policosanol: Results of a postmarketing surveillance study of 27,879 patients. *Curr Ther Res Clin Exp* **59**, 717–722.

23. Aleman, C., Puig, M. N., Elias, E. C., Ortega, C. H., Guerra, I. R., Ferreiro, R. M. & Brinis, F. (1995). Carcinogenicity of policosanol in mice: An 18-month study. *Food Chem Toxicol* **33**, 573–578.

24. Aleman, C. L., Mas, R., Hernandez, C., Rodeiro, I., Cerejido, E., Noa, M., Capote, A., Menendez, R., Amor, A., Fraga, V., Capote, A. & Jiminez, S. (1994). A 12-month study of policosanol oral toxicity in Sprague-Dawley rats. *Toxicol Lett* **70**, 77–87.

25. Mesa, A. R., Mas, R., Noa, M., Hernandez, C., Rodeiro, I., Gamez, R., Garcia, M., Capote, A. & Aleman, C. L. (1994). Toxicity of Policosanol in beagle dogs: One-year study. *Toxicol Lett* **73**, 81–90.

26. Aleman, C. L., Mas Ferreiro, R., Noa Puig, M., Rodeiro Guerra, I., Hernandez Ortega, C. & Capote, A. (1994). Carcinogenicity of policosanol in Sprague Dawley rats: A 24 month study. *Teratog Carcinog Mutagen* **14**, 239–249.

27. Valdes, S., Arruzazabala, M. L., Fernandez, L., Mas, R., Carbajal, D., Aleman, C. & Molina, V. (1996). Effect of policosanol on platelet aggregation in healthy volunteers. *Int J Clin Pharmacol Res* **16**, 67–72.

28. Rodriguez, M. D. & Garcia, H. (1998). Evaluation of peri- and post-natal toxicity of policosanol in rats. *Teratog Carcinog Mutagen,* **18**, 1–7.

29. Batista, J., Stusser, R., Saez, F. & Perez, B. (1996). Effect of policosanol on hyperlipidemia and coronary heart disease in middle-aged patients. A 14-month pilot study. *Int J Clin Pharmacol Ther* **34**, 134–137.

30. Brunton, L. L., Lazo, J. S. & Parker, K. L. (2006). *Goodman & Gilman's the Pharmacological Basis of Therapeutics*, 11th ed., McGraw-Hill, New York.

31. Katzung, B. G. (2004). *Basic and Clinical Pharmacology*, 9th ed., McGraw-Hill, Stamford, CT.

32. Molina Cuevas, V., Arruzazabala, M. L., Carbajal Quintana, D., Mas Ferreiro, R. & Valdes Garcia, S. (1998). Effect of policosanol on arterial blood pressure in rats. Study of the pharmacological interaction with nifedipine and propranolol. *Arch Med Res* **29**, 21–24.

33. Chen, J. T., Wesley, R., Shamburek, R. D., Pucino, F. & Csako, G. (2005). Meta-analysis of natural therapies for hyperlipidemia: Plant sterols and stanols versus policosanol. *Pharmacotherapy* **25**, 171–183.

34. Lin, Y., Rudrum, M., van der Wielen, R. P. J., Trautwein, E. A., McNeill, G., Sierksma, A. & Meijer, G. W. (2004). Wheat germ policosanol failed to lower plasma cholesterol in subjects with normal to mildly elevated cholesterol concentrations. *Metabolism* **53**, 1309–1314.

35. Castano, G., Fernandez, L., Mas, R., Illnait, J., Gamez, R., Mendoza, S., Mesa, M. & Fernandez, J. (2005). Effects of addition of policosanol to omega-3 fatty acid therapy on the lipid profile of patients with type II hypercholesterolaemia. *Drugs R D* **6**, 207–219.

36. Castano, G., Mas, R., Fernandez, L., Illnait, J., Mendoza, S., Gamez, R., Fernandez, J. & Mesa, M. (2005). A comparison of the effects of D-003 and

policosanol (5 and 10 mg/day) in patients with type II hypercholesterolemia: A randomized, double-blinded study. *Drugs Exp Clin Res* **31**(Suppl), 31–44.

37. Reiner, Z., Tedeschi-Reiner, E. & Romic, Z. (2005). Effects of rice policosanol on serum lipoproteins, homocysteine, fibrinogen, and C-reactive protein in hypercholesterolemic patients. *Clin Drug Invest* **25**, 701–707.
38. Wright, C. M., Zielke, J. C. & Whayne, T. F. (2005). Policosanol, an aliphatic alcohol sugarcane derivative: Use in patients intolerant of or inadequately responsive to statin therapy. *Int J Angiology* **13**, 173–175.
39. Berthold, H. K., Unverdorben, S., Degenhardt, R., Bulitta, M. & Gouni-Berthold, I. (2006). Effect of policosanol on lipid levels among patients with hypercholesterolemia or combined hyperlipidemia: A randomized controlled trial. *JAMA* **295**, 2262–2269.
40. Castano, G., Arruzazabala, M. L., Fernandez, L., Mas, R., Carbajal, D., Molina, V., Illnait, J., Mendoza, S., Gamez, R., Mesa, M. & Fernandez, J. (2006). Effects of combination treatment with policosanol and omega-3 fatty acids on platelet aggregation: A randomized, double-blind clinical trial. *Curr Ther Res* **67**, 174–192.
41. Cubeddu, L. X., Cubeddu, R. J., Heimowitz, T., Restrepo, B., Lamas, G. A. & Weinberg, G. B. (2006). Comparative lipid-lowering effects of policosanol and atorvastatin: A randomized, parallel, double-blind, placebo-controlled trial. *Am Heart J* **152**, 982e1–982e5.
42. Dulin, M. F., Hatcher, L. F., Sasser, H. C. & Barringer, T. A. (2006). Policosanol is ineffective in the treatment of hypercholesterolemia: A randomized controlled trial. *Am J Clin Nutr* **84**, 1543–1548.
43. Greyling, A., DeWitt, C., Oosthuizen, W. & Jerling, J. C. (2006). Effects of a policosanol supplement on serum lipid concentrations in hypercholesterolaemic and heterozygous familial hypercholesterolaemic subjects. *Br J Nutr* **95**, 968–975.
44. Kassis, A. M. & Jones, P. J. H. (2006). Lack of cholesterol-lowering efficacy of Cuban sugar cane policosanols in hypercholesterolemic persons. *Am J Clin Nutr* **84**, 1003–1008.
45. Cicero, A. F. G., Rovati, L. C. & Setnikar, I. (2007). Eulipidemic effects of berberine administered alone or in combination with other natural cholesterol-lowering agents: A single-blind clinical investigation. *Arzneimittel-Forschung* **57**, 26–30.
46. Murota, K., Kawada, T., Matsui, N., Sakakibara, M., Takahashi, N. & Fushiki, T. (2000). Oleyl alcohol inhibits intestinal long-chain fatty acid absorption in rats. *J Nutr Sci Vitaminol* **2000**, 302–308.
47. Castano, G., Canetti, M., Moreira, M., Tula, L., Mas, R., Illnait, J., Fernandez, L., Fernandez, J. C. & Diaz, E. (1995). Efficacy and tolerability of policosanol in elderly patients with type II hypercholesterolemia: A 12-month study. *Curr Ther Res* **56**, 819–828.
48. Ortensi, G., Julio, G., Hector, V. & Pedro, A. T. (1997). A comparative study of policosanol versus simvastatin in elderly patients with hypercholesterolemia. *Curr Ther Res* **58**, 390–401.
49. Castano, G., Mas, R., Arruzazabala, M. L., Noa, M., Illnait, J., Fernandez, J. C., Molina, V. & Menendez, A. (1999). Effects of policosanol and pravastatin on lipid profile, platelet aggregation and endothelemia in older hypercholesterolemic patients. *Int J Clin Pharmacol Res* **19**, 105–116.

50. Castano, G., Mas, R., Fernandez, J. C., Illnait, J., Fernandez, L. & Alvarez, E. (2001). Effects of policosanol in older patients with type II hypercholesterolemia and high coronary risk. *J Gerontol A Biol Sci Med Sci* **56**, M186–M192.

51. Mas, R., Castano, G., Fernandez, L., Illnait, J., Fernandez, J. & Alvarez, E. (2001). Effects of policosanol on lipid profile and cardiac events in older hypercholesterolemic patients with coronary disease. *Clin Drug Invest* **21**, 485–497.

52. Castano, G., Mas, R., Fernandez, J. C., Fernandez, L., Illnait, J. & Lopez, E. (2002). Effects of policosanol on older patients with hypertension and type II hypercholesterolemia. *Drugs R D* **3**, 159–172.

53. Castano, G., Mas, R., Fernandez, L., Illnait, J., Mesa, M., Alvarez, E. & Lezcay, M. (2003). Comparison of the efficacy and tolerability of policosanol with atorvastatin in elderly patients with type II hypercholesterolemia. *Drugs Aging* **20**, 153–163.

54. Castano, G., Mas, R., Gamez, R., Fernandez, J., Illnait, J., Fernandez, L., Mendoza, S., Mesa, M., Gutierrez, J. A. & Lopez, E. (2004). Concomitant use of policosanol and beta-blockers in older patients. *Int J Clin Pharmacol Res* **24**, 65–77.

55. Fernandez, S., Mas, R., Gamez, R., Arquimedes, D., Fernandez, J., Orta, S. D., Illnait, J., Castano, G., Mendoza, S., Valdes, F. & Alvarez, E. (2004). A pharmacological surveillance study of the tolerability of policosanol in the elderly population. *Am J Geriatr Pharmacother* **2**, 219–229.

56. United States House of Representatives Committee on Government Reform (2005). New Medicare drug plans fail to provide meaningful drug discount prices.

57. Bellosta, S., Paoletti, R. & Corsini, A. (2004). Safety of statins: Focus on clinical pharmacokinetics and drug interactions. *Circulation* **109**(Suppl III), III-50–III-57.

58. Weiss, J., Dormann, S. M. G., Martin-Facklam, M., Kerpen, C. J., Ketabi-Kiyanvash, N. & Haefeli, W. E. (2003). Inhibition of P-glycoprotein by newer antidepressants. *J Pharmacol Exp Ther* **305**, 197–204.

59. Davignon, J. (2004). Beneficial cardiovascular pleiotropic effects of statins. *Circulation* **109**(Suppl III), III-39–III-43.

60. Vaughn, C. J. (2003). Prevention of stroke and dementia with statins: Effects beyond lipid lowering. *Am J Cardiol* **91**, 23B–29B.

61. Jick, H., Zornberg, G. L., Jick, S. S., Seshadri, S. & Drachman, D. A. (2000). Statins and the risk of dementia. *Lancet* **356**, 1627–1631.

62. Young-Xu, Y., Chan, K. A., Liao, J. K., Ravid, S. & Blatt, C. M. (2003). Long-term statin use and psychological well-being. *J Am Coll Cardiol* **42**, 690–697.

63. Alsheikh-Ali, A. A., Maddukuri, P. V., Han, H. & Karas, R. H. (2007). Effect of the magnitude of lipid lowering on risk of elevated liver enzymes, rhabdomyolysis, and cancer: Insights from large randomized statin trials. *J Am Coll Cardiol* **50**, 409–418.

64. Dale, K. M., Coleman, C. I., Henyan, N. N., Kluger, J. & White, C. M. (2006). Statins and cancer risk: A meta-analysis. *JAMA* **295**, 74–80.

65. Poynter, J. N., Gruber, S. B., Higgins, P. D., Almog, R., Bonner, J. D., Rennert, H. S., Low, M., Greenson, J. K. & Rennert, G. (2005). Statins and the risk of colorectal cancer. *N Engl J Med* **352**, 2184–2192.

Chapter 8

Health Promoting Benefits of Chamomile in the Elderly Population

Janmejai K. Srivastava[1,2] and Sanjay Gupta[1,2,3]

[1]Department of Urology and Nutrition, Case Western Reserve University, Cleveland, Ohio, USA
[2]Department of Urology and Nutrition, University Hospitals Case Medical Center, Cleveland, Ohio, USA
[3]Department of Urology and Nutrition, Case Comprehensive Cancer Center, Cleveland, Ohio, USA

Abstract

Chamomile is the oldest known medicinal herb in the Western world. German Chamomile (*Chamomilla recutita*) and Roman Chamomile (*Chamaemelum nobile*) are the two most common varieties used for traditional medicine. The dried flowers of chamomile contain many terpenoids and flavonoids which are thought to contribute to the wide spectrum of medicinal effects attributed to chamomile. Chamomile preparations are commonly used for many human ailments such as hay fever, inflammation, muscle spasms, menstrual disorders, insomnia, ulcers, wounds, gastrointestinal disorders, rheumatic pain, hemorrhoids, and worm infestations. Essential oils of chamomile are used extensively in cosmetics and aromatherapy. Many different preparations of chamomile have been developed, the most popular of which is an herbal tea: more than 1 million cups of chamomile tea are consumed daily worldwide. On the basis of its longstanding widespread use in traditional medicine, chamomile has attracted considerable attention in the field of biomedical research, with regard to evaluating its curative, preventative and health-promoting properties. In addition to basic scientific research into its properties, a limited number of clinical trials have been completed or are underway currently to evaluate its usefulness in the management of inflammatory disorders, cardiovascular conditions, diarrhea, eczema, hemorrhagic cystitis, mucositis, osteoporosis, sleep disorders, sore throat, and wound healing, and to assess possible quality-of-life improvement in cancer patients and in the elderly population.

Keywords: *Chamomile, dietary agents, flavonoids, polyphenols*

Abbreviations: ACTH, Adrenocorticotropic hormone; ASA, American Society of Anesthesiologists; CAM, Complementary and alternative medicine; ESCOP, European

Scientific Cooperative for Phytotherapy; 5-FU, 5-fluorouracil; SERM, Selective estrogen receptor modulators; REM, Rapid eye movement

INTRODUCTION

The interplay of plants and human health has been documented for thousands of years [1–6]. Herbs have been integral to both traditional and non-traditional forms of medicine dating back at least 5000 years [2, 7–9]. The enduring popularity of herbal medicines may be explained by the tendency of herbs to work slowly, usually with minimal toxic side effects. This non-traditional practice of medicine has been relegated to the category of complementary and alternative medicine (CAM) [10]. The term CAM refers to therapies provided as an adjunct to mainstream medicine and intended to provide symptom relief and to improve quality of life. CAM may be a desirable addition and balance to technologically sophisticated disease care [11]. CAM therapies are often unsupported by scientific data, and some cases may produce adverse effects due to inherent toxicities [11–14]. Nonetheless, the majority of CAM therapies are beneficial to patients [15, 16]. Another important reason for the popularity of CAM is that they are usually much less costly than conventional medical treatments [17]. As many as 5% of individuals rely primarily on CAM. In a study of the use of CAM among elderly persons, it was learned that 41% of seniors reported the use of CAM to their primary care physicians. The most frequently used CAM therapies include the use of herbs (24%), chiropractic treatments (20%), massage therapy (15%), and acupuncture (14%), respectively. In this study 80% of the seniors reported that they had received substantial benefit from the use of various CAM therapies [18]. In this chapter we will discuss the use and possible merits of a common herb, chamomile, examining its historical use and recent scientific evaluations of its potential use in the management of various human ailments.

HISTORY OF CHAMOMILE

Chamomile is one of the oldest, most widely used and well documented medicinal plants in the world and has been recommended for a variety of healing applications [19]. It was described as one of the herbs of choice of Asclepiades, a physician who lived in Bithynia around 90 BC. Pliny the Elder, one of the most famous of Roman naturalists who wrote extensively on herb use, gave over his medical care to Asclepiades, because he was so skillful in prescribing herbs [20]. The history of chamomile dates even further back, at least to the time of the ancient Egyptians, when it was dedicated to their Gods for cure for the "Ague" (acute fever). Since then chamomile has been considered to be a wonderful plant and a universal cure of almost all common ailments of human beings. Today it is one of the most widely used ingredients in herbal teas worldwide [21]. It has been estimated that, on average, more than 1 million cups of chamomile tea are consumed worldwide each day [22]. As a popular remedy, chamomile may be thought of as the "European counterpart of ginseng," according to Varro Tyler, a renowned German clinician and expert in herbal medicine who call it *alles zutraut* – "capable of anything" [23]. Historically, chamomile was also known as "The Plant Doctor," because of its ability to encourage other plants to increase their essential oil content to smell stronger and more vital [24–27].

PLANT DESCRIPTION AND NOMENCLATURE

Chamomile is a native of the old World and is related to the daisy family (*Asteraceae* or *Compositae*) [28]. The hollow, bright gold cones of the flowers are packed with disc or tubular florets and are ringed with about fifteen white ray or ligulate florets, widely represented by two known varieties *viz.* German chamomile (*Matricaria chamomilla*) and Roman chamomile (*Chamaemelum nobile*) [29]. German chamomile is a sweet-scented, smooth plant and self-seeding annual herb. It is native to Europe and Western Asia, and has become widely distributed over Europe, North Africa, and the temperate region of Asia [30, 31]. Synonyms of German chamomile include *Chamomilla chamomilla*, *Chamomilla recutita*, *Matricaria chamomilla*, *and Matricaria suaveolens*. German chamomile in particular is the most common variety used for medicinal purposes. Roman chamomile is an aromatic, creeping perennial, found in dry fields and around gardens and cultivated grounds. It originated in the United Kingdom and is widely grown in American herb gardens. Roman chamomile is also known as *Anthemis nobilis*, camomile, garden camomile, ground apple, low camomile, or whig plant [32]. Chamomile was one of the first herbs evaluated and characterized by the European Scientific Cooperative for Phytotherapy (ESCOP), a coalition of scientific organizations formed to develop "harmonized" herb regulations in Europe. ESCOP produces comprehensive scientific reviews and suggested regulatory texts for herb use [33].

CHEMICAL CONSTITUENTS OF CHAMOMILE

Different classes of active constituents are present in chamomile, which have been isolated and used as medicinal preparations and cosmetics [34]. The plant contains 0.24–1.9% volatile oil, composed of a variety of separate oils. When exposed to steam distillation, the oil ranges in color from brilliant blue to deep green when fresh but turns to dark yellow after storage. Despite fading, the oil does not lose its potency. Approximately 120 secondary metabolites have been identified in chamomile, including 28 terpenoids and 36 flavonoids [33, 35–37]. The principal components of the essential oil extracted from the German chamomile flowers are the terpenoids α-bisabolol and its oxide azulenes including chamazulene and acetylene derivatives. Chamazulene and bisabolol are very unstable and are best preserved in an alcoholic tincture. The essential

oil of Roman chamomile contains less chamazulene and is mainly constituted from esters of angelic acid and tiglic acid. It also contains farnesene and
α-pinene. Roman chamomile contains up to 0.6% of sesquiterpene lactones of
the germacranolide type, mainly nobilin and 3-epinobilin. Both α-bisabolol,
bisabolol oxides A and B and chamazulene or azulenesse, farnesene and spiro-
ether quiterpene lactones, glycosides, hydroxycoumarins, flavanoids (apigenin,
luteolin, patuletin, and quercetin), coumarins (herniarin and umbelliferone),
terpenoids, and mucilage are considered to be the major bio-active ingredients
[38, 39]. Other major constituents of the flowers include several phenolic compounds, primarily the flavonoids apigenin, quercetin, patuletin as glucosides
and various acetylated derivatives. Among flavonoids, apigenin is the most
promising compound. It is present in very small quantities as free apigenin,
but predominantly exists in the form of various glycosides [40–44]. Some of
the important flavonoids identified in matricaria, such as apigenin, luteolin and
apiin, are also found in Roman chamomile, as are phenolic carboxylic acids
(caffeic, ferulic), coumarins and thiophene derivatives.

CHAMOMILE PREPARATIONS AND THEIR COMMON USES

Dry Powder of Heads

Dry powder of chamomile flower is recommended and used by many people
for traditionally established health problems. The recommended dose to achieve
therapeutic effect for adults is 2–4 g dry flower head powder 3 times daily
[45, 46].

Standardized Extract

Standardized extracts are technically and scientifically advanced herbal products. Standardization of an extract assures specific measurable levels of the
important compounds that give the product their beneficial activity [47].
Medicinal ingredients are normally extracted from the dry flowers of chamomile
by using water, ethanol, or methanol as solvents and corresponding extracts are
known as aqueous, ethanolic (alcoholic) and/or methanolic extracts. The quality
of extracts also depends on the concentrations of alcohol since water increases
the degree of enzymatic degradation. Optimum chamomile extracts in Germany
contain about 50% alcohol. Normally standardized extracts contain 1.2% of
apigenin which is one of the most effective bioactive agents. Aqueous extracts,
such as in the form of tea, contain quite low concentrations of free apigenin but
contain high levels of apigenin-7-O-glucoside. Methanol extraction provides a
better yield of apigenin; however, due to toxicity, the resulting extract can not
be used for medical purposes. The optimum extraction is achieved with 50–70%
alcohol to water, which provides the highest yield of apigenin glycosides [48].
A chamomile extract prepared from fresh flowers contains little or no apigenin.

Oral Infusion

The German Commission E dose for preparing chamomile infusion is 150 ml of boiling water poured over approximately 3 g dried flowers and steeped covered for 5–10 minutes. However, the official Swiss Tea infusion dose for the same indication is 900 mg of dried chamomile flowers [49–50].

Tea Preparation

Chamomile tea is one of the world's most popular herbal teas and about a million cups are consumed every day [51–53]. Basically, chamomile tea and chamomile infusion represent the same entity. Nowadays the word "tea" is more popular because chamomile is available in stores as "chamomile tea packs." Tea bags of chamomile are also available in the market, containing chamomile flower powder, either pure or blended with other popular medicinal herbs. According to studies by Holtzel, chamomile tea contains only 10% of the essential oil compounds and about 30% of the flavonoids. Normally dry flowers, rinsed with cold water, are added to a pot of boiling hot water. The pot is covered for 5 minutes to get the tea extracted; other herbs or fruits can be added for additional nutritional/medicinal value. Honey or sugar may be added to the tea to sweeten it. Chamomile tea should always be prepared in a covered vessel, in order to prevent the escape of steam, as the medicinal value of the flowers is to a considerable extent impaired by any evaporation.

Tincture

Chamomile tincture is prepared by mixing one part of chamomile flowers with 5 parts of 45% ethanol (w/v). The tincture can be used to correct summer diarrhea in children. Chamomile is also used with purgatives to prevent cramping. The tincture may also be prepared as one part chamomile flower in four parts of water having 12% grain alcohol [54]. The suggested dose of this preparation is 6–12 drops from 1–3 times a day. The extract, in doses of 10–15 grains, combined with myrrh and preparations of iron, also affords a powerful and convenient tonic in the form of a pill. The fluid extract of flowers is taken in doses of from 3 to 4 g; in the oil dose of 1/2 to 3 drops.

Poultice

Chamomile flowers are also extensively used alone, or combined with crushed poppy-heads, as a poultice or hot foment for inflammatory pain or congestive neuralgia, and in cases of external swelling, such as facial swelling associated with underlying infection or abscess. A suggested mixture consists of 10 parts of Chamomile flowers to 5 of poppy capsules with 100 of distilled water.

Bags may be loosely stuffed with flowers and steeped well in boiling water before being applied as a foment. The antiseptic powers of chamomile are stated to be 120 times stronger than sea-water [55].

Herb Beers and Lotion

The *whole herb* is used chiefly for making herb beers, but also for a lotion, for external application in toothache, earache, neuralgia, etc. One ounce of the dried herb is infused in 1 pint of boiling water and allowed to cool. The herb has also been employed in hot fomentations in cases of local and intestinal inflammation [55].

Bath Additive

50 g dried flower added per 10 liters (2.5 gallons) water. The water is used for a bath, and is recommended for soothing ano-genital inflammation [55, 56]. Use of soap during the bath is not advisable, as it will coat the skin and not allow the chamomile to penetrate.

Gargle

3–10 g of dry chamomile flower added to 100 ml boiling water and steeped covered, for 5–10 minutes [56]. The tea infusion is used as a wash or gargle for inflammation of the mucous membranes of the mouth and throat; an alternative mixture is 5 ml tincture poured into 100 ml warm water and gargled 3 or more times daily [57].

Inhalation

100 ml boiling water poured over 3–10 g dried flower and steeped, covered, for 5–10 minutes or 15 ml tincture poured into 0.5 liter boiled water, 1–3 times daily. Steam vapor inhaled for inflammation of the upper respiratory tract [56, 57].

Chamomile Wine

Chamomile wine is recommended for relieving upset stomach and is prepared by adding one handful of dried flowers to one bottle of white wine and allowing to steep for 7–10 days. After filtration, it is stored; a one tablespoonful dose is administered for upset stomach.

Chamomile Vapor Bath

This is used to manage lower abdomen problems, including menstrual cramps and various irritations of the anus and genitals. A hot chamomile infusion prepared from one cup of dry flowers and 1 quart water (1 US quart = 946.35 ml) is used to create a vapor bath in a shallow basin. The patient then sits over the steam, wrapped with a blanket to create a tent. Strict precautions around hot liquids are required to avoid burns. Alternatively, a cloth or towel soaked with the hot preparation can be applied to the affected area.

Homeopathic Medicine

Chamomile has many applications in the homeopathic system of medicine. Its use is often recommended for a variety of conditions, including child teething, irritability, over-sensitiveness from abuse of coffee and narcotics, pains, numbness, night-sweats, acidity, anger, asthma (with psychological basis), congestion, colic, convulsions, cramp, diarrhea, dsymenorrhea, dyspepsia, earache, fainting, fever, flatulence, gout, headache, hernia, flu, jaundice, mastitis, miscarriage, mumps, neuralgia, peritonitis, problem pregnancy, rheumatism, sciatica, ulcers, hysteria, whooping cough, etc. Chamomile is sometimes recommended for fever of unknown origin in children with one cheek red and other pale, the child is restless, thirsty, and irritable [58].

Aromatherapy and Massage Oil

Inhalation of the vaporized essential oils derived from chamomile flowers is recommended to relieve anxiety, general depression and depression associated with menopause, irritability, insomnia, hysteria, and hypersensitivity. For massage purposes, 3 oz of dried flowers are mixed with 1½ pints of olive or sweet almond or other suitable vegetable oil, placed in a glass jar, and kept in the sun for 2 weeks or more. This oil can be used for body massage for facials, masks, compresses, body wraps, bath, and hair care [59, 60].

Cosmetic Preparations

Roman chamomile is used widely in cosmetic preparations. It has a soothing and softening effect on the skin and has been used for centuries in hair preparations (shampoos and rinses) particularly for blond hair which it is said to both lighten and condition. Likewise, the water soluble fractions of the essential oil dissolved in the condensed steam from the distillation process can be utilized directly in cosmetic preparations that involve a water base, such as soaps, shampoos, and creams. This is known sometimes as "Floral Water" or "Distillation Water" of Chamomile [61–63].

Dosage Recommendation

Chamomile may be used medicinally in many forms. As an infusion, 2–3 teaspoonfuls of fresh or dried flower heads are placed in a cup of boiling water, infused for 10 minutes and taken orally three times a day. As a tincture,

1–4 ml of tincture preparations can be diluted in a cup of spring or filtered water and taken orally 3 times a day. The same preparation can be used externally as a fomentation. An infusion of 1 teaspoonful of flower heads can be given to children for pain of dentition, stomachache, earache, or neuralgic pain. In aromatherapy the essential oil of chamomile is a valued part of blended preparations and is also used as a component of massage oils [64].

USE OF CHAMOMILE IN TRADITIONAL PRACTICE

Traditionally, chamomile has been used for centuries as an anti-inflammatory, antioxidant, mild astringent, and healing medicine [65, 66]. As a traditional medicine, it is used to treat wounds, ulcers, eczema, gout, skin irritations, bruises, burns, canker sores, neuralgia, sciatica, rheumatic pain, hemorrhoids, mastitis, and other ailments [67–69]. Externally, chamomile has been used to treat diaper rash, cracked nipples, chicken pox, ear and eye infections, disorders of the eyes including blocked tear ducts, conjunctivitis, nasal inflammation, and poison ivy [70, 71]. Chamomile is widely used to treat inflammations of the skin and mucous membranes, and for various bacterial infections of the skin, oral cavity and gums, and respiratory tract. Chamomile in the form of an aqueous extract has been frequently used as a mild sedative to calm nerves and reduce anxiety, to treat hysteria, nightmares, insomnia, and other sleep problems [72]. Chamomile has been valued as a digestive relaxant and has been used to treat various gastrointestinal disturbances including flatulence, indigestion, diarrhea, anorexia, motion sickness, nausea, and vomiting [68, 73]. Other purported actions of this herb include anti-ulcer, anti-bacterial, liver stimulatory, and anti-mycotic effects. Chamomile has also been used to treat colic, croup, and fevers in children [74, 75]. It has been used as an emmenagogue and a uterine tonic in women. It is also effective in arthritis, back pain, bedsores, and stomach cramps. Chamomile's essential oil is also used as a treatment for malaria and parasitic worm infections, cystitis, as well as cold and flu symptoms [76–78].

USE OF CHAMOMILE BASED ON SCIENTIFIC EVIDENCE

Common Cold

Common cold (acute viral nasopharyngitis) is the most common human disease. It is a mild viral infectious disease of the upper respiratory system. Common cold usually lasts not more than 3 or 5 days with residual coughing and catarrh lasting approximately for 3 weeks. Typically common cold is not life-threatening, although its complications (such as pneumonia) can lead to death, if not properly treated [79, 80]. Studies indicate that inhaling steam with chamomile extract has been helpful in common cold symptoms; however, further research is needed to confirm these findings.

Cardiovascular Conditions

It has been suggested that regular use of flavonoids consumed in food may reduce the risk of death from coronary heart disease in elderly men [81]. A study assessed the flavonoid intake of 805 men aged 65–84 years who were followed up for 5 years [81]. Flavonoid intake (analyzed in tertiles) was significantly inversely associated with mortality from coronary heart disease (p for trend $= 0.015$) and showed an inverse relation with incidence of myocardial infarction, which was of borderline significance (p for trend $= 0.08$). The relative risk of coronary heart disease mortality in the highest versus the lowest tertile of flavonoid intake was 0.42 (95% CI 0.20–0.88), suggesting that flavonoid intake is inversely related to coronary heart disease mortality. In another study [82], on 12 patients with cardiac disease who underwent cardiac catheterization, hemodynamic measurements obtained prior to and 30 minutes after the oral ingestion of chamomile tea exhibited a small but significant increase in the mean brachial artery pressure. No other significant hemodynamic changes were observed after chamomile consumption. Ten of the 12 patients fell into a deep sleep shortly after drinking the beverage. A large, well-designed randomized controlled trial is needed to assess the potential value of chamomile in improving cardiac health.

Colic/Diarrhea Conditions

An apple pectin-chamomile extract may help shorten the course of diarrhea in children as well as relieve symptoms associated with the condition [83]. Two clinical trials have evaluated the efficacy of chamomile for the treatment of colic in children. Chamomile tea was combined with other herbs (German chamomile, vervain, licorice, fennel, balm mint) for administration. In a prospective, randomized, double-blind, placebo-controlled study, 68 healthy term infants who had colic (2–8 weeks old) received either herbal tea or placebo (glucose, flavoring). Each infant was offered treatment with every bout of colic, up to 150 ml/dose, no more than 3 times a day. After 7 days of treatment, parents reported that the tea eliminated the colic in 57% of the infants, whereas placebo was helpful in only 26% ($p < 0.01$). No adverse effects with regard to the number of nighttime awakenings were noted in either group [84]. In another randomized, double-blind, placebo-controlled trial, a standardized herbal preparation containing chamomile (71.1 mg/kg/day), fennel (65.7 mg/kg/day), and balm mint (38.8 mg/kg/day) was compared with a placebo in the management of colic in infants. Daily administration of the herbal preparation for 1 week reduced crying time among breastfed infants ($n = 41$) compared with a placebo ($n = 47$, $p < 0.005$). Significant results were attained within 4 days of treatment, and no side effects were observed with this dosage. Another study examined the effects of a chamomile extract and apple pectin preparation in 79 children (age 0.5–5.5 years) with acute, non-complicated diarrhea who received either the chamomile/pectin preparation ($n = 39$) or a placebo

($n = 40$) for 3 days. Diarrhea ended sooner in children treated with chamomile and pectin (85%), than in the placebo group (58%). The duration of the diarrhea was also significantly shortened by the administration of the chamomile and pectin treatment. These results provide evidence that chamomile can be used safely to treat infant colic disorders [85].

Eczema

The use of chamomile by topical application for diseases of the skin has been authorized by the German Commission E. Topical applications of chamomile have been shown to be moderately effective in the treatment of atopic eczema [86, 87]. It was found to be about 60% as effective as 0.25% hydrocortisone cream [88]. Roman chamomile of the Manzana type (Kamillosan®) may ease discomfort associated with eczema when applied as a cream containing chamomile extract. The Manzana type of chamomile is rich in active ingredients and does not exhibit chamomile-related allergenic potential [89]. In a partially double-blind, randomized study carried out as a half-side comparison, Kamillosan® cream was compared with 0.5% hydrocortisone cream and a placebo consisting only of vehicle cream in patients suffering from medium-degree atopic eczema [90]. After 2 weeks of treatment, Kamillosan® cream showed a slight superiority over 0.5% hydrocortisone and a marginal difference as compared to placebo. Further research is needed to evaluate the usefulness of topical chamomile in managing eczema.

Gastrointestinal Conditions

Chamomile is used traditionally for numerous gastrointestinal conditions, including digestive disorders, "spasm" or colic, upset stomach, flatulence (gas), ulcers, and gastrointestinal irritation [91, 92]. Chamomile is said to be especially helpful in dispelling gas, soothing the stomach, and relaxing the muscles that move food through the intestines. Chamomile tea is often recommended to treat nausea and vomiting, in the form of one to two teaspoons of dried or fresh chamomile leaves steeped in one cup of hot water for 5–10 minutes, sweetened as needed with honey, and consumed in the morning and after dinner [93]. The protective effect of a commercial preparation (STW 5, Iberogast), containing the extracts of bitter candy tuft, lemon balm leaf, chamomile flower, caraway fruit, peppermint leaf, liquorice root, Angelica root, milk thistle fruit and greater celandine herb, against the development of gastric ulcers has been previously reported [94]. STW 5 extracts produced a dose dependent anti-ulcerogenic effect associated with a reduced acid output, an increased mucin secretion, an increase in prostaglandin E(2) release and a decrease in leukotrienes. The results obtained demonstrated that STW 5 not only lowered gastric acidity as effectively as a commercial antacid, but was more effective in inhibiting secondary hyperacidity [94].

Hemorrhagic Cystitis Conditions

It has been reported that the combination of chamomile baths, chamomile bladder washes and antibiotics is superior to antibiotics alone for hemorrhagic cystitis. Anti-inflammatory agents that have been reported to be useful for the treatment of cystitis include chamomile, ginger, marshmallow, and Echinacea. Treatment takes the form of hot chamomile compresses applied over the bladder, or a chamomile hip or sitz bath [95].

Hemorrhoids

Studies suggest that chamomile ointment may improve hemorrhoids. Tinctures of chamomile can also be used in a sitz bath format. Tincture of Roman chamomile may reduce inflammation associated with hemorrhoids [96, 97].

Health Promotion

It has been claimed that consumption of chamomile tea boosts the immune system and helps fight infections associated with colds. The health promoting benefits of chamomile was assessed in a study which involved 14 volunteers who each drank 5 cups of the herbal tea daily for 2 consecutive weeks. Daily urine samples were taken and tested throughout the study, both before and after drinking chamomile tea. Drinking chamomile was associated with a significant increase in urinary levels of hippurate and glycine, which have been associated with increased antibacterial activity. Levels of both hippurate and glycine remained elevated for up to 2 weeks after the study participants stopped drinking the tea, indicating that the compounds may remain active for quite some time [98]. Additional studies are needed before a more definitive link between chamomile and its alleged health benefits can be established.

Inflammatory Conditions

Inflammation is associated with many gastrointestinal disorders complaints, such as esophageal reflux, diverticular disease, and inflammatory bowel disease [99–101]. Studies in preclinical models suggest that chamomile inhibits *Helicobacter pylori*, the bacteria that can contribute to stomach ulcers [102]. However, few studies in humans have evaluated chamomile's effects, and there is no evidence that it speeds the healing of gastric ulcers. Chamomile is believed to be helpful in reducing smooth muscle spasms associated with various gastrointestinal inflammatory disorders. Chamomile is often used to treat mild skin irritations, including sunburn, rashes, sores, and even eye inflammations [103–107], but its value in treating these conditions has not been shown with evidence-based research.

Mucositis

Mouth ulcers are a common condition with a variety of etiologies [108]. Stomatitis is a major dose-limiting toxicity from bolus 5-fluorouracil-based (5-FU) chemotherapy regimens. A double-blind, placebo-controlled clinical trial including 164 patients was conducted [109]. Patients were entered into the study at the time of their first cycle of 5-FU-based chemotherapy. All patients received oral cryotherapy for 30 minutes with each dose of 5-FU. In addition, each patient was randomized to receive a chamomile or placebo mouthwash thrice daily for 14 days. There was no suggestion of any stomatitis difference between patients randomized to either protocol arm. There was also no suggestion of toxicity. Subset analysis did reveal unsuspected differential effects between males and females that could not be explained by reasons other than chance. This suggested that a chamomile mouthwash might ameliorate this toxicity, and a prospective trial was developed to test chamomile in this situation. Data obtained from this clinical trial did not support the pre study hypothesis that chamomile could decrease 5-FU-induced stomatitis. The results of other similar studies are conflicting, and it remains unclear if chamomile is helpful in this situation.

Osteoporosis

Osteoporosis is a metabolic bone disease resulting from low bone mass (osteopenia) due to excessive bone resorption. Sufferers are prone to bone fractures from relatively minor trauma. Agents which include selective estrogen receptor modulators or SERMs, biphosphonates, calcitonin are frequently used to prevent bone loss. To prevent bone loss that occurs with increasing age, chamomile extract was evaluated for its ability to stimulate the differentiation and mineralization of osteoblastic cells. Chamomile extract was shown to stimulate osteoblastic cell differentiation and to exhibit an anti-estrogenic effect, suggesting an estrogen receptor-related mechanism [110]. However, further studies are needed before it can be considered for clinical use.

Sleep Aid/Sedation

Traditionally, chamomile preparations such as tea and essential oil aromatherapy have been used to treat insomnia and to induce sedation (calming effects). Chamomile is widely regarded as a mild tranquillizer and sleep-inducer. Sedative effects may be due to the flavonoid, apigenin that binds to benzodiazepine receptors in the brain [111]. Studies in preclinical models have shown anticonvulsant and central nervous system (CNS) depressant effects respectively. Clinical trials are notable for their absence, although 10 cardiac patients are reported to have immediately fallen into a deep sleep lasting for 90 minutes after drinking chamomile tea [112]. Although randomized, placebo-controlled studies have been conducted to evaluate a few compounds, rigorous scientific data supporting a beneficial effect have not been found for the majority of available herbal or dietary supplements [113]. Studies are limited by small numbers of participants and, in some instances, inadequate design, lack of statistical analysis, and sparse use of objective measurements. Little or no scientific data is available to assess the efficacy of most products as hypnotics. Investigations on the hypnotic activities of chamomile and passiflora extracts using sleep-disturbed preclinical model demonstrated a significant decrease in sleep latency observed with chamomile extract at a dose of 300 mg/kg, while passiflora extract showed no effects on sleep latency even at a dose of 3000 mg/kg. No significant effects were observed with both herbal extracts on total times of wakefulness, non-rapid eye movement (non-REM) sleep, and REM sleep. Flumazenil, a benzodiazepine (BDZ) receptor antagonist, at a dose of 3 mg/kg showed a significant antagonistic effect on the shortening in sleep latency induced by chamomile extract. No significant effects were observed with chamomile and passiflora extracts on delta activity during non-REM sleep. In conclusion, chamomile extracts exhibit benzodiazepine-like hypnotic activity [114]. In another study, inhalation of the vapor of chamomile oil reduced a stress-induced increase in plasma adrenocorticotropic hormone (ACTH) levels. Diazepam, co-administered with the chamomile oil vapor, further reduced ACTH levels, while flumazenile, a BDZ antagonist blocked the effect of chamomile oil vapor on ACTH. According to Paladini *et al.* [115], the separation index (ratio between the maximal anxiolytic dose and the minimal sedative dose) for diazepam is 3 while for apigenin it is 10. Compounds, other than apigenin, present in extracts of chamomile can also bind BDZ and GABA (gamma-aminobutyric acid) receptors in the brain and are thought to be responsible for some of the sedative effect; however, many of these compounds are as yet unidentified.

Sore Throat/Hoarseness

The efficacy of lubrication of the endo-tracheal tube cuff with chamomile before intubation on postoperative sore throat and hoarseness was determined in a randomized double-blind study. One hundred and sixty one patients whose American Society of Anesthesiologists physical status was I or II, and undergoing elective surgical, orthopedic, gynecological or urological surgeries were divided in two groups. The study group received 10 puffs of chamomile extract (Kamillosan M spray, total 370 mg of chamomile extract) at the site of the cuff of the endotracheal tube for lubrication, while the control group did not receive any lubrication before intubations. Standard general anesthesia with tracheal intubations was given in both groups. Forty one out of 81 patients (50.6%) in the chamomile group reported no postoperative sore throat in the post-anesthesia care unit compared with 45 out of 80 patients (56.3%) in the control group. Postoperative sore throat and hoarseness both in the post-anesthesia care unit and at 24 hours post-operation were not statistically different. Lubrication of endo-tracheal tube cuff with chamomile extract spray before intubations can not prevent postoperative sore throat and hoarseness [116]. Similar results were obtained in another double-blind study [117].

Vaginitis

Vaginal inflammation is common in women of all ages. Vaginitis is associated with itching, vaginal discharge, or pain with urination. Atrophic vaginitis most commonly occurs in menopausal and postmenopausal women, and its occurrence is often associated with reduced levels of estrogen. Chamomile douche may improve symptoms of vaginitis with few side effects. Because infection (including sexually transmitted diseases), poor hygiene, or nutritional deficiencies can cause vaginitis, medical attention should be sought by people with this condition [118]. There is insufficient research data to allow conclusions concerning possible potential benefits of chamomile for this condition.

Wound Healing

The efficacy of topical use of chamomile to enhance wound healing was evaluated in a double-blind trial on 14 patients who underwent dermabrasion of tattoos. The effects on drying and epithelialization were observed, and chamomile was judged to be statistically efficacious in producing wound drying and in speeding epithelialization [119]. Another study evaluated the wound healing activity in animals using excision, incision, and production of dead space wounds. The test animals were treated with aqueous extract of *Matricaria recutita* (120 mg/kg/day) mixed in their drinking water where as the control animals were given plain drinking water. Healing was assessed by the rate of wound contraction, period of epithelialization, wound-breaking strength, granulation tissue weight and hydoxyproline content. Antimicrobial activity of the extract against various microorganisms was also assessed. The test group, on day 15, exhibited a greater reduction in the wound area when compared with the controls (61% versus 48%), faster epithelialization and a significantly higher wound-breaking strength ($p < 0.002$). In addition, wet and dry granulation tissue weight and hydroxyproline content were significantly higher. The increased rate of wound contraction, together with the increased wound-breaking strength, hydroxyproline content and histological observations, support the use of *M. recutita* in wound management [120]. However, further studies are needed before it can be considered for clinical use.

Anticancer Activity

Most evaluations of tumor growth inhibition by chamomile involve studies of apigenin, one of the bioactive constituents of chamomile. Studies on preclinical models of skin, prostate, breast, and ovarian cancer have shown promising growth inhibitory effects [121–128]. In a recently conducted study, chamomile extracts were shown to cause minimal growth inhibitory effects on normal cells, but showed significant reductions in cell viability in various human cancer cell lines. Chamomile exposure induced apoptosis in cancer cells but not in normal cells at similar doses [44]. Further investigations through well-deigned clinical studies of chamomile are warranted in evaluating the potential usefulness of this herbal remedy in the management of cancer patients.

Quality of Life in Cancer Patients

Essential oils obtained from Roman chamomile are the basic ingredients of aromatherapy. A recently conducted research study on cancer patients has assessed the positive effect of aromatherapy/massage on the psychological morbidity, distress, or quality of life [129]. The results suggested that the most consistent beneficial effect of massage or aromatherapy massage was on anxiety, with four of the trials (a total of 207 patients) reporting a reduction in anxiety. It is unclear whether aromatherapy, when added to massage therapy, provided additional benefit in reducing anxiety. Of three trials that examined depression in cancer patients, only one reported significant differences. Two trials reported a reduction in nausea and three reported a reduction in pain. Clinical trials of aromatherapy in cancer patients have shown no statistically significant differences between treated and untreated patients [130]. Another pilot study investigated the effects of aromatherapy massage on the anxiety and self-esteem experience in Korean elderly women. A quasi-experimental, control group, pretest–posttest design used 36 elderly females: 16 in the experimental group and 20 in the control group. Aromatherapy massage using lavender, chamomile, rosemary, and lemon was given to the experimental group only. Each massage session lasted 20 minutes, and was performed 3 times per week for two 3-week periods with an intervening 1-week break. The intervention produced significant differences in the anxiety and self-esteem and no significant differences in blood pressure or pulse rate between the two groups. These results suggest that aromatherapy massage exerts positive effects on anxiety and self-esteem [131–133]. However, more objective, clinical measures should be applied in a future study with a randomized placebo-controlled design.

ADVERSE EFFECTS, ALLERGIC REACTIONS, AND SAFETY ISSUES

A relatively low percentage of people are sensitive to chamomile and develop allergic reactions [134]. People sensitive to ragweed and chrysanthemums or other members of the *Compositae* family are more prone to develop contact allergies to chamomile, especially if they take other drugs that help to trigger the sensitization. A large-scale clinical trial was conducted in Hamburg, Germany, between 1985 and 1991 to study the development of contact dermatitis secondary to exposure to a mixture of components derived from the

Compositae family. Twelve species of the *Compositae* family, including German chamomile, were selected and tested individually when the mixture induced allergic reactions. During the study, 3851 individuals were tested using a patch with the plant extract [135]. Of these patients, 118 (3.1%) experienced an allergic reaction. Further tests revealed that feverfew elicited the most allergic reactions (70.1% of patients) followed by chrysanthemums (63.6%) and tansy (60.8%). Chamomile fell in the middle range (56.5%). A study involving 686 subjects exposed either to a sesquiterpene lactone mixture or a mixture of *Compositae* extracts led to allergic reactions in 4.5% of subjects [136]. In another study it was shown that eye washing with chamomile tea in hay fever patients who have conjunctivitis exacerbates the eye inflammation, whereas no worsening of eye inflammation was noted when chamomile tea was ingested orally [137]. There are rare reports of persons who experienced an anaphylactic reaction to ingestion of chamomile tea [138]. All such patients suffered from hay fever and one of them had bronchial asthma caused by a variety of pollens. One patient additionally ingested aspirin, which may have triggered the anaphylactic shock [139]. Chamomile is listed on the FDA's GRAS (generally recognized as safe) list. It has been reported that chamomile can cause severe allergic reactions in persons who are allergic to ragweed; however, there is no convincing data to show that chamomile is more allergenic than other known allergenic plant [140]. It is possible that some reports of allergic reactions to chamomile may be due to contamination of chamomile by "dog chamomile," a highly allergenic and bad-tasting plant of similar appearance. It is notable that coumarin, a natural blood thinner, is present in chamomile, and it has been reported that a patient taking therapeutic doses of warfarin and also ingesting chamomile experienced excessive "blood thinning," which led to internal bleeding [141]. Evidence of cross-reactivity of chamomile with other drugs is not well documented, and further study of this issue is needed prior to reaching conclusions. Safety in young children, pregnant or nursing women, or those with liver or kidney disease has not been established, although there have not been any credible reports of toxicity caused by this common beverage tea.

CONCLUSIONS

Chamomile has been used as an herbal medication since ancient times, is still popular today and probably will continue to be used in the future. Establishing whether or not CAM therapies are beneficial to patients will require research and generation of scientific evidence. Without such evidence, it will remain unclear whether these untested and unproven medical treatments are truly beneficial to patients. Clearly, some patients report improvements, but it remains unclear whether the improvements can be attributed to medication effect, spontaneous disease remission, or placebo effect. Scientists play an important role in conducting studies and in helping the public understand the benefits of CAM therapies. Very few CAM therapies have undergone rigorous scientific testing. Clinicians should await reports of well-conducted scientific research, including clinical studies of various herbs that clearly demonstrate the efficacy of CAM before recommending such treatments to their patients. Chamomile, a herb that has been familiar to practitioners and in common use for centuries in traditional herbal medicine, has recently been receiving attention from the scientific community with regard to more clearly defining its potential usefulness as a therapeutic entity for a variety of maladies.

ACKNOWLEDGMENTS

The original work from author's laboratory outlined in this chapter was supported by United States Public Health Service Grants RO1 CA108512 and RO1 AT002709.

REFERENCES

1. Newman, D. J., Cragg, G. M. & Snader, K. M. (2000). The influence of natural products upon drug discovery. *Nat Prod Rep.* **17**, 215–234.
2. Newman, D. J., Cragg, G. M. & Snader, K. M. (2003). Natural products as sources of new drugs over the period 1981–2002. *J Nat Prod.* **66**, 1022–1037.
3. Koehn, F. E. & Carter, G. T. (2005). The evolving role of natural products in drug discovery. *Nat Rev Drug Discov.* **4**, 206–220.
4. Paterson, I. & Anderson, E. A. (2005). The renaissance of natural products as drug candidates. *Science* **310**, 451–453.
5. Balunas, M. J. & Kinghorn, A. D. (2005). Drug discovery from medicinal plants. *Life Sci* **78**, 431–441.
6. Jones, W. P., Chin, Y. W. & Kinghorn, A. D. (2006). The role of pharmacognosy in modern medicine and pharmacy. *Curr Drug Targets* **7**, 247–264.
7. Philip, R. B. (2004). Herbal remidies: The good, the bad, and the ugly. *J Comp Integ Med.* **1**, 1–11.
8. Fabricant, D. S. & Farnsworth, N. R. (2001). The value of plants used in traditional medicine for drug discovery. *Environ Health Perspect* **109**, 69–75.
9. Hadley, S. K. & Petry, J. J. (2003). Medicinal herbs: A primer for Primary Care. *Hosp Prac*, 1–14.
10. Pearson, N. J. & Chesney, M. A. (2007). The CAM Education Program of the National Center for Complementary and Alternative Medicine: An overview. *Acad Med* **82**, 921–926.
11. N.I.H. Publication (2005). Thinking about complementary and alternative medicine – a guide for people with cancer. NIH publication no. 05–5541, Sept. 2–13.
12. Ernst, E. (2002). The risk-benefit of commonly used herbal therapies: Ginko, St. John's wort, ginseng, Echinacea, saw palmetto and kawa. *Ann Intern Med.* **136**, 42.
13. Jonas, W. B. (1998). Alternative medicine-learning from the past, examining the present, advancing to the future. *JAMA* **280**, 1616–1618.
14. Philp, R. B. (2004). *Herb drug interactions and adverse effects (an evidence-based quick reference guide)*, Appendix, McGraw-Hill, New York.

15. Kemper, K. J. & Shannon, S. (2007). Complementary and alternative medicine therapies to promote healthy moods. *Pediatr Clin North Am* **54**, 901–926.
16. Astin, J. A. (1998). Why patients use alternative medicine: Results of a national study. *JAMA* **279**, 1548–1553.
17. Eisenberg, D. M., Kessler, R. C., Foster, C., Norlock, F. E., Calkins, D. R. & Delbanco, T. L. (1993). Unconventional medicine in the United States. Prevalence, costs, and patterns of use. *N Engl J Med.* **328**, 246–252.
18. Astin, J. A., Pelletier, K. R., Marie, A. & Haskell, W. L. (2000). Complementary and alternative medicine use among elderly persons: One year analysis of Blue Shield medicare supplement. *J Gerontol* **55A**, M4–M9.
19. Salamon, I. (1992). Chamomile, a medicinal plant: The herb, spice, and medicinal plant. *Digest* **10**, 1–4.
20. Savage, F. G. (1923). *The Flora and Folk Lore of Shakespeare*, Shakespeare Press, Stratford-on-Avon.
21. Mark, T. S. (2005). Chamomile Tea: New evidence supports health benefits (http://www.eurekalert.org/pub_release/2005-01/acs-tn010405.php)
22. Chamomile (*Matricaria recutita*) – Chamomile benefits (2007) (www.herbwisdom.com)
23. Tyler, V. E. (1994). *Herbs of Choice – The Therapeutic Use of Phytomedicinals*, Binghamton, Pharmaceutical Products Press, New York.
24. Holtom, J. & Hylton. W. (1979). *"Complete Guide to Herbs" – A Good Herbal.* Rodale Press ISBN 0-87857-262-7.
25. Hatfield., A. W. (1977). *How to Enjoy your Weeds.* Frederick Muller Ltd. ISBN 0-584-10141-4.
26. Allardice. P. (1993). *A–Z of Companion Planting.* Cassell Publishers Ltd. ISBN 0-304-34324-2.
27. Bown. D. (1995). *Encyclopaedia of Herbs and their Uses.* Dorling Kindersley, London. ISBN 0-7513-020.
28. Castleman, M. (1991). Chamomile: Pretty flowers, potent medicine. In *The Healing Herbs*, pp. 158–163, Bantam books Doubleday Dell Publishing Group, New York.
29. Grieve, M. (1931). Chamomiles-Herb Profile and Information: "A Modern Herbal" (http://www.botanical.com/botanical/mgmh/c/chammo49.html).
30. Jackson, T. (2001). Medical Attributes of Matricaria chamomilla – Chamomile (http://klemow.wilkes.edu/Matricaria.html).
31. Cole, S. (2007). Chamomile: Farm & Garden (http://www.farm-garden.com/node/975).
32. Foster, S. (1991). *Chamomile, Botanical Series, No. 307*, American Botanical Council, Austin, Texas.
33. E.S.C.O.P (1990). *Proposal for a European Monograph on the Medicinal Use of Matricariae Flos (Chamomile Flowers)*, ESCOP, Brussels.
34. Der, M. A. & Liberti, L. (1988). *Natural Product Medicine: A Scientific Guide to Foods, Drugs, Cosmetics*, George F. Stickley Co, Philadelphia.
35. Mann, C. & Staba, E. J. (1986). *In* Herbs, Spices and Medicinal Plants: Recent Advances in Botany, Horticulture and Pharmacology (L. E. Craker & J. E. Simon, Eds.), pp. 235–280, Oryx Press, Phoenix, Arizona, 1:235.
36. McKay, D. L. & Blumberg, J. B. (2006). A review of the bioactivity and potential health benefits of chamomile tea (*Matricaria recutita* L.). *Phytother Res* **20**, 519–530.

37. Carnat, A., Carnat, A. P., Fraisse, D., Ricoux, L. & Lamaison, J. L. (2004). The aromatic and polyphenolic composition of Roman camomile tea. *Fitoterapia* **75**, 32–38.
38. Lemberkovics, E., Kéry, A., Marczal, G., Simándi, B. & Szöke, E. (1998). Phytochemical evaluation of essential oils, medicinal plants and their preparations. *Acta Pharm Hung* **68**, 141–149.
39. Baser, K. H., Demirci, B., Iscan, G., Hashimoto, T., Demirci, F., Noma, Y. & Asakawa, Y. (2006). The essential oil constituents and antimicrobial activity of *Anthemis aciphylla* BOISS. var. discoidea BOISS. *Chem Pharm Bull (Tokyo)* **54**, 222–225.
40. Babenko, N. A. & Shakhova, E. G. (2006). Effects of *Chamomilla recutita* flavonoids on age-related liver sphingolipid turnover in rats. *Exp Gerontol* **41**, 32–39.
41. Redaelli, C., Formentini, L. & Santaniello, E. (1981). Reversed-phase high-performance liquid chromatography analysis of apigenin and its glucosides in flowers of *Matricaria chamomilla* and chamomile extracts. *Planta Med* **42**, 288–292.
42. Avallone, R., Zanoli, P., Puia, G., Kleinschnitz, M., Schreier, P. & Baraldi, M. (2000). Pharmacological profile of Apigenin, a flavnoid isolated from *Matricaria chamomilla*. *Bioch Pharmacol* **59**, 1387–1394.
43. Svehliková, V., Bennett, R. N., Mellon, F. A., Needs, P. W., Piacente, S., Kroon, P. A. & Bao, Y. (2004). Isolation, identification and stability of acylated derivatives of apigenin 7-O-glucoside from chamomile (*Chamomilla recutita* [L.] Rauschert). *Phytochemistry* **65**, 2323–2332.
44. Srivastava, J. K. & Gupta, S. (2007). Antiproliferative and apoptotic effects of chamomile extract in various human cancer cells. *J Agric Food Chem* **55**, 9470–9478.
45. Bradley, P. (1992). *In* British Herbal Compendium (), Vol. 1, pp. 154–157, British Herbal Medicine Association, Bournemouth, UK. 45.
46. Central Council for Research in Unani Medicine (CCRUM) (1992). *Standardisation of Single Drugs in Unani Medicine*, Part II, pp. 141–147, New Delhi, India: CCRUM Ministry of Health & Family Welfare Government of India.
47. Michael, T. (1999). Why standardized extracts? An Herbalist's Perspective (www.planetherbs.com)
48. Chamomillae, Flos (1999). World Health Organization, Geneva, pp. 86–94.
49. Chamomile- Medicinal Parts (http://www.innvista.com/health/herbs/chamomil.htm)
50. Roman Chamomile (*Anthemis nobilis*) – Herbs 2000.com. (http://www.herbs2000.com/herbs/herbs_chamomile_rom.htm)
51. Chamomile (2003). Elix Relaxation Herb (http://www.elixnow.com/html/relaxation.htm)
52. Michael, B. (2005). Chamomile tea: New evidence supports health benefits. American Chemical Society, 2005 (http://www.eurekalert.org/pub_releases/2005-01/acs-tn010405.php)
53. Carnat, A., Carnat, A. P., Fraisse, D., Ricoux, L. & Lamaison, J. L. (2004). The aromatic and polyphenolic composition of Roman camomile tea. *Fitoterapia* **75**, 32–38.
54. Steve, M. (2008). Chamomile – Medicinal Uses, Interactions, Dosage (http://ezinearticles.com/?Chamomile---Medicinal-Uses,-Interactions,-Dosage&id=446977).

55. Blumenthal, M., Gruenwald, J., Hall, T. & Rister, R. S. (Eds.) (1998). The Complete German Commission E Monographs, American Botanical Council, Austin, Texas.
56. Braun, R., Surmann, P., Wendt, R. et al. (Eds.) (1996). Standardzulassungn for fertgarzneimittel – Text and Kommentar, Deutscher Apotheker Verlag, Stuttgart, Germany.
57. Asta Medica (1998). *Fachinformation: Kamillosan® Konzentrat*, Asta Medica AG, Frankfurt, Germany.
58. Sidney, S. (2001). *An Introduction to Homeopathic Medicine in Primary Care*, an ASPEN Publication, Chapter 6: Chamomilla pp. 62–64.
59. Anderson, C., Lis-Balchin, M. & Kirk-Smith, M. (2000). Evaluation of massage with essential oils on childhood atopic eczema. *Phytother Res* **14**, 452–456.
60. Wilkinson, S., Aldridge, J., Salmon, I., Cain, E. & Wilson, B. (1999). An evaluation of aromatherapy massage in palliative care. *Palliat Med* **13**, 409–417.
61. Potting, C. M., Uitterhoeve, R., Op Reimer, W. S. & Van Achterberg, T. (2006). The effectiveness of commonly used mouthwashes for the prevention of chemotherapy-induced oral mucositis: A systematic review. *Eur J Cancer Care* **15**, 431–439.
62. Scala, G. (2006). Acute, short-lasting rhinitis due to camomile-scented toilet paper in patients allergic to compositae. *Int Arch Allergy Immunol* **139**, 330–331.
63. Thornfeldt, C. (2005). Cosmeceuticals containing herbs: Fact, fiction, and future. *Dermatol Surg* **7**, 873–880.
64. Nemecz, G. (2002). Herbal Pharmacy: Chamomile, US Pharmacist – a Jobson Publication (http://www.uspharmacist.com/oldformat.asp?url=newlook/files/alte/acf2fb5.htm)
65. Weiss, R. F. (1998). *In* Herbal Medicine (A. B. Arcanum, Ed.), pp. 22–28, Beaconsfield publishers, Beaconsfield, UK.
66. Hansel, R. & Sticher, O. (2002). *Pharmakognosie, Phytopharmazie*, Springer-Verlag, Heidelberg, Germany.
67. Rombi, M. (1993). *Cento Piante Medicinali*, Nuovo Insttuto d'Arti Grafiche, Bergamo, Italy, pp. 63–65.
68. Tyler, V. E. (1993). *In* The Honest Herbal (F. George, Ed.), 3rd ed., Stickley Co., Philadelphia.
69. Medicine Plus (2007). Herbs and Supplements: Chamomile (*Matricaria recutita, Chamaemelum nobile*): A Service of the U.S. National Library of Medicine and National Institutes of Health (http://www.nlm.nih.gov/medlineplus/druginfo/natural/patient-chamomile-.html)
70. Martens, D. (1995). Chamomile: The herb and remedy, power. *Chiropra Acad Homeopathy* **6**, 15–18.
71. Newall, C. A., Anderson, L. A. & Phillipson, J. D. (1996). *Herbal Medicine: A Guide for Health Care Professionals*, Vol ix, pp. 296, Pharmaceutical Press, London.
72. LHTP Publication on Chamomile (2002). In depth monograph and clinician information summary on chamomile (*Matricaria recutita, Anthemis nobilis*) (http://www.longwoodherbal.org/chamomile/chamomile.pdf)
73. Forster, H. B., Niklas, H. & Lutz, S. (1980). Antispasmodic effects of some medicinal plants. *Planta Med* **40**, 309–319.

74. Crotteau, C. A., Wright, S. T. & Eglash, A. (2006). Clinical inquiries. What is the best treatment for infants with colic? *J Fam Pract* **55**, 634–636.
75. Linda, B. & Sunny, M. (1999). Fever in children: A blessing in disguise. *Mothering Magazine* (*online*) (http://www.mothering.com/articles/growing_child/child_health/fever.html)
76. Achterrath-Tuckermann, U., Kunde, R., Flaskamp, E., Isaac, O. & Thiemer, K. (1980). Pharmacological investigations with compounds of chamomile. V. Investigations on the spasmolytic effect of compounds of chamomile and Kamillosan on the isolated guinea pig ileum. *Planta Med* **39**, 38–50.
77. Gupta, S., Afaq, F. & Mukhtar, H. (2002). Involvement of nuclear factor−κB, Bax and Bcl-2 in induction of cell cycle arrest and apoptosis by apigenin in human prostate carcinoma cells. *Oncogene* **21**, 3727–3738.
78. Al-Jubouri, H. H. F., Al-Jalil, B. H., Farid, I. et al. (1990). The effect of chamomile on hyperlipidemias in rats. *J Fac Med Baghdad* **32**, 5–11.
79. Chamomile (*Matricaria recutita, Chamaemelum nobile*), Medline Plus: (http://www.nlm.nih.gov/medlineplus/druginfo/natural/patient-chamomile.html)
80. McKesson Health Solutions LLC (2003). *Chamomile natural remedy – patient handout*, MD Consult, Elsevier Publication, St. Louis.
81. Hertog, M. G., Feskens, E. J., Hollman, P. C., Katan, M. B. & Kromhout, D. (1993). Dietary antioxidant flavonoids and risk of coronary heart disease: The Zutphen Elderly Study. *Lancet* **342**, 1007–1011.
82. Gould, L., Reddy, C. V. & Gomprecht, R. F. (1973). Cardiac effects of chamomile tea. *J Clin Pharmacol* **11**, 475–479.
83. Natural Standard: The Authority on Integrative Medicine (http://www.naturalstandard.com/index-abstract.asp?create-abstract=/monographs/news/news200609012.asp)
84. Gardiner, P. (2007). Complementary, holistic, and integrative medicine: Chamomile. *Pediat Rev* **28**, 16–18.
85. Kell, T. (1997). More on infant colic. *Birth Gaz. Spring* **13**, 3.
86. Nissen, H. P., Blitz, H. & Kreyel, H. W. (1988). Prolifometrie, eine methode zur beurteilung der therapeutischen wirsamkeit kon Kamillosan®-Salbe. *Z Hautkr* **63**, 84–90.
87. Aergeers, P., Albring, M., Klaschka, F. et al. (1985). Vergleichende prüfung von Kamillosan®-creme gegenüber seroidalen (0.25% hydrocortison, 0.75% flucotinbutylester) und nichseroidaseln (5% bufexamac) externa in der erhaltungsterpaie von ekzemerkrankungen. *Z Hautkr* **60**, 270–277.
88. Albring, M., Albrecht, H., Alcorn, G & Lüker, P. W. (1983). The measuring of the anti-inflammatory effect of a compound on the skin of volunteers. *Meth Find Exp Clin Pharmacol* **5**, 75–77.
89. Eczema: University of Maryland Medical Centre – Complementary Medicine (http://www.umm.edu/altmed/articles/eczema-000054.htm)
90. Patzelt-Wenczler, R. & Ponce-Pöschl, E. (2000). Proof of efficacy of Kamillosan® cream in atopic eczema. *Eur J Med Res* **5**, 171–175.
91. Fundamentals: Dyspepsia (indigestion) – Mcadams Health Int. Inc. Livingston (http://www.bloodrootproducts.com/dyspepsia.htm)
92. Kroll, U. & Cordes, C. (2006). Pharmaceutical prerequisites for a multi-target therapy. *Phytomedicine* **5**, 12–19.

93. Gastrointestinal (GI) Tips – Herb Research Foundation (http://www.meredy.com/nursetips/gastrointestinaltips.html)
94. Khayyal, M. T., Seif-El-Nasr, M., El-Ghazaly, M. A., Okpanyi, S. N., Kelber, O. & Weiser, D. (2006). Mechanisms involved in the gastro-protective effect of STW 5 (Iberogast) and its components against ulcers and rebound acidity. *Phytomedicine* **13**, 56–66.
95. Mary Ann Copson, Herbs & Urinary Tract Infections (http://evenstaronline.com/articles/urinary.html)
96. Lyseng-Williamson, K. A. & Perry, C. M. (2003). Micronised purified flavonoid fraction: A review of its use in chronic venous insufficiency, venous ulcers, and haemorrhoids. *Drugs* **63**, 71–100.
97. Misra, M. C. & Parshad, R. (2000). Randomized clinical trial of micronized flavonoids in the early control of bleeding from acute internal haemorrhoids. *Br J Surg* **87**, 868–872.
98. Wang, Y., Tang, H., Nicholson, J. K., Hylands, P. J., Sampson, J. & Holmes, F (2005). A metabonomic strategy for the detection of the metabolic effects of chamomile (*Matricaria recutita* L.) ingestion. *J Agric Food Chem* **53**, 191–196.
99. Ramos-e-Silva, M., Ferreira, A. F., Bibas, R. & Carneiro S. (2006). Clinical evaluation of fluid extract of *Chamomilla recutita* on oral aphthae. *J Drugs Dermatol* **5**, 612–617.
100. Wu, J. (2006). Treatment of rosacea with herbal ingredients. *J Drugs Dermatol* **5**, 29–32.
101. Graf, J. (2000). Herbal anti-inflammatory agents for skin disease. *Skin Therapy Lett* **5**, 3–5.
102. Weseler, A., Geiss, H. K., Saller, R. & Reichling, J. A. (2005). Novel colorimetric broth microdilution method to determine the minimum inhibitory concentration (MIC) of antibiotics and essential oils against *Helicobacter pylori*. *Pharmazie* **60**, 498–502.
103. Fugh-Berman, A. (2002). Herbal supplements: Indications, clinical concerns, and safety. *Nutr Today* **37**, 122–124.
104. Wechselberger, G., Schoeller, T., Otto, A., Obrist, P., Rumer, A. & Deetjen, H. (1998). Total gluteal pouching with pseudoanus caused by burn injury: Report of a case. *Dis Colon Rectum* **41**, 929–931.
105. Tubaro, A., Zilli, C., Redaelli, C. & Della, L. R. (1984). Evaluation of anti-inflammatory activity of chamomile extract after topical application. *Planta Med* **50**, 359.
106. Fugh, B. A. (2002). Herbal supplements: Indications, clinical concerns, and safety. *Nutr Today* **37**, 122–124.
107. Michel, D. & Zäch, G. A. (1997). Antiseptic efficacy of disinfecting solutions in suspension test *in vitro* against methicillin-resistant *Staphylococcus aureus*, *Pseudomonas aeruginosa* and *Escherichia coli* in pressure sore wounds after spinal cord injury. *Dermatology* **195**, 36–41.
108. Prevention and Treatment of Oral Mucositis in Cancer Patients; The Joanna Briggs Institute. (http://www.joannabriggs.edu.au/best_practice/bp5.php)
109. Fidler, P., Loprinzi, C. L., O'Fallon, J. R., Leitch, J. M., Lee, J. K., Hayes, D. L., Novotny, P., Clemens-Schutjer, D., Bartel, J. & Michalak, J. C. (1996). Prospective evaluation of a chamomile mouthwash for prevention of 5-FU-induced oral mucositis. *Cancer* **77**, 522–525.

110. Kassi, E., Papoutsi, Z., Fokialakis, N., Messari, I., Mitakou, S. & Moutsatsou, P. (2004). Greek plant extracts exhibit selective estrogen receptor modulator (SERM)-like properties. *J Agric Food Chem* **52**, 6956–6961.

111. Avallone, R., Zanoli, P., Corsi, L., Cannazza, G. & Baraldi, M. (1996). Benzodiazepine compounds and GABA in flower heads of matricaria chamomilla. *Phytother Res* **10**, 177–179.

112. Gould, L., Reddy, C. V. R. & Comprecht, R. F. (1973). Cardiac effect of Chamomile tea. *J Clin Pharmacol* **13**, 475–479.

113. Meolie, A. L., Rosen, C., Kristo, D., Kohrman, M., Gooneratne, N., Aguillard, R. N., Fayle, R., Troell, R., Townsend, D., Claman, D., Hoban, T. & Mahowald, M. (2005). Oral nonprescription treatment for insomnia: An evaluation of products with limited evidence. *J Clin Sleep Med* **1**, 173–187.

114. Shinomiya, K., Inoue, T., Utsu, Y., Tokunaga, S., Masuoka, T., Ohmori, A. & Kamei, C. (2005). Hypnotic activities of chamomile and passiflora extracts in sleep-disturbed rats. *Biol Pharm Bull* **28**, 808–810.

115. Paladini, A. C., Marder, M., Viola, H., Wolfman, C., Wasowski, C. & Medina, J. H. (1999). Flavonoids and the central nervous system: From forgotten factors to potent anxiolytic compounds. *J Pharm Pharmacol.* **51**, 519–526.

116. Charuluxananan, S., Sumethawattana, P., Kosawiboonpol, R., Somboonviboon, W. & Werawataganon, T. (2004). Effectiveness of lubrication of endotracheal tube cuff with chamomile-extract for prevention of postoperative sore throat and hoarseness. *J Med Assoc Thai* **87**(Suppl 2), S185–S189.

117. Kyokong, O., Charuluxananan, S., Muangmingsuk, V., Rodanant, O., Subornsug, K. & Punyasang, W. (2002). Efficacy of chamomile-extract spray for prevention of post-operative sore throat. *J Med Assoc Thai* **85**(Suppl 1), S180–S185.

118. Benetti, C. & Manganelli, F. (1985). Clinical experiences in the pharmacological treatment of vaginitis with a camomile-extract vaginal douche. *Minerva Ginecol* **37**, 799–801.

119. Glowania, H. J., Raulin, C. & Swoboda, M. (1987). Effect of chamomile on wound healing: A clinical double-blind study. *Z Hautkr* **62**(1262), 1267–1271.

120. Nayak, B. S., Raju, S. S. & Rao, A. V. (2007). Wound healing activity of *Matricaria recutita* L. extract. *J Wound Care* **16**, 298–302.

121. Iwashita, K., Kobori, M., Yamaki, K. & Tsushida, T. (2000). Flavonoids inhibit cell gowth and induce apoptosis in B16 melanoma 4A5 cells. *Biosci Biotechnol Biochem* **64**, 1813–1820.

122. Caltagirone, S., Rossi, C., Poggi, A., Ranelletti, F. O., Natali, P. G., Brunetti, M., Aiello, F. B. & Piantelli, M. (2000). Flavonoids apigenin and quercetin inhibit melanoma growth and metastatic potential. *Int J Cancer* **87**, 595–600.

123. Way, T. D., Kao, M. C. & Lin, J. K. (2004). Apigenin induces apoptosis through proteasomal degradation of HER2/neu in HER2/neu-overexpressing breast cancer cells via the phosphatidylinositol-3'-kinase/Akt-dependent pathway. *J Biol Chem* **279**, 4479–4489.

124. Birt, D. F., Mitchell, D., Gold, B., Pour, P. & Pinch, H. C. (1997). Inhibition of ultraviolet light induced skin carcinogenesis in SKH-1 mice by apigenin, a plant flavonoid. *Anticancer Res* **17**, 85–91.

125. Wang, W., Heideman, L., Chung, C. S. et al. (2000). Cell-cycle arrest at G2/M and growth inhibition by apigenin in human colon carcinoma cell lines. *Mol Carcinog* **28**, 102–110.

126. Patel, D., Shukla, S. & Gupta, S. (2007). Apigenin and cancer chemoprevention: Progress, potential and promise (review). *Int J Oncol* **30**, 233–245.

127. Gates, M. A., Tworoger, S. S., Hecht, J. L., De Vivo, I., Rosner, B. & Hankinson, S. E. (2007). A prospective study of dietary flavonoid intake and incidence of epithelial ovarian cancer. *Int J Cancer* **121**, 2225–2232.

128. Shukla, S., Mishra, A., Fu, P., MacLennan, G. T., Resnick, M. I. & Gupta, S. (2005). Up-regulation of insulin-like growth factor binding protein-3 by apigenin leads to growth inhibition and apoptosis of 22Rv1 xenograft in athymic nude mice. *FASEB J* **19**, 2042–2044.

129. Fellowes, D., Barnes, K. & Wilkinson, S. (2004). Aromatherapy and massage for symptom relief in patients with cancer. *Cochrane Database Syst Rev (2)*, CD002287.

130. Wilcock, A., Manderson, C., Weller, R. et al. (2004). Does aromatherapy massage benefit patients with cancer attending a specialist palliative care day centre? *Palliat Med* **18**, 287–290.

131. Soden, K., Vincent, K., Craske, S. et al. (2004). A randomized controlled trial of aromatherapy massage in a hospice setting. *Palliat Med* **18**, 87–92.

132. Graham, P. H., Browne, L., Cox, H. et al. (2003). Inhalation aromatherapy during radiotherapy: Results of a placebo-controlled double-blind randomized trial. *J Clin Oncol* **21**, 2372–2376.

133. Hadfield, N. (2001). The role of aromatherapy massage in reducing anxiety in patients with malignant brain tumours. *Int J Palliat Nurs* **7**, 279–285.

134. Budzinski, J. W., Foster, B. C., Vandenhoek, S. et al. (2000). An *in vitro* evaluation of human cytochrome P450 3A4 inhibition by selected commercial herbal extracts and tinctures. *Phytomedicine* **7**, 273–282.

135. Hausen, B. M. (1996). A 6-year experience with compositae mix. *Am J Contact Dermat* **7**, 94–99.

136. Paulsen, E., Andersen, K. E. & Hausen, B. M. (1993). Compositae dermatitis in a Danish dermatology department in one year (I). Results of routine patch testing with the sesquiterpene lactone mix supplemented with aimed patch testing with extracts and sesquiterpene lactones of Compositae plants. *Contact Dermatitis* **29**, 6–10.

137. Subiza, J., Subiza, J. L., Alonso, M., Hinojosa, M., Garcia, R., Jerez, M. & Subiza, E. (1990). Allergic conjunctivitis to chamomile tea. *Ann Allergy* **65**, 127–132.

138. Subiza, J., Subiza, J. L., Hinojosa, M., Garcia, R., Jerez, M., Valdivieso, R. & Subiza, E. (1989). Anaphylactic reaction after the ingestion of chamomile tea: A study of cross-reactivity with other composite pollens. *J Allergy Clin Immunol* **84**, 353–358.

139. Reider, N., Sepp, N., Fritsch, P., Weinlich, G. & Jensen-Jarolim, E. (2000). Anaphylaxis to camomile: Clinical features and allergen cross-reactivity. *Clin Exp Allergy* **30**, 1436–1443.

140. Paulsen, E. (2002). Contact sensitization from Compositae-containing herbal remedies and cosmetics. *Contact Dermatitis* **47**, 189–198.

141. Segal, R. & Pilote, L. (2006). Warfarin interaction with *Matricaria chamomilla*. *CMAJ* **174**, 1281–1282.

Chapter 9

Bamboo Extract in the Prevention of Diabetes and Breast Cancer

Jun Panee

Department of Cell and Molecular Biology, John A. Burns School of Medicine,
University of Hawaii at Manoa, Honolulu, HI, USA and Cancer Research
Center of Hawaii, University of Hawaii, Honolulu, HI, USA

Abstract

Bamboo plants are a fast growing, widely distributed and renewable natural resource that has been used both in daily life and for medicinal purposes for centuries in China and other Asian countries. Recent scientific research has demonstrated multiple health benefits from varied extracts from bamboo. The studies carried out in our laboratory have shown that an ethanol/water extract from bamboo *Phyllostachys edulis* significantly reduced fatty acid – induced lipotoxicity and high fat diet-induced adiposity, hyperinsulinemia, and hyperglycemia. Most strikingly, it also inhibited the development of chemically induced breast cancer. Bamboo extract holds a high promise as a complementary and alternative approach for the prevention of diabetes and breast cancer, two major epidemic diseases threatening lives in the developed countries.

Keywords: *Obesity, diabetes, breast cancer, inflammation*

Abbreviations: AUC, area under curve; BEX, bamboo extract; DMBA, 7,12–Dimethy lbenz[a]anthracene; DMSO, dimethyl sulfoxide; E2, 17β-estradiol; FA, fatty acid; GST, Glutathione-*S*-transferases; IL-6, interleukin 6; PA, palmitic acid; PAH, polycyclic aromatic hydrocarbon; PCB, polychlorinated biphenyl; SD rats, Sprague-Dawley rats; SULT, Sulfotransferase; T2DM, type 2 diabetes mellitus; TNF-α, tumor necrosis factor alpha; UGT, UDP-glucuronosyltransferase.

INTRODUCTION

The close relationship between bamboo and the daily life of Chinese people was vividly described by William E. Geil in his book *A Yankee on the Yangtze* over a century ago: "A man can sit in a bamboo house under a bamboo roof, on a bamboo chair at a bamboo table, with a bamboo hat on his head and bamboo sandals on his feet. He can at the same time hold in one hand a bamboo bowl, in the other hand bamboo chopsticks and eat bamboo sprouts. When through with his meal, which has been cooked over a bamboo fire, the table may be washed with a bamboo cloth, and he can fan himself with a bamboo fan, take a siesta on a bamboo bed, lying on a bamboo mat with his head resting on a bamboo pillow. He might then take a walk over a bamboo suspension bridge, drink water from a bamboo ladle, and scrape himself with a bamboo scraper (handkerchief)." However, what was not touched in the description is the medicinal use of the bamboo plants. In fact different parts of bamboo have been traditionally used in Asian countries to treat hypertension, arteriosclerosis, cardiovascular disease, and certain forms of cancer. The earliest scientific research on the health benefiting effect of bamboo extracts traceable in the Pubmed online resources was carried out in Japan in early 1960s [1], followed by a series of studies performed by Shibata *et al.* in Japan in the 1970s [2–6]. The research in this area was relatively sparse during the 80s and 90s [7–9], but has been enjoying increased popularity since the beginning of the 21st century in both Asian countries such as China, Korea, and Japan, and western countries such as the US and Canada [10–19]. The bamboo extracts were found to be rich in antioxidants, and had preventive or therapeutic effects on inflammation, fatigue, cancer, hyperlipidemia, and hypertension. Extracts from bamboo leaves were found to be non-toxic to rodents [20, 21].

In the past decades, dramatic changes in life style and diet, together with other factors such as environmental pollution, have caused significant increases in the incidences of several diseases including obesity, type 2 diabetes mellitus (T2DM), and breast cancer. Between 1980 and 2002, obesity rates in the United States doubled in adults and tripled in children and adolescents [22]. As a result, in 2003–2004, 17.1% of US children and adolescents were overweight and 32.2% of adults were obese [23]. Similarly, the prevalence of diagnosed diabetes among US adults has increased by 40% in 10 years from 4.9% in 1990 to 6.9% in 1999 [24]. This number is expected to increase by 165% between 2000 and 2050 [25]. Worldwide breast cancer rates have been rising steadily since the 1940s with over a million new cases diagnosed each year. In the United States, a woman's lifetime risk of breast cancer has nearly tripled during the past four decades, making this the most prevalent cancer in American women [26]. In 2005, an estimated 211,240 women in United States were diagnosed with invasive breast cancer, and more than 40,000 cases were metastatic and lethal [27].

Our research team explores the biological functions of an ethanol/water extract from bamboo *Phyllostachys edulis*, commonly known as "Moso." We have observed significant protective effects of this bamboo extract (BEX) on high fat diet-induced obesity, diabetes, and chemically induced breast cancer. These results indicate the potential of BEX as a cost-effective health benefiting neutraceutical.

OBESITY, LIPOTOXICITY, DIABETES AND THE PREVENTIVE EFFECTS OF BEX

In subjects with high risk of T2DM, the earliest detectable abnormality is insulin resistance in skeletal muscle. Obesity is a causative factor to insulin resistance, as evidenced by both human and animal studies demonstrating that weight loss/gain correlates closely with increasing/decreasing insulin sensitivity [28–31]. Obesity induces insulin resistance through pathways such as (i) exerting lipotoxicity to muscle cells [32]; (ii) altering the profile of adipokines such as leptin, adiponectin, and resistine [33]; and (iii) inducing chronic inflammation in fat tissues, characterized by the increased secretion of pro-inflammation factors such as tumor necrosis factor α (TNF-α) and interleukin 6 (IL-6) from fat tissues [34].

Lipotoxicity refers to the tissue disease that may occur when fatty acid (FA) spillover in excess of the oxidative needs of those tissues enhances metabolic flux into harmful pathways of non-oxidative metabolism [35]. Exposure to high concentrations (70–1000 μM) of long-chain saturated FA induce apoptosis in varied types of cells, including cardiomyocyte [36], pancreatic β-cells [37], fibroblasts, endothelial cell monolayers [38, 39], ventricular cells [40], retinal pericytes [27], and skeletal muscle cells [41]. Skeletal muscles in lipotoxic conditions contribute to the majority of insulin resistance triggered by hyperlipidemia [42].

The protective effect of BEX on palmitic acid (PA) induced lipotoxicity in mouse myoblast C2C12 cells and other cell lines has been studied in our laboratory [43]. The raw BEX was produced in Hunan province in China using ethanol/water extraction in close accordance to a patented procedure (publication number: CN 1287848A). Leaves and small branches were used in this extraction. The raw extract, upon arriving in the laboratory, was further freeze dried and ground into fine powder. The fine powder was extracted with 100% ethanol (100 mg/ml) at room temperature for 3 hours, followed by centrifugation. The supernatant containing ethanol soluble portion of the raw extract was used in this study. This final extract was added to cell culture media for up to 0.5% (v/v) to test its lipo-detoxification function. Equal amount of ethanol or dimethyl sulfoxide (DMSO) was added to media as solvent control.

C2C12 cells were exposed to 0.4 mM PA in the presence of either BEX or ethanol at different dosages. After 26 hours of treatment without BEX protection, most of the cells died, regardless of the volume of ethanol applied (represented in Fig. 9.1B). In contrast, BEX protected the cells in a dose-dependent manner (Fig. 9.1C and 9.1D). The same protective effects were observed regardless of the solvents (ethanol or DMSO) used to reconstitute BEX, indicating that the lipo-detoxification function of BEX was independent on the solvent used. Similar protective effects of BEX were observed in myotubes differentiated from C2C12 cells and monkey kidney Vero cells under the challenge of PA. Cell viabilities of different cells co-incubated with BEX or ethanol during the PA treatment were analyzed using MTT assay and are shown in Figs 9.2A and 9.2B.

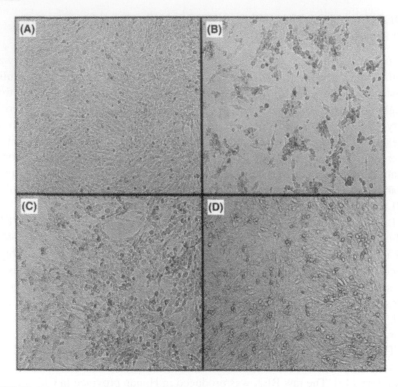

FIGURE 9.1 The morphology of C2C12 cells after exposure to 0.4 mM PA for 26 hours. (A) PA free medium + 0.3% (v/v) ethanol as control, (B) 0.4 mM PA + 0.3% ethanol, (C) 0.4 mM PA + 0.3% BEX, and (D) 0.4 mM PA + 0.5% BEX.

The apoptotic status of the cells were analyzed using Vybrant Apoptosis Assay Kit #2 (Invitrogen, Carlsbad, CA) after incubating C2C12 cells with 0.4 mM PA in combination with BEX or ethanol for 16 hours. Figure 9.3 shows that 16 hour of PA treatment induced about 30% of apoptosis in C2C12 cells, adding 0.2–0.5% of ethanol has no significant effect, but addition of 0.2% BEX decreased the apoptotic rate to 17.3%, and 0.5% BEX brought the rate further down to 5.6%.

Furthermore, we investigated the inhibitory effect of BEX on high fat diet-induced obesity and diabetes in C57/BL6J mice. The BEX powder was sent to Research Diets (New Brunswick, NJ) to be incorporated into a high fat diet (45 Kcal% lard fat, catd D12451) at a ratio of 10 g dry mass per 4057 Kcal. Before BEX supplementation, the diet did not contain plant-derived material, therefore are free of phytochemicals. The high fat diet without BEX supplementation was used as c ontrol. Male C57BL/6J mice 3 weeks of age were purchased from the Jackson Laboratory (Bar Harbor, MN) and hosted at University of Hawaii Laboratory Animal Services facilities. The

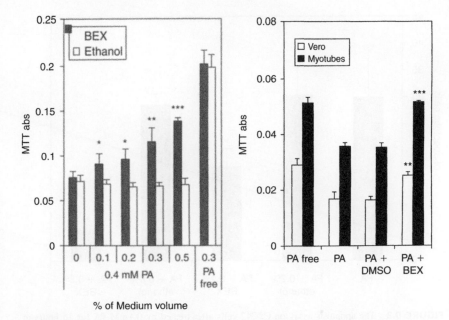

% of Medium volume

FIGURE 9.2 The MTT-based cell viability of C2C12, Myotubes differentiated from C2C12, and Vero cells after PA treatment. (A) C2C12 cells exposed for 26 hours to 0.4 mM PA in combination with 0–0.5% (v/v) of BEX or ethanol; PA-free medium + 0.3% BEX or ethanol were used as control. Average ± SD, $N = 3$. Samples treated with BEX are compared to those treated with ethanol at the same concentration. (B) Myotubes differentiated from C2C12 cells and Vero cells were treated for 24 hours with PA-free media, media containing 0.4 mM PA, or 0.4 mM PA in combination with 0.5% BEX or DMSO. Average ± SD, $N = 3$. Samples treated with PA and BEX are compared to those treated with PA and DMSO.

experimental procedure has been approved by the Institutional Animal Care and Use Committee of the University of Hawaii. The mice were hosted 2–3/cage, with free access to food and water. After acclimation with standard laboratory rodent chow for 1 week, the mice were assigned to the BEX diet or the control diet. The dietary regime was maintained throughout the rest of the experiment.

Mice were closely monitored during the experiment. The appearance and behavior of all mice appeared normal; no adverse effect of BEX supplementation was observed.

Food consumption in each cage and the body weight of each mouse was monitored throughout the experiment. The average daily food intake of the BEX group was 2.48 ± 0.44 g, slightly higher than that of the control group which was 2.28 ± 0.56, indicating BEX may marginally increase the consumption of food with high fat content. However, regardless of the increased food intake, mice in the BEX group started to gain less weight than those in the control group after 7 weeks on special diets ($p < 0.001$, t-test, Day 49 to Day 167), as shown in Fig. 9.4.

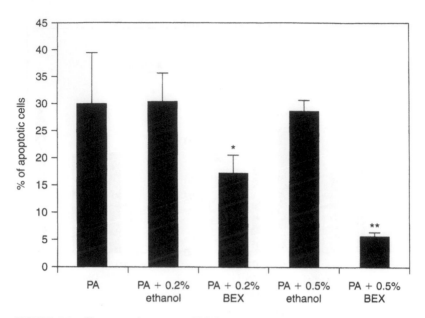

FIGURE 9.3   The apoptosis assay on C2C12 cells after treated by 0.4 mM PA for 16 hours in presence of 0.2–0.5% of BEX or ethanol (control). The cells were stained by Annexin V label with fluorophore and the fluorescence intensity of the cells was measured by flow cytometer. Average ± SD, $N = 3$. Samples treated with BEX are compared to those treated with ethanol at the same concentration.

Blood glucose was measured by OneTouch Ultra Glucose Meter (LifeScan, Milpitas, CA) after 3 hours of fasting (the fasting, usually starting around 10 am). Table 9.1 shows that long-term high-fat diet increased blood glucose in mice and BEX supplementation inhibited this trend ($p = 0.077$, t-test). Glucose tolerance of the mice was also measured. D-(+)-glucose (Sigma, St. Louis, MO) was dissolved in sterile water and delivered to each mouse via intraperitoneal (ip) injection at a dosage of 1 g/kg body weight after 3 hours of fasting. Blood glucose level was monitored at time points 0, 0.5, 1, 1.5, and 2 hours. Glucose tolerance was indicated by the total area under curve (AUC). In comparison to controls, glucose tolerance in the mice on BEX diet was improved by 6% at day 50 ($p = 0.063$), 19% at day 150 ($p = 0.0062$) and 16% at day 180 ($p = 0.012$), as shown in Table 9.1.

After 6 months of high fat diet treatment, the mice were sacrificed and the blood was collected from heart puncture. Insulin and TNF-α levels in serum were measured using mouse insulin ELISA (enzyme-linked immunosorbent assay) kits (Mercodia AB, Uppsala, Sweden) and mouse TNF-α ELISA kits (eBioscience, San Diego, CA), respectively. Table 9.2 shows that BEX supplementation dramatically decreased insulin and TNFα levels by 40% ($p = 0.038$) and 77% ($p = 0.0027$), respectively.

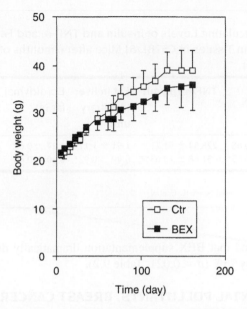

FIGURE 9.4 Average body weight of the mice on high fat diet with and without BEX supplementation. $N = 8$ for BEX group and $N = 7$ for control group. Day 0 in the figure corresponds to the first day of the special diet regime. Average and SD are shown.

TABLE 9.1 Blood Glucose and Glucose Tolerance in C57BL/6J Mice on High Fat Diet

Parameter	Diet	Day 50	Day 150	Day 180
Blood glucose (mg/dl)	Control	197 ± 41.1	234 ± 30.8	290.9 ± 44.4
	BEX	186 ± 30.5	202.5 ± 30.5	254 ± 40.9
Glucose tolerance (AUC, h mg/dl)*	Control	661.8 ± 71.5	775.3 ± 108.0	794.0 ± 77.8
	BEX	585.5 ± 24.0	628.3 ± 56.8**	666.8 ± 89.4*

*$0.01 < p \leq 0.05$.
**$0.001 < p \leq 0.01$, in comparison to the Control.

The epididymal fat pad was excised from each mouse after sacrifice, and the weight was measured. The average weight of epididymal fat was decreased by 37% in mice on the BEX diet (Table 9.2). Livers were embedded in paraffin and processed into slide sections of 5 μm. Fat accumulation was detected by Oil Red O staining. The area of positive staining was quantitated using ImageJ software downloaded from the National Institute of Health (NIH) website, and the total positive staining area represents the amount of fat deposited in the

TABLE 9.2 Circulating Levels of Insulin and TNF-α, and Fat Accumulation in Tissues in C57BL/6J Mice after 6 months of High Fat Diet Treatment

Diet	Insulin (μg/l)	TNF-α (pg/ml)	Fat in liver (Arbitrary unit)	Epididymal fat (g)	Epididymal fat/body weight (%)
Control	1.93 ± 0.68	228.54 ± 91.21	1.91 ± 1.17	1.27 ± 0.69	3.49 ± 0.019
BEX	1.17 ± 0.65*	51.68 ± 14.63**	0.49 ± 0.92*	0.80 ± 0.40	2.33 ± 0.010

*$0.01 < p \leq 0.5$.
**$0.001 < p \leq 0.01$, in comparison to the Control.

liver. It was found that BEX supplementation dramatically decreased the fat content in liver by 75% ($p = 0.021$, Table 9.2).

ENVIRONMENTAL POLLUTANTS, BREAST CANCER, AND THE PREVENTIVE EFFECT OF BEX

A comprehensive review sponsored by the Susan G. Komen Breast Cancer Foundation has recently revealed evidence of increased risk of breast cancer associated with exposure to polychlorinated biphenyls (PCBs) in genetically susceptible women and to polycyclic aromatic hydrocarbons (PAHs) [44]. PCBs have been widely used in electrical equipment and other products since the 1930s because of their excellent electrical and temperature insulating abilities, but were banned by the Environmental Protection Agency in 1978. Although PCBs can still challenge human health through professional exposure or accidental spills, the threat of this group of chemicals to the majority population is under control. On the other hand, PAHs are ubiquitous environmental contaminants resulting from incomplete combustion of organic matter, such as wood, coal, and diesel [45]. Since human civilization relies heavily on combustion, PAHs are inevitably linked to our energy production. Human exposure to PAHs is mainly through polluted air, diet (polluted food and grilled meat), and tobacco smoking [46, 47].

Several members of the PAH family have been demonstrated as mammary carcinogens through animal studies [48]. 7,12-Dimethylbenz[a]anthracene (DMBA) is a synthetic chemical in the PAH family and can efficiently induce breast cancer in rodents [49]. Oral delivery of DMBA to rats, a model that closely mimics the dietary intake of carcinogens in humans, has been intensively used for carcinogenic studies since the 1960s.

DMBA causes breast cancer through mutagenic effect. After entering a cellular environment, DMBA is metabolically activated by the phase I enzyme, cytochrome P450-dependent monooxygenase 1A1 (CYP1A1), to covalently bind to

DNA, forming DNA adducts [50–52]. Both the liver and mammary glands are capable of metabolizing DMBA to reactive bay-region diol-epoxides [53–55]. The anti-diol-epoxide: deoxyguanosine adduct is the major adduct formed in rat mammary tissue *in vivo* following DMBA administration [56]. Maximum DNA binding in the mammary tissue of Sprague-Dawley (SD) rats have been detected 24–48 hours after DMBA treatment [57, 58]. The metabolites formed by phase I enzymes can be detoxified by phase II enzymes, which conjugate the genotoxic intermediate to endogenous polar substrates to further increase its water solubility therefore excretability. Glutathione-S-transferases (GST) constitute a major group of phase II enzymes that use glutathione as a substrate. The expression of GST is controlled by multiple transcription factors and is highly inducible by dietary components [59]. Polymorphisms of GSTs have been found correlated with elevated carcinogen-DNA adducts in human breast tissue and incidence and mortality of breast cancer [60, 61]. UDP-glucuronosyltransferase (UGT) is another group of phase II enzymes transferring a nucleotide sugar to small, hydrophobic molecules. Several of the UGTs are integral in the conjugation and excretion of steroid hormones, for example UGT1A1 conjugates 17β-estradiol (E2), and UGT2B15 conjugates androgens [62]. Polymorphorisms in UGT1A1 and UGT2B15 have been associated with higher serum estradiol concentrations in post-menopausal women [63]. Sulfotransferase (SULT) is a family of phase II enzymes transferring a sulfate group from 3′-phosphoadenylyl sulfate to the hydroxyl group of an acceptor. SULT metabolizes estrone, E2, and catecholestrogens [64], with SULT1E1 having the highest affinity for these substrates [65]. SULT1E1 is expressed in the liver and breast, but not in malignant breast cells, potentially signaling that SULT is vital for normal cellular proliferation and lack or absence of SULT may be integral to estrogen-mediated carcinogenesis [66].

We tested the protective effect of BEX on the development of DMBA-induced breast cancer in SD rats [67]. The BEX was incorporated into a standard diet (10 Kcal% fat, Cat# D12450B, Research Diets) at a dosage of 10 g dry mass per 4057 Kcal. Before BEX supplementation, the diet did not contain plant-derived material and is therefore free from phytochemicals. Female SD rats 3 weeks of age were purchased from Charles River Laboratories (Wilmington, MA). After 1 week of acclimation with standard laboratory rodent chow, the rats were assigned to either a BEX-supplemented diet or a control diet. Three weeks after the special diets, all the rats were treated with DMBA (75 mg/kg body weight) via intragastric injection. The rats were fasted overnight before and further fasted for 4 hours after DMBA treatment. The dietary regimens were maintained throughout the experimental period.

The food intake and body weight of the SD rats were recorded during the experimental period, and no significant difference between the two groups was observed. The onset of mammary tumors was monitored by palpation weekly, and it was found that BEX supplementation delayed the onset of mammary tumors by 1 week, decreased the tumor incidence by 44% and decreased tumor multiplicity by 67% 11 weeks after DMBA treatment (Figs 9.5A and 9.5B).

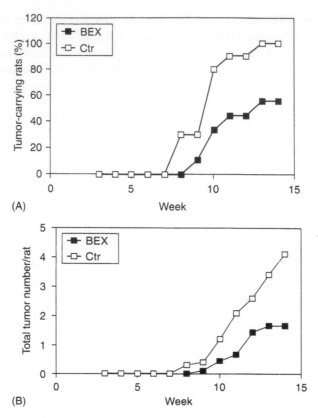

FIGURE 9.5 The inhibitory effect of BEX supplementation on DMBA-induced breast cancer in SD rats. (A) BEX delayed the onset of mammary tumor and decreased the incidence. (B) BEX decreased the tumor multiplicity. $N = 9$ for BEX and $N = 10$ for Control.

The activities of different families of phase II enzyme were analyzed in rat livers. These included SULT [68,69], UGT [70], and GST [71,72]. BEX increased the total activity of SULT by 63% ($p = 0.011$), slightly increased UGT activity by 14%, and did not change GST activity. The increases of the activities of estrogen metabolizing enzymes such as SULT and UGT indicate that enhanced estrogen detoxification may be one of the pathways through which BEX exerts anti-breast cancer function.

LINKS BETWEEN OBESITY AND BREAST CANCER AND HYPOTHESES ON MORE FUNCTIONS OF BEX

Numerous studies have demonstrated that obesity is positively associated with the risk of breast cancer in post-menopausal women [73–75]. Central obesity has been reported to increase the risk of breast cancer in pre-menopausal women [76]. Obesity is also associated with increased breast cancer recurrence and death in both pre- and post-menopausal women [75]. The mechanisms by which body weight and obesity affect the risk of breast cancer have been related to estrogenic activity.

E2 has been widely used as a carcinogen in rodent tumor models since the 1930s. Recent cohort studies revealed strong relationships between elevated levels of circulating estrogens and the risk of breast cancer in humans [77–83]. E2 has a dual role in the carcinogenesis of breast cancer [84, 85]. It is a carcinogen that becomes genotoxic after metabolic activation [86]. Phase I enzymes convert E2 into semiquinone derivatives [87] and then to quinone derivatives that can form DNA adducts and initiate breast cancer [88]. The E2-activating phase I enzymes are CYP1A1, CYP3A4, and CYP1B1 [89–91]. E2 also interacts with estrogen receptors (ER) to stimulate the proliferation of mammary epithelial cells thereby enhancing the mutagenesis of DNA damage [92–94].

Three pathways have been proposed in the molecular links between obesity and breast cancer [95]:

(i) Obesity elevates circulating estrogens from peripheral aromatization of androgens. Estrogen biosynthesis is catalyzed by aromatase. In obese, post-menopausal women, adipose tissues are the main sites of estrogen biosynthesis. The aromatase levels in adipose tissues increase with age and Body Mass Index [96].

(ii) Obesity induces insulin resistance and increases the circulating level of insulin. Hyperinsulinemia has been correlated with risk of breast cancer recurrence and mortality in both pre- and post-menopausal women [97]. Hyperinsulinemia results in decreased concentrations of sex-hormone-binding globulin that binds testosterone and E2 [98, 99], therefore increasing the bioavailability of circulating E2.

(iii) Adipokines and pro-inflammatory factors secreted by adipocytes affect tumorigenesis. For example, TNF-α not only contributes to the development of insulin resistance [100], but also enhances aromatase expression in adipose tissue [101, 102]. The gene expression of TNF-α markedly increases in obese subjects [103]. IL-6 promotes cell migration, inhibit cell apoptosis, and facilitates metastatic growth [104]. High circulating levels of IL-6 are associated with poor outcome in advanced metastatic breast cancer [105]. IL-6 also stimulates aromatase expression in adipose tissue thereby stimulating estrogen biosynthesis [101, 102]. The synthesis of IL-6 is regulated by TNF-α [106] and increases in obese and insulin resistant subjects [107, 108].

We have observed the following effects of BEX and from these observations posit hypotheses regarding the function of BEX in the inhibition of breast cancer in obese subjects: (i) BEX inhibited high fat diet-induced weight gain and fat deposition in the abdominal cavity indicating that BEX may decrease the expression of aromatase in fat tissues. (ii) BEX also inhibited hyperinsulinemia, therefore it may decrease the bioavailability of circulating estrogen. (iii) BEX dramatically decreased the circulating level of TNF-α in high fat diet-treated mice, indicating that it may also decrease the circulating level of IL-6 through the regulation of TNF-α, and subsequently inhibit the development and metastasis of breast cancer. Taken together, it is likely that BEX is able to decrease the risk and improve the prognosis of breast cancer in obese human subjects.

SUMMARY

Bamboo *Phyllostachys edulis* is one of the fastest growing land plants in the world. It can grow 1–1.6 feet per day during the initial growth phase, is a "running bamboo" that can be easily propagated, and is also a tolerant plant adaptable to five of the eight climate zones. Our research has shown that an ethanol/water extract from this bamboo significantly reduced fatty acid-induced lipotoxicity and high fat diet-induced adiposity, hyperinsulinemia, hyperglycemia and also inhibited chemically induced breast cancer. It is likely that BEX is also able to reduce the risk and improve the prognosis of breast cancer in obese subjects. In summary, bamboo extract is a highly promising anti-diabetic and anti-breast cancer nutraceutical.

ACKNOWLEDGMENTS

I would like to thank my mentor Dr. Marla J. Berry for her encouragement and continuous support on my research on the health benefiting effects of bamboo extract. I also would like to thank my husband Brian K. Panee for his generous and constant support on my research and his editing contribution to this chapter. These studies were made possible by Grant numbers R21 AT003874-01 and -02 (Panee) from the National Center for Complementary and Alternative Medicine (NCCAM). The contents are solely the responsibility of the authors and do not necessarily represent the official views of the NCCAM, or the National Institute of Health.

REFERENCES

1. Sakai, S., Saito, G., Sugayama, J., Kamasuka, T., Takada, S. & Takano, T. (1963). [on the Anticancer Action of Bamboo Extract.]. *J Antibiot [B]* **16**, 387–391.
2. Shibata, M., Yamatake, Y., Sakamoto, M., Kanamori, M. & Takagi, K. (1975). [Phamacological studies on bamboo grass (1). Acute toxicity and anti-inflammatory and antiulcerogenic activities of water-soluble fraction (Folin) extracted from
Sasa albomarginata Makino et Shibata]. *Nippon Yakurigaku Zasshi* **71**, 481–490.
3. Shibata, M., Kubo, K. & Onoda, M. (1976). [Pharmacological studies on bamboo grass. (2) Central depressant and antitoxic actions of a water-soluble fraction

(folin) extracted from Sasa albomarginata Makino et Shibata]. *Nippon Yakurigaku Zasshi* **72**, 531–541.

4. Shibata, M., Kubo, K. & Onoda, M. (1978). [Pharmacological studies on bamboo grass. III. Effects on cardiovascular and isolated organs of water-soluble fraction extracted from Sasa albomarginata Makino et Shibata (Bambusaceae) (author's transl)]. *Yakugaku Zasshi* **98**, 1436–1440.

5. Shibata, M., Fojii, M. & Yamaguchi, R. (1979). [Pharmacological studies on bamboo grass. IV. Toxicological and pharmacological effects of the extract (FIII) obtained from Sasa albomarginata Makino et Shibata (author's transl)]. *Yakugaku Zasshi* **99**, 663–668.

6. Okabe, S., Takeuchi, K., Takagi, K. & Shibata, M. (1975). Stimulatory effect of the water extract of bamboo grass (Folin solution) on gastric acid secretion in pylorus-ligated rats. *Jpn J Pharmacol* **25**, 608–609.

7. Sato, T., Tsuchiya, A., Kobayashi, N., Kimura, J., Hayashi, H., Kobayashi, H., Hobo, R. & Kamoi, K. (1986). [The use in periodontal therapy of a bamboo leaf extract solution]. *Nippon Shishubyo Gakkai Kaishi* **28**, 752–757.

8. Otani, K., Yanaura, S., Yuda, Y., Kawaoto, H., Kajita, T., Hirano, F., Osawa, F. & Inouye, S. (1990). Histo-chemical studies on the anti-ulcer effect of bamboo grass in rats. *Int J Tissue React* **12**, 319–332.

9. Tsunoda, S., Yamamoto, K., Sakamoto, S., Inoue, H. & Nagasawa, H. (1998). Effects of Sasa health, extract of bamboo grass leaves, on spontaneous mammary tumourigenesis in SHN mice. *Anticancer Res* **18**, 153–158.

10. Hu, C., Zhang, Y. & Kitts, D. D. (2000). Evaluation of antioxidant and prooxidant activities of bamboo Phyllostachys nigra var. Henonis leaf extract *in vitro*. *J Agric Food Chem* **48**, 3170–3176.

11. Kweon, M. H., Hwang, H. J. & Sung, H. C. (2001). Identification and antioxidant activity of novel chlorogenic acid derivatives from bamboo (Phyllostachys edulis). *J Agric Food Chem* **49**, 4646–4655.

12. Kim, K. K., Kawano, Y. & Yamazaki, Y. (2003). A novel porphyrin photosensitizer from bamboo leaves that induces apoptosis in cancer cell lines. *Anticancer Res* **23**, 2355–2361.

13. Ren, M., Reilly, R. T. & Sacchi, N. (2004). Sasa health exerts a protective effect on Her2/NeuN mammary tumorigenesis. *Anticancer Res* **24**, 2879–2884.

14. Zhang, Y., Wu, X., Ren, Y., Fu, J. & Zhang, Y. (2004). Safety evaluation of a triterpenoid-rich extract from bamboo shavings. *Food Chem Toxicol* **42**, 1867–1875.

15. Kurokawa, T., Itagaki, S., Yamaji, T., Nakata, C., Noda, T., Hirano, T. & Iseki, K. (2006). Antioxidant activity of a novel extract from bamboo grass (AHSS) against ischemia-reperfusion injury in rat small intestine. *Biol Pharm Bull* **29**, 2301–2303.

16. Lu, B., Wu, X., Shi, J., Dong, Y. & Zhang, Y. (2006). Toxicology and safety of antioxidant of bamboo leaves. Part 2: Developmental toxicity test in rats with antioxidant of bamboo leaves. *Food Chem Toxicol* **44**, 1739–1743.

17. Zhang, Y., Yao, X., Bao, B. & Zhang, Y. (2006). Anti-fatigue activity of a triterpenoid-rich extract from Chinese bamboo shavings (Caulis bamfusae in taeniam). *Phytother Res* **20**, 872–876.

18. Jiao, J., Zhang, Y., Lou, D., Wu, X. & Zhang, Y. (2007). Antihyperlipidemic and antihypertensive effect of a triterpenoid-rich extract from bamboo shavings

and vasodilator effect of friedelin on phenylephrine-induced vasoconstriction in thoracic aortas of rats. *Phytother Res* **21**, 1135–1141.

19. Park, H. S., Lim, J. H., Kim, H. J., Choi, H. J. & Lee, I. S. (2007). Antioxidant flavone glycosides from the leaves of Sasa borealis. *Arch Pharm Res* **30**, 161–166.

20. Lu, B., Wu, X., Shi, J., Dong, Y. & Zhang, Y. (2006). Toxicology and safety of antioxidant of bamboo leaves. Part 2: Developmental toxicity test in rats with antioxidant of bamboo leaves. *Food Chem Toxicol* **44**, 1739–1743.

21. Lu, B., Wu, X., Tie, X. & Zhang, Y. (2005). Toxicology and safety of anti-oxidant of bamboo leaves. Part 1: Acute and subchronic toxicity studies on anti-oxidant of bamboo leaves. *Food Chem Toxicol* **43**, 783–792.

22. Hedley, A. A., Ogden, C. L., Johnson, C. L., Carroll, M. D., Curtin, L. R. & Flegal, K. M. (2004). Prevalence of overweight and obesity among US children, adolescents, and adults, 1999–2002. *JAMA* **291**, 2847–2850.

23. Ogden, C. L., Carroll, M. D., Curtin, L. R., McDowell, M. A., Tabak, C. J. & Flegal, K. M. (2006). Prevalence of overweight and obesity in the United States, 1999–2004. *JAMA* **295**, 1549–1555.

24. Mokdad, A. H., Ford, E. S., Bowman, B. A., Nelson, D. E., Engelgau, M. M., Vinicor, F. & Marks, J. S. (2000). Diabetes trends in the U.S.: 1990–1998. *Diabetes Care* **23**, 1278–1283.

25. Boyle, J. P., Honeycutt, A. A., Narayan, K. M., Hoerger, T. J., Geiss, L. S., Chen, H. & Thompson, T. J. (2001). Projection of diabetes burden through 2050: Impact of changing demography and disease prevalence in the U.S. *Diabetes Care* **24**, 1936–1940.

26. Parkin, D. M., Bray, F., Ferlay, J. & Pisani, P. (2005). Global cancer statistics, 2002. *CA Cancer J Clin* **55**, 74–108.

27. Cacicedo, J. M., Benjachareowong, S., Chou, E., Ruderman, N. B. & Ido, Y. (2005). Palmitate induced apoptosis in cultured bovine retinal pericytes: Roles of NAD(P)H oxidase, oxidant stress, and ceramide. *Diabetes* **54**, 1838–1845.

28. Sims, E. A., Danforth, E., Horton, E. S., Bray, G. A., Glennon, J. A. & Salans, L. B. (1973). Endocrine and metabolic effects of experimental obesity in man. *Recent Prog Horm Res* **29**, 457–496.

29. Beck-Nielsen, H., Pedersen, O. & Lindskov, H. O. (1979). Normalization of the insulin sensitivity and the cellular insulin binding during treatment of obese diabetics for one year. *Acta Endocrinol (Copenh)* **90**, 103–112.

30. Freidenberg, G. R., Reichart, D., Olefsky, J. M. & Henry, R. R. (1988). Reversibility of defective adipocyte insulin receptor kinase activity in non-insulin-dependent diabetes mellitus. Effect of weight loss. *J Clin Invest* **82**, 1398–1406.

31. Bak, J. F., Moller, N., Schmitz, O., Saaek, A. & Pedersen, O. (1992). *In vivo* insulin action and muscle glycogen synthase activity in type 2 (non-insulin-dependent) diabetes mellitus: Effects of diet treatment. *Diabetologia* **35**, 777–784.

32. Unger, R. H. (2002). Lipotoxic diseases. *Annu Rev Med* **53**, 319–336.

33. Dyck, D. J., Heigenhauser, G. J. & Bruce, C. R. (2006). The role of adipokines as regulators of skeletal muscle fatty acid metabolism and insulin sensitivity. *Acta Physiol (Oxf)* **186**, 5–16.

34. Tilg, H. & Moschen, A. R. (2006). Adipocytokines: Mediators linking adipose tissue, inflammation and immunity. *Nat Rev Immunol* **6**, 772–783.
35. Unger, R. H. & Zhou, Y. T. (2001). Lipotoxicity of beta-cells in obesity and in other causes of fatty acid spillover. *Diabetes* **50**(Suppl 1), S118–121.
36. Frustaci, A., Kajstura, J., Chimenti, C., Jakoniuk, I., Leri, A., Maseri, A., Nadal-Ginard, B. & Anversa, P. (2000). Myocardial cell death in human diabetes. *Circ Res* **87**, 1123–1132.
37. Shimabukuro, M., Zhou, Y. T., Levi, M. & Unger, R. H. (1998). Fatty acid-induced beta cell apoptosis: A link between obesity and diabetes. *Proc Natl Acad Sci U S A* **95**, 2498–2502.
38. Rosenthal, M. D. (1981). Accumulation of neutral lipids by human skin fibroblasts: Differential effects of saturated and unsaturated fatty acids. *Lipids* **16**, 173–182.
39. Zhang, C. L., Lyngmo, V. & Nordoy, A. (1992). The effects of saturated fatty acids on endothelial cells. *Thromb Res* **65**, 65–75.
40. de Vries, J. E., Vork, M. M., Roemen, T. H., de Jong, Y. F., Cleutjens, J. P., van der Vusse, G. J. & van Bilsen, M. (1997). Saturated but not mono-unsaturated fatty acids induce apoptotic cell death in neonatal rat ventricular myocytes. *J Lipid Res* **38**, 1384–1394.
41. Rachek, L. I., Musiyenko, S. I., LeDoux, S. P. & Wilson, G. L. (2007). Palmitate induced mitochondrial deoxyribonucleic acid damage and apoptosis in l6 rat skeletal muscle cells. *Endocrinology* **148**, 293–299.
42. Perseghin, G., Scifo, P., De Cobelli, F. *et al.* (1999). Intramyocellular triglyceride content is a determinant of in vivo insulin resistance in humans: A 1H- 13C nuclear magnetic resonance spectroscopy assessment in offspring of type 2 diabetic parents. *Diabetes* **48**, 1600–1606.
43. Panee, J., Liu, W., Lin, Y., Gilman, C. & Berry, M. J. (2008). A novel function of bamboo extract in relieving lipotoxicity. *Phytother Res*, **22**, 675–80.
44. Brody, J. G., Moysich, K. B., Humblet, O., Attfield, K. R., Beehler, G. P. & Rudel, R. A. (2007). Environmental pollutants and breast cancer: Epidemiologic studies. *Cancer* **109**, 2667–2711.
45. Phillips, D. H. (1983). Fifty years of benzo(a)pyrene. *Nature* **303**, 468–472.
46. Phillips, D. H. (1999). Polycyclic aromatic hydrocarbons in the diet. *Mutation Res* **443**, 139–147.
47. Menzie, C. A., Potocki, B. B. & Santodonato, J. (1992). Exposure to carcinogenic PAHs in the environment. *Environ Sci Technol* **26**, 1278–1284.
48. Rudel, R. A., Attfield, K. R., Schifano, J. N. & Brody, J. G. (2007). Chemicals causing mammary gland tumors in animals signal new directions for epidemiology, chemicals testing, and risk assessment for breast cancer prevention. *Cancer* **109**, 2635–2666.
49. Heimann, R., Heuson, J. C. & Coune, A. (1968). Tumors developing in oophorectomized Sprague-Dawley rats after a single gastric instillation of 7,12-dimethylbenz(a)anthracene. *Cancer Res* **28**, 309–313.
50. Kleiner, H. E., Vulimiri, S. V., Hatten, W. B., Reed, M. J., Nebert, D. W., Jefcoate, C. R. & DiGiovanni, J. (2004). Role of cytochrome P450 1 family members in the metabolic activation of polycyclic aromatic hydrocarbons in mouse epidermis. *Chem Res Toxicol* **17**, 1667–1674.

51. Han, E. H., Kim, J. Y. & Jeong, H. G. (2006). Effect of biochanin A on the aryl hydrocarbon receptor and cytochrome P450 1A1 in MCF-7 human breast carcinoma cells. *Arch Pharm Res* **29**, 570–576.

52. Granberg, L., Ostergren, A., Brandt, I. & Brittebo, E. B. (2003). CYP1A1 and CYP1B1 in blood-brain interfaces: CYP1A1-dependent bioactivation of 7,12-dimethylbenz(a)anthracene in endothelial cells. *Drug Metab Dispos* **31**, 259–265.

53. Dipple, A., Cheng, S. C. & Bigger, C. A. H. (1990). Polycyclic aromatic hydrocarbon carcinogens. *Prog Clin Biol Res* **347**, 109–127.

54. Vater, S. T., Baldwin, D. M. & Warshawsky, D. (1991). Hepatic metabolism of 7,12-dimethylbenz(a)anthracene in male, female, and ovariectomized Sprague-Dawley rats. *Cancer Res* **51**, 492–498.

55. Moore, C. J., Tricomi, W. A. & Gould, M. N. (1988). Comparison of 7, 12-dimet hylbenz(a)anthracene metabolism and DNA binding in mammary epithelial cells from three rat strains with differing susceptibilities to mammary carcinogenesis. *Carcinogenesis* **9**, 2099–2102.

56. Singletary, K. W., Parker, H. M. & Milner, J. A. (1990). Identification and in vivo formation of 32P-postlabeled rat mammary DMBA-DNA adducts. *Carcinogenesis* **11**, 1959–1963.

57. Daniel, F. B. & Joyce, N. J. (1983). DNA adduci formation by 7,12-dimethylbenz (a)anthracene and its noncarcinogenic 2-fiuoro analogue in female Sprague-Dawley rats. *J Natl Cancer Inst* **70**, 111–118.

58. Singletary, K. W. (1990). Effect of dietary butylated hydroxytoluene on the *in vivo* distribution, metabolism, and DNA-binding of 7.12-dimethylbenz(a)anthracene. *Cancer Lett* **49**, 187–193.

59. Pool-Zobel, B., Veeriah, S. & Bohmer, F. D. (2005). Modulation of xenobiotic metabolizing enzymes by anticarcinogens – focus on glutathione *S*-transferases and their role as targets of dietary chemoprevention in colorectal carcinogenesis. *Mutat Res* **591**, 74–92.

60. Rundle, A., Tang, D., Zhou, J., Cho, S. & Perera, F. (2000). The association between glutathione *S*-transferase M1 genotype and polycyclic aromatic hydrocarbon- DNA adducts in breast tissue. *Cancer Epidemiol Biomarkers Prev* **9**, 1079–1085.

61. Chang, T. W., Wang, S. M., Guo, Y. L., Tsai, P. C., Huang, C. J. & Huang, W. (2006). Glutathione *S*-transferase polymorphisms associated with risk of breast cancer in southern Taiwan. *Breast* **15**, 754–761.

62. Lampe, J. W. (2007). Diet, genetic polymorphisms, detoxification, and health risks. *Altern Ther Health Med* **13**, S108–111.

63. Sparks, R., Ulrich, C. M., Bigler, J. *et al.* (2004). UDP-glucuronosyltransferase and sulfotransferase polymorphisms, sex hormone concentrations, and tumor receptor status in breast cancer patients. *Breast Cancer Res* **6**, R488–498.

64. Weinshilboum, R. M., Otterness, D. M., Aksoy, I. A., Wood, T. C., Her, C. & Raftogianis, R. B. (1997). Sulfation and sulfotransferases 1: Sulfotransferase molecular biology: cDNAs and genes. *FASEB J* **11**, 3–14.

65. Adjei, A. A. & Weinshilboum, R. M. (2002). Catecholestrogen sulfation: Possible role in carcinogenesis. *Biochem Biophys Res Commun* **292**, 402–408.

66. Falany, J. L. & Falany, C. N. (1996). Expression of cytosolic sulfotransferases in normal mammary epithelial cells and breast cancer cell lines. *Cancer Res* **56**, 1551–1555.

67. Lin, Y., Collier, A., Liu, W., Berry, M. J. & Panee, J. (2007). The inhibitory effect of bamboo extract on the development of 7,12-Dimethylbenz[a]anthracene

(DMBA)-induced breast cancer and its regulatory effect on sulfotransferase activity. *Phytother Res*, In press.

68. Mulder, G. J. & Van Doorn, A. B. D. (1975). A rapid NAD + − linked assay for microsomal uridine diphosphate glucuronosyl transferase of Rat liver and some observations on substrate specificity of the enzyme. *Biochem J* **151**, 131–140.

69. Tabrett, C. A. & Coughtrie, M. W. (2003). Phenol sulfotransferase 1A1 activity in human liver: Kinetic properties, interindividual variation and re-evaluation of the suitability of 4-nitrophenol as a probe substrate. *Biochem Pharmacol* **66**, 2089–2097.

70. Collier, A. C., Tingle, M. D., Keelan, J. A., Paxton, J. W. & Mitchell, M. D. (2000). A highly sensitive fluorescent microplate method for the determination of UDP-glucuronosyl transferase activity in tissues and placental cell lines. *Drug Metabol Disp* **28**, 1184–1186.

71. Gonzalez, P., Tunon, M. J., Manrique, V., Garcia-Pardo, L. A. & Gonzalez, J. (1989). Changes in hepatic cytosolic glutathione-*S*-transferase enzymes induced by clotrimazole treatment in rats. *Clin Exp Pharmacol Physiol* **16**, 867–871.

72. Habig, W. H., Pabst, M. J. & Jakoby, W. B. (1974). Glutathione-*S*-Transferases. *J Biol Chem* **249**, 7130–7139.

73. Friedenreich, C. M. (2001). Review of anthropometric factors and breast cancer risk. *Eur J Cancer Prev* **10**, 15–32.

74. Stephenson, G. D. & Rose, D. P. (2003). Breast cancer and obesity: an update. *Nutr Cancer* **45**, 1–16.

75. Carmichael, A. R. (2006). Obesity and prognosis of breast cancer. *Obes Rev* **7**, 333–340.

76. Harvie, M., Hooper, L. & Howell, A. H. (2003). Central obesity and breast cancer risk: A systematic review. *Obes Rev* **4**, 157–173.

77. Toniolo, P. G., Levitz, M., Zeleniuch-Jacquotte, A., Banerjee, S., Koenig, K. L., Shore, R. E., Strax, P. & Pasternack, B. S. (1995). A prospective study of endogenous estrogens and breast cancer in post-menopausal women. *J Natl Cancer Inst* **86**, 1076–1082.

78. Berrino, F., Muti, P., Micheli, A., Bolelli, G., Krogh, V., Sciajno, R., Pisani, P., Panico, S. & Secreto, G. (1996). Serum sex hormone levels after menopause and subsequent breast cancer. *J Natl Cancer Inst* **88**, 291–296.

79. Shimizu, H., Ross, R. K., Bernstein, L., Pike, M. C. & Henderson, B. E. (1990). Serum oestrogen levels in postmenopausal women: Comparison of American whites and Japanese in Japan. *Br J Cancer* **62**, 451–453.

80. Bernstein, L., Ross, R. K., Pike, M. C., Brown, J. B. & Henderson, B. E. (1990). Hormone levels in older women: A study of post-menopausal breast cancer patients and healthy population controls. *Br J Cancer* **61**, 298–302.

81. Bernstein, L., Yuan, J. M., Ross, R. K., Pike, M. C., Hanisch, R., Lobo, R., Stanczyk, F., Gao, Y. T. & Henderson, B. E. (1990). Serum hormone levels in pre-menopausal Chinese women in Shanghai and white women in Los Angeles; results from two breast cancer case-control studies. *Cancer Causes Control* **1**, 51–58.

82. Feigelson, H. S. & Henderson, B. E. (1996). Estrogens and breast cancer. *Carcinogenesis* **17**, 2279–2284.

83. Bernstein, L. (1998). The epidemiology of breast cancer. *LOWAC J* **1**, 7–13.

84. Liehr, J. G. (2000). Is estradiol a genotoxic mutagenic carcinogen? *Endocr Rev* **21**, 40–54.

85. Yager, J. D. & Davidson, N. E. (2006). Estrogen carcinogenesis in breast cancer. *N Engl J Med* **354**, 270–282.

86. Mitrunen, K. & Hirvonen, A. (2003). Molecular epidemiology of sporadic breast cancer. The role of polymorphic genes involved in oestrogen biosynthesis and metabolism. *Mutat Res* **544**, 9–41.

87. Thompson, P. A. & Ambrosone, C. (2000). Molecular epidemiology of genetic polymorphisms in estrogen metabolizing enzymes in human breast cancer. *J Natl Cancer Inst Monogr* **27**, 125–134.

88. Cavalieri, E. L., Stack, D. E., Devanesan, P. D., Todorovic, R., Dwivedy, I. & Higginbotham, S. (1997). Molecular origin of cancer: Catechol estrogen-3,4-quinones as endogenous tumor initiators. *Proc Natl Acad Sci USA* **94**, 10937–10942.

89. Kisselev, P., Schunck, W. H., Roots, I. & Schwarz, D. (2005). Association of CYP1A1 polymorphisms with differential metabolic activation of 17 beta-estradiol and estrone. *Cancer Res* **65**, 2972–2978.

90. Symonds, D. A., Miller, K. P., Tomic, D. & Flaws, J. A. (2006). Effect of methoxychlor and estradiol on cytochrome P450 enzymes in the mouse ovarian surface epithelium. *Toxicol Sci* **89**, 510–514.

91. Spink, D. C., Katz, B. H., Hussain, M. M., Pentecost, B. T., Cao. Z. & Spink, B. C. (2003). Estrogen regulates Ah responsiveness in MCF-7 breast cancer cells. *Carcinogenesis* **24**, 1941–1950.

92. Katzenellenbogen, B. S. (1996). Estrogen receptors: Bioactivity and interactions with cell signaling pathways. *Biol Reprod* **54**, 287–293.

93. Liehr, J. G., Sirbasku, D. A., Jurka, E., Randerath, K. & Randerath, E. (1988). Inhibition of estrogen-induced renal carcinogenesis in male Syrian hamsters by Tamoxifen without decrease in DNA adduct levels. *Cancer Res* **48**, 779–783.

94. Wani, M. A., Zhu, Q., El-Mahdy, M., Venkatachalam, S. & Wani, A. A. (2000). Enhanced sensitivity to anti-benzo(a)pyrene-diol-epoxide DNA damage correlates with decreased global genomic repair attributable to abrogated p53 function in human cells. *Cancer Res* **60**, 2273–2280.

95. Lorincz, A. M. & Sukumar, S. (2006). Molecular links between obesity and breast cancer. *Endocr Relat Cancer* **13**, 279–292.

96. Grodin, J. M., Siiteri, P. K. & MacDonald, P. C. (1973). Source of estrogen production in postmenopausal women. *J Clin Endocrin Metab* **36**, 207–214.

97. Goodwin, P. J., Ennis, M., Pritchard, K. I., Trudeau, M. E., Koo, J., Madarnas, Y., Hartwick, W., Hoffman, B. & Hood, N. (2002). Fasting insulin and outcome in early-stage breast cancer: results of a prospective cohort study. *J Clin Oncol* **20**, 42–51.

98. Pugeat, M., Crave, J. C., Elmidani, M., Nicolas, M. H., Garoscio-Cholet, M., Lejeune, H., Dechaud, H. & Tourniaire, J. (1991). Pathophysiology of sex hormone binding globulin (SHBG): Relation to insulin. *J Steroid Biochem Mol Biol* **40**, 841–849.

99. McTiernan, A., Rajan, K. B., Tworoger, S. S. *et al.* (2003). Adiposity and sex hormones in postmenopausal breast cancer survivors. *J Clin Oncol* **21**, 1961–1966.

100. Hotamisligil, G. S. (2003). Inflammatory pathways and insulin action. *Int JObes Relat Metab Disord* **27**, S53–S55.

101. Purohit, A., Newman, S. P. & Reed, M. J. (2002). The role of cytokines in regulating estrogen synthesis: Implications for the etiology of breast cancer. *Breast Cancer Res* **4**, 65–69.

102. Purohit, A. & Reed, M. J. (2002). Regulation of estrogen synthesis in postmenopausal women. *Steroids* **67**, 979–983.
103. Hotamisligil, G. S., Shargill, N. S. & Spiegelman, B. M. (1993). Adipose expression of tumor necrosis factor-alpha: Direct role in obesity-linked insulin resistance. *Science* **259**, 87–91.
104. Grano, M., Mori, G., Minielli, V., Cantatore, F. P., Colucci, S. & Zallone, A. Z. (2000). Breast cancer cell line MDA-231 stimulates osteoclastogenesis and bone resorption in human osteoclasts. *Biochem Biophys Res Comm* **270**, 1097–1100.
105. Bachelot, T., Ray-Coquard, I., Menetrier-Caux, C., Rastkha, M., Duc, A. & Blay, J. Y. (2003). Prognostic value of serum levels of interleukin 6 and of serum and plasma levels of vascular endothelial growth factor in hormone-refractory metastatic breast cancer patients. *Br J Cancer* **88**, 1721–1726.
106. de Nascimento, C. O., Hunter, L. & Trayhurn, P. (2004). Regulation of haptoglobin gene expression in 3T3-L1 adipocytes by cytokines, catecholamines, and PPARgamma. *Biochem Biophys Res Comm* **313**, 702–708.
107. Vozarova, B., Weyer, C., Hanson, K., Tataranni, P. A., Bogardus, C. & Pratley, R. E. (2001). Circulating interleukin-6 in relation to adiposity, insulin action, and insulin secretion. *Obesity Res* **9**, 414–417.
108. You, T., Yang, R., Lyles, M. F., Gong, D. & Nicklas, B. J. (2005). Abdominal adipose tissue cytokine gene expression: Relationship to obesity and metabolic risk factors. *Am J Physiol Endocrinol Metabol* **288**, E741–E747.

Chapter 10

Cranberry and Other Dietary Supplements for the Treatment of Urinary Tract Infections in Aging Women

Lynn Stothers

Department of Urology, Bladder Care Centre, University of British Columbia, Vancouver, BC, Canada

Abstract

A wide range of herbal remedies and complementary medicine regimes are used in traditional medicine for the prevention and treatment of urinary tract infections (UTIs). There is now good evidence in the literature that cranberry products of all types (juice, juice cocktail, tablets, and dried sweetened berries) prevent adhesion of *Escherichia coli* to uroepithelial cells. The evidence is becoming more convincing that cranberry products are effective in preventing UTIs. The evidence supporting the use of other *Vaccinium* family berries, such as blueberries, lingonberries and huckleberries is mounting. However, it is less clear whether cranberry products are effective in the treatment of UTIs. Other herbal remedies that may contribute to the prevention or treatment of UTIs in adults include bearberry (uva-ursi), forskolin (coleus), berberine (from goldenseal or other plants), juniper oil, and St. John's wort. Products described to a lesser degree in the scientific literature include buchu, vitamin A, vitamin C, bromelain, nettle, Oregon grape, plantain, horsetail, horseradish, and green tea.

Keywords: *UTI, cranberry, vaccinium, herbal, anthocyanidin, prevention and treatment, urology, bladder*

INTRODUCTION

Urinary tract infections (UTIs) are one of the most common problems presenting in physicians' offices, clinics and emergency departments [1], with an estimated 8 million visits per year in the United States [2]. This is equivalent to about one in four adult women being affected at some point in their lifetime, at an annual cost of 1 billion dollars [3]. The incidence among young, sexually active women is approximately 0.5 person-years [4], equivalent to about 0.1–0.15 person-years for the total population. The incidence of UTIs is much lower in men. Age and sexual activity are significant risk facts in adult women.

The incidence of UTIs increases in women with advancing age although the mechanisms underlying this are not entirely understood [5]. Among healthy women age 55–75, the incidence of community-acquired UTI is about 7/100 person-years among non-diabetic women and 12/100 person-years among those with diabetes [6]. These rates are about 10% of the incidence rates in younger, more sexually active women [5]. Several factors seem to increase the risk of UTI in older women, including estrogen deficiency, prior urogenital surgery, incontinence, cystocele, incomplete bladder emptying, lifetime history of UTI (more than six UTIs throughout lifetime), and being a non-secretor of ABO histo-blood group antigens, a genetically determined characteristic. Non-secretors of these antigens have increased adherence of *E. coli* to uroepithelial cells [5]. After menopause, there is a change in the vaginal pH and thus the vaginal flora, which allows bacteria such as *E. coli* to grow, and subsequently colonize the urinary tract.

Estrogen has a role in maintaining normal vaginal flora, thus reducing the risks of UTI, but if levels are too high, the risk of UTI may increase by facilitating adherence of bacteria to uroepithelial cells [7]. Also, vaginal creams may increase the risk of UTI by increasing the delivery of infective agents to the vagina [6].

MECHANISMS OF LOWER URINARY TRACT INFECTION

Most lower UTIs in women are caused by ascending organisms. The infection begins with vaginal colonization by bacteria from feces, usually *E. coli*. The bacteria colonize the area around the meatus and the distal urethra. The colonization then moves up the urethra to the bladder. Bladder colonization and infection begins with binding of bacteria to the epithelial tissues of the bladder wall. This is an important distinction, in that bacteria in the urinary tract (bacteriuria) may be present in the urine, unbound and without symptoms (asymptomatic bacteriuria). To create an infection of the bladder, itself the bacteria have various adhesive organelles on the surface which facilitate adhesion, and subsequent invasion of the bladder epithelial cells [7].

After the bacteria enter the uroepithelial cells, they divide rapidly and form small clusters, or intracellular bacterial communities. Ultimately, the bacteria form biofilms, or communities of bacteria attached to each other, and there is community behaviour. Biofilms protect the communities from environmental changes and insults, and result in the bacteria being resistant to the efforts of the host cells to attack, because the bacteria are hidden inside the matrix of the biofilm.

Eventually, the bacteria detach from the biofilm and rebind to another uroepithelial site to form another generation and another reservoir of bacteria. The infection may remain asymptomatic for weeks in this latent stage. Thus an infection can remain present, despite antibiotic treatment, for protracted periods.

An alternative mechanism of infection is a rare condition in which the bladder becomes infected directly from adjacent organs, such as a vesicoenteric fistula. In this case, multiple organisms, rather than a single organism, can often be identified in the urine culture.

DESIRE FOR NON-ANTIBIOTIC INTERVENTIONS FOR PREVENTION OR MANAGEMENT

Women who experience recurrent UTIs are often prescribed low-level prophylactic antibiotic regimens in an effort to attack bacteria in the bladder, but increasingly, there are reports of antibiotic-resistant bacterial strains [8]. Thus, an agent such as an herbal product that is not specific to a particular bacterial strain is desirable if it can be shown to be effective.

Cranberries

Cranberries have long been thought to be useful in the prevention and treatment of UTIs. The plant is a low growing shrub with evergreen leaves. The berry is initially white, and harvest of the berry at this point produces the white cranberry juice that is commercially available. As the berry ripens, it turns red due to the presence of anthocyanins, which are flavonoid pigments.

For centuries, cranberries (*Vaccinium macrocapon*) and cranberry juice have been used by Native Americans as a food source and for medicinal purposes including treatment of bladder and kidney disease. Once introduced to Europe, they were used in the treatment of stomach ailments, blood disorders, liver problems, fevers and scurvy. In the late 1800s and early 1900s, cranberries were described as a treatment for bladder disorders including bladder "gravel" and "blood toxins" [9].

The mechanism of therapeutic action of cranberries in the prevention and treatment of UTIs continues to be investigated at a basic science level. In 1923, researchers demonstrated that consumption of cranberries resulted in acidification of the urine, and made the theoretical leap that it was the hippuric acid in the berries that provided the curative effect [10], but this was refuted in 1959 [11]. In 1984, Sobota reported that cranberry juice interfered with the attachment of bacteria to uroepithelial cells, and thus had potential in the treatment of UTI [12, 13]. Recent work supports the theory that it is interference with bacterial attachment that provides therapeutic effect. Interference with attachment has been documented with *E. coli*, *Proteus*, *Klebsiella*, *Enterobacter*, and *Pseudomonas*. Several molecules have been proposed as the source of the interference: hippuric acid [14], fructose [15], ascorbic acid [16], and anthocyanidins/proanthocyanidins [17, 18].

Vaccinium species, which include cranberries and blueberries, are unique in their high concentrations of quinic acid, which is aromatized to benzoic acid, and with the addition of glycine, is changed to hippuric acid. Hippuric acid is found in the urine following consumption of cranberries, and has been shown to interfere with bacterial attachment [19]. Fructose, found in all fruit, prevents adhesion of type 1-fimbriated bacteria [15].

Proanthocyanidins found in cranberries have been shown to prevent attachment of P-fimbriated *E. coli* to cellular surfaces [15, 18]. Although proanthocyanidins are likely absorbed and metabolized, there is evidence that they have high bioavailability in humans [20]. Proanthocyanidins can be subject to degradation over time when exposed to light and heat, particularly at pH greater than 5 [21]. Keeping juice at cool temperatures and away from light may help to maintain these levels. Levels of proanthocyanidins have been shown to vary widely in commercially available products (Table 10.1) [21].

Cranberries and *Prevention* of UTIs

Cranberries are one of five the most-commonly used herbal remedies for the prevention and treatment of UTIs [8]. However, the evidence supporting the use of cranberries in the prevention of UTI was not strong until recent randomized controlled trials of adequate power and design were reported [22].

TABLE 10.1 Anthocyanin content of some commercially-available cranberry products

Cranberry material	Total anthocyanins (mg/g)	Estimated daily consumption (mg/dosage recommended on packaging)
Raw	0.7	3.5 (125 ml = 50 g)
Capsule/tablet product 1	6.3	no recommendation
Capsule/tablet product 2	1.3	no recommendation
Capsule/tablet product 3	1.3	no recommendation
Capsule/tablet product 4	1.8	no recommendation
Capsule/tablet product 5	1.2	no recommendation
Cranberry beverages	Total anthocyanins (ppm) (mg/l)	
Juice 1, pasteurized	116	29 (8 oz)
Juice 2, pasteurized	208	52 (8 oz)
Cranberry Cocktail 1	9	2 (8 oz)
Cranberry Cocktail 2	23	6 (8 oz)

A 2004 Cochrane systematic review of the literature on cranberries for the prevention of UTIs [9] found seven trials, four of which were cross-over studies, and three of which were parallel group studies. Two of the studies were good quality randomized controlled trials, both of which showed reduction in the incidence of symptomatic UTIs. However, the dropout and withdrawal rates were high, and side effects, primarily gastric, were common.

Among older women, one randomized double-blind study [19] demonstrated that drinking 300 ml of cranberry cocktail daily reduced the incidence of UTIs in elderly women by almost 50%. Unfortunately, there were significant baseline differences between the two groups in this study. In a second study [23], reported only in a letter, data on only 7 of the 38 patients initially enrolled in the study were included in the analysis.

Since the Cochrane review, there have been few additional reports of studies of cranberry juice in the *prevention* of UTI. In one open-label study of women aged 25–70 with recurrent UTI (minimum of six UTIs in the preceding year), women taking two capsules of concentrated cranberry extract (standardized to 30% phenolics) experienced no UTIs during treatment [24]. In a randomized, placebo-controlled, double-blind study assessing the efficacy of 300 ml of sweetened cranberry juice cocktail in older people in hospital, the overall infection rate was lower than anticipated, and the study lacked power [25]. The study did find that, although 3% of patients were regular consumers of cranberry products (and were therefore eliminated from the study), over 30% refused to participate in the study because they did not like the cranberry juice flavor. There are several important randomized controlled trials underway, funded by the National Center for Complementary and Alternative Medicine (NCCAM) branch of the National Institutes of Health NCCAM [26].

The evidence that ingestion of cranberry products, including unsweetened juice [27], juice cocktails [25], lite (calorie-reduced) cocktails [25], dried cranberry (Craisins™) [28], dried cranberry juice [29], and even cranberry sauce [30], prevents UTIs is mounting. Further research is needed to determine the amount of cranberry product required to be effective, and to standardize methods for reporting the products' active components. Cranberry juice as a pure unsweetened juice is tart and therefore patients are more likely to regularly consume cranberry juice cocktail. These preparations typically include dilute juice sweetened with fructose, which has also been shown to have a therapeutic effect on UTIs.

Cranberries and *Treatment* of UTIs

A Cochrane systematic review of the literature (initially performed in 1998 and updated in 2004) on cranberries for the treatment of UTIs found no trials meeting the inclusion criteria [31]. One study in people with spinal cord injuries and indwelling catheters who had proven UTIs prior to beginning treatment found no difference in outcome of 6 months of treatment with cranberry compared with placebo [32]. However, many women continue to claim that taking cranberry products when they first experience the symptoms of a urinary tract infection (i.e., as treatment of the infection) is curative and studies are needed to assess this.

OTHER HERBS OR VITAMINS

- *Other members* of the Vaccinium *family*: The fact that many people dislike the flavor of cranberry products [25] has encouraged the investigation of the potential of other *Vaccinium* berries to prevent or treat UTIs. Blueberries, bilberries, lingonberry, and huckleberries, all of which are members of the *Vaccinium* family may also be effective in prevention of UTIs [32]. These berries have the benefit of being generally held as more palatable in their full fruit form compared to cranberries. Blueberries are only about 1/3 as effective as cranberries because more of the proanthocyanidins in blueberries are B-linked than A-linked, the more anti-adhesive type of proanthocyanidins [33]. However, because they are much more palatable, consumption is likely to be higher, possibly balancing the difference in effectiveness. Also, different blueberry species have different levels of proanthocyanidins, with the wild low-bush blueberries having higher levels than commercially grown high-bush blueberries [33]. Currently, blueberry products are generally less available, but as demand increases, availability is also increasing [33]. No studies have been done on blueberries, but one study on lingonberry showed that the juice is effective in preventing UTIs [34]. Studies are needed on the potential of blueberries and other *Vaccinium* products to prevent or treat UTIs.
- *Arctostaphylos uva-ursi* (bearberry or umbabazane) leaf extracts contain arbutin, which has been shown to kill bacteria in the urine [35]. Arbutin is metabolized to hydroquinone and hydroquinone derivatives that make it potentially useful for urinary conditions. It has been approved for treating inflammation of the lower urinary tract by Commission E of the German Federal Institute for Drugs and Medical Devices, which is the German governmental agency that evaluates the safety and effectiveness of herbal products [36].
- *Forskolin*, an herbal medicine made from the Asiatic coleus plant (*Plectranthus barbatus*), raises levels of cAMP which might help move bacterial colonies out of the cells and into the bladder where antibiotics or antiadhesives can be effective [37, 38].
- *Hypericum perforatum* (St. John's Wort) is recommended by herbalists for viral and bacterial infections. An *in vitro* study showed that the extracts have antibacterial activity against *E. coli* but it is not known whether this effect is passed into the urine [39].
- *Berberine*: Berberine-containing plants include goldenseal root (*Hydrastis Canadensis*), goldenthread (*Coptis chinensis*), Oregon grape (*Berberis*

aquifolium), barberry (*Berberis vulgaris*), and tree tumeric (*Berberis aristata*). These plants have been used for hundreds of years in Ayurvedic and Chinese medicine, and berberine is used in almost all traditional medicine systems [40]. Extracts have been shown to have antimicrobial activity against bacteria, viruses, fungi, protozoans, helminthes, and Chlamydia. Isolates have shown low antibiotic activity, and initially it was believed that this indicated that berberine was not an effective antibiotic. However, recent work indicates that there are other chemicals in the plant that work symbiotically with the berberine, allowing it to enter the bacteria where it can be effective [41]. Further studies are needed.

- *Juniper*: Juniper oil has been shown *in vitro* to have antibiotic characteristics against several gram negative and gram positive bacteria, including *E. coli in vitro* [42]. Some extracts or decoctions use the berries and some use the leaves. Different species differ in the specific components or ratios of the compound believed to have antimicrobial activity (36). Testing *in vivo* is needed before any recommendations can be made.

- *Agathosma betulina* (buchu) has been used by the natives of the Western Cape of Southern Africa for many centuries. Early Dutch settlers used buchu to make a brandy tincture and Boegoebrandewyn (buchu brandy) is still used today to treat many disorders. Buchu is described as a urinary antiseptic and diuretic [43]. However, it has been shown to have very low activity against *E. coli*, so there is little potential for the oils to be used as antimicrobial agents [44].

- *Other agents* that have been suggested (from various sites on the World Wide Web), but for which there is either little scientific evidence or minimal health benefits include, but are not limited to, vitamin A, vitamin C, bromelain, nettle, Oregon grape, plantain, horsetail, horseradish, and green tea. Rigorous studies investigating the antimicrobial activity of these are needed before comments can be made.

POTENTIAL FOR ADVERSE SIDE EFFECTS

Cranberries

Complications reported with the use of cranberry as an herbal medication are rare. There have been rare reports of allergic reaction.

There have been several reports of cranberry appearing to increase the anticoagulant effect of warfarin [45, 46], possibly secondary to the presence of naturally occurring salicylic acid in cranberries, but studies designed to investigate the interaction have found no adverse effects [47–50]. Nevertheless, recommendations are that physicians monitor closely patients taking both warfarin and cranberry products [51, 52].

Although there is evidence that cyclosporine interacts with pomelo juice, no evidence has been found to indicate that it interacts with cranberry [53].

Cranberry contains high levels of oxalates, raising concern that it might increase the risk of renal stones [54]. However, other studies have suggested that cranberry consumption decreases the risk of renal stones, and components of the juice have been described as a treatment modality for renal stones [55, 56].

Others

The adverse effects and potential for interactions with drugs have not been well-investigated for most herbal products. However, over 10% of women in Canada report using herbal products in the previous 2 days so the issue of interactions is of concern [57]. Older women use herbal products more often than younger women, and more often than men. They also often use them in combination with conventional medications [58], with more than half of women reporting herbal use also reporting that they took conventional medications in the same 2-day period. Physicians should be careful to inquire specifically about the use of herbal products and document usage.

There have been some reports in the medical literature of adverse effects with some of the supplements suggested for UTIs. These include bull's-eye maculopathy with bearberry (uva-ursi) use [59] and contact dermatitis from coleus (forskolin) [60]. There is one report in the literature of an allergic reaction to lignonberry [61].

One plant assessed extensively, because of its utility in treating depression is St. John's wort. It has been shown to have a low incidence of adverse effects. Reversible photosensitivity may occur [62]. There is one report of convulsions following an overdose of St. John's wort [63].

POTENTIAL SUPPLEMENTARY BENEFITS OF CRANBERRIES

Apart from the urinary tract benefits of cranberry, cranberries have been suggested to have *cardioprotective* potential and to reduce low-density lipoprotein (LDL) levels [64, 65]. They have also been shown to provide antioxidants that likely contribute to cardiovascular health [66–68]. Cranberry and blueberry products have been described as a treatment for *Helicobacter pylori* infection [69], and to increase the effectiveness of current treatment modalities [70].

The use of cranberry has been investigation for other diseases that commonly affect the elderly. One study of the neuropsychologic effects of cranberry consumption in older cognitively intact, community-dwelling adults found that cranberry improved self-reported memory compared to placebo [71]. *Rheumatoid arthritis*, a disease primarily affecting older women, is now believed to be initiated by sub-clinical UTIs with *Proteus mirabilis* microbes, and thus, particularly in the early stages, be amenable to treatment with cranberry products [72, 73]. This concept is at the hypothesis stage, and assumes efficacy of cranberry products in treatment (rather than prevention) of UTIs, and also assumes efficacy against *Proteus* rather than *E. coli*.

Cranberry has also been shown to have antimicrobial activity against *Streptococcus mutans*, the bacteria responsible for dental caries [74]. Gingivitis, another disease that increases in prevalence with age, has been shown to be responsive to cranberry products [75].

Cranberry products have also been clearly shown in both *in vitro* and *in vivo* studies to have anti-proliferative activity, both by inhibiting growth and by stimulating apoptosis, and are described in the prevention and management of various cancers [67, 68, 76, 77]. Cranberry has also been shown in *in vitro* studies to have antimicrobial activity against bacteriophages and rotaviruses and thus may play a role in treatment of viral infections [78].

SUMMARY

A wide range of herbal remedies and other complementary medicine regimes are used in traditional medicine for the prevention and treatment of UTIs. There is now good evidence in the literature that cranberry products of all types (juice, juice cocktail, tablets, and dried sweetened berries) prevent adhesion of *E. coli* to uroepithelial cells. The evidence is becoming more convincing that cranberry products are effective in preventing UTIs. There are several randomized clinical trials (RCTs) being conducted with NCCAM funding to verify this. The evidence supporting the use of other *Vaccinium* family berries, such as blueberries, lingonberries, huckleberries, is mounting. However, it is less clear whether cranberry products are effective in the treatment of UTIs. Other herbal remedies that may contribute to the prevention or treatment of UTIs include bearberry (uva-ursi), forskolin (coleus), berberine (from goldenseal or other plants), juniper oil, and St. John's wort. Products for which there is little evidence include buchu, vitamin A, vitamin C, bromelain, nettle, Oregon grape, plantain, horsetail, horseradish, and green tea.

REFERENCES

1. Hooten, T. M. (2000). Pathogenesis of urinary tract infections: An update. *J Antimicr Chem* **46**(Suppl S1), 1–7.
2. National Institutes of Health (1990). *The National Kidney and Urological Diseases Advisory Board 1990 Long-Range Plan-Window on the 21st Century.* Pub no.90-583, NIH, Bethesda Maryland.
3. Johnson, J. R. & Stamm, W. E. (1987). Diagnosis and treatment of acute urinary tractions. *Infect Dis Clin North Am* **1**, 773–791.
4. Hooten, T. M., Scholes, D., Hughes, J. P., Winter, C., Roberts, P. L., Stapleton, A. E. *et al.* (1996). A prospective study of risk factors for symptomatic urinary tract infection in young women. *New Eng J Med* **335**, 468–474.
5. McLaughlin, S. P. & Carson, C. C. (2004). Urinary tract infections in women. *Med Clin North Am* **88**(2), 417–429.
6. Jackson, S. L., Boyko, E. J., Scholes, D., Abraham, L., Gupta, K. & Fihn, S. (2004). Predictors of urinary tract infection after menopause: A prospective study. *Am J Med* **117**, 903–911.

7. Franco, A. V. M. (2005). Recurrent urinary tract infections. *Best Practice Res Clin Obs Gynecol* **19**(6), 861–873.
8. Bennett, J. & Brown, C. M. (2000). Use of herbal remedies by patients in a health maintenance organization. *J Am Pharm Assoc (Wash)* **40**(3), 349–351.
9. Jepson, R. G., Mihaljevic, L. & Craig, J. (2000). Cranberries for preventing urinary tract infections (Review). *Cochrane Database Syst Rev* **2**, CD001321.
10. Blatherwick, N. R. & Long, M. L. (1923). Studies on urinary acidity. The increased acidity produced by eating prunes and cranberries. *J Biol Chem* **57**, 815–818.
11. Bodel, P. T., Cotran, R. & Kass, E. H. (1959). Cranberry juice and the antibacterial action of hippuric acid. *J Lab Clin Med* **54**, 881–888.
12. Sobota, A. E. (1984). Inhibition of bacterial adherence by cranberry juice: Potential use for the treatment of urinary tract infections. *J Urol* **131**(5), 1013–1016.
13. Schmidt, D. R. & Sobota, A. E. (1988). An examination of the anti-adherence activity of cranberry juice on urinary and non-urinary bacterial isolates. *Microbios* **55**, 173–182.
14. Kinney, A. B. & Blount, M. (1979). Effect of cranberry juice on urinary pH. *Nurs Res* **28**(5), 287–290.
15. Foo, L. Y., Yu, Y., Howell, A. B. & Vorsa, N. (2000). A-type proanthocyanidin trimers from cranberrry that inhibit adherence of uropathogenic P-fimbriated *Escherichia coli*. *J Nat Prod* **63**, 1225–1228.
16. Habash, M. B., VanderMei, H. C., Busscher, H. J. & Reid, G. (1999). The effect of water, ascorbic acid, and cranberry derived supplementation on human urine and uropathogen adhesion to silicone rubber. *Can J Microbiol* **45**(8), 691–694.
17. Zafriri, D., Ofek, I., Adar, R., Pocino, M. & Sharon, N. (1989). Inhibitory activity of cranberry juice on adherence of type I and type P fimbriated *Escherichia coli* to eucaryotic cells. *Antimicrob Agents Chemother* **33**(1), 92–98.
18. Howell, A. B., Vorsa, N., Marderosian, A. D. & Foo, L. Y. (1998). Inhibition of the adherence of P-fimbriated *Escherichia coli* to uroepithelial surfaces by proanthocyanidin extracts from cranberries. *N Engl J Med* **339**, 1085–1086.
19. Avorn, J., Monane, M., Gurwitz, J. H., Glynn, R. J., Choodnovskiy, I. & Lipsitz, L. A. (1994). Reduction of bacteriuria and pyuria after ingestion of cranberry juice. *JAMA* **272**(8), 588–589.
20. Packer, L., Rimbach, G. & Virgili, F. (1999). Antioxidant activity and biologic properties of a procyanidin-rich extract from pine (*Pinus martima*) bark, Pycnogenol. *Free Rad Biol Med* **27**(5/6), 704–724.
21. Brown, P. & Stothers, L. (2005). The effects of pH and light on important naturopathic compounds found in commercially-available cranberry products used in the prevention of urinary tract infection. Presented at Western Section of American Urologic Assoc Meeting, August 2005.
22. Stamm, W. E., McKevitt, M. & Roberts, P. L. (1991). White NJ: Natural history of recurrent urinary tract infections in women. *Rev Infect Dis* **13**(5), 1024–1025.
23. Haverkorn, M. J. & Mandigers, J. (1994). Reduction of bacteriuria and pyuria using cranberry juice [letter]. *J Am Med Assoc* **272**(8), 590.
24. Bailey, D. T., Dalton, C., Daugherty, F. J. & Tempesta, M. S. (2007). Can a concentrated cranberry extract prevent recurrent urinary tract infections in women? A pilot study. *Phytomedicine* **14**, 237–241.
25. McMurdo, M. E. T., Bissett, L. Y., Price, R. J. G., Phillips, G. & Crombie, I. K. (2005). Does ingestion of cranberry juice reduce symptomatic urinary tract

infections in older people in hospital? A double-blind, placebo-controlled trial. *Age and Aging* **34**, 256–261.

26. http://clinicaltrials.gov/search/term=(NCCAM)+%5BSPONSOR%5D (cranberry)+%5BTREATMENT%5D?recruiting=false.

27. Stothers, L. (2002). A randomized trial to evaluate effectiveness and cost effectiveness of naturopathic cranberry products as prophylaxis against urinary tract infections in women. *Can J Urol* **9**(3), 1558–1562.

28. Greenberg, J. A., Newmann, S. J. & Howell, A. B. (2005). Consumptions of sweetened dried cranberries verus unsweetened raising for inhibition of uropathogenic *Escherichia coli* adhesion in human urine. A pilot study. *J Altern Complem Med,* **11**(5), 875–878.

29. Valentova, K., Stejskal, D., Bednar, P., Vostalova, J., Cihalik, C., Vecerova, R., Koukalova, D., Lokar, M., Reichenback, R., Sknouril, L., Ulrichova, J. & Simanek, V. (2007). Biosafety, antioxidant status, and metabolites in urine after consumption of dried cranberry juice in health women. A pilot double-blind placebo-controlled trial. *J Acric Food Chem* **55**, 3217–3224.

30. Howell, A. B. (2007). Bioactive compounds in cranberries and their role in prevention of urinary tract infections. *Mol Nutr Food Res* **51**, 732–737.

31. Jepson, R. G., Mihaljevic, L. & Craig, J. C. (1998). Cranberries for treating urinary tract infections. *Cochrane Data System Rev*, CD001322.

32. Ofek, I., Goldhar, J. & Sharon, N. (1996). Anti-*Escherichia coli* adhesion activity of cranberry and blueberry juices. *Adv Exp Med Miol* **408**, 179–183.

33. Schmidt, B. M., Howell, A. B., McEniry, B., Knight, C. T., Seigler, D., Erdman, J. W., Jr. & Lila, M. A. (2004). Effective separation of potent antiproliferation and antiadhesion components from wild blueberry (*Vaccinium angustifolium* AIT.) fruits. *J Acric Food Chem* **51**, 6433–6442.

34. Kontiokari, T., Sundqvist, K., Nuutinen, M., Pokka, T., Koskela, M. & Uhari, M. (2001). Randomised trial of cranberry-lingonberry juice and *Lactobacillus* GG drink for the prevention of urinary tract infections in women. *Br Med J* **30**(7302), 1571, 322.

35. Frohne, D. (1970). The urinary disinfectant effect of extract from leaves uva ursi. *Planta Med* **18**(1), 1–25.

36. Yarnell, E. (2002). Botanical medicines for the urinary tract. *World J Urol* **20**, 285–293.

37. Bishop, B. L., Duncan, M. J., Song, J., Li, G., Zaas, D. & Abraham, S. N. (2007). Cyclic AMP-regulated exocytosis of *Escherichia coli* from infected bladder epithelial cells. *Nature Med* **13**(5), 625–630.

38. Monograph (2006). Coleus forskohlii. *Alt Med Rev* **11**(1), 47–51.

39. Cecchini, C., Cresci, A., Coman, M. M., Ricciutelli, M., Sagratini, G., Vittori, S., Lucarini, D. & Maggi, E. (2007). Antimicrobial activity of seven *Hypericum* entities from central Italy. *Planta Med* **73**(6), 564–566.

40. Birdsall, T. C. & Kelly, G. S. (1997). Berberine: Therapeutic potential of an alkaloid found in several medicinal plants. *Alt Med Rev* **2**(2), 94–103.

41. http://www.biology.neu.edu/faculty03/lewis03.html

42. Schelz, Z., Molnar, J. & Hohmann, J. (2006). Antimicrobial and antiplasmid activities of essential oils. *Fitoterapia* **77**, 279–285.

43. http://www.bcdex.com/herbalremedies/utinfection.html

44. Lis-Balchin, M., Hart, S. & Simpson, E. (2001). Buchu (*Agathosma betulina* and *A. crenulata*, Rutaceae) essential oils: Their pharmacological action on guinea

pig ileum and antimicrobial activity on microorganisms. *J Pharm Pharacol* **53**(4), 579–582.

45. Pham, D. Q. & Pham, A. Q. (2007). Interaction potential between cranberry juice and warfarin. *Am J Health-Sys Pharm* **64**(1), 490–494.
46. Suvarna, R., Piromahamed, M. & Henderson, L. (2003). Possible interaction between warfarin and cranberry juice. *BMJ* **327**, 1454.
47. Ridone, J. P. & Murphy, T. W. (2006). Warfarin–cranberry juice interaction resulting in profound hypothrombinemia and bleeding. *Am J Ther* **13**(3), 283–284.
48. Wittkowsky, A. N. (2007). Dietary supplements, herbs and oral anticoagulants: The nature of the evidence. *J Thromb Thrombolysis*, Sep. 29 (Epub).
49. Ansell, J., McDonough, M., Harmatz, J. S. & Greenblatt, D. J. (2007). A randomized, double-blind trial of the interaction between cranberry juice and warfarin. *J Thromb Throbolysis*, Nov. 8 (Epub).
50. Lilja, J. J., Backman, J. T. & Neuvonen, P. J. (2007). Effects of daily ingestion of cranberry juice on the pharmacokinetics of warfarin, tizanidine, and midazolam – probes of CYP2C9, CYP1A2, and CYP3A4. *Clin Pharacol Therapeut* **81**(6), 833–839.
51. Sylvan, L. & Justice, N. P. (2005). Possible interaction between warfarin and cranberry juice, Letter to the Editor. *Am Fam Phys* **72**(6), 1000.
52. Paeng, C. H., Sprague, M. & Jackevicius, C. A. (2007). Interaction between warfarin and cranberry juice. *Clin Ther* **29**(8), 1730–1735.
53. Grenier, J., Gradette, C., Morelli, G., Merritt, G. J., Vrandierick, M. & Ducharme, M. P. (2006). Pomelo juice, but not cranberry juice, affects the pharmacokinetics of cyclosporine in humans. *Clin Pharmacol Ther* **79**(3), 255–262.
54. Terris, M. K., Issa, M. M. & Tacker, J. R. (2001). Dietary supplementation with cranberry concentrate tablets may increase the risk of nephrolithiasis. *Urology* **57**, 26–29.
55. McHarg, T., Rodgers, A. & Charlton, K. (2003). Influence of cranberry juice on the urinary risk factors for calcium oxalate kidney stone formation. *BJU Int* **92**(7), 765–768.
56. Kessler, T., Jansen, B. & Hesse, A. (2002). Effect of blackcurrant-, cranberry- and plum juice consumption on risk factors associated with kidney stone formation. *Eur J Clin Nutr* **56**(10), 1020–1023.
57. Singh, S. R. & Levine, M. A. (2006). Natural health product use in Canada. Analysis of the National Population Health Survey. *Can J Clin Pharacol* **13**(2), Epub.
58. Gunther, S., Patterson, R. E., Kristal, A. R., Stratton, K. L. & White, E. (2004). Demographic and health-related correlates of herbal and specialty supplement use. *J Am Diet Assoc* **104**, 27–34.
59. Wang, L. & Del Priore, L. V. (2004). Bull's-eye maculopathy secondary to herbal toxicity from uva ursi. *Am J Ophthalmol* **137**(6), 1135–1137.
60. Bryld, L. E. (1997). Airborne contact dermatitis from Coleus plant. *Am J Contact Dermat* **8**(1), 8–9.
61. Matheu, V., Baeza, M. L., Zubeldia, J. M. & Barrios, Y. (2004). Allergy to lingonberry: A case report. *Clin Mol Allergy* **2**, 2–5.
62. Schulz, V. (2006). Safety of St. John's Wort extract compared to synthetic antidepressants. *Phyomedicine* **13**, 199–204.

63. Karalapillai, D. C. & Bellomo, R. (2007). Convulsions associated with an overdose of St. John's wort. *Med J Aust* **186**(4), 213–214.

64. Ruel, G., Pomerleau, S., Couture, P., Lemiuex, S., Lamarche, B. & Couillard, C. (2007). Low-calorie cranberry juice supplementation reduces plasma oxidized LDL and cell adhesion molecule concentrations in men. *Br J Nutr* **29**, 1–8.

65. Ruel, G. & Couillard, C. (2007). Evidences of the cardioprotective potential of fruits. The case of cranberries. *Mol Nutr Food Res* **51**(6), 692–701.

66. Zafra-Stone, S., Yasmin, T., Bagchi, M., Chatterjee, A., Vinson, J. A. & Bagchi, D. (2007). Berry anthocyanins as novel antioxidants in human health and disease prevention. *Mol Nutr Food Res* **51**, 675–683.

67. Neto, C. C. (2007). Cranberry and blueberry: Evidence for protective effects against cancer and vascular diseases. *Mol Nutr Food Res* **51**, 652–664.

68. Duthie, S. J., Jenkinson, A. M., Crozier, A., Mullen, W., Pirie, L., Kyle, J., Yap, L. S., Christen, P. & Duthie, G. G. (2006). The effects of cranberry juice consumption on antioxidant status and biomarkers relating to heart disease and cancer in healthy human volunteers. *Eur J Nutr* **45**, 113–122.

69. Zhang, L., Ma, J., Pan, K., Go, V. L. W., Chen, J. & You, W.-C. (2005). Efficacy of cranberry juice on *Helicobacter pylori* infection: A double-blind, randomized placebo-controlled trial. *Helicobacter* **10**(2), 139–145.

70. Shmuely, H., Yahav, J., Samra, Z., Chodick, G., Koren, R., Niv, Y. & Ofek, I. (2007). Effect of cranberry juice on eradication of *Helicobacter pylori* in patients treated with antibiotics and a proton pump inhibitor. *Mol Nutr Food Res* **51**, 746–751.

71. Crews, W. D., Harrison, D. W., Griffin, M. L., Addison, K., Yount, A. M., Giovenco, M. A. & Hazell, J. (2005). A double-blind, placebo-controlled, randomized trial of the neuropsychologic efficacy of cranberry juice in a sample of older adults: Pilot study findings. *J Altern Complement Med* **11**(2), 305–309.

72. Ebringer, A. & Rashid, T. (2006). Rheumatoid arthritis is an autoimmune disease triggered by Proteus urinary tract infection. *Clin Dev Immunol* **13**(1), 41–48.

73. Ebringer, A., Rashid, T. & Wilson, C. (2003). Rheumatoid arthritis: Proposal for the use of anti-microbial therapy in early cases. *Scand J Rheumatol* **32**(1), 2–11.

74. Gregoir, S., Singh, A. P., Vorsa, N. & Koo, H. (2007). Influence of cranberry phenolics on glucan synthesis by glucosyltransferases and *Streptococcus mutans* acidogenicity. *J Appl Microbiol* **103**(5), 1960–1968.

75. Yamanaka, A., Kouchi, T., Kasai, K., Kata, T., Ishihara, K. & Okuda, K. (2007). Inhibitory effect of cranberry polyphenol on biofilm formation and systeine proteases of *Porphyromonas gingivalis*. *J Periodontal Res* **42**(6), 589–592.

76. Seeram, N. P., Adams, L. S., Zhang, Y., Lee, R., Sand, D., Scheuller, H. S. & Heber, D. (2006). Blackberry, black raspberry, blueberry, cranberry, red raspberry and strawberry extracts inhibit growth and stimulate apoptosis of human cancer cells *in vitro*. *J Agric Food Chem* **54**, 9329–9339.

77. Seeram, N. P., Adams, L. S., Hardy, M. L. & Heber, D. (2004). Total cranberry extract vs its phytochemical constituents: Antiproliferative and syndergistic effects against human tumor cell lines. *J Agric Food Chem* **52**, 2512–2517.

78. Lipson, S. M., Sethi, L., Cohen, P., Gordon, R. E., Tan, I. P., Burdowski, A. & Stotzky, G. (2007). Antiviral effects on bacteriophages and rotavirus by cranberry juice. *Phytomedicine* **12**, 23–30.

Chapter 11

Black Cohosh: Chemopreventive and Anticancer Potential

Linda Saxe Einbond

Department of Rehabilitation Medicine, Columbia University College of Physicians and Surgeons, New York, NY, USA

Abstract

Extracts and purified components of black cohosh (*Actaea racemosa* L. syn. *Cimicifuga racemosa* Nutt), a North American perennial used for centuries to treat inflammatory and female health conditions, may be able to prevent and treat breast and other cancers. Many women use the herb today to alleviate the symptoms of menopause. Epidemiological studies suggest that such menopausal treatment is correlated with reduced breast cancer risk. Numerous *in vitro* studies indicate that the herb has a significant effect on growth inhibition and other physiological processes related to carcinogenesis. Black cohosh suppresses tumor development in certain mouse models of carcinogenesis. The rhizomes and roots of the plant contain two major classes of secondary metabolites, triterpene glycosides and phenylpropanoids. Scientific knowledge of related compounds suggests that actein and functionally similar triterpene glycosides isolated from the plant may represent new lead compounds for the synthesis of potent derivatives. Black cohosh is, in sum, a promising agent, but with many unknowns – including its primary molecular target, off-target effects, bioavailability, safety, toxicity, impact on different types and stages of carcinogenesis and tumor-initiating subpopulations, as well as unique effects on aging men and women. Once these questions are satisfactorily addressed, scientifically controlled black cohosh extracts or components can be advanced for cancer prevention or therapy.

Keywords: *Actaea racemosa, actein, black cohosh, Cimicifuga, cimigenol, phenylpropanoid, triterpene glycoside, unfolded protein response*

Abbreviations: ACCX, 25-acetylcimigenol xylopyranoside; CDDO, 2-cyano-3,12-dioxooleana-1,9-dien-28-oic acid; EBV-EA, Epstein-Barr virus early antigen; ER$^{+/-}$, Estrogen Receptor$^{+/-}$; HPLC, High performance liquid chromatography; HRS, hormone-related supplements; iCR, isopropanolic extract of *Actaea (=Cimicifuga) racemosa;* ISR, integrated stress response; SO, synthetic oleanane triterpenes; TNM, classification of malignant tumors; TPA, 12-*O*-tetradecanoylphorbol-13-acetate; UPR, unfolded protein response.

INTRODUCTION

This chapter will review the evidence for a chemopreventive and anticancer role for black cohosh, a North American perennial that has been used to treat inflammatory and female health conditions and is now sought out as an alternative medicine to alleviate menopausal symptoms. Black cohosh is primarily used by midlife and older women, a population segment that is at relatively high risk for developing cancer.

Breast cancer and colorectal cancer have been associated with mutations in 189 genes (average of 11 per tumor). These numbers do not include mutations in non-coding genes, non-coding regions of coding genes, nor deletions, insertions, amplifications or translocations [1, 2]. The optimal treatment for cancer, it can be reasoned, most likely requires an agent or combination of agents that can correctly target multiple pathways with minimal toxicity. As studies have already shown for the related synthetic oleanane triterpenes (SOs) [2], the triterpene glycosides in black cohosh may be multifunctional, relatively nontoxic agents and thus useful for the prevention and treatment of cancer.

Numerous studies indicate that extracts and purified components from black cohosh inhibit the growth of human breast, prostate, oral and skin cancer cells. However, there are only a limited number of patient and animal studies to support these findings, and a mechanism of action has not been established (Table 11.1).

This chapter will address the following about black cohosh:

- Properties
- Chemical constituents
- Evidence of a role in cancer prevention and treatment
- Mode of action of extracts and components
- Comparison to the mode of action of other triterpene glycosides and aglycones
- Bioavailability, metabolites, safety and toxicity of extracts and components

Since most studies involving black cohosh have targeted breast cancer, this review will concentrate on this research and also include studies on prostate, skin and oral cancers.

BACKGROUND

Historical Use

Black cohosh (*Actaea racemosa* L. syn. *Cimicifuga racemosa* {L} Nutt) is a North American perennial in the buttercup family (Ranunculaceae) used for hundreds of years by Native Americans for a variety of purposes, including inflammatory conditions, stimulation of menstrual flow, dysmenorrhea, cough suppression, diarrhea, rheumatism, arthritis and muscle pain [3]. Traditionally,

TABLE 11.1 Black Cohosh's Role in Chemoprevention and Anticancer Activity

Positive evidence	• Black cohosh appeared to reduce the risk of primary breast cancer [23], and prevent its recurrence [22] in patients
	• An aqueous/ethanolic extract of black cohosh inhibited the development of prostate cancer in a mouse xenograft model [57], and purified triterpenes inhibited the initiation and promotion of skin cancer in a two-stage model of mouse skin carcinogenesis [41, 42]
	• Extracts and purified components of black cohosh consistently inhibited the growth of human breast [24, 28–33], prostate [37, 53], oral [40] and skin [41, 42] cancer cells. Black cohosh extracts enhanced the effects of chemotherapy agents on mouse [8] and human breast cancer cells, and actein enhanced the effects on human breast cancer cells [43, 66]
	• An isopropanolic extract and fractions of black cohosh inhibited the invasiveness of breast cancer cells [36]
	• Nonmalignant breast and oral cells were more resistant to the inhibitory effects of triterpene glycosides and an ethyl acetate extract of black cohosh than malignant cells [33, 40]
	• The growth inhibitory effect of 100% methanolic and lipophilic extracts and actein from black cohosh on human breast cancer was associated with the activation of stress response pathways [18, 64, 92]
	• Synthetic oleanane triterpenes, which are structurally related to the triterpenes in black cohosh, have been shown to affect multiple pathways and to be relatively nontoxic [2]. These findings may lend insight into the mode of action of black cohosh
Precautions	• An extract of black cohosh increased the rate of lung metastases in a MMTV-neu mouse model of mammary carcinoma [58]
	• Little is known about the metabolites, bioavailability or toxicity of black cohosh. There have been isolated reports of co-occurring liver toxicity [105, 106].

black cohosh has served as an herbal remedy for female conditions, as the native name "squaw root" implies. It has also been known as black snakeroot, macrotys, bugbane, bugwort, rattleroot and rattleweed. "Cohosh" is an Algonquin word which means "it is rough," with hairs [4]. The plant grows in the understory of hardwood forests east of the Mississippi River, from Georgia to Ontario. Early settlers used it as a sedative and muscle relaxant [5]. From 1820 to 1926, black cohosh was an official drug of the US Pharmacopoeia, under the name "black snakeroot." The eclectic John King (in 1832) reported that the medical effects resembled, but were not as strong as, those of digitalis [4]. In 1848, the American Medical Association "uniformly found *Macrotys* to lessen

the frequency and force of the pulse, to soothe pain and to allay irritability."
Related Asian species have been employed in Traditional Chinese Medicine to
treat infectious diseases [6].

Current Use

Black cohosh has been used in Europe for the last 50 years as a natural alternative to hormone replacement therapy and for other gynecological conditions [7].
It has recently been prescribed by physicians and examined in clinical studies as
an alternative therapy for menopausal symptoms that include hot flashes, night
sweats and vaginal dryness [3]. In the United States, women have increasingly
turned to black cohosh as a "more natural" alternative to estrogen replacement
therapy, in the belief that its has the benefits, without the risks, of estrogen therapy [8, 9]. Interest in the herb particularly increased since the Women's Health
Initiative published findings indicating that hormone replacement therapy may
increase the risk of cardiovascular diseases and breast cancer [10].

A standardized black cohosh extract (Remifemin®), has been developed
and manufactured in Germany for over 40 years, and more recent preparations
have been studied both in animals and in short-term clinical trials of menopausal women. The studies have yielded contradictory results regarding its ability
to alleviate menopausal symptoms, particularly hot flashes [10–13]. This could
be related to differences in the preparations, doses, durations of treatment and
outcomes measured. For instance, the preparation and recommended doses of
Remifemin® have been altered during the last 20 years [14]. The drug was
originally prepared as a liquid ethanol extract and then changed to an isopropa-
nol extract in pill form. It is also unclear if it contained 20 or 40 mg of extract
or extract from 20 to 40 mg of plant material.

Chemical Constituents

The roots and rhizomes of black cohosh are used for medicinal purposes.
These contain two major classes of secondary metabolites: triterpene glycosides (such as actein) and phenylpropanoids (such as fukinolic acid) (Table 11.2;
Fig. 11.1). Both of the novel classes of compounds – triterpene glycosides and
phenylpropanoids – have been shown to exhibit significant anticancer effects
in vitro [15, 16], but little is known about how these and other compounds in
black cohosh are metabolized *in vivo*.

Black cohosh can contain more than 42 triterpene glycosides [17], one
of which is actein, constituting about 2.3% of a methanolic extract of black
cohosh [18]. The total percent of triterpenes in this extract is greater than 10.5%
and the total percent of phenylpropanoids exceeds 4%. The composition of the
extract can be affected by the source, solvent and ratio of material to solvent in
the preparations, as well as the presence of contaminants therein. For instance,
HPLC (high performance liquid chromatography) analysis of black cohosh

TABLE 11.2 Constituents of Black Cohosh [3, 4, 17, 44][a,b,c]

Class	Compounds
Triterpene glycosides	Actein; 26-deoxyacein, 23-epi-26-deoxyactein (formerly 27-deoxyactein[b]);12-acetylactein; cimifugoside (aglycone: cimigenol), cimiracemoside C
Phenylpropanoids	Aromatic acids such as isoferulic, ferulic, caffeic, salicyclic, fukiic, piscidic and cinnamic acid; aromatic acid esters such as fukinolic acid, cimicifugic acids A, B, E, F, G
Alkaloids	Cimipronidine[c]
Lignans	Actaealactone [44]
Other constituents	Tannins, sugars, resins; fatty acids

[a]Zheng, Q. Y., He, K., Pilkington, L., Yu, S. and Zheng, B.(2000) CimiPure (Cimicufuga racemosa): a standardized black cohosh extract with novel triterpene glycosides for menopausal women. Phytochem Phytopharm, 360–370.
[b]Chen, S. N., Li, W., Fabricant, D. S., Santarsiero, B. D., Mesecar, A., Fitzloff, J. F., Fong, H. H. & Farnsworth, N. R. (2002). Isolation, structure elucidation, and absolute configuration of 26-deoxyactein from Cimicifuga racemosa and clarification of nomenclature associated with 27-deoxyactein. J Nat Prod **65**, 601–5.
[c]Fabricant, D., Nikolic, D., Lankin, D., Chen, S., Jaki, B., Krunic, A., van Breemen, R., Fong, H., Farnsworth, N. and Pauli, G. (2005) Cimipronidine, a cyclic guanidine alkaloid from Cimicifuga racemosa. J Nat Prod **68**, 1266–1270.

collected in various regions of Appalachia and extracted using different material-to-solvent ratios revealed different triterpene patterns. No triterpenes were detected in a plant that had been growing on a rock [19], indicating that the source of the plant can affect its constituents. It is essential, therefore, to preserve root and rhizome samples from each source for later assay.

Black cohosh can be distinguished from related Asian species by the presence of cimiracemoside C, while cimifugin is characteristic of Asian species [17].

Extracts Vs. Pure Compounds

Studies of the chemopreventive and anticancer properties of black cohosh have employed extracts and purified components. Arguments can be put forth for the use of either extracts or pure compounds for chemoprevention and cancer therapy. One advantage of using pure compounds is that it is simpler to define a mode of action for a pure compound than an extract. Different extracts may contain different chemicals. An extract also must be carefully standardized as to source and method of preparation. One solution is to use a defined mixture; a paradigm for this is the extract polyphenone E from green tea, which contains a defined mixture of green tea polphenols [20].

Studies of extracts are nevertheless essential because a majority of black cohosh consumers ingest extracts of the herb, not pure compounds.

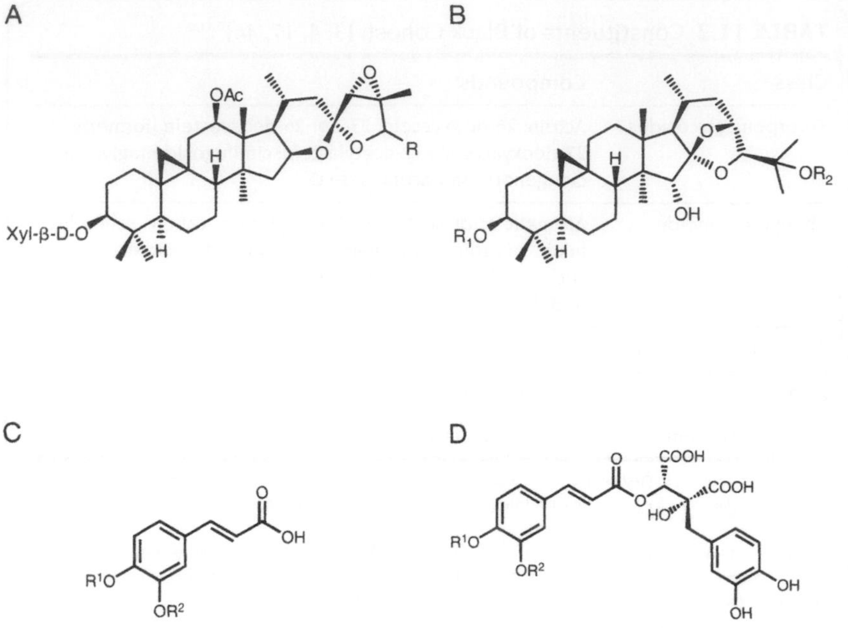

Structure	Compound	R-groups
(A)	Actein	R=OH
	23-epi-26-deoxyactein	R=H
(B)	Cimiracemoside C	R1=α-L-arabinoside, R2=H
	Cimigenoside	R1=β-D-xyloside, R2=H
	25-acetylcimigenol xylopyranoside (ACCX) [56]	R1=β-D-xyloside, R2=Ac
(C)	Caffeic acid	R^1=H, R^2=H
	Ferulic acid	R^1=H, R^2=CH$_3$
	Isoferulic acid	R^1=CH$_3$, R^2=H
(D)	Fukinolic acid	R^1=H, R^2=H
	Cimicifugic acid A	R^1=H, R^2=CH$_3$
	Cimicifugic acid B	R^1=CH$_3$, R^2=H

FIGURE 11.1   Chemical structures of the triterpene glycosides (A, B) and phenylpropanoids (C, D).

Since cancer affects multiple genes, one can argue, the optimal treatment may require mixtures, including extracts, containing multiple components that can target multiple pathways. For example, a study of the effect of tomato extract and lycopene on the development of prostate cancer indicates that the extract, but not lycopene, inhibited carcinogenesis; it is also possible that lycopene is only one of numerous components responsible for the effects [21].

Epidemiologic, *in vitro*, and animal studies provide evidence that both extracts and pure compounds from black cohosh have chemopreventive and anti-cancer potential. Where possible we have indicated the source, solvent and dose of the black cohosh extract used in the experiments discussed in this review.

EPIDEMIOLOGIC STUDIES

Two recent case-control studies suggest that black cohosh may generate chemopreventive activity. A retrospective cohort study tracked 18,862 breast cancer patients over a mean time of 3.6 years [22]. After being diagnosed, 1102 patients were given a prescription for the iCR (isopropanolic extract of *Actaea* (=*Cimicifuga*) *racemosa*) therapies Remifemin® or Remifemin® plus. The study indicates that use of iCR was associated with prolonged recurrence-free survival after breast cancer. The rate of recurrence was 14% after two years for the control group, whereas the treated group reached this rate after 6.5 years. The Cox regression model, with control for age and other confounding factors, such as tamoxifen usage and natureopathic therapy, indicated a 17% decrease in the rate of recurrence. iCR also increased the time of recurrence-free survival when used in combination with tamoxifen, compared to tamoxifen alone.

Age did not significantly influence the effectiveness of iCR in prolonging recurrence-free survival after breast cancer; iCR reduced recurrence risk similarly in those women above and below age 55. The mean age at diagnosis was 61.4 years. Data was accessed from IMS's Disease Analyzer MediPlus database, one of the largest medical databases worldwide and the only European database that registers links between diagnoses and therapies. Patients were excluded if they used black cohosh other than as Remifemin® or Remifemin® plus.

The importance of the study is supported by a number of objective factors in its approach: (1) the investigators were blinded to the iCR status of the patients; (2) the use of strict inclusion criteria for breast cancer diagnosis; and (3) the duration of follow-up, which was 3.6 years. However, several relevant variables, including receptor and TNM (classification of malignant tumors) status, were not available.

In a population-based case control study of 2473 women (949 breast cancer cases and 1524 controls), the use of hormone-related supplements (HRS), taken at least 3 times a week for 1 month or more, was shown to reduce breast cancer risk [23] (Table 11.3). The incidence of breast cancer was significantly lower for women who reported use of any of the HRS, including soy, dong quai or ginseng, versus women who reported no use (adjusted OR 0.65,

TABLE 11.3 Association of Hormone-Related Supplement (HRS) Use and Breast Cancer in a Population-Based Sample of Women in the Philadelphia Metropolitan Area [23] (© 2007; reprinted with permission of Wiley-Liss, Inc., a subsidiary of John Wiley & Sons, Inc.)

Exposure	Use in European Americans		Use in African Americans		Ever use of specific herb vs. never use of specific HRS, OR[1]	Ever use of specific herb vs. never use of any HRS, OR[1]
	Cases (N = 677)	Controls (N = 905)	Cases (N = 272)	Control (N = 619)		
Any HRS	77 (11.4)[2]	155 (17.2)	46 (16.9)	125 (20.2)	0.65 [0.49–0.87][3]	0.65 [0.49–0.87]
Any phytoestrogen	20 (3.0)	44 (4.9)	20 (7.4)	46 (7.4)	0.76 [0.48–1.21]	0.69 [0.43–1.11]
Any Isoflavone or genistein	9 (1.3)	19 (2.1)	2 (0.7)	8 (1.3)	0.74 [0.32–1.67]	0.67 [0.29–1.53]
Isoflavone	9 (1.3)	17 (1.9)	0	5 (0.8)	ND[4]	ND[4]
Genistein	0	2 (0.2)	2 (0.7)	3 (0.5)	ND[4]	ND[4]
Red clover	2 (0.3)	8 (0.9)	13 (4.8)	29 (4.7)	0.78 [0.38–1.61]	0.70 [0.33–1.47]
Soy medications	11 (1.6)	21 (2.3)	6 (2.2)	14 (2.2)	0.81 [0.39–1.67]	0.69 [0.33–1.44]
Black cohosh or Remifemin®	15 (2.2)	36 (4.0)	10 (3.7)	40 (6.5)	0.47 [0.27–0.82]	0.44 [0.25–0.77]
Black cohosh	13 (1.9)	34 (3.8)	9 (3.3)	39 (6.3)	0.39 [0.22–0.70]	0.37 [0.20–0.66]
Remifemin®	3 (0.4)	6 (0.7)	2 (0.7)	2 (0.3)	ND[4]	ND[4]
Biestrogen	0	1 (0.1)	0	0	ND[4]	ND[4]
DHEA	8 (1.2)	16 (1.8)	2 (0.7)	4 (0.7)	ND[4]	ND[4]
Dong quai	12 (1.8)	21 (2.3)	9 (3.3)	20 (3.2)	0.83 [0.43–1.59]	0.75 [0.39–1.45]
Estrovin	3 (0.4)	4 (0.4)	3 (1.1)	7 (1.1)	ND[4]	ND[4]
Ginseng	41 (6.1)	84 (9.3)	31 (11.4)	80 (12.9)	0.74 [0.53–1.06]	0.75 [0.53–1.06]
Promensil	1 (0.2)	4 (0.4)	0	2 (0.3)	ND[4]	ND[4]
Rejuvex	7 (1.0)	10 (1.1)	2 (0.7)	8 (1.3)	ND[4]	ND[4]
Steroid creams	6 (0.9)	13 (1.4)	1 (0.4)	3 (0.5)	ND[4]	ND[4]
Yam creams	5 (0.7)	10 (1.1)	1 (0.4)	4 (0.7)	ND[4]	ND[4]

[a]The odds ratio (OR) represents the relationship of herbal exposure and breast cancer risk as estimated from conditional logistic regression matched on age and race, and adjusted for the following variables: (i) education (less than high school, high school, greater than high school but not a college graduate, or college graduate or higher). (ii) age at first full-term pregnancy (nulliparous vs. age of first live birth <20 vs. age at first live birth 20–24 vs. age of first live birth 25–29 vs. age of first live birth >30). (iii) menopause status (known natural, assumed natural at reference age of 50 if menopausal status is unknown, and induced), (iv) family history of breast cancer (any vs. none). (v) time from diagnosis/ascertainment to interview (<86 days vs. 87–135 days vs. 136–208 days vs. >209 days), (vi) reference age as a continuous variable and (vii) ever use of hormone replacement therapy. [b]Values within parentheses indicate percentages. [c]Values within square brackets indicate 95% CIs. [d]Odds ratio associations not undertaken due to limited number of women who used this preparation. *

95% CI: 0.49, 0.87). Of these HRS, only black cohosh (Remifemin® or other black cohosh preparations) appeared to reduce the incidence of breast cancer (adjusted OR 0.39, 95% CI: 0.22, 0.70), especially PR positive tumors.

The results of the study are encouraging, but there are numerous potential confounding factors, including: (1) unspecified content and dose of black cohosh preparations; (2) differential recall bias between cases and control; (3) no data on timing of exposure; and (4) other factors that could influence the results, such as diet, physical exercise, or the use of antibiotics. It is possible that women who use black cohosh may have healthier diets and lifestyles.

Nevertheless, these studies lend credence to the theory that nontoxic, menopausal doses of black cohosh may also be chemopreventive. The epidemiological evidence is critical as a hypothesis generator and is consistent with numerous *in vitro* and *in vivo* studies indicating that black cohosh may be effective as a chemopreventive and anticancer agent.

IN VITRO STUDIES

Studies have shown that extracts, fractions and purified compounds from black cohosh inhibit various types of carcinogenesis, *in vitro*.

Growth Inhibitory Effects on Breast Cancer

Though it was once thought to have estrogenic effects, most recent data suggest that black cohosh does not stimulate breast cancer cell growth *in vitro* or *in vivo* [3, 24, 25]. A review of 15 animal and 15 *in vitro* studies indicated that the effects of black cohosh are central, rather than hormonal [26]. Neither a 50% ethanolic extract nor phenolic esters (at 10^{-8} to 10^{-6} M), obtained from the rhizomes of black cohosh, significantly increased the proliferation of MCF7 cells [27].

Instead, crude extracts of black cohosh have been shown to inhibit the *in vitro* growth of a variety of breast cancer cell lines, as discussed later in this chapter [24, 28–33]. Extracts of black cohosh (ethanol extract, 0.1% v/v) suppressed the growth of serum-stimulated T-47D (estrogen receptor (ER$^+$), Her2 low) breast cancer cells [28] and also slowed the proliferation of the MDA-MB-435 cancer cell line [29]. Isopropanolic extracts of black cohosh reduced MCF7 (ER$^+$, Her2 low) cell proliferation and estrogen-induced proliferation of MCF7 cells [24], and enhanced the inhibitory effect of tamoxifen [30]. The methanolic extract has been shown to be more active than both the ethanolic and isopropanolic extracts, in inhibiting the proliferation of MDA-MB-453 (ER$^-$, Her2 overexpressing) breast cancer cells [18].

Purified triterpene glycosides and aglycones have also been shown to suppress the growth of various types of cancer cells, *in vitro*. Actein and related triterpene glycosides inhibited the proliferation of MCF7 and MDA-MB-453 breast cancer cells [33]. MCF7 cells transfected for Her2 (MCF7/Her2-18, 45-fold increase Her2) [34] were more sensitive than the parental MCF7 cells to the growth-inhibitory effects of actein. This indicates that Her2 plays a role in the action of actein [35]. In these studies, 25-acetyl-7,8-didehydrocimigenol 3-O-β-D-xylopyranoside, isolated from *Cimicifuga acerina*, was about twice as active as the parent compound 7,8-didehydrocimigenol 3-O-β-D-xylopyranoside or actein. Thus, the acetyl group at position C-25 enhanced growth inhibitory activity. The order of decreasing activity of the triterpene glycosides tested on MCF7 human breast cancer cells was actein, cimifugoside, 23-epi-26-deoxy-actein and cimiracemoside [33]. Nonmalignant mammary epithelial cells appeared to be less sensitive to the growth limiting effects of the ethyl acetate fraction or actein than breast cancer cells, indicating that these agents possess specificity and may have limited toxicity, *in vivo*.

Anti-Angiogenic Effects on Breast Cancer

Black cohosh extract (iCR) and two major fractions, triterpene glycosides and caffeic acid esters, inhibited the invasiveness of breast cancer cells assayed by cell invasion through a Matrigel matrix [36]. The assay correlates with the progression of cancer to a more aggressive state. iCR and the two fractions suppressed MDA-MB-231 breast cancer cell invasion at doses that did not inhibit proliferation. The iCR extract (77.4 μg/ml) induced the maximal effect, 50% inhibition – comparable to the effects of paclitaxel or doxycycline. The two fractions, triterpene glycosides and caffeic acid esters, were less active, inducing the greatest inhibition, 34% and 25.5%, respectively, at 5 μg/ml. It is possible that different doses may alter the properties of the cellular membrane, and be less effective at higher doses.

Growth Inhibitory Effects on Prostate Cancer

Another hormone-dependent malignancy, prostate cancer, appears to be suppressed by extracts and purified components from black cohosh. An isopropanolic extract of black cohosh dose-dependently inhibited the growth of androgen-responsive (LNCaP) and unresponsive (PC-3 and DU145) prostate cancer cells and increased M30 antigen level in these cell lines [37]. Similarly, the *Cimicifuga racemosa* (CR) extract BNO 1055 (aqueous/ethanolic, 50%) subdued the growth of the prostate cancer cell line LNCaP [38]. The effect may be mediated by the aryl hydrocarbon receptor since the extract reduced tracer binding to the receptor to 71%.

The phenylpropanoid petasiphenone, isolated from an ethanolic extract of black cohosh, alone and combined with estradiol or dihydrotestosterone, also inhibited the growth of the prostate cancer cell line LNCaP [39]. It did not affect the secretion of prostate specific antigen. Petasiphenone is a structural homologue of petasiphenol, which has been shown to inhibit the proliferation of human leukemia cell lines by inhibiting the activity of DNA polymerase lambda, an enzyme that mediates DNA repair. Petasiphenone does not appear to have growth inhibitory effects on MCF7 human breast cancer cells [27]; the compound's activity may, therefore, be due to a mechanism specific to prostate cancer cells, or the anti-proliferative activity may vary for different cell lines.

Growth Inhibitory Effects on Oral Cancer

In a study that tested the growth inhibitory effects of 12 cycloartane glycosides, isolated from the rhizomes of black cohosh, on oral squamous cell carcinoma (HSC-2) cells and nonmalignant gingival fibroblasts (HGF), the cycloartane glycosides were found to slow the increase of HSC-2 cells [40]. The most active compound tested was cimiracemoside G, a minor component, with an IC_{50} value of $18\,\mu M$. Among the cimiacerogenin derivatives, the 7(8) dehydro-saponins were more active than the corresponding saturated saponins.

The second most active was 25-O-methoxycimigenol-3-O-α-L-arabino-pyranoside ($IC_{50} = 30\,\mu M$), while the parent compound, cimigenol-3-O-α-L-arabinopyranoside, was inactive. Actein, the C-26 hydroxyl derivative of 23-epi-26-deoxyactein, was more active ($IC_{50} = 44\,\mu M$) than the parent compound ($IC_{50} = 211\,\mu M$) in inhibiting the growth of HSC-2 oral squamous carcinoma cells. Thus the structure of the triterpene skeleton influenced the activity and potency of the compounds.

It is notable that the compounds were all more active on malignant HSC-2 than nonmalignant HGF cells. The ratio of activity on malignant vs. nonmalignant cells was about 15.6-fold for cimiracemoside G and about 3.2-fold for actein.

Effects on EBV-EA: Structure–Activity Relations

The ability of compounds to inhibit Epstein-Barr virus early antigen (EBV-EA) activation by tumor promoters correlates with their ability to inhibit tumor promotion *in vivo* [41]. Cimigenol (an acid- and base-stable compound) and related compounds, as well as isoferulic acid, isolated from *Cimicifuga* species, inhibited EBV-EA activation induced by the cocarcinogen 12-O-tetradecanoylphorbol-13-acetate (TPA) in Raji cells [41, 42]. The most active compounds (100% inhibition of activation at 1000 mol ratio/TPA) were cimigenol, cimigenol-3-one, cimigen-3,15-dione, 12-hydroxycimigenol, 15-deoxycimigenol, 7β-hydroxycimigenol [41] and isoferulic acid [42]. Their activity was greater than the activity of the strong antitumor promoter glycyrrhetic acid. In most instances, the addition of sugars or an acetyl group to the 3- or 25-hydroxyl groups decreased activity. The presence of 16,23; 16,24-diepoxy and hydroxyl or carbonyl groups at positions 3 and 25 in the 9,19-cycloartane skeleton appeared to be related to antitumor promotion activity.

Thus, the inhibitory effects of *Cimicifuga* components on EBV-EA activation, as well as cancer cell growth, point to a relationship between the triterpene structures and their anticancer activity. Investigators in one group of studies conjectured that the 9,19-cycloartane triterpenes could be divided into four structural groups: cimigenol, cimifugoside, hydroshengmanol and actein/deoxy-actein compounds [42]. The cimigenol and cimifugoside compounds were, in general, more active than the latter two classes of compounds. Of the cimifugosides, the H-4 and H-2 possessed more activity than the H-1 compounds. The activity, therefore, appeared to be related to the triterpene structure, especially the D ring side chain. With the exception of cimigenol, the xylosides exhibited slightly greater or equal activity compared to the corresponding aglycones. The dimethyl succinyl diesters were less active than the aglycones. Cimigenol and 25-O-acetylcimigenol were more active than the C-3 ketone derivatives and cimigenol and cimigenol-3-one were more active than their esters. The presence of more hydroxyl groups increased activity. The activity *in vitro* and *in vivo* could also be dependent on the metabolic changes of the compounds [42].

Growth Inhibitory Effects in Combination with Chemotherapy Agents

The optimal treatment for breast cancer most likely requires a combination of agents or modalities [2], Since extracts of black cohosh are used by breast cancer patients [8], it is important to determine whether there are synergistic, additive or antagonistic effects exhibited by extracts, in combination with chemotherapy agents.

Extracts of black cohosh enhanced the efficacy or toxic side effects of the chemotherapy agents adriamycin (doxorubicin) and taxotere on EMT6 mouse breast cancer cells [8]. The extract protected the cells from cisplatin and did not alter the effect of radiation or 4-hydroxycyclophosphamide. The absence of an effect on radiation suggests that the extract may affect drug uptake or efflux.

In agreement with these findings, a partially purified ethyl acetate extract of black cohosh enhanced the effects of doxorubicin on MDA-MB-453 human breast cancer cells [43]. Actein also: (1) exerted a synergistic effect on growth inhibition when combined with doxorubicin or 5-flourouracil; (2) increased the percentage of cells in the G1 phase of the cell cycle and had a similar effect when combined with 5-flourouracil or doxorubicin; and (3) enhanced the induction of apoptosis by paclitaxel, 5-flourouracil or doxorubicin.

Relatively low concentrations of actein or the ethyl acetate fraction of black cohosh appear to cause synergistic inhibition of breast cancer cell proliferation when combined with different classes of chemotherapy agents. The ethyl acetate fraction exerted a synergistic effect even though actein constitutes only about 2.5% of the extract; the compound or compounds responsible for synergy are not known. The activity of this fraction could be due to the presence of other triterpene glycosides (13.9%), aglycones or other compounds, such as phenylpropanoids (2.5%), but a study suggested that some phenylpropanoids may have little activity [44].

In sum, extracts and purified components from black cohosh, alone and in combination with chemotherapy agents, exhibited significant growth inhibitory activity on breast, prostate and oral cancer cells. Additional studies are required to determine the effects on tumour-initiating subpopulations [45].

Effects of Black Cohosh Extracts and Components on Other Biological Activties

Studies have shown that black cohosh has effects on other biological activities that are thought to be related to carcinogenesis.

Anti-Inflammatory Activity

Black cohosh has been traditionally used to treat inflammation. Studies have shown a correlation between the inflammatory process and carcinogenesis, and attributed the linkage to the transcription factor nuclear factor-kappaB (NF-κB) pathway [46, 47]. This key interrelationship between inflammation and cancer suggests that a study of the anti-inflammatory activity of black cohosh components would be fruitful. Fukinolic acid (2-E-caffeoylfukiic acid) has been shown to inhibit the activity of neutrophil elastase, which is involved in the inflammatory process [48]. Ferulic and isoferulic acid inhibited murine interleukin-8 synthesis, induced by infection with influenza virus *in vitro* and *in vivo* [49]. This evidence suggests that black cohosh may inhibit a process that, in turn, can lead to cancer.

Anti-Oxidant Activity

Reactive oxygen species induce DNA damage, which may result in the development of cancer. The anti-oxidant activity of certain compounds in black cohosh is another characteristic that may help explain the ability of the herb to help prevent cancer. Bioactivity-guided fractionation of the methanolic extract resulted in the isolation of nine anti-oxidant compounds, of which methyl caffeate was the most active in reducing menadione (a cytotoxic derivative of vitamin E)-induced DNA damage in cultured S30 breast cancer cells [50]. None of the compounds were cytotoxic to S30 cells. The findings of a second study support these results [44]: a new lignan, actaealactone, and a new phenylpropanoid ester derivative, cimicifugic acid G, displayed anti-oxidant activity in the 1,1-diphenyl-2-picrylhydrazyl (DPPH) free-radical assay with IC_{50} values of 26 and 37 μM, respectively. Other anti-oxidants identified from *A. racemosa* included cimicifugic acid A, cimicifugic acid B, the most active with an IC_{50} value of 21 μM and fukinolic acid.

Anti-HIV Activity

A methanolic extract of black cohosh, in which actein was the active principal, was shown to inhibit HIV activity [51]. Among 83 related saponins isolated from various plant species, the tetracyclic triterpenes exhibited the greatest anti-HIV activity. The most potent compound was actein, with an EC_{50} of 0.375 µg/ml and a therapeutic index (TI) of 144. The TI is the ratio of IC_{50}, the dose of the agent that induced 50% cell killing of the mock-infected H9 cells, to EC_{50}, the dose that suppressed HIV replication by 50%. The anti-HIV activity of actein may be related to anticancer potential since the SO 2-cyano-3,12-dioxooleana-1,9-dien-28-oic acid (CDDO), discussed later, inhibits HIV replication by inhibiting the expression of p21 [2].

Serotonergic, Dopaminergic and Opioid Activity

Extracts of black cohosh have been reported to have serotonergic, dopaminergic and opioid activity which could contribute to its vasomotor (menopausal) effect. Extracts of the plant appear to bind to the two serotonin receptors $5\text{-}HT_7$ and $5\text{-}HT_{1A}$. The methanolic extract has been shown to be the most active, exhibiting a higher binding affinity to these serotonin receptors than the 2-propanolic (40%) or ethanolic (75%) extracts [52]. It also possessed the greatest growth inhibitory activity on MDA-MB-453 breast cancer cells [18]. In studies using a dopamine D2 receptor assay, the black cohosh CR extract BNO 1055 (contained in Klimadynon and Menofem) induced dopaminergic activity [53]. Black cohosh extracts also appear to act as mixed competitive ligands of the human µ opiate receptor; the most active extract is the clinically used 75% ethanolic extract [54].

Osteoclastogenesis

Black cohosh has been shown to induce osteoprotective effects, especially in osteoblasts. The CR extract BNO 1055, given to ovariectomized rats for 3 months- at a dose of 33 mg/day, reduced the loss of bone mass density in tibia and serum osteocalcin levels [55]. Estrogenic effects were observed in the bone and fat tissue, but not the uterus of ovariectomized rats.

Of 48 compounds from black cohosh screened for an effect on *in vitro* osteoclastogenesis, 25-acetylcimigenol xylopyranoside (ACCX) was the most active, with an IC_{50} value of 5 µM, followed by cimigenol, actein and cimiracemoside B [56]. ACCX blocks osteoclastogenesis induced by the cytokines RANKL or TNF-α, resulting in inhibition of the NF-κB or ERK pathways, respectively. ACCX also reduced TNF-α induced bone loss in mice. The specific target in the NF-κB pathway is not known, but may be upstream of IκBα phosphorylation.

This correlation of affected activities and pathways is not only evidence of black cohosh's potential to inhibit carcinogenesis, but also opens a portal into its mechanism of action, which is discussed later in the chapter.

IN VIVO STUDIES

In vivo studies on the effects of black cohosh in mouse models of carcinogenesis lend support to the epidemiological and *in vitro* studies, but the animal studies are limited. *In vivo* studies on prostate and skin cancer present strong evidence

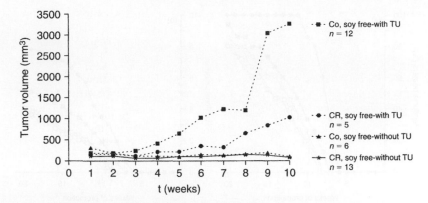

FIGURE 11.2 Tumor volume in male CD1 nu/nu mice after s.c. inoculation of LNCaP cells ($n = 18$/group). Development of subcutaneous tumors after inoculation with LNCaP cells. The apparent tumor volume in animals without tumor is due to the size of the scar that developed following inoculation of the cells. Note the dramatically increased number and size of tumors in the control animals in comparison to the CR-treated animals [57] (© 2006; reprinted with permission of Georg Thieme Verlag KG Stuttgart, New York).

that black cohosh extracts or components exert an anticancer role [41, 42, 57]. But a recent breast cancer study found contradictory evidence and raises a red light which warns that the effects of black cohosh are still unknown [58].

Effects on Prostate Cancer

In an animal model of prostate cancer, the CR extract BNO 1055 inhibited development, proliferation, size and malignancy of tumors induced by LNCaP cells in immunodeficient mice [57]. After subcutaneous inoculation of 1 million cells in immunodeficient nu/nu mice, 12/18 control mice developed tumors, whereas 5/18 treated mice developed tumors. The treated animals developed smaller tumors and less overall tumor tissue, which was mostly confined to connective tissue (Fig. 11.2). The tumors in the treated animals thus appeared to be less malignant than those in the untreated animals, indicating that black cohosh components may inhibit the progression, as well as the development of tumors.

In another study, mixtures of herbs which contained black cohosh inhibited the growth of xenografts of CWR22R and PC3 human prostate cancer cells in athymic mice. Inhibition may involve anti-angiogenic mechanisms, but the nature of the active extracts or components is not known [59].

Effects on Skin Cancer

Components from *Cimicifuga* species have potent antitumor initiating and promoting activities in an animal model of skin cancer [41, 42]. Previous studies [42]

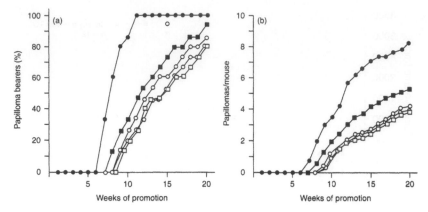

FIGURE 11.3 Inhibition of peroxynitrite/TPA-induced tumor promotion by multiple application of cimigenol (**1**), cimigenol-3,15-dione (**2**), EGCG and tocinol (topical administration). All mice were carcinogenically initiated with peroxynitrite (390 nmol) and promoted with 1.7 nmol of T1PA given twice weekly starting 1 week after initiation. (A) Percentage of mice bearing papillomas; (B) average number of papillomas per mouse [42] (© 2005; reprinted with permission of Elsevier BV).
(-●-): positive control, peroxynitrite (390 nmol) + TPA (1.7 nmol): group I
(-○-): peroxynitrite (390 nmol) + 0.0025% of cimigenol (2 weeks) + TPA (1.7 nmol): group II
(-○-): peroxynitrite (390 nmol) + 0.0025% of cimigenol-3,15-dione (2 weeks) + TPA (1.7 nmol): group III
(-□-): peroxynitrite (390 nmol) + 0.0025% of ECGC (2 weeks) + TPA (1.7 nmol): group IV
(-■-): peroxynitrite (390 nmol) + 0.0025% of Tocinol (2 weeks) + TPA (1.7 nmol): group V
At 20 weeks of promotion, groups II, III, IV and V were significantly different from group I ($p < 0.05$) on papillomas per mouse.

indicated that the inhibitory effects of other herbal components on EBV-EA induction by tumor promoters were related to antitumor promoting activity. Two of the most active compounds from *Cimicifuga* species in this assay (EBV-EA), cimigenol and cimigenol-3,15-dione, inhibited mouse skin tumor promotion [41, 42] in a 2-stage mouse skin carcinogenesis model that used the carcinogen DMBA as an initiator and TPA as a promoter. Cimigenol, applied before each TPA treatment, delayed and reduced the development of tumors. It reduced the incidence of papilloma-bearing mice from 100% of the positive control to 27% and 93% at 10 and 20 weeks, respectively and the average number of tumors per mouse from 4.8 and 9.1 in the positive control to 1.0 and 4.3 at 10 and 20 weeks, respectively.

To assess an effect on tumor initiation, a two-stage mouse skin carcinogenesis model that used the carcinogen peroxynitrite as an initiator and TPA as a promoter was employed [42] (Fig. 11.3A). When administered orally 1 week before and 1 week after initiation, cimigenol and cimigenol-3,15-dione (0.0025%) increased the latent period compared to the parent group and reduced the incidence and multiplicity of tumors. Cimigenol reduced the incidence of tumor-bearing mice from 100% of the positive control to 27% and 80% after 11 and 20 weeks of promotion, respectively. The average number of papillomas per mouse was reduced by one-half, with respect to the controls (from 8 in the positive control to 4) at 20 weeks. Indeed, cimigenol and cimigenol-3,15-dione had antitumor initiating activity commensurate with EGCG, suggesting a chemopreventive role for these compounds (Fig. 11.3B).

Effects on Breast Cancer

The few studies that have evaluated the effects of black cohosh on breast cancer in animal models have reported contradictory results.

An unpublished study of black cohosh performed using MMTV-neu transgenic mice yielded alarming results: The spontaneous activation of the proto-oncogene neu (erb2, Her2), the most common oncogene in breast cancer, in MMTV-neu female mice, results in primary and metastatic mammary tumors. The herb was included in the diet of the mice from 2 to16 months, at a dose equivalent to the dose given to women for relief of menopausal symptoms. It did not affect the incidence or number of mammary tumors in the mice, but did increase the rate of lung metastases [58]. The percentage of mice with detectable lung tumors at necropsy increased, compared to those on a control diet (27.1%, $n = 96$, vs. 10.9%, $n = 110$, of females with primary mammary tumors). Furthermore, the number of lung tumors/female was increased after long-term exposure to black cohosh. Survival time was not altered, even though metastatic disease increased in the mice [60].

The study, however, suffers from several problems. The duration of exposure lasted from adolescence until death, a treatment period that is atypical for humans taking black cohosh [60]. The more significant problem is that the promoter is hormone-responsive and can respond to a number of conditions, including pregnancy, as well as glucocorticoids and progestins. Black cohosh could have activated the promoter used in this mouse model, so that it is possible that the murine model of carcinogenesis may not yield effects relevant to breast cancer [61]. Given the widespread use of black cohosh, it is imperative to confirm these results and clarify the effects of black cohosh extracts on human breast cancer, before these results are accepted.

Manipulating the TGFβ pathway can induce a similar pattern of effects. A decrease in tumor metastases was observed in an MMTV-neu animal model with impaired TGFβ signaling [62]. An increase in TGFβ signaling resulted in a decrease in the formation or growth of primary mammary tumors, but an increase in metastatic growth in the lungs [63]. Both methanolic extract (100%) of black cohosh and actein have been shown to activate the expression of genes in the TGFβ pathway, such as ATF3 and MIC-1 [18, 64]; this finding may, in part, account for the stimulation of lung metastases.

Other studies suggest that black cohosh has a protective or no effect on breast cancer. An isopropanolic extract of black cohosh did not stimulate the growth of mammary tumors induced by 7,12-dimethylbenz[a]anthracene (forms DNA adducts) [65]. In fact, the extract slightly reduced the growth of tumors that remained after ovariectomy.Consistent with these results, black cohosh and tamoxifen have synergistic effects in an animal model of mammary carcinoma [66]. Compared to animals that received only tamoxifen, black cohosh increased the number of animals without tumors from 20% to 50%, and retarded neoplastic growth. The results of necropsy confirmed that the tumor burden was reduced by 50%. However, no synergistic effects were observed when iCR (60 mg/kg) was combined with two low doses of the aromatase inhibitor, formestane, in a rat model of chemically induced mammary carcinoma [67].

In contrast to the findings in a mouse model of breast cancer, in-uterus derived tissue (an *in vivo* tumor model of implanted RUCA-1 rat endometrial adenocarcinoma cells) an isopropanolic black cohosh extract did not increase or antagonize the tumor-promoting effects of high doses of tamoxifen (200 mg/km), but slightly decreased the metastases rate to the lung and abdomen [68].

Summary of Animal Studies

While the findings that black cohosh extracts and compounds decrease some instances of tumor growth suggest that the herb may be a promising chemopreventive agent, it is premature to draw conclusions about its effectiveness and safety, especially in view of the conflicting study results. It is important to note that the studies were few in number and performed with different black cohosh preparations. Furthermore, animal models are limited because they cannot replicate and therefore adequately predict all aspects of the disease. The xenograft model is limited in its ability to predict anticancer activity in that the hosts lack a normal immune response, and the epithelial breast cancer cells are transplanted to a foreign environment and cannot coevolve with the surrounding stromal cells [45, 69]. To resolve the conflicting results, it is important to replicate existing studies and examine the effects of black cohosh on different stages of carcinogenesis as well as before the development of mammary and other tumors, using varied animal models of carcinogenesis such as genetically engineered mouse models of breast cancer [70]. It will also be important to examine the effects of black cohosh on models that replicate tumor-initiating subpopulations [45].

MODE OF ACTION

Effects of Extracts and Components on Apoptosis and the Cell Cycle

Studies suggest that the growth inhibitory activity of black cohosh on various breast and prostate cancer cell lines may be due to induction of apoptosis and caspase action. Isopropanolic and ethanolic extracts of black cohosh inhibited the proliferation of ER^+ MCF7 and ER^- MDA-MB-231 breast cancer cells by induction of apoptosis and the action of caspases, which cleave intermediate filament CK 18 in epithelial cells – detected by an increase in reactivity of the M30 monoclonal antibody [31]. Similar effects were observed in hormone responsive and unresponsive prostate cancer cells [37]. Pretreatment of the isopropanolic black cohosh extract with rat liver microsomal S9 fraction containing P450 enzymes did not affect cell killing or apoptosis. The two major fractions of black cohosh, the triterpene glycosides or the cinnamic acid esters, did inhibit cell growth and induce apoptosis at concentrations lower than those required for cell killing [32].

Other studies have examined the effect of black cohosh on cell cycle control. An ethanolic extract of black cohosh inhibited the activity of the cyclin D1 promoter and increased the activity of the p21^{cip1} promoter in the ER$^-$ human breast cancer cell line T-47D [71]. The ethyl acetate partition of the methanol/water (80%) extract of black cohosh inhibited growth of MCF7 and MDA-MB-453 cells; the nonmalignant cells were the least sensitive and the Her2 over-expressing MDA-MB-453 cells were the most sensitive to the growth inhibitory effects of black cohosh. In MCF7 cells, the extract induced cell cycle arrest at G1 after treatment with 30 μg/ml and at G2/M after treatment with 60μg/ml [33]. This suggests that the fraction contained a mixture of components with the more active or more abundant component causing G1 arrest and the less active causing G2/M arrest, and/or that individual component(s) in the fraction exerted different effects at different concentrations. Possibly, at high concentrations the fraction affects proteins that regulate phases later in the cell cycle.

Molecular Effects of Triterpene and Cardiac Glycosides

How triterpene glycosides act is not known with certainty. Triterpene molecules, structurally related to steroids, are synthesized by the cyclization of squalene. This can occur by approximately 100 different folding patterns [2]. Over millions of years, some of the molecules may have evolved to interact with receptors on animal cells. These may have less inherent toxicity than totally synthetic drugs. When cells are injured, hydrophobic areas of lipid and proteins may be exposed in individual proteins or cell membranes. Triterpenes are hydrophobic structures that can interact with these portions and prevent or repair such injury. It is notable that most of the targets of triterpenes protect cells from injury or repair the injury.

For insight into the mode of action of triterpene glycosides from black cohosh, it is useful to consider the mode of action of triterpenes and cardiac glycosides from other plant species. Avicins, triterpenoid saponins from the plant *Acacia victoriae* (Bentham), are potent inhibitors of the transcription factor NF-κB and act by inhibiting its translocation to the nucleus and its capacity to bind DNA, perhaps by altering sulfhydryl groups critical for NF-κB activation [72]. Betulinic acid, a pentacyclic triterpene in the bark of white birch trees, is a selective inhibitor of melanoma and induces apoptosis by a direct effect on mitochondria in neuroectodermal tumors [73]. It also suppresses NF-κB activation induced by carcinogens and inflammatory stimuli [74]. Betulinic acid and boswellic acid, also a pentacyclic terpenoid, from *Boswellia serratia*, have both been shown to inhibit Topoisomerase I [75, 76].

Cardiac glycosides bind to the alpha subunit of the Na^+/K^+-ATPase; they act as potent and highly selective inhibitors of the active transport of Na^+ and K^+ across cell membranes [77]. This leads to a small increase in intracellular Na^{-+} and a large increase in intacellular Ca^{2+}. In heart muscle, this enhances the force of contraction. Recent studies indicate that extracts of foxglove and cardiac glycosides also inhibit the growth of breast and other cancer cells [78]. Moreover, digitalis is selective for malignant vs. non-malignant cells [79].

Cardiac glycosides appear to alter multiple pathways. The ability of cardiac glycosides to induce apotptosis may be related to the abilty to generate an increase in Ca^{2+} and a decrease in K^+. BCL-2 family members may play a role [80]. The cardiac glycoside ouabain affects both the ion pumping function and the signal transducing function of the Na^+/K^+ ATPase in the heart and in human breast cancer cells; doses that inhibit breast cancer growth also induce Src, activate the EGFR and, in turn, activate Erk1/2 and p21^{cip1} [81]. The K_i for inhibition of pumping is amplified 7.2-fold for inhibition of cell signaling [82]. The ability of cardiac glycosides to inhibit cancer cell growth may be related to the ability to inhibit topoisomerase activity, FGF-2 and NF-κB [83]. Digitoxin appears to block phosphorylation of IκBκ, the inhibitor of NF-κB, in cultures of cystic fibrosis lung epithelial cells [84]. Digitoxin and other cardiac glycosides also inhibit TNF-α/NF-κB signaling by blocking recruitment of the TNF receptor-associated death domain (TRADD) to the TNF receptor [85].

Triterpene glycosides from black cohosh have been shown to inhibit growth of MCF7 (ER$^+$, Her2 low) and MDA-MB-453 (ER$^-$, Her2 overexpressing) breast cancer cells and induce cell cycle arrest at G1 [33]. The most potent component tested in this study, actein, decreased the levels of cyclin D1, cdk4, pEGFR and the hyperphosphorylated form of pRb and increased the level of the Cdk inhibitory protein p21^{cip1} in MCF7 cells. These are changes which may contribute to the arrest in G1.

Actein induced an increase in caspase 3 activity [43], consistent with the finding that an isopropanolic or an ethanolic fraction of black cohosh induces apoptosis in MCF7 cells, which lack caspase 3, by the activation of caspases, such as caspase 7 [32].

Effects of Actein and the Methanolic Extract on the Unfolded Protein Response

Knowledge of the mode of action of black cohosh could help determine how to optimally customize the agent to target a particular cancer or patient. Gene expression allows a comprehensive view of an agent's pattern of gene effects. Gene expression analysis of the molecular effects of a methanolic extract (100%) and actein, on MDA-MB-453 and MCF7 breast cancer cells has revealed significant effects on genes that respond to diverse cellular stresses [18, 64], in particular, the unfolded protein response (UPR). This finding lends support to the hypothesis that triterpenes may protect cells from or repair cell injury.

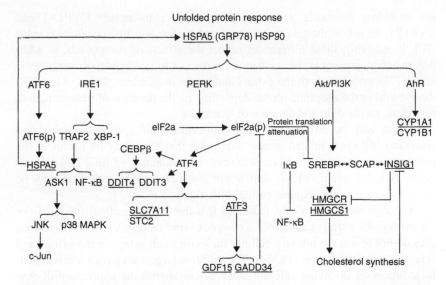

Unfolded protein response

FIGURE 11.4 Cellular responses to diverse stresses including the integrated stress response (ISR), unfolded protein response (UPR), endoplasmic reticulum (ER), stress response, cholesterol and NF-κB pathways. The responses to stress are integrated in this diagram: the ISR is adapted from Wek *et al.*[1], the UPR from Benjamin and Xu *et al.* [87, 88], the cholesterol and NF-κB pathway from Harding *et al.* [86] and the ATF3 pathway from Jiang *et al.*[2] The underlined genes are those whose expression was significantly altered in the RT-PCR analyses, when the cells were treated with the methanolic extract [18] (© 2007; reprinted with permission of Dr. John G. Delinassios).
[1] Wek, R. C., Jiang, H. Y. & Anthony, T. G. (2006). Coping with stress: eIF2 kinases and translational control. *Biochem Soc Trans* **34**, 7–11.
[2] Jiang, H. Y., Wek, S. A., McGrath, B. C., Lu, D., Hai, T., Harding, H. P., Wang, X., Ron, D., Cavener, D. R. & Wek, R. C. (2004). Activating transcription factor 3 is integral to the eukaryotic initiation factor 2 kinase stress response. *Mol Cell Biol* **24**, 1365–1377.

Different types of stress are known to induce four mammalian protein kinases to phosphorylate the eukaryotic initiation factor (eIF2). The response, referred to as the integrated stress reponse (ISR) [86] results in repair or apoptosis. The ISR is one of three signaling pathways that comprise the UPR; the other two signaling pathways are inositol-requiring enzyme 1 (IRE1)/XBP1 and ATF6 [87–89] (Fig. 11.4).

Actein induced four genes that mediate the ISR, including activating transcription factor 4 (ATF4), GRP78, a calcium dependent endoplasmic reticulum stress molecular chaperone, PERK and GADD34 [64]. Both the extract and actein appear to induce the expression of the stress gene GRP78, apoptotic gene GDF15 and lipid biosynthetic genes at 6 hours and to repress the expression of cell cycle related genes (HELLS and MCM10) and RNA metabolism gene RIBC2 at 24 hours [18, 64]. Both the extract and actein increased the level of the apoptotic stress protein DDIT3. Unique to the extract was induction of the multidrug resistance gene ABCC3 and the cytochromes CYP1A1 and CYP1B1, an action thought to be generated by the aryl hydrocarbon receptor [90]. Presumably, these differences reflect the effects of compounds, in addition to actein, present in the methanolic extract or to synergistic or antagonistic effects. Nevertheless, both the extract and actein induce two phases of the ISR, the survival or the apoptotic phase, depending on the duration of treatment; and, for actein, on the dose and duration of treatment.

Actein and the extract activated transcription of apoptotic factors and repressed cell-cycle related genes, indicating that they may be useful in the prevention and treatment of breast cancer. The induction of lipid biosynthetic genes and, for actein, VEGF, which can enhance angiogenesis [91] may be cause for concern and requires further investigation.

Although the above results indicated that the exposure of cells to actein or the methanolic extract can induce a complex array of cellular stress responses, they do not reveal the primary cellular molecules that actein or the extract and related compounds target [18, 64]. The putative targets may play a role in cellular processes involving calcium since actein altered the expression of several genes involved in calcium homeostasis, including GRP78, STC2, ADPN, JAG2, CALML5 and TRAM2.

The effects of actein and the extract on the expression of genes related to the ISR are not cell type specific since similar effects were observed on the ER^+ breast cancer cell line MCF7. Treatment of this cell line with actein also induced increased expression of ATF4, DDIT3, GDF15, SLC7A11 and CYP1A1 [64].

Consistent with these findings, a lipophilic extract of black cohosh rhizome activated the expression of stress response genes (DDIT4, HIF1A, VEGF, HMOX1, DNAJB4) and enriched the expression of anti-proliferative genes (cell cycle, CCNE2, CCNG2; transcription regulators, PCNA, E2F2) in the Erα positive breast cancer cell line MCF7, as assayed by gene expression analysis [92]. The apoptotic genes (BIRC5, GADD45A, GDF15) also displayed an enriched expression. The extract induced the expression of several oxidoreductases, including the cytochrome P450 family genes CYP1A1 and CYP1B1. The most highly upregulated gene was CYP1A1. CYP1A1 converts estrogen (E2) to non-carcinogenic 2-hydroxy-E2, whereas CYP1B1 metabolizes E2 to the carcinogenic compound 4-hydroxy-E2. Since the ratio of CYP1A1 to CYP1B1 was greater than one, this effect could contribute to the anticancer activity of black cohosh. The expression of the aryl hydrocarbon receptor (AhR), which has been shown to induce CYP1A1, was also upregulated. Transcripts coding for tumor promoting activity, such as S100P, as well as transcripts coding for antitumor activity, were altered. RT-PCR analysis indicated that the triterpene glycoside actein and a triterpene aglycon mixture displayed patterns similar to those of the extract on transcripts representing six regulated functional categories: apoptosis, proliferation, general growth, signaling and transport and metabolism and others. This suggests that these may be the active agents.

With respect to proliferation and cell survival genes, the pattern induced by the extract resembles that induced by tamoxifen, but is opposite to that of estradiol. The extract did not alter the expression of estrogen regulated genes, except for ERα and VEGF. However, these genes could be induced by the hypoxia response. The extract induced more genes than E2 or tamoxifen, indicating that the response is more complex. It is neither estrogenic nor antiestrogenic, but multifaceted.

Comparison to the Mode of Action of Synthetic Oleananes

To better understand the mode of action of actein and related compounds from black cohosh, it is useful to consider the mode of action of SOs, especially the highly potent triterpene CDDO, because these have been extensively studied in both animal and *in vitro* systems.

Suh *et al.* [93] have generated a series of derivatives of the triterpenes oleanic and ursolic acids that are highly potent in suppressing the expression of inducible nitric oxide synthase and cyclooxygenase-2 in primary mouse macrophages. Indeed, the derivative CDDO is 1000 times more potent than oleanic acid in this cell system [16]. CDDO also displays potent differentiating, anti-proliferative and anti-inflammatory activities [94]. It induces apoptosis by a caspase-8-dependent mechanism [95, 96] and inhibits NF-κB-mediated gene expression at a point after translocation of the activated form to the nucleus [97]. This compound is a ligand for the peroxisome proliferator activated receptor-γ [98]. CDDO-imizadole has been shown to induce cytoprotective genes through KEAP1-NRF2 anti-oxidant response element (ARE) signaling [99]; the transcription factor NRF2 binds to and activates the ARE, a cis-acting sequence found in the 5′ flanking region of genes encoding many cytoprotective enzymes, including NAD(P)H:quinine oxidoreductase (NQO1).

In a similar manner to actein, CDDO activates the expression of stress-related genes in MCF7 breast cancer and MDA-MB-435 cells [100]. The primary cellular target of CDDO and related SOs that mediate the above biologic effects is not known. SOs are not targeted therapeutics with a single high-affinity receptor-ligand, but rather they appear to target multiple pathways [2] by altering regulatory proteins that control the activity of transcription factors. Molecular targets include KEAP1 (NRF2 pathway), IKK (NF-κB pathway), TGFβ signaling and STAT.

SOs appear to interact with sulfhydryl groups on specific cysteine residues. The accessibility of the residues is an important factor. The mechanism appears to be mediated by Michael addition (the reaction of a nucleophile with an α,β unsaturated carbonyl compound yielding an addition product) to an active nucleophilic group on proteins, such as the SH groups on cysteine residues. A major complication is the reversible nature of the formation of Michael adducts.

The binding affinity of drugs that react by Michael addition may vary for different protein targets. The affinity may be high for some, such as KEAP1, resulting in the release of NRF2, and activating phase 2 enzymes, and low for other targets, such as tubulin or IKK, resulting in inhibiton of cell proliferation and apoptosis. Thus the response to SOs could be dose dependent: low doses may result in survival and high doses may result in apoptosis.

Selective apoptosis of cancer cells may result from their higher levels of oxidative stress. Cells that are already stressed are susceptible to cell-killing by SOs, which further increase reactive oxygen species production. It is significant that SOs induce apoptosis in cancer cells that are resistant to conventional chemotherapeutic agents.

Analogous to SOs, the ketal-hemiacetal and epoxide grouping of actein suggest that the agent would readily react with nucleophiles. The activity of actein resembles that of CDDO in that it induces two phases of the ISR, the survival or apoptotic phase, depending on the dose and duration of treatment. Similar to CDDO, actein activated the expression of the phase 2 gene HMOX. At 24 hours after treatment with actein at $40\,\mu g/mL$, HMOX1 was the most highly upregulated gene [64]. Both compounds are selective for malignant vs. nonmalignant cells.

SAFETY

Bioavailability

Bioavailability studies of black cohosh are limited, and most remain unpublished. It is essential to determine the bioavailability of black cohosh in preclinical or human studies to ascertain its anticancer and chemopreventive potential. Important considerations in assessing chemopreventive activity are whether sufficient blood and tissue levels can be achieved following oral administration and whether the agent exerts significant toxicity.

While doses prescribed for menopausal therapy may also be sufficient for chemoprevention [22, 23], the optimal dose to prevent or treat cancer may be higher or lower. Further studies are required to determine these doses.

Relatively low concentrations of actein or the ethyl acetate extract of black cohosh ($0.2\,\mu g/ml$ to $2\,\mu g/ml$ ($3\,\mu M$)) have been shown to cause synergistic inhibition of the proliferation of breast cancer cells when combined with chemotherapy agents [43]. In this study, the exposure time was only 96 hours; it is possible that during continuous administration to patients the effective concentration might be even lower because of cumulative effects and because of the compound's possible concentration in specific tissues. This seems likely since other natural products, like extracts of green tea, have antitumor effects in rodent models [101], even though the oral doses would predict very low blood levels [102]. It may also be possible to synthesize derivatives of black cohosh components, such as actein or other triterpene glycosides that are more potent inhibitors of breast cancer cells.

Clinical Studies

Isopropanolic and ethanolic extracts of black cohosh have been in use for over 40 years in Europe with few reported toxic effects [3]. The side effects reported were relatively mild, except for recent reports of co-occurring hepatotoxicity [103, 104]. Liver toxicity is often the major reason drugs are withdrawn. It is not clear, however, whether black cohosh was responsible. The reports of liver toxicity all involved middle-aged and older women and it is possible that black cohosh may have precipitated a pre-existing hepatic problem. Since most studies of black cohosh have been performed for the relief of menopausal symptoms in women in midlife [105], the results may have been influenced by changes in hormone levels. Although most studies of black cohosh and menopause report that isopropanolic and ethanolic extracts of the herb are free of significant side effects, they have not been sufficiently long – greater than 6 months – to determine safety. Additional studies are required to establish the safety of higher doses, as well as other extracts and pure compounds.

Studies have disagreed on the effects of the agent on lipid levels. Administering the CR extract BNO 1055 at 40 mg for 3 months resulted in a statistically significant increase in TTG, but no effects on total, LDL or HDL cholesterol [106]. A randomized, placebo-controlled trial using the same extract at a higher dose, 120 mg/kg for 12 weeks, showed no effect on either cholesterol or TTG [105]. Yet, another study demonstrated that black cohosh administered at 40 mg for 52 weeks without a placebo control increased both TTG and cholesterol (HDL-cholesterol) while lowering LDL-cholesterol [107].

These apparently contradictory results could be due to the use of different preparations, isolates of the same preparation or to chance [105]. It is important to resolve the effects of black cohosh on lipid and other physiological parameters before it is used for chemoprevention or therapy.

Animal Studies

Animal studies indicate that black cohosh extracts do not induce toxic, mutagenic or carcinogenic effects [3]. Wistar rats given 5 g/kg of Remifemin® granulate for 26 weeks did not show any organ or chemical toxicity [108] nor was toxicity observed in dogs given 400 mg/kg/day of black cohosh for 26 weeks [109]. The LD_{50} (lethal dose) of a black cohosh preparation in mice was 7.7 g/kg (intragastric) and 1.1 g/kg (intravenous). Results of the Ames test for a 40% 2-propanol extract were negative.

A study of the hepatic effects of black cohosh indicated that an ethanolic extract of black cohosh given to female Wistar rats (at doses greater than 500 mg/kg) induced hepatic mitochondrial toxicity; this was evidenced by microvesicular steatosis [110]. Black cohosh reduced mitochondrial β-oxidation starting at 10 μg/ml in freshly isolated rat liver mitochondria; since this effect was pronounced, and was detected at a lower dose than other effects on mitochondria, it could be the primary effect. Blockage of β-oxidation can result in the accumulation of long-chain acyl CoA's, which may induce liver damage and apoptosis. Indeed, the extract induced a dose dependent increase in early apoptotic HepG2 liver cancer cells. However, the dose required to cause microvesicular steatosis in rats was significantly higher than human doses, suggesting that black cohosh is safe.

In Vitro Studies

Moderate doses of black cohosh appear to be safe, with respect to the formation of quinoid metabolites [19, 109]. Black cohosh catechols are converted (by metabolism or chemicals) to electrophilic quinones *in vitro*. The catechols do not appear to be absorbed across the intestinal epithelium, whereas the triterpenoids are absorbed. No catechols were detected in the blood or urine of 10 women who ingested 40, 80 or 120 mg of black cohosh for 1 week. In addition, there was no change in liver enzymes from 6 women in this study. Quinones were not detected in the urine of women who ingested up to 256 mg of a standardized ethanolic extract of black cohosh (70% prepared by Pure World Botanicals). However, metabolic activation could be a hazard at higher doses.

A number of findings may be a cause for concern: (1) cimifugoside and actein inhibited thymidine transport into phytohemagglutinin-stimulated lymphocytes; (2) actein and cimigenol appear to be immunosuppressive in PHA-stimulated lymphocytes *in vitro* [111]; (3) black cohosh may interact with CYP2D6 substrates [112]; and (4) commercially available black cohosh, whose active constituents were identified as triterpene glycosides, inhibited CYP3A4 in intestinal epithelium [113]; black cohosh may thus increase the bioavailability of a variety of CYP3A4 substrates. These diverse findings require further investigation.

Extracts and components of black cohosh have been shown to preferentially inhibit the growth of malignant breast and oral cells, but not nonmalignant cells, as discussed earlier. It is therefore likely that actein, cycloartane glycosides and fractions of black cohosh will have limited toxicity *in vivo*.

CONCLUSIONS

Recent case control studies suggest that black cohosh can help to prevent primary and recurrent breast cancer. These studies are consistent with numerous *in vitro* findings indicating that black cohosh has powerful growth inhibitory capabilities and limited toxicity, and with some animal studies indicating that black cohosh can suppress tumor development and malignancy. Research has begun to explain the herb's mode of action and identify its most active components. This will open the possibility of synthesizing more potent anticancer compounds based on the structure of actein and related triterpene glycosides from black cohosh.

These successes show that further research of this remarkable herb is a necessary and worthwhile pursuit. Questions remain about the herb's bioavailability, safety, toxicity, mode of action, effect on various cancers, stages of carcinogenesis and unique effects on older men and women. It will be important to examine the effect of black cohosh on models that replicate tumor-initiating subpopulations of cells. If these issues are adequately addressed, various forms of black cohosh may be identified in the near future as useful agents for chemoprevention and cancer therapy.

ACKNOWLEDGMENTS

I thank Erica Cruz for excellent assistance in the preparation of this chapter; Dr. Bei Jiang for drawing the chemical structures and a thorough reading of the manuscript; Dr. I. Bernard Weinstein for a constructive critique; and Laura Chen for assisting in literature research.

REFERENCES

1. Sjoblom, T., Jones, S., Wood, L., Parsons, D., Lin, J., Barber, T., Mandelker, D., Leary, R., Ptak, J., Silliman, N., Szabo, S., Buckhaults, P., Farrell, C., Meeh, P., Markowitz, S., Willis, J., Dawson, D., Willson, J., Gazdar, A., Hartigan, J., Wu, L., Liu, C., Parmigiani, G., Park, B., Bachman, K., Papadopoulos, N., Vogelstein, B., Kinzler, K. & Velculescu, V. (2006). The consensus coding sequences of human breast and colorectal cancers. *Science* **314**, 268–274.
2. Liby, K., Yore, M. & Sporn, M. (2007). Triterpenoids and rexinoids as multifunctional agents for the prevention and treatment of cancer. *Nat Rev Cancer* **7**, 357–369.
3. Foster, S. (1999). Black cohosh: *Cimicifuga racemosa*. A literature review. *HerbalGram* **45**, 35–49.
4. Upton, R. (2002). Black Cohosh Rhizome. *American Herbal Pharamacopoeia and Therapeutic Compendium. American Herbal Pharmacopoeia.*
5. Low Dog, T. (2002). Black Cohosh. In *7th Annual Course Botanical Medicine in Modern Clinical Practice*, pp. 556, New York.
6. Hsu, H.-Y., Chen, Y.-P., Hsu, C.-S., Shen, S.-J., Chen, C.-C. & Chang, H.-C. (1986). *Oriental Materia Medica: A Concise Guide*, Keats Publishing, Inc, New Canaan.
7. McKenna, D. J., Jones, K., Humphrey, S. & Hughes, K. (2001). Black cohosh: Efficacy, safety, and use in clinical and preclinical applications. *Altern Ther Health Med* **7**, 93–100.
8. Rockwell, S., Liu, Y. & Higgins, S. A. (2005). Alteration of the effects of cancer therapy agents on breast cancer cells by the herbal medicine black cohosh. *Breast Cancer Res Treat* **90**, 233–239.
9. Jacobson, J. & Granny, V. (2004). Can an herbal agent replace estrogen for hot flashes. *Cancer Invest* **22**, 645–647.
10. Reed, S. D., Newton, K. M., Lacroix, A. Z., Grothaus, L. C., Grieco, V. S. & Ehrlich, K. (2007). Vaginal, endometrial, and reproductive hormone

findings: Randomized, placebo-controlled trial of black cohosh, multibotanical herbs, and dietary soy for vasomotor symptoms: the Herbal Alternatives for Menopause (HALT) Study. *Menopause.*

11. Lehmann-Willenbrock, E. & Riedel, H. H. (1998). Clinical and endocrinological examinations concerning therapy of climacteric symptoms following hysterectomy with remaining ovaries. *Z Gynaekologe* **110**, 611–618.

12. Stoll, W. Phytotherapy influences atrophic vaginal epithelium: Double-blind study – Cimicifuga vs. estrogenic substances. *Therapeuticum*, **1**, 23–31.

13. Cheema, D., Coomarasamy, A. & El-Toukhy, T. (2007). Non-hormonal therapy of post-menopausal vasomotor symptoms: A structured evidence-based review.

14. Farnsworth, N. (2004). Black Cohosh: What Do We Know About This Botanical? Preparation and Possible Adulteration and Contamination. Workshop on the Safety of Black Cohosh in Clinical Studies, Bethesda, Maryland, National Institutes of Health.

15. Luo, J., Soh, J. W., Xing, W. Q., Mao, Y., Matsuno, T. & Weinstein, I. B. (2001). PM-3, a benzo-gamma-pyran derivative isolated from propolis, inhibits growth of MCF-7 human breast cancer cells. *Anticancer Res* **21**, 1665–1671.

16. Sporn, M. B. & Suh, N. (2000). Chemoprevention of cancer. *Carcinogenesis* **21**, 525–530.

17. Jiang, B., Kronenberg, F., Nuntanakorn, P., Qiu, M. H. & Kennelly, E. J. (2006). Evaluation of the botanical authenticity and phytochemical profile of black cohosh products by high-performance liquid chromatography with selected ion monitoring liquid chromatography-mass spectrometry. *J Agric Food Chem* **54**, 3242–3253.

18. Einbond, L. S., Su, T., Wu, H. A., Friedman, R., Wang, X., Jiang, B., Hagan, T., Kennelly, E. J., Kronenberg, F. & Weinstein, I. B. (2007). Gene expression analysis of the mechanisms whereby black cohosh inhibits human breast cancer cell growth. *Anticancer Res* **27**, 697–712.

19. Bolton, J. (2004). Black Cohosh: What Do We Know About This Botanical? Mechanism of Action, Estrogenic Activity, and *In Vitro* Toxicology Screening Assays. Workshop on the Safety of Black Cohosh in Clinical Studies, Bethesda, Maryland, National Institutes of Health.

20. Shimizu, M., Deguchi, A., Lim, J. T., Moriwaki, H., Kopelovich, L. & Weinstein, I. B. (2005). (–)-Epigallocatechin gallate and polyphenon E inhibit growth and activation of the epidermal growth factor receptor and human epidermal growth factor receptor-2 signaling pathways in human colon cancer cells. *Clin Cancer Res* **11**, 2735–2746.

21. Boileau, T., Liao, Z., Kim, S., Lemeshow, S., Erdman, J. J. & Clinton, S. (2003). Prostate carcinogenesis in N-methyl-N-nitrosourea (NMU)-testosterone-treated rats fed tomato powder, lycopene, or energy-restricted diets. *J Natl Cancer Inst* **95**, 1578–1586.

22. Zepelin, H. H., Meden, H., Kostev, K., Schröder-Bernhardi, D., Stammwitz, U. & Becher, H. (2007). Isopropanolic black cohosh extract and recurrence-free survival after breast cancer. *Clin Pharmacol Ther* **45**, 143–154.

23. Rebbeck, T. R., Troxel, A. B., Norman, S., Bunin, G. R., DeMichele, A., Baumgarten, M., Berlin, M., Schinnar, R. & BL., S. (2007). A retrospective case-control study of the use of hormone-related supplements and association with breast cancer. *Int J Cancer* **120**, 1523–1528.

24. Bodinet, C. & Freudenstein, J. (2004). Influence of marketed herbal menopause preparations on MCF-7 cell proliferation. *Menopause* **11**, 281–289.
25. Low Dog, T., Powell, K. L. & Weisman, S. M. (2003). Critical evaluation of the safety of *Cimicifuga racemosa* in menopause symptom relief. *Menopause* **10**, 299–313.
26. Borrelli, F., Izzo, A. A. & Ernst, E. (2003). Pharmacological effects of *Cimicifuga racemosa*. *Life Sci* **73**, 1215–1229.
27. Stromeier, S., Petereit, F. & Nahrstedt, A. (2005). Phenolic esters from the rhizomes of *Cimicifuga racemosa* do not cause proliferation effects in MCF-7 cells. *Planta Med* **71**, 495–500.
28. Dixon-Shanies, D. & Shaikh, N. (1999). Growth inhibition of human breast cancer cells by herbs and phytoestrogens. *Oncol Rep* **6**, 1383–1387.
29. Nesselhut, T., Schellhase, C., Dietrich, R. & Kuhn, W. (1993). Studies on mamma carcinoma cells regarding the proliferative potential of herbal medications with estrogen-like effects. *Arch Gynecol Obstet* **254**, 817–818.
30. Bodinet, C. & Freudenstein, J. (2002). Influence of *Cimicifuga racemosa* on the proliferation of estrogen receptor-positive human breast cancer cells. *Breast Cancer Res Treat* **76**, 1–10.
31. Hostanska, K., Nisslein, T., Freudenstein, J., Reichling, J. & Saller, R. (2004). *Cimicifuga racemosa* extract inhibits proliferation of estrogen receptor-positive and negative human breast carcinoma cell lines by induction of apoptosis. *Breast Cancer Res Treat* **84**, 151–160.
32. Hostanska, K., Nisslein, T., Freudenstein, J., Reichling, J. & Saller, R. (2004). Evaluation of cell death caused by triterpene glycosides and phenolic substances from *Cimicifuga racemosa* extract in human MCF-7 breast cancer cells. *Biol Pharm Bull* **27**, 1970–1975.
33. Einbond, L. S., Shimizu, M., Xiao, D., Nuntanakorn, P., Lim, J. T., Suzui, M., Seter, C., Pertel, T., Kennelly, E. J., Kronenberg, F. & Weinstein, I. B. (2004). Growth inhibitory activity of extracts and purified components of black cohosh on human breast cancer cells. *Breast Cancer Res Treat* **83**, 221–231.
34. Benz, C., Scott, G., JC, S., Johnson, R., Tripathy, D., Coronado, E., Shepard, H. & Osborne, C. (1992). Estrogen-dependent, tamoxifen-resistant tumorigenic growth of MCF-7 cells transfected with HER2/neu. *Breast Cancer Res Treat*, 1–10.
35. Einbond, L. S., Wen-Cai, Y., He, K., Wu, H., Cruz, E., Roller, M. & Kronenberg, F. (2007). Growth inhibitory activity of extracts and compounds from Cimicifuga species on human breast cancer cells. *Phytomedicine*, [Epub ahead of print].
36. Hostanska, K., Nisslein, T., Freudenstein, J., Reichling, J. & Saller, R. (2007). Inhibitory effect of an isopropanolic extract of black cohosh on the invasiveness of MDA-MB 231 human breast cancer cells. *In Vivo* **21**, 349–355.
37. Hostanska, K., Nisslein, T., Freudenstein, J. & Saller, R. (2005). Apoptosis of human prostate androgen-dependent and -independent carcinoma cells induced by an isopropanolic extract of black cohosh involves degradation of cytokeratin (CK) 18. *Anticancer Res* **25**, 151–160.
38. Jarry, H., Thelen, P., Christoffel, V., Spengler, B. & Wuttke, W. (2005). *Cimicifuga racemosa* extract BNO 1055 inhibits proliferation of the human prostate cancer cell line LNCaP. *Phytomedicine* **12**, 178–182.
39. Jarry, H., Stromeier, S., Wuttke, W. & Nahrstedt, A. (2007). Petasiphenone, a phenol isolated from *Cimicifuga racemosa*, *in vitro* inhibits proliferation of the human prostate cancer cell line LNCaP. *Planta Med* **73**, 184–187.

40. Watanabe, K., Mimaki, Y., Sakagami, H. & Sashida, Y. (2002). Cycloartane glycosides from the rhizomes of *Cimicifuga racemosa* and their cytotoxic activities. *Chem Pharm Bull (Tokyo)* **50**, 121–125.

41. Sakurai, N., Kozuka, M., Tokuda, H., Nobukuni, Y., Takayasu, J., Nishino, H., Kusano, A., Kusano, G., Nagai, M., Sakurai, Y. & Lee, K. H. (2003). Antitumor agents 220. Antitumor-promoting effects of cimigenol and related compounds on Epstein-Barr virus activation and two-stage mouse skin carcinogenesis. *Bioorg Med Chem* **11**, 1137–1140.

42. Sakurai, N., Kozuka, M., Tokuda, H., Mukainaka, T., Enjo, F., Nishino, H., Nagai, M., Sakurai, Y. & Lee, K. H. (2005). Cancer preventive agents. Part 1: Chemopreventive potential of cimigenol, cimigenol-3,15-dione, and related compounds. *Bioorg Med Chem* **13**, 1403–1408.

43. Einbond, L. S., Shimizu, M., Nuntanakorn, P., Seter, C., Cheng, R., Jiang, B., Kronenberg, F., Kennelly, E. J. & Weinstein, I. B. (2006). Actein and a fraction of black cohosh potentiate antiproliferative effects of chemotherapy agents on human breast cancer cells. *Planta Med* **72**, 1200–1206.

44. Nuntanakorn, P., Jiang, B., Einbond, L. S., Yang, H., Kronenberg, F., Weinstein, I. B. & Kennelly, E. J. (2006). Polyphenolic constituents of *Actaea racemosa*. *J Nat Prod* **69**, 314–318.

45. Vargo-Gogola, T. & Rosen, J. (2007). Modeling breast cancer: One size does not fit all. *Nat Rev Cancer* **7**, 659–672.

46. Karin, M. (2006). Nuclear factor-kappaB in cancer development and progression. *Nature* **441**, 431–436.

47. Kundu, J. K. & Surh, Y. J. (2005). Breaking the relay in deregulated cellular signal transduction as a rationale for chemoprevention with anti-inflammatory phytochemicals. *Mutat Res* **591**, 123–146.

48. Loser, B., Kruse, S., Melzig, M. & Nahrstedt, A. (2000). Inhibition of neutrophil elastase activity by cinnamic acid derivatives from *Cimicifuga racemosa*. *Planta Med* **66**, 751–753.

49. Hirabayashi, T., Ochiai, H., Sakai, S., Nakajima, K. & Terasawa, K. (1995). Inhibitory effect of ferulic acid and isoferulic acid on murine interleukin-8 production in response to influenza virus infections *in vitro* and *in vivo*. *Planta Med.* **6**, 221–226.

50. Burdette, J., Chen, S., Lu, Z., Xu, H., White, B., Fabricant, D., Liu, J., Fong, H., Farnsworth, N., Constantinou, A., Van Breemen, R., Pezzuto, J. & Bolton, J. (2002). Black Cohosh (*Cimicifuga racemosa* L.) protects against Menadione-induced DNA damage through scavenging of reactive oxygen species: Bioassay-directed isolation and characterization of active principles. *J Agric Food Chem*, 7022–7028.

51. Sakurai, N., Wu, J. H., Sashida, Y., Mimaki, Y., Nikaido, T., Koike, K., Itokawa, H. & Lee, K. H. (2004). Anti-AIDS agents. Part 57: Actein, an anti-HIV principle from the rhizome of *Cimicifuga racemosa* (Black cohosh), and the anti-HIV activity of related saponins. *Bioorg Med Chem Lett* **14**, 1329–1332.

52. Burdette, J., Liu, J., Chen, S., Fabricant, D., Piersen, C., Barker, E., Pezzuto, J., Mesecar, A., Van Breemen, R., Farnsworth, N. & Bolton, J. (2003). Black cohosh acts as a mixed competitive ligand and partial agonist of the serotonin receptor. *J Agric Food Chem*, 5661–5670.

53. Jarry, H., Metten, M., Spengler, B., Christoffel, V. & Wuttke, W. (2003). *In vitro* effects of the *Cimicifuga racemosa* extract BNO 1055. *Maturitas*, S31–S38.

54. Rhyu, M. R., Lu, J., Webster, D. E., Fabricant, D. S., Farnsworth, N. R. & Wang, Z. J. (2006). Black cohosh (*Actaea racemosa*, *Cimicifuga racemosa*) behaves as a mixed competitive ligand and partial agonist at the human mu opiate receptor. *J Agric Food Chem* **54**, 9852–9857.

55. Seidlová-Wuttke, D., Jarry, H., Becker, T., Christoffel, V. & Wuttke, W. (2003). Pharmacology of *Cimicifuga racemosa* extract BNO 1055 in rats: Bone, fat and uterus. *Maturitas* **14**, S39–S50.

56. Qiu, S. X., Dan, C., Ding, L. S., Peg, S., Chen, S. N., Farnsworth, N. R., Nolta, J., Gross, M. L. & Zhou, P. (2007). A triterpene glycoside from black cohosh that inhibits osteoclastogenesis by modulating RANKL and TNFalpha signaling pathways. *Chem Biol* **14**, 860–890.

57. Seidlova-Wuttke, D., Thelen, P. & Wuttke, W. (2006). Inhibitory Effects of a Black Cohosh (Cimicifuga racemosa) Extract on Prostate Cancer. *Planta Med* **72**, 521–526.

58. Davis, V. L., Jayo, M. J., Hardy, M. L., Ho, A., Lee, H., Shaikh, F., Foster, W. G. & Hughes, C. L. (2003). Effects of black cohosh on mammary tumor development and progression in MMTV-neu transgenic mice. *Proceedings of the American Association of Cancer Research* XLIV, 181.

59. Ng, S. S. & Figg, W. D. (2003). Antitumor activity of herbal supplements in human prostate cancer xenografts implanted in immunodeficient mice. *Anticancer Res* **23**, 3585–3590.

60. Davis, V. (2004). Black Cohosh, Breast Cancer, and Metastases to Lung: Data from the Mouse Model. Workshop on the Safety of Black Cohosh in Clinical Studies, Bethesda, Maryland, National Institutes of Health.

61. Green, J. E. (2004). Discussion. Workshop on the Safety of Black Cohosh in Clinical Studies, Bethesda, Maryland, National Institutes of Health.

62. Siegel, P. M., Shu, W., Cardiff, R. D., Muller, W. J. & Massague, J. (2003). Transforming growth factor beta signaling impairs Neu-induced mammary tumorigenesis while promoting pulmonary metastasis. *Proc Natl Acad Sci USA* **100**, 8430–8435.

63. Muraoka, R. S., Koh, Y., Roebuck, L. R., Sanders, M. E., Brantley-Sieders, D., Gorska, A. E., Moses, H. L. & Arteaga, C. L. (2003). Increased malignancy of Neu-induced mammary tumors overexpressing active transforming growth factor beta1. *Mol Cell Biol* **23**, 8691–8703.

64. Einbond, L. S., Su, T., Wu, H. A., Freidman, R., Wang, X., Ramirez, A., Kronenberg, F. & Weinstein, I. (2007). The growth inhibitory effect of actein on human breast cancer cells is associated with activation of stress response pathways. *Int J Cancer* **121**, 2073–2083.

65. Freudenstein, J., Dasenbrock, C. & Nisslein, T. (2002). Lack of promotion of estrogen-dependent mammary gland tumors *in vivo* by an isopropanolic *Cimicifuga racemosa* extract. *Cancer Res*, 3448–3452.

66. Freudenstein, J., Dasenbrock, C. & Nisslein, T. Lack of promotion of mammary gland tumors in vivo by an isopropanolic black cohosh extract. *Phytomedicine* 7 Suppl 2, 13.

67. Nisslein, T. & Freudenstein, J. (2007). Coadministration of the aromatase inhibitor formestane and an isopropanolic extract of black cohosh in a rat model of chemically induced mammary carcinoma. *Planta Med.* **73**, 318–322.

68. Nisslein, T. & Freudenstein, J. (2004). Concomitant administration of an isopropanolic extract of black cohosh and tamoxifen in the *in vivo* tumor model

of implanted RUCA-I rat endometrial adenocarcinoma cells. *Toxicol Lett* **150**, 271–275.

69. Sikder, H., Huso, D. L., Zhang, H., Wang, B., Ryu, B., Hwang, S. T., Powell, J. D. & Alani, R. M. (2003). Disruption of Id1 reveals major differences in angiogenesis between transplanted and autochthonous tumors. *Cancer Cell* **4**, 291–299.

70. Miller, H., Dobs, A. & Chesney, M. (2004). Summary and Next Steps. Workshop on the Safety of Black Cohosh in Clinical Studies, Bethesda, Maryland, National Institutes of Health.

71. Garita-Hernandez, M., Calzado, M. A., Caballero, F. J., Macho, A., Munoz, E., Meier, B., Brattstrom, A., Fiebich, B. L. & Appel, K. (2006). The growth inhibitory activity of the *Cimicifuga racemosa* extract Ze 450 is mediated through estrogen and progesterone receptors-independent pathways. *Planta Med* **72**, 317–323.

72. Haridas, V., Higuchi, M., Jayatilake, G. S., Bailey, D., Mujoo, K., Blake, M. E., Arntzen, C. J. & Gutterman, J. U. (2001). Avicins: Triterpenoid saponins from *Acacia victoriae* (Bentham) induce apoptosis by mitochondrial perturbation. *Proc Natl Acad Sci U S A* **98**, 5821–5826.

73. Pisha, E., Chai, H., Lee, I.-S., Chagwedera, T. E., Farnsworth, N. R., Cordell, G. A., Beecher, C. W. W., Fong, H. H. S., Kinghorn, A. D., Brown, D. M., Wani, M. C., Wall, M. E., Hieken, T. J., Das Gupta, T. K. & Pezzuto, J. M. (1995). Discovery of betulinic acid as a selective inhibitor of human melanoma that functions by induction of apoptosis. *Nat Med* **1**, 1046–1051.

74. Takada, Y. & Aggarwal, B. B. (2003). Betulinic acid suppresses carcinogen-induced NF-kappa B activation through inhibition of I kappa B alpha kinase and p65 phosphorylation: Abrogation of cyclooxygenase-2 and matrix metalloprotease-9. *J Immunol* **171**, 3278–3286.

75. Chowdhury, A., Mandal, S., Mittra, B., Sharma, S., Mukhopadhyay, S. & Majumder, H. (2002). Betulinic acid, a potent inhibitor of eukaryotic topoisomerase I: Identification of the inhibitory step, the major functional group responsible and development of more potent derivatives. *Med Sci Monit* **8**, 254–265, BR.

76. Wang, L. G., Liu, X. M. & Ji, X. J. (1991). Determination of DNA topoisomerase II activity from L1210 cells – a target for screening antitumor agents. *Zhongguo Yao Li Xue Bao* **12**, 108–114.

77. Goodman, G. (1996). *Goodman and Gilman's The Pharmacological Basis of Therapeutics* (9 ed.), (H. A. Limbird, Ed.).

78. Lopez-Lazaro, M. (2007). Digitoxin as an anticancer agent with selectivity for cancer cells: Possible mechanisms involved. *Expert Opin Ther Targets* **11**, 1043–1053.

79. Haux, J. (1999). Digitoxin is a potential anticancer agent for several types of cancer. *Med Hypothese* **53**, 543–548.

80. McConkey, D., Lin, Y., Nutt, L., Ozel, H. & Newman, R. (2000). Cardiac glycosides stimulate $Ca2^+$ increases and apoptosis in androgen-independent, metastatic human prostate adenocarcinoma cells. *Cancer Res* **60**, 3807–3812.

81. Kometiani, P., Liu, L. & Askari, A. (2004). Digitalis-induced signaling by Na^+/K^+-ATPase in human breast cancer cells. *Mol Pharmacol* **December**, 929–936.

82. Liu, L. & Askari, A. (2006). On the importance and mechanism of amplification of digitalis signal through Na^+/K^+-ATPase. *Cell Molec Biol (Noisy-le-grand)* **52**, 28–30.

83. Winnicka, K., Bielawski, K. & Bielawska, A. (2006). Cardiac glycosides in cancer research and cancer therapy. *Acta Pol Pharm* **63**, 109–115.

84. Srivastava, M., Eidelman, O., Zhang, J., Paweletz, C., Caohuy, H., Yang, Q., Jacobson, K., Heldman, E., Huang, W., Jozwik, C., Pollard, B. & Pollard, H. (2004). Digitoxin mimics gene therapy with CFTR and suppresses hypersecretion of IL-8 from cystic fibrosis lung epithelial cells. *Proc Natl Acad Sci U S A* **101**, 7693–7698.

85. Yang, Q., Huang, W., Jozwik, C., Lin, Y., Glasman, M., Caohuy, H., Srivastava, M., Esposito, D., Gillette, W., Hartley, J. & Pollard, H. B. (2005). Cardiac glycosides inhibit TNF-alpha/NF-kappaB signaling by blocking recruitment of TNF receptor-associated death domain to the TNF receptor. *Proc Natl Acad Sci USA* **102**, 9631–9636.

86. Harding, H. P., Zhang, Y., Zeng, H., Novoa, I., Lu, P. D., Calfon, M., Sadri, N., Yun, C., Popko, B., Paules, R., Stojdl, D. F., Bell, J. C., Hettmann, T., Leiden, J. M. & Ron, D. (2003). An integrated stress response regulates amino acid metabolism and resistance to oxidative stress. *Mol Cell* **11**, 619–633.

87. Benjamin, I. J. (2006). Viewing a stressful episode of ER: Is ATF6 the triage nurse. *Circ Res* **98**, 1120–1122.

88. Xu, C., Bailly-Maitre, B. & Reed, J. C. (2005). Endoplasmic reticulum stress: Cell life and death decisions. *J Clin Invest* **115**, 2656–2664.

89. Zhang, K. & Kaufman, R. J. (2006). The unfolded protein response: A stress signaling pathway critical for health and disease. *Neurology* **66**, S102–S109.

90. Delescluse, C., Lemaire, G., Dde Sousa, G. & Rahmani, R. (2000). Is CYP1A1 induction always related to AHR signaling pathway. *Toxicology* **153**, 73–82.

91. Millauer, B., Shawver, L. K., Plate, K. H., Risau, W. & Ullrich, A. (1994). Glioblastoma growth inhibited *in vivo* by a dominant-negative Flk-1 mutant. *Nature* **367**, 576–579.

92. Gaube, F., Wolfl, S., Pusch, L., Kroll, T. & Hamburger, M. (2007). Gene expression profiling reveals effects of *Cimicifuga racemosa* (L.) Nutt. (Black cohosh) on the estrogen receptor positive human breast cancer cell line MCF-7. *BMC Pharmacol* **7**, 11.

93. Suh, N., Honda, T., Finlay, H., Barchowsky, A., Williams, C., Benoit, N., Xie, O. W., Nathan, C., Gribble, G. & Sporn, M. B. (1998). Novel triterpenoids suppress inducible nitric oxide synthase (iNOS) and inducible cyclooxygenase (COX-2) in mouse macrophages. *Cancer Res* **58**, 717–723.

94. Suh, N., Wang, Y., Honda, T., Gribble, G. W., Dmitrovsky, E., Hickey, W. F., Maue, R. A., Place, A. E., Porter, D. M., Spinella, M. J., Williams, C. R., Wu, G., Dannenberg, A. J., Flanders, K. C., Letterio, J. J., Mangelsdorf, D. J., Nathan, C. F., Nguyen, L., Porter, W. W., Ren, R. F., Roberts, A. B., Roche, N. S., Subbaramaiah, K. & Sporn, M. B. (1999). A novel synthetic oleanane triterpenoid, 2-cyano-3,12-dioxoolean-1,9-dien-28-oic acid, with potent differentiating, antiproliferative, and anti-inflammatory activity. *Cancer Res* **58**, 336–341.

95. Ito, Y., Pandey, P., Sporn, M. B., Datta, R., Kharbanda, S. & Kufe, D. (2001). The novel triterpenoid CDDO induces apoptosis and differentiation of human osteosarcoma cells by a caspase-8 dependent mechanism. *Mol Pharmacol* **5**, 1094–1099.

96. Pedersen, I. M., Kitada, S., Schimmer, A., Kim, Y., Zapata, J. M., Charboneau, L., Rassenti, L., Andreeff, M., Bennett, F., Sporn, M. B., Liotta, L. D., Kipps, T. J. & Reed, J. C. (2002). The triterpenoid CDDO induces apoptosis in refractory CLL B cells. *Blood* **8**, 2965–2972.

97. Stadheim, T. A., Suh, N., Ganju, N., Sporn, M. B. & Eastman, A. (2002). The novel triterpenoid 2-cyano-3,12-dioxooleana-1,9-dien-28-oic acid (CDDO) potently enhances apoptosis induced by tumor necrosis factor in human leukemia cells. *J Biol Chem* **19**, 16448–16455.

98. Wang, Y., Porter, W. W., Suh, N., Honda, T., Gribble, G. W., Leesnitzer, L. M., Plunket, K. D., Mangelsdorf, D. J., Blanchard, S. G., Willson, T. M. & Sporn, M. B. (2000). A synthetic triterpenoid, 2-cyano-3,12-dioxooleana-1,9-dien-28-oic acid (CDDO), is a ligand for the peroxisome proliferator-activated receptor gamma. *Mol Endocrinol* **14**, 1550–1556.

99. Yates, M. S., Tauchi, M., Katsuoka, F., Flanders, K. C., Liby, K. T., Honda, T., Gribble, G. W., Johnson, D. A., Johnson, J. A., Burton, N. C., Guilarte, T. R., Yamamoto, M., S, M. B. & Kensler, T. W. (2007). Pharmacodynamic characterization of chemopreventive triterpenoids as exceptionally potent inducers of Nrf2-regulated genes. *Mol Cancer Ther* **6**, 154–162.

100. Lapillonne, H., Konopleva, M., Tsao, T., Gold, D., McQueen, T., Sutherland, R. L., Madden, T. & Andreeff, M. (2003). Activation of peroxisome proliferator-activated receptor gamma by a novel synthetic triterpenoid 2-cyano-3,12-dioxooleana-1,9-dien-28-oic acid induces growth arrest and apoptosis in breast cancer cells. *Cancer Res* **63**, 5926–5939.

101. Chow, H., Cai, Y., Hakim, I., Crowell, J., Shahi, F., Brooks, C., Dorr, R., Hara, Y. & Alberts, D. (2003). Pharmacokinetics and safety of green tea polyphenols after multiple-dose administration of epigallocatechin galate and polyphenon e in healthy individuals. *Clin Cancer Res* **9**, 3312–3319.

102. Swezey, R. R., Aldridge, D. E., LeValley, S. E., Crowell, J. A., Hara, Y. & Green, C. E. (2003). Absorption, tissue distribution and elimination of 4-[(3)h]-epigallocatechin gallate in beagle dogs. *Int. J. Toxicol.* **22**, 187–193.

103. Cohen, S., O'Connor, A., Hart, J., Merel, N. & Te, H. (2004). Autoimmune hepatitis associated with the use of black cohosh: A case study. *Menopause* **11**, 575–577.

104. Kerlin, P. (2004). Herbal Hepatitis – Black Cohosh. Workshop on the Safety of Black Cohosh in Clinical Studies, Bethesda, Maryland, National Institutes of Health.

105. Spangler, L., Newton, K. M., Grothaus, L. C., Reed, S. D., Ehrlich, K. & LaCroix, A. Z. (2007). The effects of black cohosh therapies on lipids, fibrinogen, glucose and insulin. *Maturitas* **57**, 195–204.

106. Wuttke, W., Gorkow, C. & Seidlova-Wuttke, D. (2006). Effects of black cohosh (*Cimicifuga racemosa*) on bone turnover, vaginal mucosa, and various blood parameters in postmenopausal women: A double-blind, placebo-controlled, and conjugated estrogens-controlled study. *Menopause* **13**.

107. Raus, K., Brucker, C., Gorkow, C. & Wuttke, W. (2006). First-time proof of endometrial safety of the special black cohosh extract (*Actaea* or *Cimicifuga racemosa* extract) CR BNO 1055. *Menopause* **13**, 678–691.

108. Liske, E. (1998). Therapeutic efficacy and safety of *Cimicifuga racemosa* for gynecologic disorders. *Adv Ther* **15**, 45–53.

109. Johnson, B. & Van Breemen, R. (2003). *In vitro* formation of quinoid metabolites of the dietary supplement *Cimicifuga racemosa* (Black cohosh). *Chem Res Toxicol* **16**, 838–846.

110. Lude, S., Torok, M., Dieterle, S., Knapp, A., Kaeufeler, R., Jaggi, R., Spornitz, U. & Krahenbuhl, S. (2007). Hepatic effects of Cimicifuga racemosa extract in vivo and in vitro . *Cell Mol Life Sci* 2848–2857.

111. Hemmi, H., Kitame, F., Ishida, N., Kusano, G., Kondo, Y. & Nozoe, S. (1979). Inhibition of thymidine transport into phytohemagglutinin-stimulated lymphocytes by triterpenoids from *Cimicifuga* species. *J. Pharmacobio-Dyn* **2**, 339–349.

112. Gurley, B. J., Gardner, S. F., Hubbard, M. A., Williams, D. K., Gentry, W. B., Khan, I. A. & Shah, A. (2005). *In vivo* effects of goldenseal, kava kava, black cohosh, and valerian on human cytochrome P450 1A2, 2D6, 2E1, and 3A4/5 phenotypes. *Clin Pharmacol Ther* **77**, 415–426.

113. Tsukamoto, S., Aburatani, M. & Ohta, T. (2005). Isolation of CYP3A4 inhibitors from the Black cohosh (*Cimicifuga racemosa*). *Evidence-based complementary and alternative medicine: eCAM* **2**, 223–226.

Chapter 12

Integrating Comprehensive and Alternative Medicine into Stroke

Herbal Treatment of Ischemia

Baowan Lin

Cerebral Vascular Disease Research Center, Department of Neurology, University of Miami Miller School of Medicine, Miami, FL, USA

Abstract

Plants manufacture their own compounds to protect themselves against dangers and illness. Those defenders turn out to protect humans against diseases. Chinese herbs have been used to treat humans' illness for thousands of years. This chapter reports that one specific nine-herb combination, believed to be effective in mitigating ischemic stroke injury in patients in China, protected the brain from focal and global ischemia in animal studies, demonstrated by behavioral and histopathological tests. Daily administration of the nine-herb cocktail soup by gavage, initiated at 4 hours after ischemia, reduced the infarct volume by 53 and 62%, compared to nontreated groups, at days 3 and 28, encouraged neurological function recovery, prevented brain cavitation and enhanced the self-repair in brain infarcts; the therapy reduced neuronal death in hippocampal CA1 and striatum in the acute stage, prevented the delayed encephalopathy and improved coordination at the chronic stage after global ischemia. This chapter documents 2 formulas and 19 single herbs which have been used applying to treat ischemia in China for centuries. All of these herbs are nontoxic. Their dosages and disease-fighting compounds are depicted.

Keywords: *Brain, infarction, ischemia, neuroprotection, herb*

INTRODUCTION

Stroke Treatment in Western Medicine (Orthodox Medicine)

Stroke is the third leading cause of death in industrialized countries and a major cause of permanent disability. With the increase of aging population, stroke becomes a major health problem. One in three North Americans will suffer a stroke, becomes demented, or both [1]. Most strokes (~80%) are cerebral focal ischemia, that is brain infarction, resulting from occlusion of a major cerebral artery by thrombus or embolus blocking blood flow to a specific brain region [2].

Thrombolysis of clots in occluded arteries in order to restore blood supply to the affected territory is the current and standard therapy for limiting brain infarction [3]. Tissue-plasminogen activator (t-PA) is the only thrombolytic drug that has been approved to treat the acute brain infarction by blood clot resolution, but, t-PA is restricted to administration within 3 hours after the clot formation, and has a risk to induce brain hemorrhage [3]. No effective conventional pharmacotherapy or approved treatment has been established in humans to increase brain repair, to reduce infarct volume or to prevent neurological deficits [3, 4]. In the last decade, stem cell and gene therapy have become the two hottest topics in the stroke field. However, transforming the information obtained from animal studies into the clinic faces many huge challenges. Therefore, the viewpoint is shifting to combine therapies to reduce neuronal damage and enhance endogenous neurogenesis to replace the damaged neurons [5] because neurogenesis exists in human brain [6].

Stroke Treatment of Comprehensive and Alternative Medicine (CAM)

Complementary and alternative medicine (CAM) may offer a way to combat stroke. Traditional Chinese medicine (TCM), based on herbal medicine, is ancient but still vital. It is an important element in the treatment of brain ischemia in clinic in China, Korea, and Japan [7, 8]. Many people including doctors have turned to TCM to help stroke victims because cerebral ischemia is not responsive to the current Western medicine (WM). In Korea, 25% of stroke patients visit traditional medicine doctors [8]. In China, about one third of brain ischemia patients are treated with TCM [9]. The Chinese government encourages integrating TCM into WM to serve patients better because some diseases not responsive to WM may be cured by TCM. Bedside herbal treatment has been present in WM hospitals in China since 1960s. Meanwhile, the Chinese government continuously provides huge financial support to the science research of TCM.

The theory of, and formulas for, *enhancing the circulation to encourage self-repair* by TCM were conceived and tested clinically long ago, long before the establishment of laboratory studies of disease models in the United Kingdom and United States of America. Today, experimental animal studies can be used to explain why and how medications are effective. The experimental study on Chinese medicine combating stroke in the United States started in 1998 in the Cerebral Vascular Disease Research Center, Department of Neurology, University of Miami, School of Medicine, in Miami, Florida.

A formula consisting of nine specific herbs has been demonstrated to possess significant neuroprotection by our experimental studies, including decreasing infarct volume, preventing cavitation, enhancing self-repair, accelerating functional recovery in brain focal ischemia and attenuating neuronal injury, preventing delayed encephalopathy and maintaining good coordination in global forebrain ischemia. Other effective formulas and herbs were reported by bench studies from many labs. Phytochemical efforts to identify the herbs' active ingredients and to investigate each ingredient's properties are now being conducted in laboratories around the world in the recent decade.

This chapter will review the functions of formulas and herbs that have been demonstrated for neuroprotection in ischemic stroke including disease-fighting compounds and their properties. Since formulas are usually more effective than single herbs in mitigating diseases, thus, 2 formulas are introduced first and, then, 19 herbs in this chapter.

BRAIN ISCHEMIA

Several hypotheses and theories are involved in the mechanism of ischemic damage development. However, this chapter will focus on the histopathology following ischemia.

Focal Brain Ischemia

Cerebral blood vessel occlusion impedes or blocks the focal cerebral blood flow (CBF) resulting in focal brain ischemia, infarction. Infarction happens if the CBF drops below 25% of normal. The initial CBF reduction determines the area of the latter infarct [2]. In humans, brain infarction is characterized by coagulative necrosis and inflammation with neutrophil infiltration in the first 3 days. Monocytes emigrate later; necrotic tissue is liquefied by lytic enzymes released from leukocytes; infarct progresses to re-sorption at around 1 month with neovascularization, cavitation, and ultimately becomes a cavity in most cases [10]. Infarct volume is related to the functional status after middle cerebral artery stroke [11]. About 25% of patients develop dementia in 3 months [12, 13]. Both β amyloid precursor protein (βAPP) and amyloid β peptide (Aβ), the prominent feature of Alzheimer's disease (AD), are deposited in cortical and subcortical areas in the brains of non-dementia patients following stroke [14].

The process of focal ischemia in animals is similar to humans. Delayed neuronal death and continuous change exist until the end of the 4th week; necrotic neurons are still visible in both striatum and cortex at this time [15]; brain infarction induces neurodegeneration in remote region, including thalamus and hippocampus [16, 17].

Endothelial damage in the infarcted region is prominent [18, 19]. The endothelial injury results in (1) blood–brain barrier (BBB) disruption leading to release of potentially toxic chemicals in the plasma into the brain parenchyma to induce destruction and inflammation, and (2) a 2-week secondary CBF decline via vasoconstriction and micro-thrombosis [20–23], which may promote the death of injured neurons in the penumbra. Leukocyte-platelet aggregates are increased two-fold in peripheral blood vessels and adhered to cerebral microcirculation to result in significant postischemic CBF decrease [24]. Endothelin-1 (ET-1) over-formation by injured endothelia leads to water accumulation and brain edema [25].

Many articles reported that endogenous neurogenesis exists in the brain including humans after ischemia. However, the brain's atrophy and cavity make repair unrealistic; detrimental inflammation and inadequate blood supply *in situ* cause massive loss of newborn neurons [26].

Global Forebrain Ischemia

Global cerebral ischemia is the consequence of cardiac arrest, and may occur after heart surgery. Delayed encephalopathy characterized by dementia and ataxia, associated with parenchymal lesions and damage in white matter emerges after a symptom-free period following an initial recovery [27]. The encephalopathy is not uncommon after brief cardiac arrest and surgery [27–29]. About one third of survivors from resuscitation have the significant neurological dysfunction [30]. Two main types of irreversible brain lesions exist in humans: (1) acidophilic neurons with consecutive neuronal loss and reactive astroglial activation in the brain regions vulnerable to ischemia and in the micro-infarcts or (2) perivascular and diffuse tissue sponginess without the gliosis. The primary injury is neuronal death in the form of acidophilic neurons, necrosis, in the hippocampal CA1 sector, the area vulnerable to ischemia. The second injury, delayed encephalopathy, occurs later, including macro- and micro-infarcts or confluent areas of pan-necrosis associated with perivascular and diffuse tissue sponginess [31]. Lesion exists in the watershed zones of parietoocipitotemporal cortex, basal ganglia, thalamus, hippocampus, pons as well as cerebellum, are in a progressively changing manner [27, 31]. Such lesions are associated with diffuse brain atrophy in patients having persistent vegetative state [27–29, 32]. Beta-amyloid protein (Aβ) also is deposited in the brain after cardiac arrest [33]. Platelets contribute to the cerebral Aβ deposition in humans [34, 35].

Previous animal studies demonstrated such two kinds of damage existing in the brain after a brief forebrain ischemia [36] and revealed the mechanisms of the damage [36–38]. Brief transient ischemia results in necrosis [39] and triggers slowly progressive pathological alterations in rat brains at 4–10 weeks [36]. Components of this delayed secondary injury are: (a) endothelial degeneration associated with thrombosis, infarction and perivascular neurodegeneration and spongy change; and (b) the abnormal cerebral accumulation of βAPP and Aβ emerged at 2 months, concentrated in perivascular regions and released from blood vessels. βAPP and Aβ induce neuronal shrinkage and disappearance. Therefore, cerebral endothelia play a key role in the chronic neuronal injury development [36, 37, 40]. Platelet activity and aggregation associated with thrombi significantly increase for 1 year after global ischemia [41].

BASIC THEORY ABOUT STROKE IN TCM

Traditional Chinese medicine is a coherent and independent medicine system to WM. It has a totally different process from WM on critical thinking, extensive clinical observation and testing. Because my medical training was in WM, as a neurologist, I originally speculated that the effect of herbs was an accident from the viewpoint of WM whenever I saw that diseases were cured by herbs. Later, I was convinced by the facts of clinical outcomes that some severe syndromes were certainly healed by herbs. I came to our lab to investigate the herbal efficacy with experimental studies. The studies revealed that the bedside therapy of the nine-herb evidently protected the brain from ischemia and eliminated doubts about the potential of phytomedicine. Now we are trying to integrate TCM into WM.

The TCM theory about ischemic stroke will be simply depicted below.

TCM Emphasizes that Blood Supply Decline Causes Ischemia, Wind Stroke

The character of stroke, including a sudden onset, quick change of the severe multiple-symptoms and the strong destruction in the human body, is comparable to the character of a wind-gust in nature: a sudden and strong rush associated with violent and fast direction shifting. Thus, brain ischemia is called *wind stroke* in TCM [42].

Blockage of blood supply results in the *endogenous wind* to induce stroke. Prompting blood circulation to relieve the stroke symptoms and encourage brain's repair is the therapeutic strategy. Some specific herbs have been extensively used to improve blood circulation, to relieve stroke symptoms and to encourage self-healing. Combining one major active herb and several supporting ones to synergize the pharmacodynamic action has been the philosophy underlying prescribing practice in TCM and is supported by the knowledge accumulated during centuries.

Strategy of Treatment: Prompting Blood Circulation and Rebalancing Yin and Yang in Liver and Kidney

TCM considers that unbalance of *Yin* and *Yang* breaks body's harmony to induce diseases. To rebuild the body's harmony is the principle to treat diseases. Disturbance of blood circulation are caused by hypertension, arteriosclerosis, decreased body function due to aging, overwork and mental stress [42]. TCM terms hypertension and arteriosclerosis as *exuberant Yang* in *liver* and *deficient Yin* in *liver*. In addition, TCM realizes the importance of hormones. When people are aged, formation of sexual hormone in the body is decreased. TCM calls this *Yin deficiency* in *kidney*. The imbalance of *Yin* and *Yang* in the "*liver* and *kidney*" induces the *internal wind* to cause the stroke. The rebalance of *Yin* and *Yang* in *liver* and *kidney* prevents the new *internal wind* production. Some herbs are able to increase the *liver Yin* or decrease the *liver Yang* and other herbs increase the *kidney Yin*. Such herbs are given to patients in chronic stage.

Liver and *kidney* in TCM have a different conception from WM. The *liver* in TCM includes liver and involves part of the central nervous system, the vegetative nervous system, retina, and blood vessels. The *kidney* includes part of the endocrine system and nervous system, reproductive system, kidney, and urinary system.

FORMULAE AND MAJOR HERBS FOR ISCHEMIA TREATMENT

During my 15-year practice as an academic neurologist of WM in Beijing, I observed that drinking a specific nine-herb cocktail soup relieved the symptoms of ischemic stroke without adverse effects. We demonstrated the neuroprotection of the nine-herb cocktail-therapy in our lab and will report the efficacy in this chapter.

Formulae

Formulae, consisting of several herbs with many functions work synergistically, are employed to treat diseases because a single herb is usually less effective than expected, or has no efficacy at all [8, 43].

Specific Nine-herb Modified Buyang Huanwu Tang (Decoction)

The present studies, the first time, provided experimental evidence for the known protective efficacy of the nine-herb formula on humans' brain ischemia by means of an animal model of ischemia with behavioral and histological studies. Tang means decoction in Chinese language.

The combination of nine herbs consists of *Ligusticum wallichii*, *Angelica sinensis*, *Carthamus tinctorius*, *Prunus persica*, *Astragali*, *Paeonia veitchii*, *Scutellaria baicalensis*, *Paeonia suffruticosa*, and *Glycyrrhiza*. Their LD_{50} responses were tested and reveal no toxicity [44–46]. These 9 herbs are safe and documented in *Pharmacopoeia of P. R. China*.

Decoction leads to a better bioavailability since aqueous extracts are absorbed quickly by the gastrointestinal tract, give a rapid onset of action, and provide longer and higher efficacy than other preparations and administration including intravenous injection [42, 47–50]. The aqueous extracts of the nine herbs are rapidly absorbed [44, 47, 50]. The amount of baicalin is about 10-fold of the baicalein in *Scutellaria baicalensis*. Baicalin rapidly appears in plasma to exist for 24 hours after oral administration and metabolizes into baicalein, in part, by bacteria prior to intestinal absorption [47], and subsequently metabolizes into baicalein in the human body [49]. *Glycyrrhiza* enhances the absorption of other herbs and leads to higher bioavailability in the body [50, 51]. Thus, oral administration provides longer and higher efficacy.

Phytochemical studies found that these herbs are multi-functional. The nine herbs and their compounds work as neuroprotectant, antioxidant, anti-inflammatory, and antithrombotic agents, as well as vasoconstriction antagonists (see Section "Herbs"). Their known disease-fighting compounds are flavonoids, saponins, and 1,2,3,4,6-penta-O-galloyl-beta-D-glucose (PGG), etc., including baicalin, baicalein, wogonin, oroxylin A, and Skullcapflavone II in *Scutellaria*, astragalus saponins in *Astragalas,* tetramethylpyrazine (TMP) in *Ligusticum*, vitamin E and ferulic acid in *Angelica*, safflower yellow in *Carthamus*, PGG and paeonol in *Paeonia veitchii* and *Paeonia suffruticosa,* as well as glycyrrhizin in *Glycyrrhiza* [44, 52, 53]. Baicalein, baicalin and TMP, readily cross the BBB and become evenly distributed throughout the intact rat brain in 20 minutes after oral administration [44, 54–56], and the onset of their action is rapid [47, 57].

We designed two experiments, supported by National Institutes of health (NIH)/National Center for Complementary and Alternative Medicine (NCCAM) grant AT001598-01, to investigate whether the nine-herb formula works on brain infarction and global ischemia. Animals were given the herbal cocktail soup in the same manner given to patients including dosage and administration. Histopathology and behavioral tests were employed to test neuroprotection as the most important and the key methods. Bromodeoxyuridine (BrdU) was precluded owing to BrdU injection is beyond the treatment to humans and because it would be improper to test the herbal therapy's efficacy since BrdU may produce cell toxicity and unspecific labeling [58, 59]. Water-maze test was not employed owing to swimming does not apply in the clinic. To prevent the influence of postischemic change of estrogen on the outcome, the use of female lab animals was avoided.

Experiment 1 (Focal cerebral ischemia) and Experiment 2 (Global forebrain ischemia)

Decoction Preparation

Each dry herb was individually weighed into 10 g (0.2 g/kg/day) amounts for each of Ligusticum wallichii, Angelica sinensis, Carthamus tinctorius, Prunus persica, Astragalas, Scutellaria, Paeonia veitchii, and Paeonia suffruticosa, and 3 g for Glycyrrhiza (0.07 g/kg/day), same as the dosage for one adult Chinese per day. Herbs were macerated together in cold drinkable water and boiled for 45 minutes, and then the decoction was filtered. The procedure was repeated 3 times. The three filtered decoctions were mixed and concentrated to yield a final volume of 750 ml. The decoctions were tested by HPLC (high performance liquid chromatography), and the extraction is reproducible (see chromatographs in Fig. 12.1). The amount of baicalin was ~0.65 mg/ml. The decoction was stored at −20°C

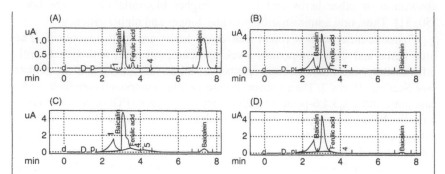

FIGURE 12.1   Chromatographs of standard solution (A) and of 3 decoctions (B, C, D).

until for administration. Contamination-free herbs were obtained from Mayway Co., Oakland, CA.

Experiment 1 (Focal cerebral ischemia)

Materials and Method

Animal Preparation and Production of Cerebral Ischemia
Thirty-nine male Sprague-Dawley rats weighing 280–350 g participated in the focal cerebral ischemia study. Brain infarction was produced by a 2-hour middle cerebral artery occlusion (MCAo) by intraluminal suture insertion following one overnight fast [18]. A 3–0 monofilament, poly-L-lysine-coated nylon suture inserted under anesthesia conducted with halothane (induced at 2%, maintained at 1%) into the internal carotid artery and advanced a distance of 20–23 mm to block the MCA. Rectal temperature was monitored and maintained at 36.5–37°C, the cranial temperature was at 36–36.5°C. Rectal temperature was measured during the first 3 days of survival. All of the physiological variables during surgery were controlled in normal ranges. The rats were sacrificed for histopathological assessment on day 3 or day 28.

Medicine Treatment
The rats in the treated groups received the nine-herb cocktail soup (HC) daily up to 28 days by gavage, started at 2 hours after recirculation. The 15 ml/kg/day, that is 6 ml/day, of decoction were administered in two divided doses. The dosage of baicalin in the decoction given to the rats is 10 mg/kg/day. Rats were allowed to survive for 3 days ($n = 9$) and 28 days ($n = 11$). The rats in the control groups received drinkable water (DW, $n = 10$ and 9 respectively).

Neurobehavioral Testing and Evaluation
A standard neurobehavioral test battery was employed to assess the brain deficits [60]. *Postural reflex test* detects both cortical and striatal lesions. Five *forelimb placing tests* reflect sensorimotor integration, assessing the forelimb response to visual, tactile and proprioceptive stimuli. The total deficit score ranges from 0 to 12, designating normal to maximal deficit. All of the rats received the behavioral tests before surgery and at 60 and 110 minutes, days 1, 2, 3, 14, and 28 after MCAo.

Histology

Histopathological exams were on days 3 or 28 after the ischemic insult. Under halothane anesthesia, rats were perfused via the ascending aorta with FAM (a mixture of 40% formaldehyde, glacial acetic acid, and methanol, 1:1:8 by volume) for 20 minutes following a 2-minutes initial perfusion with physiological saline. The head was immersed in FAM at 4°C for 1 day. The brain was removed and placed in FAM for an additional day. Coronal brain blocks were embedded in paraffin. Rats' brains were cut into 10-μm thick sections from 5.5 mm to −7.5 mm from bregma at nine standard levels to cover the whole infarcted areas. The sections were stained with hematoxylin and eosin (H&E) to determine the infarct volume or processed for immunohistochemical studies.

Immunohistochemistry

Consecutive sections were obtained at the nine standard intervals. Expression of the targeted proteins was visualized by routine immunoperoxidase techniques. Primary antibodies were: anti-rat endothelial barrier antigen (EBA) for normal endothelia (SMI 71, 1: 2000; Sternberger Monoclonals, Lutherville, MD) [18], NeuN (MAB377, 1: 400; Chemicon) for mature neurons [61], anti-βIII tubulin (TUJ1, 1: 400; Sigma Chemical Corp.) for developing neurons [62], doublecortin (DCX, 1: 200, Santa Cruz Biotech.) for migrating neurons [63], BS-1 isolectin B_4 (GSA1-B_4, 1:200, Sigma, St. Louis, MO) for active microglia, antiglial fibrillary acidic protein (GFAP, 1:1500, Dako Corp.) for active astrocytes, anti-human myeloperoxidase (MPO, 1:1000; Dako Corp., Carpenteria, CA) for neutrophils, ED-1 (MCA 341R, 1: 400; Serotec, Raleigh, NC) for macrophage, and anti-COX2 (Cat # 160126, 1: 400; Cayman Chemicals, Ann Arbor, MI) for cyclooxygenase-2 [64]. As negative controls, sections were incubated in mouse IgG1 or rabbit Immunoglobulin fraction (X0931, X0903, Dako Corp.). The Vectastain ABC method (Vector Labs, Burlingame, CA) and 3,3′-diaminobenzidine (DAB) were used for visualization of primary antibody binding. Specific staining was identified by the dark-brown appearance.

Image Analysis and Cell Counting

Infarct volume analysis was conducted with the MCID system (Imaging Research, Inc., St. Catherine's, ON, Canada). The volumes of infarcts were computed on the nine sections across the nine standard coronal levels stained by H&E with numerical integration using Simpson's method. Quantitative histopathological infarct frequency maps were computer-generated for each group with image analysis methods [65]. Sections were examined and analyzed under a computer-assisted light microscope connected to the imaging system. Cell counting was performed on sections spaced at bregma level − 0.3 mm. Counting of neutrophil, macrophage and normal endothelia was conducted on the infarcted hemispheres, and positive-stained cells were digitized under microscope (10-fold objective) [18]. Image analysis was conducted under a blind manner.

Statistical Analysis

Results were presented as mean±SD. Data were analyzed by one-way analysis of variance (ANOVA) followed by Dunn's test for multiple comparisons. Significance was accepted as $p < 0.05$.

TABLE 12.1 Physiological variables (Values are means ± S.D. MABP means arterial blood pressure)

	Herbal cocktail soup (HC)		Drinkable water (DW)	
	3-Day $n = 9$	4-Week $n = 11$	3-Day $n = 10$	4-Week $n = 9$
Before MCAo (15 minutes)				
Body weight (g)	320 ± 24	320 ± 27	314 ± 30	318 ± 23
MABP (mm Hg)	117 ± 7	117 ± 14	114 ± 5	119 ± 24
Arterial pH	7.44 ± 0.07	7.439 ± 0.05	7.448 ± 0.05	7.453 ± 0.03
$PaCO_2$ (mm Hg)	39.6 ± 0.8	37.5 ± 4.3	37.2 ± 6.2	36.7 ± 4.1
PaO_2 (mm Hg)	141 ± 43	118 ± 24	172 ± 66	147 ± 42
Plasma glucose (mg/dl)	157 ± 28	150 ± 40	159 ± 38	132 ± 27
During MCAo (15 minutes)				
MABP (mm Hg)	119 ± 3	113 ± 39	119 ± 14	125 ± 15
Arterial pH	7.407 ± 0.07	7.432 ± 0.04	7.451 ± 0.05	7.421 ± 0.04
$PaCO_2$ (mm Hg)	40.7 ± 7	39.3 ± 3	36.6 ± 4	39.1 ± 5
PaO_2 (mm Hg)	139 ± 29	132 ± 17	152 ± 38	147 ± 46
Plasma glucose (mg/dl)	164 ± 46	153 ± 23	149 ± 53	133 ± 18
After MCAo (2 hours)				
Plasma glucose (mg/dl)	218 ± 87	218 ± 70	193 ± 48	187 ± 32
Rectal temperature (°C)	37.2 ± 0.6	36.8 ± 1.2	37.8 ± 1.0	37.3 ± 1.2
During survival				
Rectal temperature (°C), day 1	37.5 ± 0.8	37.5 ± 0.8	37.8 ± 1.0	37.8 ± 0.7
Rectal temperature (°C), day 2	37.7 ± 0.7	37.2 ± 0.5	37.5 ± 0.6	37.7 ± 0.3
Rectal temperature (°C), day 3	37.5 ± 0.6	37.3 ± 0.5	37.5 ± 0.6	36.5 ± 1.0

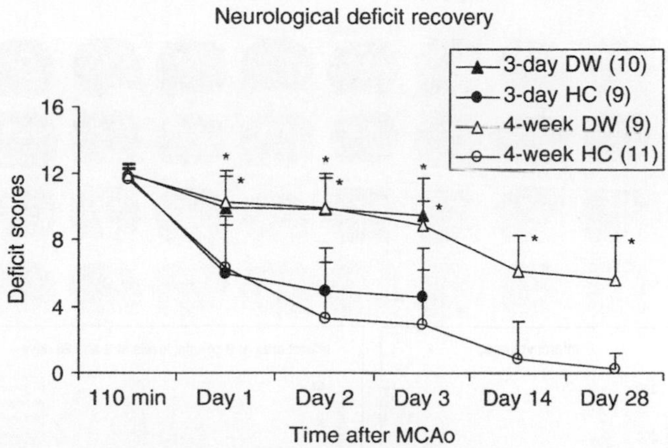

Neurological deficit recovery

FIGURE 12.2 Neurobehavioral scores (mean±SD) for the 3-day and 28-day studies after 2-hours MCAo. The HC animals showed a significant improvement, compared to DW groups, from day 1 to day 28 (* denotes $p < 0.01$).

Results

Physiological variables: Physiological variables including arterial blood gases, plasma glucose, mean arterial blood pressure (MABP) rectal and cranial temperatures at the time of surgery and after were in the normal range in all groups, and no inter-group differences existed (Table 12.1).

Behavioral analysis: All rats were normal before surgery, and displayed marked neurological deficits at 110 minute after MCAo. Significant neurological-functional recovery began at 24 hours and continued up to 28 days, which was completely recovered in all HC rats while some deficits persisted in DW rats. Deficit scores were more markedly reduced in HC groups than DW rats (Fig. 12.2).

Histopathology: The infarct volumes of HC groups decreased by 53% |194 ± 70 (DW, $n = 10$) vs. $91 ± 69$ mm³ (HC, $n = 9$) ($p = 0.01$)| at day 3, and by 62% |101 ± 51 (DW, 9) vs. 38 ± 22 mm³ (HC, 11) ($p < 0.01$)| at day 28. The protection was present in penumbra, infarct periphery (Figs. 12.3 and 12.4).

At day 3, 8 of 10 DW rats had massive hemorrhagic infarcts in dorsal lateral striatum. In contrast, seven of nine HC rats displayed very small peri-arterial hemorrhages. Five of 10 DW rats displayed many eosinophilic and shrunken neurons in ipsilateral thalamus; one DW rat had necrosis in ipsilateral hippocampus. HC rats showed no injury in the two regions.

At day 28, frank cavities were seen in 8 of 9 brains in DW group, with smaller cavities in 2 of 11 HC rats (Fig. 12.3A). Several neurons were scattered at the edge of infarct in the striatum of DW rats (Fig. 12.5A). Many neurons, including spindle-like neurons, were distributed along the edge of the infarct in the striatum in HC rats (Fig. 12.5B), which was different from the distribution of neurons in DW rat (Fig. 12.5A) and in the contralateral striatum of the HC rats (Fig. 12.5C). While massive proliferation was seen in the subventricular zone (SVZ) of the lateral ventricle ipsilateral to MCAo in nontreated (DW) rats (Fig. 12.5D), mild genesis showed in this region in HC treated rats (Fig. 12.5G), which was astrocytic gliosis

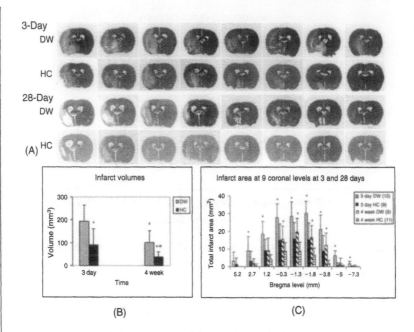

FIGURE 12.3 (A) Low-power photographs of H&E-stained coronal sections at the 5th level of the central lesion (bregma ~−1.3 mm) in DW and HC rats. Eight brains in each group are ranked in descending order of ipsilateral hemisphere tissue injury. At day 3, seven DW rats displayed typical infarction occupying the whole territory of the MCA and midline shifting toward the contralateral hemisphere indicates severe hemisphere enlargement. Smaller infarcts were seen in eight HC rats. At day 28, eight DW rats showed cavitation and evident infarct, while only two HC rats had smaller cavities and all eight brains present much milder damage. (B) Herbal treatment reduces infarct volume. The herbal cocktail therapy begun at 4 h after initiation of ischemia reduced infarct size as measured by H&E staining. The infarct volume in HC groups was 53 and 62% less than that of DW groups at days 3 and 28. * indicates significant difference from the corresponding value in DW groups ($p < 0.01$). Infarct volume at 4 weeks was smaller than day 3. # represents the significant difference from day 3 in DW group ($p < 0.005$); @ denotes significant difference from day 3 in HC group ($p < 0.05$; error bars represent SD). (C) HC treatment significantly reduced infarct size in 8 of 9 levels at day 3 and in 4 of 9 levels at day 28. * indicates significant difference from HC group in the same time ($p < 0.05$).

confirmed by GFAP immunostaining. We investigated the source of the migrating neurons, spindle-like neurons, adjacent to the lesion in the inferior striatum. Unexpectedly we found the source in the rostrum of 3rd ventricle, distant from infarct, where young (presumably newly produced) neurons, that is spindle-like neurons, and mature neurons were apparently existed in the HC rat (Figs. 12.5H and 12.5I) and confirmed by NeuN-immunostaining (Fig. 12.5K). Such neuronal proliferation was not present in DW rats (Figs. 12.5E, 12.5F and 12.5J).

The peri-infarct zone had abundant ghost neurons and obvious inflammation in three of nine DW rats (Fig. 12.6A). However, the peri-infarct injury ceased and

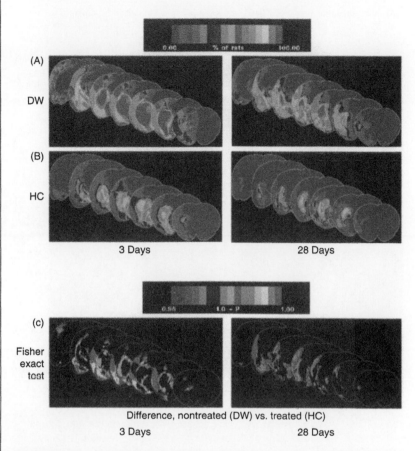

FIGURE 12.4 Distributions of infarction frequency and comparisons. Color-coded computerized image figures show the percentages of animals with infarcted tissue at 8 rostro-caudal coronal levels in DW and HC rats. Red = 95% of rats' infarcts in panels A and B. Panel C shows the comparison between panels A vs. B on a pixel-basis by Fisher's exact test. Color bar depicts $(1-p)$, where p is the significance level of inter-group statistical significance. The lower threshold of the color bar has been set to $1-p = 0.95$, so as to highlight those pixels with $p < 0.05$. The figures reveal that the majority of neuroprotection of the therapy presents in the penumbra (A, B) and exists in the cortex (C).

normal neurons remained in this region in all 11 HC rats (Fig. 12.6B). Meanwhile, no neurons were seen in the lesions in DW rats while many normal neurons existed in the infarcted regions in all HC rats. NeuN-immunoreactivity was completely lost in the infarct in all DW rats (Fig. 12.6C) but numerous NeuN-labeled neurons were seen in the lesion, in the core (Fig. 12.6D) and the border (Fig. 12.6E) in all HC rats. They were distributed in different sites along or around blood vessels. Many neurons in the infarct had long and short processes, resembling axons and dendrites; these processes extended and reached other neurons

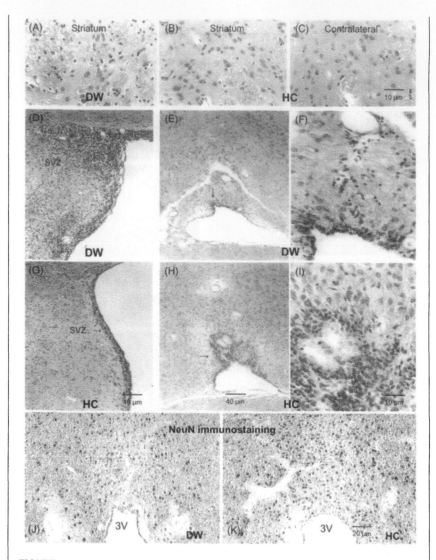

FIGURE 12.5 A few neurons appear in the edge of the striatal infarct in DW rat at day 28 after MCAo. (A). More neurons are seen in the border zone of the striatal infarct of HC rat; some spindle-like neurons is distributed along the boundary of the infarct (B). Neurons appear oval in shape in intact contralateral striatum of the HC rat (C). Cell proliferation exists in the SVZs of lateral ventricles ipsilateral to MCAo in DW and HC rats (D, G). Prominent cell proliferation is seen in the rostrum of 3rd ventricle in HC rat (H), but not in DW rat (E). The views of the regions (arrows) in panels E and H are magnified (F, I). NeuN-labeling shows some neurons existing in the rostrum in the adjacent section of the DW rat (J), numerous neurons in the same HC rat (K).

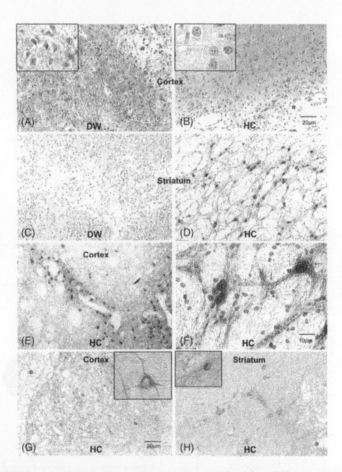

FIGURE 12.6 Neuronal injury in infarction at day 28 after 2-hour MCA occlusion. At day 28, in cortex, the peri-infarct zone of DW rat is fully filled by ghost neurons and inflammatory cells with no normal neurons (* indicates infarct) (A); while the extent of inflammation is apparently less and a high-density of neurons persist in this zone in the HC rat (B). The corners images are magnified views of the histological changes. NeuN immunoreactivity is absent in the infarct core in striatum (C) and in the inner boundary zone in cortex (not present) in DW rats. In HC rat, many NeuN+ neurons are observed in the injured region closed to cavity in striatum (D) and in the inner border zone of infarct in cortex (E). Clusters of neurons are gathered around and along the blood vessels from border toward the core (E). A magnified view of neurons in panel D is presented. The neurons have long processes morphologically resembling axons and dendrites (arrows) (F). βIII Tubulin (TUJ1) immunostaining is seen in the infarct next to the cavity in cortex (G) and striatum (H) of HC rats. The TUJ1+ neurons have shorter processes. The corner images are the magnified views of the immature neurons exhibiting TUJ1 in cytoplasm of soma and processes (* denotes infarct).

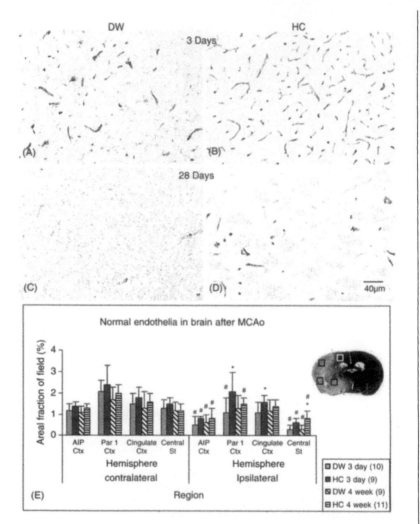

FIGURE 12.7 EBA immunoreactivity in cerebral microvessels after MCAo. Normal endothelia are detected in the ipsilateral parietal cortex part I in DW (A) and HC (B) rats at day 3; and in striatum, the center of infarct, on day 28 after MCAo in DW (C) and HC (D) rats. (E) The normal endothelia (NE) labeled by anti-EBA in the anatomic regions of interest (ROIs) marked by rectangles in the hemisphere ipsilateral to MCAo and the corresponding regions of the contralateral hemisphere in the diagram were quantitatively assessed. The area of each ROI is 0.27 mm^2. Amount of NE at day 3 in DW rats decreases in the ipsilateral agranular insular cortex (AIP), zone 1 of parietal cortex (Par 1), cingulate cortex, and striatum, compared to contralateral hemisphere. The amount of NE in Par 1 and cingulate cortex in HC group is significantly higher than DW rats. On day 28, NE was significantly increased in central striatum of HC rats. * indicates significant difference from corresponding value in DW groups at the same time (error bars denote SD; $p \leq 0.01$). # presents significant difference from contralateral hemispheres ($p < 0.05$).

in four HC rats (Figs. 12.6D and 12.6F); the long process is the sign of new mature neurons [61, 66]. The numbers of neuroblasts labeled by βIII Tubulin were 60 ± 50 (DW) vs. 140 ± 100 (HC) (sum of three bregma levels ~1.2, −1.3 and −3.8 mm; p = 0.02). The therapy prevented neuronal degeneration in the infarct. The study demonstrated that this nine-herb treatment successfully reduced the brain injury.

Endothelial injury was detected by endothelial barrier antigen (EBA) (Fig. 12.7). EBA-immunoreactivity is a reliable index of intact endothelial function (e.g., BBB intactness, recovery from inflammation or injury), and is performed in all of normal endothelia in rat brains except those in the choroid plexus. The absence of EBA-immunostaining is the sign of endothelial injury induced by ischemia, edema, and inflammation in the injured area and the adjacent zone in rat brain [18, 67, 68].

On day 3, more normal endothelia were observed in the infarcted hemisphere of the HC rats (Figs. 12.7B and 12.7D). The proportional area occupied by normal endothelia profiles in the field were 0.8 ± 0.4% (DW) vs. 1.5 ± 0.4% (HC) in the whole ipsilateral cortex, 1.0 ± 1.0 (DW) vs. 2.1 ± 1.0% (HC) in zone 1 of parietal cortex, and 1.1 ± 0.5 (DW) vs. 1.6 ± 0.3% (HC) in the cingulate cortex ($p ≤ 0.01$) at day 3, and 0.3 ± 0.02 % (DW) vs. 0.8 ± 0.4% (HC) in the central striatum (p = 0.001) at day 28. Normal endothelia increased in the infarct core in HC group at day 28. Quantitation of EBA immunoreactivity is shown in Fig. 12.7E. The treatment significantly protected endothelia.

At day 3, neuronal COX2 expression was scattered in cortical layers II and III in both groups. Massive peri-infarct neuronal COX2 overexpression was detected in the normal-appearance neurons and in the necrotic neurons in the penumbra, not in the core, in DW rats (Figs. 12.8A and 12.8C). Overexpression was not seen in HC rats (Figs. 12.8B and 12.8D). The treatment inhibited the early peri-infarct neuronal COX2 expression.

Quantitative counts of neutrophils labeled by MPO were 1343 ± 413 (DW) vs. 548 ± 252 (HC) ($p < 0.01$); macrophages marked by ED-1 were 7374 ± 1824 (DW) vs. 4485 ± 1487 (HC) ($p < 0.05$) in the lesioned hemisphere in bregma level ~−0.3 mm at day 3. The treatment inhibited inflammation inside the infarct and in the peri-infarct zone (Figs. 12.8E and 12.8F). The numbers of the two kinds of inflammatory cells were significantly decreased in the HC group. At day 28, numerous monocytes appeared inside the infarct in DW rats (Fig. 12.8G), but only a few monocytes were seen in HC rats (Fig. 12.8H).

Discussion

This study, for the first time, provides experimental support for the protective efficacy of the nine-herb formula in human infarcted brain by means of an animal model of focal ischemia with behavioral-histological studies. The daily treatment of the nine-herb combination, initiated at 2 hours after recirculation, reduced the infarct volume by 53–62% at days 3 and 28 respectively, compared to control groups. The treatment improved neurological deficits and protected endothelia, inhibited inflammation, decreased the risk of hemorrhage, prevented cavitation and alleviated infarct-periphery destruction in rat brains. Many normal neurons existed in the infarcts in all of the treated rats, and these neurons settled along and around the blood vessels in the peri-infarct inner zone while no normal neurons were seen in the infarcts in the nontreated rats at day 28. Many neurons

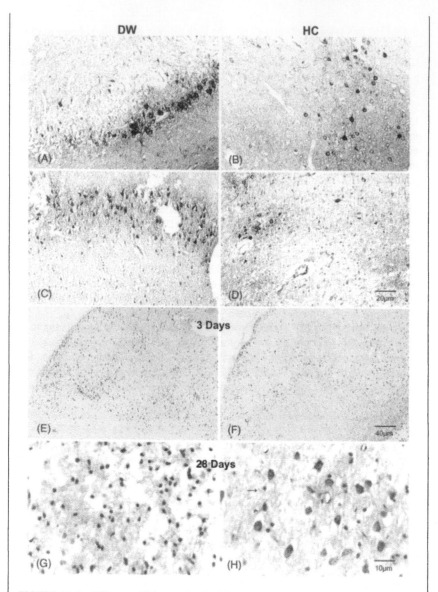

FIGURE 12.8 DW rats exhibit cytoplasmic COX2 overexpression in numerous normal-like neurons in the peri-infarct region (A) and in shrunken neurons in the penumbra (C) at day 3 after MCAo. HC rats display scattered COX2-positive neurons in the infarct periphery (B, D). Massive macrophage migration in cortical infarct is more prominent in DW rat (E) than in HC rat (F) at day 3. Inflammation in striatal infarct is characterized by intensive monocyte infiltration associated with neuronal disappearance in DW rat (G), whereas inflammation involves only a few monocytes (arrow), and many neurons are seen in HC rat (H) at day 28.

even formed long processes resembling axons which indicated they were newly matured. More neuroblasts, more normal blood vessels and less inflammation coexisted in the lesions at day 28 in treated rats.

Reactive oxygen species (ROS) markedly increase in the postischemic recirculation and inflammation; and antioxidants prevent ROS injuring the mitochondrial membrane of neurons and endothelia, thus, decreasing infarct volume [69,70]. Seven herbs in the formula are antioxidants. *Scutellaria* and its five flavonoids are the most powerful antioxidants [71–74]. *Ligusticum* via TMP reduces ROS formation in infarct [75]. *Angelica, Astragali, Carthamus, Paeonia veitchii* and *Paeonia suffruticosa* are strong antioxidants because they contain vitamin E, astragalus saponins, safflower yellow, paeoniflorin and PGG [44,53,76]. Thus, this therapy targets ROS to ameliorate ischemic injury.

Neuroprotection: *Scutellaria* and baicalein protect neurons from lethal damage in ischemia [71]. Five flavonoids of *Scutellaria* are 5- and 12-lipoxygenase (LO) inhibitors, and protect neuronal and mitochondrial membranes by effectively inhibiting lipid peroxidation [71, 73]. Baicalin [77], wogonin [78], TMP [75], paeonol [79] and *Angelica* [80] reduce infarct volume. Safflower yellow protects against neuronal degeneration caused by ischemia [53, 81, 82]. *Angelica sinensis* reduces apoptotic neurons by prohibiting protein BAX expression [80].

Our study shows that the treated rats had mature neurons and more newborn neurons inside the infarcts. Numerous studies have reported endogenous neurogenesis following brain ischemia. Newly generated neurons migrate into the severely damaged striatum and cortex at 1–6 weeks after MCAo [61, 63, 66]. Newborn neurons marked by βIII tubulin peak at day 21 [83], grow to have multiple processes [63, 66], and finally express NeuN to differentiate into mature neurons with formation of long processes at week 5 [61, 66]. However, detrimental inflammation and inadequate blood supply to the infarct core cause massive loss of neuroblasts [61]. Our results are similar to the information reported by these recent studies. The density of new matures and neuroblasts increased, vascularization improved and inflammation was mitigated inside the infarcted area simultaneously at day 28 in the treated rats, which indicates an adequate environment for survival and growth of neuroblasts.

Endothelial protection: The treatment protected endothelia, as evidenced by more normal endothelia in the penumbra at day 3 and in the core at day 28, coexisted with neuroprotection and ameliorated inflammation.

The nine-herb combination is able to protect endothelia because *Scutellaria* [84] and PGG [85] inhibit the expression of endothelial leukocyte adhesion molecule-1 (ELAM-1) and intercellular adhesion molecule-1 (ICAM-1) to suppress vascular inflammation. The cocktail therapy might prevent CBF decline owing to TMP, *Angelica* and *Carthamus* [44] antagonist platelet aggregation, inhibit synthesis of thromboxane A2 (TXA$_2$) and endothelin-1 (ET-1) to prevent vasoconstriction and dilate blood vessels. In addition, the combination of *Ligusticum, Angelica, Astragalas, Carthamus,* and *Prunus persica* encourages capillary angiogenesis via basic fibroblast growth factor (bFGF) [86, 87]. This is very important for patients because sprouting angiogenesis is involved in the brain recovery and the increase of neovascularization is correlated with longer survival of patients [88].

Broad anti-inflammatory effects: Necrotic tissue is liquefied by lytic enzymes released from leukocytes. Acute inflammation may be healed without consequences if inflammation mediators are no longer secreted [89]. COX2 is the key inflammation mediator and converts the released arachidonic acid (AA) to prostaglandins (PGs) [90]. Toxic PGs instigate tissue damage [70, 90]. Neuronal COX2 overexpression exhibits in the peri-infarct zone [64, 91]; and inhibiting COX2 expression reduces infarct volume [91]. Our treatment prevented the early neuronal COX2 overexpression in the peri-infarct zone. In the therapy, wogonin, oroxylin A, and PGG enable the inhibition of COX2 expression and PGs formation [52, 85].

The herbal cocktail possibly inhibited inflammation by: (1) protecting endothelia to reduce BBB disruption, (2) binding to inflammatory cytokines interleukin (IL)-1β, -6, and tumor necrosis factor-α (TNF-α) to abolish their function by baicalin and *Astragali* [92–94], (3) decreasing neutrophils migration into the lesions by TMP [75], and decreasing macrophages' immigration by wogonin [78], and paeonol [79], to reduce the tissue destruction and prevent cavitation in the infarct. Baicalein reduced the microglia-mediated neuronal degeneration [95].

A combination of six of the nine herbs and earthworm, *Buyang Huanwu* Tang, is for treating brain infarction after the acute stage in TCM. However, postischemic treatment with *Buyang Huanwu* decoction has not been reported to reduce infarct volume by animal experiments yet. In the present study, adding *Scutellaria, Paeonia suffruticosa,* and *Glycyrrhiza* to enhance inhibition of COX2 and inflammation alleviated infarction. Taken together, the nine-herb formula confers multiple salutary actions: neuroprotection, endothelia-protection, and inflammation inhibition.

In conclusion, the nine-herb treatment accelerated neurological functional recovery, reduced infarct volume, prevented cavitation and encouraged brain repair.

Experiment 2 (Global forebrain ischemia)

Materials and Method

Global Ischemia Production

Sixty-seven male Wistar rats weighing 256–405 g and aged 2.8 ± 0.6 months and 9 aged male Wistar rats weighing 478–567 g and aged 10 ± 2 months were subjected to 12.5-minute global forebrain ischemia produced by common carotid arteries occlusion plus systemic hypotension (40–50 mm Hg) following an overnight fast. Blood was withdrawn into a heparinized syringe to reduce the systemic blood pressure to 40–50 mm Hg. After 12.5-minute ischemia, the carotid ligatures were removed, and the warmed shed blood was re-infused to restore blood pressure to normal. The physiological monitoring was continued for 3 hours into the postischemic period. After the experiment finished, the wounds were infiltrated with 1% lidocaine. Rats were placed in cages at room temperature with free access to water and food. Sham rats received similar surgery but not ischemia [36].

Medicine Treatment

Rats in the treated groups received the herbal cocktail (HC) decoction throughout survival. Gavage was used to daily administer the decoction 6 ml/day in 2 divided doses, began at 4 hours after reperfusion. Nontreated rats received vehicle, drinkable water (DW). Rats were allowed to survive for 3, 7, 28 and 56 days. Sham rats had drinkable water.

Behavioral Test

Rats were trained to walk on the 1.5 cm wide, 95 cm long beam at 62 cm high to assess the rats' ability to maintain balance during walking before the surgery. While arriving at traverse without slips, time to traverse was recorded with stopwatch. The test detects the deficits of coordination and integration of motor movement.

Histopathological Studies

The 10-µm sections at bregma levels ∼−0.2, −3.3, and −4.8 mm were stained with hematoxylin and eosin (H&E) to determine ischemic injury, displaying necrotic neurons, or processed for immunohistochemical studies. Expression of the targeted proteins was visualized by routine immunoperoxidase techniques. Adjacent sections were stained by H&E and were reacted for the histochemical visualization of active microglia with BS-I isolectin B4. Primary antibodies for immunocytochemical visualization were: anti-GFAP for activated astrocytes, anti-COX2 for COX2, and ED-1 for macrophage.

The striatum and hippocampus were examined in a blind manner. Cell counts of normal neurons, necrotic neurons, $COX2^+$ neurons, lectin$^+$ microglia and macrophages were carried out in a standardized, consistently located high-power microscopic field in the dorsolateral striatum and central striatum (bregma −0.2 mm), and in the pyramidal cell layer of the hippocampal CA1 sector (bregma −3.3 mm). Both hemispheres were counted and the results were averaged. Cell counting in striatum was counted at ×400; cell counting in the hippocampus was performed at ×100. Normal neurons were defined as those having normal properties, nucleus and nucleolus.

Results

Physiological Variables: Preischemic physiological variables were in the normal range in all groups, and no significant inter-group differences existed (Table 12.2).

All animals gained weight over the chronic survival period and all treated rats had white shining hairs while nontreated rats showed brown-yellow rough hairs on the back at day 56.

Behavioral analysis: Time to traverse the beam at day 56 by the rats were 12 ± 5.9 (DW group, $n = 7$) vs. 4.4 ± 1.6 (HC, $n = 6$) seconds ($p < 0.01$), 5.2 ± 0.86 seconds in sham rats ($n = 4$). The nine-herb therapy encouraged rats' coordination performance and neurological function recovery.

Neuronal Histopathology

Striatum: All of the rats showed mild ischemic changes in the dorsolateral striatum and several rats had mild damage in the central striatum at days 3–7. The necrotic injury disappeared at days 28 and 56. Quantitative cell counting revealed that necrotic neurons in dorsolateral striatum were 56 ± 27 (DW, $n = 10$) via 20 ± 17 (HC, $n = 12$) per field ($p = 0.0001$) at day 3, and more normal neurons in dorsolateral striatum in HC groups days 3–56 (Fig. 12.9). Aged rats sustained severe histopathological change and more neuronal loss in striatum. The injury was much severer and extended into central striatum. H&E staining revealed these zones were demarcated and pale. GFAP staining showed large numbers of reactive

TABLE 12.2 Physiological Variables in Rats Subjected to Global Brain Ischemia (values are mean ± SD)

Group	n	Weight (g)	Age (month)	MABP (mm Hg)	pH unit	pCO$_2$ (mm Hg)	pO$_2$ (mm Hg)	Glucose (mg/dl)
3 Day								
DW	10	365±10	3.4±0.4	127±12	7.390±.04	41±3	124±24	160±17
HC	12	337±31	3.2±0.5	128±11	7.395±.03	39±4	136±30	143±29
7 Day								
DW	8	322±49	3.0±0.4	125±11	7.374±.04	41±4	148±29	145±15
HC	7	308±24	2.9±0.3	125±14	7.406±.05	39±3	140±35	152±22
4 Week								
DW	6	288±29	2.7±0.2	133±12	7.374±.04	40±4	145±18	144±24
HC	6	271±25	2.5±0.1	132±8	7.400±.03	39±4	141±31	151±25
8 Week								
DW	7	319±46	2.7±0.5	129±10	7.428±.08	38±3	126±17	139±23
HC	6	324±17	3.1±0.5	133±10	7.391±.05	40±4	137±19	141±25
Sham	5	304±23	2.7±0.4	137±11	7.395±.05	40±4	157±16	142±14
Aged								
DW	5	522±35	10±1.3	134±9	7.441±.04	39±4	109±2	141±17
HC	4	527±19	10±1.6	136±6	7.470±.01	37±2	127±16	143±31

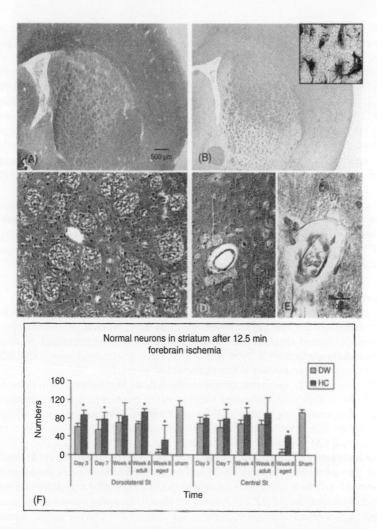

FIGURE 12.9   Sections of striata in DW rats studied 8 weeks following 12.5 minutes of forebrain ischemia. Sections stained with H&E (A, C–E) and GFAP (B). Discrete striatal lesion characterized by pallor on H&E stain (A) and associated with GFAP immunoreactivity (B). Up-corner image magnified the view of the striatum processes. Severe and evident spongy changes present in striata (C, D) and next to enlarged perivascular space (D). Thrombus associated with enlarged perivascular space is noticed in striatum (E). Numbers of normal neurons in striatum (St) in HC groups are higher than DW groups at days 3–56 following ischemia ($p < 0.05$) (F).

astrocytes in these foci. Normal neurons in the 5 aged DW rats had almost disappeared. However, the HC group had fivefold normal neurons compared to the DW group. The large incomplete infarcts presented in 10 of 10 striata of the aged DW rats at day 56 (Figs. 12.9A and 12.9B), and 2 of 8 striata in the HC group had small infarcts. Sponginess in striatum was present at day 56: severe or moderate sponginess in five adult DW rats, and mild spongy damage in one HC rat (Figs. 12.9C and 12.9D).

Hippocampal CA1: Numbers of normal CA1 pyramidal neurons significantly reduced at days 3–56; micro-infarction was seen in CA1 at day 56 (Figs. 12.10 and 12.11). At days 7–56, the numbers of normal CA1 neurons of treated groups were 3–4-fold of the nontreated groups. Associated with this neuronal loss were the massive increase of neuronal COX2 protein expression, the increase of reactive microglia and macrophages in CA1 at day 3. The therapy significantly decreased the neuronal necrosis, inhibited the neuronal COX2 expression and reduced the inflammation in the hippocampus CA1 sector at day 3 (Figs. 12.10G and 12.10H).

Significantly apoptotic neurons were seen in the brains including midbrain at day 56. The numbers of apoptotic neurons of cortex (sum in the three standard levels) were 62 ± 44 (HC, $n = 6$) and 213 ± 140 (DW, 7) at day 56 ($p < 0.05$), 89 ± 44 in sham group ($n = 5$). These data indicate that the nine-herb therapy reduced neuronal necrosis and prevented neurodegeneration.

Discussion

This present study reported, for the first time, that the postischemic daily cocktail treatment of the specific nine-herb up to 56 days, initiated at 4 hours after ischemia, protected striatum and hippocàmpal CA1 from the acute and delayed injury including infarction in 3–56 days. The therapy ameliorated neuronal COX2 expression and inflammation in hippocampal CA1 at day 3.

The present study found that severe neuronal death in striatum and in hippocampal CA1 at days 3–56 associated with macro- or micro-infarction and sponginess in the brain at day 56 after 12.5-minute transient forebrain ischemia, which is consistent with previous study [36]; increase of neuronal COX2 expression in hippocampal CA1 at day 3 are similar to other reports [96, 97].

Antioxidants and other protection: Seven herbs in the treatment are antioxidants, thus were able to scavenge ROS and reduce ROS production in the present experiment. *Scutellaria baicalensis* is defined as the most powerful antioxidant owing to its five compounds [71, 72, 74]. *Angelica, Carthamus, Astragalas, Paeonia veitchii,* and *Paeonia suffruticosa* are strong antioxidants via vitamin E, safflower yellow, astragalus saponins, paeoniflorin and PGG [44, 53, 76]. Therefore, this therapy could target ROS to ameliorate neuronal peroxidation to reduce necrosis in the study. The five compounds of *Scutellaria baicalensis* are 5- and 12-LO inhibitors and protect cellular and mitochondrial membranes by effectively inhibiting neuronal lipid peroxidation to protect neurons [71, 72]; paeoniflorin and PGG protect neurons via heme oxygenase-1 induction [76]; paeoniflorin blocks the sodium current influxes into neurons after ischemia [98].

Neuronal death and COX2 expression in hippocampus CA1: Neuronal death of CA1 is delayed, does not appear in the first 24 hours after ischemia in both humans [99] and animals [100]. COX2 is critical to the delayed neuronal death [96, 101]. COX2 activity has been considered one of mechanisms of the neuronal injury in CA1 following the ischemia [96, 97].

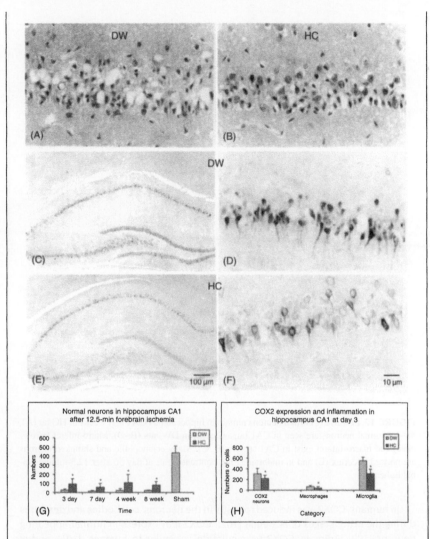

FIGURE 12.10 Neuropathological changes in hippocampus CA1 3 days following ischemia. Significant reduction of normal CA1 neurons, H&E stained (A, B), and COX2 expression (C–F) are present in hippocampus. Almost all of the normal neurons in CA1 disappear in DW rats (A) while numerous normal neurons remaining in HC rats (B). Nontreated-ischemic brain shows dense COX2 immunostaining in cell layers of CA1 sector (C), and high-intensity cytoplasmic immunoreactivity within widespread shrunken neurons' soma and axons (D); the treated brain displays lower COX2 immunostaining in CA1 (E), and low-density COX2 immunoreactivity is seen in apparently normal neurons and shrunken neurons of CA1 (F). The therapy reduces the neuronal death, COX2 expression and inflammation in CA1 ($p < 0.05$) (G, H).

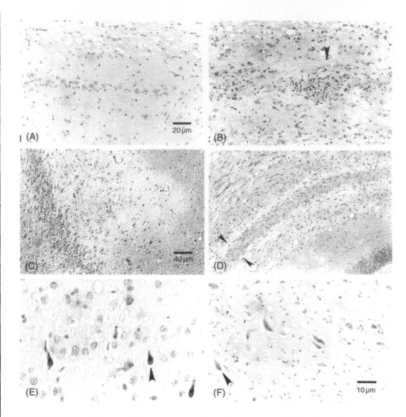

FIGURE 12.11   Many normal neurons remain in hippocampus CA1 at 8 weeks in HC rat (A), but no normal neurons are seen in CA1 (arrowheads) in DW rats (B–D). Micro-infarct (arrowhead) and macro-infarct exist in CA1 sectors (B, C). Many eosinophilic and shrunken neurons are noticed in cortex (E) and in midbrain (F) in nontreated rats at day 56 after 12.5-minute global ischemia.

In humans, COX2 was induced robustly in the neurons' cell bodies and dendrites during the acute stages of ischemia [102]. COX2 may express in normal-appearing neurons [102]. Animals' COX2 up-regulation is similar to humans' [101], and is rapidly induced in the neurons of hippocampal CA1 [97, 101, 102]. Our study is consistent with the previous studies.

Stress leads TNF-α releasing to activate nuclear factor NF-kappa B (NF-κB) to result in COX2 induction to cause the great portion of neuronal damage [103]. The enzyme COX2 converts the released AA from ischemia to PGs, including TXA$_2$ [101, 102]. COX2 leads to tissue damage through ROS and PGE2 to mediate lipid peroxidation [104]. Inhibiting COX2 expression ameliorates the neuronal death in CA1 [96].

Scutellaria baicalensis [105], oroxylin A [106] and paeoniflorin [98] protect neurons in CA1 after global ischemia. Wogonin and oroxylin A block NF-κB activation to prevent COX2 expression |52, 106, 107|. PGG inhibits COX2 activity |109|; astragalus saponins inhibit PGE2 production |92|. Therefore, the therapy is able to protect neurons and inhibit COX2 expression in CA1.

Inflammatory inhibition might ameliorate ischemic injury in the present study. Wogonin |108| and baicalein |95| are neuroprotective via inhibiting inflammatory activation of microglia. Astragalus saponins |92|, wogonin |107|, and baicalin |94| bind to inflammatory cytokines IL-1β, -6 and TNF-α to inhibit inflammation.

This study substantiated that herbal therapy attenuated the neuronal apoptosis during the chronic stage. TMP, ferulic acid in *Angelica*, and *Carthamus* protect against neuronal degeneration caused by ischemia |53, 98|.

Platelet aggregation and activity contribute to ischemic injury: The fact that occasional nontreated animals showed a delayed appearance of focal ischemic pathology at week 8 in our study, suggests that a delayed secondary insult occurred. Vascular damage associated with thrombosis and infarction was noticed. These phenomena are consistent with our previous report. Platelet aggregation and thrombosis are found in large- and micro-vessels associated with infarction in the brain for 4–10 weeks after transient forebrain ischemia |36|. Platelet aggregation exists in the brain for 1 year and is more widespread in the basal ganglia and hippocampus |41|. Platelets and leukocytes accumulated in micro-vessel branches or vessel bifurcations which are correlated with BBB alterations |36, 41|. Thus, platelet aggregation and accumulation are one of the major causes which induce the chronic injury.

We did not find a right antibody to detect the platelets with immunostaining in rat brain. However, the therapy has the ability to inhibit platelet aggregation because PGG |109|, TMP |110, 111|, *Angelica sinensis*, *Carthamus* |44| antagonist platelet aggregation. In addition, *Scutellaria* |84| and PGG |109| inhibit the expression of ELAM-1 and ICAM-1 to suppress vascular coagulation.

Preischemic treatment of *Buyang Huanwu* decoction for 7 days has been reported to ameliorate neuronal death in hippocampal CA1 at days 3–7 after global ischemia |45|. Efficacy of its postischemic treatment has not been reported yet. In the present study, adding *Scutellaria*, *Paeonia suffruticosa*, and *Glycyrrhiza* to enhance the inhibiting COX2 expression and inflammation leads to a strong neuroprotection, even the treatment started 4 hours after ischemia.

The neuropathological changes following both focal and forebrain ischemia in rats are comparable to the humans. Oral administration of the nine-herb decoction provides neuroprotection in both focal and global cerebral ischemia, and inhibiting neuronal COX2 activity involved in the protection. However, much information is still not available or understood. Phytochemistry is only beginning to reveal the herbal components, functions and the synergistic effects because Phytomedicine has largely been abandoned in the USA in the last century.

Shengmai San (生脉散 *or* 生脉饮)

Shengmai San consists of *Panax ginseng* (*Ginseng*), *Ohiopogon japonicus* (*Mai Don*), and *Fructus schisandra chineses* (*Wu Wei Zi*). This formula has been applied to acute myocardiac infarction associated with shock in the clinic in China. This therapy was reported to elevate the blood pressure, and improve the blood microcirculation and cardiac function in 829 cases [112]. If blood pressure is maintained at 60 mm Hg during resuscitation, brain injury significantly decreases in patients [113]. Recently, *Shengmai San* was reported to prevent the progression of injury in brain infarction by animal experimental study [114–116]. The mechanism is not clear. The combination of *Fructus Schisandra chineses* and *Ginseng* has been found beneficial in memory consolidation of humans [44]. *Ginseng* extract is effective in inhibiting the increase in capillary permeability, reducing inflammation, and improves healing of wounds [44]. *Ginsenoside Rb*$_1$ effectively prevents the delayed neuronal death, stabilizes the mitochondrial structure in hippocampal neurons, and reduces the degenerative process of aging [44].

Herbs

The principle to treat ischemia is to promote blood circulation plus anti-inflammation in the acute stage, for instance, adding the anti-inflammatory agent *Scutellaria baicalensis* to the treatment to inhibit and clean the inflammation if the patient has fever and adding the herbs which depress *liver Yang* as well as increase *kidney Yin* to the formula to rebuild *Yin-Yang* balance at the chronic stage. The herbs listed below are neuroprotectant, antioxidant, anti-inflammatory agents, and anti-coagulant.

Improve Blood Circulation

Sprouting angiogenesis is involved in brain recovery in humans after stroke; an increase of neovascularization is correlated with longer survival of the patients [88]. Five herbs, including *Ligusticum wallichii* (*Chuan Xiong*), *Angelica sinensis* (*Dang Gui*), *Radix Astragali membranaceus* (*Huang Qi*), *Carthamus tinctorius* (*Hong Hua*) that is saffron, and seed of *Prunus persica*, that is peaches (*Tao Ren*) are the core to treat ischemia and routinely used in TCM.

Ligusticum wallichii (川芎, Chuan Xiong)

The root of *Ligusticum wallichii* is the part used for medicine. Dosage: dried crude herb 3–9 g day/adult patient. Nontoxic; LD_{50} is 65.9 ± 31.3 g/kg. Alkaloids tetramethylpyrazine (TMP) is the main active principle [44, 117]. It also contains ferulic acid [44]. *Ligusticum wallichii* protects endothelial cells against reperfusion injury, improves the microcirculation [118], promotes blood flow and removes blood stasis [44] as well as prevents proliferation of vascular smooth muscle cells [46, 119]. *Ligusticum* and TMP have been used in treatment of ischemic stroke and angina pectoris in China since the 1960s. TMP has been used to work in three ways: as *antithrombotic agent, antagonist of vasoconstriction, and anti-inflammatory compound.*

TMP reduces the infarct volume via scavenging free radicals and prohibiting neutrophil migration [75]. It releases the vascular resistance to abolish coronary vasoconstriction and increase blood circulation by reducing plasma endothelin-1 (ET-1) levels during and after acute ischemia [120, 121] and by inhibiting platelet aggregation and decreasing the synthesis of ET-1 and TXA_2 in endothelia [44, 122, 123]. Inhibiting ET-1 production from endothelia [122] lowers the vascular resistance and increases CBF [44, 120, 121, 124].

TMP has antithrombotic effects [110] by inhibiting platelet activity in humans [111, 120, 125]. In addition, TMP is an inflammatory inhibitor [75], antioxidant [126], and calcium antagonist [127]. TMP readily crosses the BBB and is evenly distributed throughout the intact rat brain in 20 minutes after oral administration [55, 56]. LD_{50} of TMP is 239 mg/kg i.v. [44]. In addition, ferulic acid also inhibits inflammation after ischemia [128].

Angelica sinensis (当归, Dang Gui)

The root is the medical part of the plant and contains significant quantities of vitamin B12 and E, folic acid, biotin, ferulic acid, succinic acid, nicotinic acid, uracil, adenine, and ligustilide [44]. Dosage: 6–15 g/day/adult. Nontoxic; no LD_{50}. It dilates coronal arteries and increases coronal blood flow [42, 44]. The water-extract of *Angelica sinensis* markedly inhibits platelet action to decrease 5-HT release and TXA_2 and ET-1 formation, reduces myocardial injury from ischemia, lowers blood cholesterol and reduces atherosclerosis formation [44]. *Angelica sinensis* decreases the infarct volume in brain and reduces neuronal apoptosis after brain ischemia via prohibiting protein BAX expression after MCAo [80]. *Angelica* protects human's vascular endothelia [129], and relaxes arteries [130]. Vitamin E is a major endogenous antioxidant and an inhibitor of intracellular phospholipases A2 (PLA2) [131–133]. In addition, *Angelica sinensis* stimulates hematopoiesis in bone marrow because of its high vitamin B12 content (0.25–0.4 µg/100 g dried root) as well as the content of folic acid and biotin [44].

Astragalas membranaceus (黄芪, Huang Qi)

The root of *Astragalas* is the medical portion and called as *Radix Astragali*. Dosage: 10–15 g/day/adult. Nontoxic; LD_{50} is tested and none. The active principles are astragalus saponins, flavonoids, and polysaccharide [44, 134].

Water extract of *Astragali* dilates coronal arteries [42]. *Astragali Radix* promotes DNA synthesis, inhibits platelet aggregation [44] and protects neurons from anoxic damage [135]. *Astragali* has a broad anti-inflammatory effect since *Astragalus saponins* strongly inhibit production of IL-6 and PGE2, and block the effect of IL-1β [92], decrease the formation of TNF-α and scavenge free radicals [93]. It inhibits fibrosis progression via decrease of transforming growth factor β1 (TGF-β1) [93]. While *Astragali radix* works together with *Angelica*, estrogenic and anti-platelet aggregation activities are inserted [136], and good angiogenesis of capillaries is enhanced [87].

Astragalus saponins are antioxidant to scavenge free-radicals [134], and promote DNA synthesis [44]. Astragaloside IV upregulates t-PA expression in human endothelia after ischemia [137], thus it is a fibrinolytic potential agent.

Carthamus tinctorius (红花, Hong Hua)

Saffron flower's stigma is the working part of *Carthamus tinctorius*, saffron. Dosage: 3–9 g/day/adult. Nontoxic; LD_{50} is tested and saffron flower's stigma has no LD_{50}. The principle active component is safflower yellow [124, 137]. *Carthamus tinctorius* is a strong antioxidant and a potent Ca^{2+} channel antagonist [44, 124, 137]. The water extract of *Carthamus tinctorius* dilates arteries to increase the cells' tolerance to oxygen deprivation and lower blood pressure, inhibits platelet aggregation and prevents blood coagulation [44, 124]. It protects against neuronal degeneration caused by ischemia [42, 53, 81, 82], and alleviates retinal ischemic damage [82]. It lowers plasma cholesterol and triglyceride level [44]. In China it is used to treat cerebral thrombosis and angina pectoris to increase the coronary circulation [44]. Safflower yellow protects against neuronal degeneration caused by ischemia *in vivo* [53].

Prunus persica (桃仁, Tao Ren)

The kernel in the seed is believed to be the most powerful herb in improving circulation and maintaining the endothelial integrity, although its exact mechanism of action is still unknown. Dosage: 6–9 g/day/adult. Nontoxic; LD_{50}: 222.5 ± 7.5 g/kg. It inhibits platelet aggregation and coagulation, dilates blood vessels, increases cerebral blood flow (CBF), decreases capillary permeability and inhibits inflammation while orally administered [46]. However, *Prunus persica* is active only by oral administration. *Prunus persica* contains vitamin B1 [46] and a lot of oil to solve constipation [42]. Overdosage can cause cyanide intoxication [42].

These five herbs: *Astragali*, *angelica*, *Ligusticum*, *Carthamus tinctorius*, and *Prunus persica*, are the most important components of the common formula used to treat brain ischemia by inhibiting platelet activity, preventing thrombosis, dilating and protecting blood vessels, and maintaining BBB integrity [42, 46]. They promote circulation by inhibiting blood aggregation, maintaining vascular integrity, vasodilatation and encouraging self-healing. The combination of these five herbs works more favorably and effectively than any single one of them [42, 134, 138, 139], and encourages angiogenesis [86, 87].

Cinnamomum cassia (桂枝, Gui Zhi)

The twig is the medical portion in the plant. Dosage: 3–10 g/day/adult. Nontoxic; LD_{50} is not available. The ingredients are cinnamic aldehyde and cinnamyl acetate. *Cinnamomum cassia* has antioxidant [140], antibacterial, and vasodilatation functions [42, 44]. Working together with *Prunus persica* and *Paeonia suffruticosa* will get a better effect. Attention: Do not give *Cinnamomum cassia* to patients who have fever.

Ginseng (人参)

Ginseng is the root of *Panax ginseng* C.A. Mey. Dosage: 3–9 g/day/adult. Nontoxic; LD_{50}: 5 g/kg. It is the most valued herb and widely used in China, Korea, and Japan, and among the overseas Chinese in the United States. For thousands of years, ginseng has been used by the common people as a tonic and in emergency medicine to rescue dying patients, and by the rich and emperors as a revitalizing agent. Ginseng contains multiple active elements. The research on Ginseng started in the early 19th century. Some of its chemical structures have been well studied and recognized, but many are not yet fully understood. Its component saponins, that is ginsenosides are the principles. It contains maltol, salicylic and vanillic acid, three antioxidants, and vitamins. Extract of ginseng lowers serum cholesterol levels and prevents atherosclerosis [44].

Ginsenosides increase learning performance, improve memory and movement activity, increase protein in the brain, stabilize the membrane structure of mitochondria of neurons in the hippocampus, reduce the degeneration of aging, and prevent delayed neuronal death. Ginsenosides enhance the biosynthesis of DNA and protein in the brain, bone marrow, testis, and increase sex hormone production. Such increase in biosynthesis of DNA and protein exert some indirect action in prolonging cell life [44]. Ginsenosides increase the synthesis of high-density lipids (HDL) in serum [44]. Rb_1, one of ginsenosides, is the principle for neuroprotective action [42, 44]. Rb_1 effectively prevents delayed neuronal death, and reduces the degenerative process of aging [44]. However, ginseng should not give to patients who have high fever or hypertension.

Fructus *Crataegus pinnatifida* (山楂, Shan Zha, Haw Fruit)

It is the dried fruit of *Crataegus pinnatifida*, nontoxic and sold on street corners as a popular snack food in North China. Dosage: 10–15 g/day/adult. Nontoxic; LD_{50}: 33.8 ml/kg of 10% water extract. The active principles are chlorogenic acid, caffeic acid, citric acid, crataegolic acid, maslinic acid, ursolic acid, and some saponins. The herb lowers blood cholesterol by increasing cholesterol's catabolism to help the surface of the atherosclerotic area in the arterial wall to shrink and become smoother. It increases myocardial contractility, and promotes coronary circulation via increase of blood flow. This reduces the oxygen consumption and protects against myocardiac ischemia. In addition, it is very good to help in digesting meat [42, 44].

Ginkgo biloba (银杏叶, Yin Xing Ye)

The leaf of *Ginkgo biloba* has been used for circulatory disorders to increase peripheral and cerebral blood follow for decades. Nontoxic; LD_{50}: 7725 mg. Leaf of *Ginkgo biloba* has several flavone glucosides, including ginkgolide

A and B, and bilobalide. It improves the contractile function of the ischemic heart, exerts a protective effect on myocardium and increase cerebral blood flow in animals. *Ginkgo* extract showed neuroprotection on hippocampus neurons [44].

Inflammation Antagonists

Scutellaria baicalensis (黄芩, Huang Qin)

The root of *Scutellaria baicalensis* is used as medicine. Dosage: 3–9 g/day/adult. Nontoxic; LD_{50} is tested, none. *Scutellaria baicalensis* is a very well-known anti-inflammatory agent widely used in oriental medicine. *Scutellaria* is multi-functional: antioxidant, anti-inflammatory, and antithrombic agent, as well as neuroprotectant according to recent studies. *Baicalin, baicalein, wogonin, oroxylin A*, and *Skullcapflavone II* are the active compounds: strong antioxidants, lipoxygenase inhibitors, anti-inflammatory, and anti-coagulation agents [44, 74, 106, 141, 142]. Baicalein and baicalin decrease blood cholesterol [124].

Scutellaria is defined as the most powerful antioxidant owing to these five compounds [71, 72, 143–146]. It protects neurons in CA1 *in vivo* [71, 105] and *in vitro* [71, 72, 145] from lethal oxidant damage in ischemia/reperfusion. Baicalin and baicalein directly scavenge and quench superoxide, hydrogen peroxide, and hydroxyl radicals [71, 73, 147], and inhibit hydroxyl radical production to protect cellular and mitochondrial membranes [71, 73, 144, 147–149]. Baicalin improves the cellular repair potential of oxidatively damaged DNA [150].

These five flavonoids are 5- and 12-lipoxygenase (LO) inhibitors [72, 142] to protect neuronal and mitochondrial membranes by effectively inhibiting lipid peroxidation [71, 73, 144, 147, 149]. In addition, baicalin and baicalein inhibit $(Ca^{2+})_i$ elevations [151] to protect neurons from ischemia [71–73, 95, 144, 147], and prevent neurotoxicity induced by glutamate [152]. Wogonin protects neurons from lethal damage in ischemia/reperfusion [152, 153] and decreases the infarct volume [78].

Scutellaria has strong anti-inflammatory actions [94, 154]. It is used in the acute stage of ischemia if patients have fever and acts powerfully against bacteria to treat infection in the respiratory system. Baicalin, baicalein, and wogonin are strong inflammation inhibitor [154].

Wogonin inhibits COX2 expression, and reduces synthesis of PGE2 by retarding arachidonic acid release following ischemia [52, 106, 149, 151] and blocking nuclear NF-kB activation [52, 106, 107, 155]. Wogonin markedly reduces the microglia activation and macrophages in the infarct [78]. Baicalin binds inflammatory cytokines IL-1β, -6, and TNF-α to limit their biological functions and inhibits their production [44, 94, 105]. Baicalein and baicalin inhibit fibrillation and disaggregate the existing fibrils in the brain [156].

Scutellaria baicalensis protects vascular endothelia and prevents thrombotic tendencies by inhibiting TXA_2 release to inhibit arterial vasoconstriction [157], preventing platelet aggregation [151, 158], decreasing expression of ELAM-1 and ICAM-1 [84, 159], reducing $[Ca^{2+}]$ elevation [160], and pre-venting the decrease of t-PA production [161]. Part of cerebral $A\beta$ deposition is released from platelets in humans [34, 35]. Baicalein and baicalin inhibit COX2/LO from human platelets [142] and protect neurons from $A\beta$ toxicity-induced apoptosis [162, 163].

Scutellaria is nontoxic when given orally and absorbed fast by the gastroin-testinal tract [44, 47, 54]. The amount of baicalin in *Scutellaria* is 10-fold of baicalein; baicalin is metabolized into baicalein in human body [57] and by bacteria prior to intestinal absorption and subsequently metabolized into bai-calein [49]. Baicalein, baicalin, and wogonin, the aqueous extracts are absorbed immediately, onset action quickly, and provide longer and higher efficacy by oral administration [47, 57, 164]. Baicalin rapidly appears in plasma and exists for 24 hours [47], and enter brain parenchyma: cortex, hippocampus, striatum, thalamus, and brain stem [77, 165]. Baicalein crosses BBB quickly and evenly distribute in intact rat brain in 20 minutes [44, 54].

Paeonia veitchii (赤芍, Chi Shao) and Paeonia suffruticosa (牡丹皮, Mu Dan Pi)

The roots of *Paeonia veitchii* and the bark of rhizome of *Paeonia suffruticosa* are the portion for medicine. Dosages: 6–12 g/day/adult. Nontoxic; LD_{50}: none for *Paeonia veitchii*, 3.43 g/kg for *Paeonia suffruticosa*. They are important agents to decrease inflammation and reduce capillary permeability to inhibit tis-sue swelling in TCM. *Paeonia veitchii* and *Paeonia suffruticosa* have paeonol, paeonoside, paeoniflorin, and PGG as the active compounds [44, 76, 124].

Both *Paeonia veitchii* and *Paeonia suffruticosa* inhibit COX2 activities and inflammation [109], prevent fibrosis [44, 124], and are antioxidant [140] to protect neurons from ROS-mediated death [76]. In addition, *Paeonia veitchii* increases endothelium-dependent relaxation, and *Paeonia suffruticosa* antag-onizes platelet aggregation, thus inhibiting TXA_2 production [166]. They are absorbed quickly from the gastrointestinal tract [51, 167].

Paeonol reduces cerebral infarction via scavenging superoxide anion and inhibiting activated microglia and macrophages in the infarct [79]. Paeoniflorin and PGG reduce capillary permeability [44]. Paeoniflorin and PGG pro-tect neurons by induction of heme oxygenase-1 (HO-1) and scavenging free radicals against ischemic stress [76]. Blocking Na^+ channels is considered as a target for protecting brain damage. Paeoniflorin blocks sodium channels in hippocampal neurons to prevent sodium current into neurons after ischemia [98], and upregulates heat shock protein (HSP) expression, the lifeguard against proteotoxic stresses, to protect neurons [168]. PGG inhibits COX2 activity [109], prevents NF-κB translocation induced by TNF-α in human endothelia, and suppresses ELAM-1 and ICAM-1 expression to inhibit vas-cular inflammation [85]. PGG inhibits platelet aggregation and the synthesis of TXA_2 and ET-1 to prevent vasoconstriction and dilate blood vessels, thus, PGG is a vasorelaxant [85].

Glycyrrhiza uralensis (甘草, Gan Cao)

Its root is used to treat diseases. Dosage: 3–6 g/day/adult. Nontoxic; LD_{50}: none. The major active compounds are glycyrrhizin, flavonoid licorice, and ferulic acid [169]. *Glycyrrhiza* is an antioxidant [140] and enhances the absorption of the constituents of *Scutellaria baicalensis*, *Paeonia veitchii*, and *Paeonia suffruticosa* to lead to a higher bioavailability of baicalin in the body [50, 51, 164]. Glycyrrhizin is an antioxidant and inflammatory inhibitor [44, 169]. Licorice reduces capillary permeability [44]. Since gycyrrhizin is about 170% sweeter than cane sugar, glycyrrhiza is the principal adjuvant in formulae [44].

Anemarrhena asphodeloides Bunge (知母, Zhi Mu)

The medical part is the rhizome. Dosage: 3–15 g/day/adult. Nontoxic; LD_{50} is not available. Recent studies reported that *Anemarrhena asphodeloides* decreases the infarct volume through inhibiting neutrophils migrating into injured brain cortex in the early stage after ischemia [170]. Its active principle timosaponin lowers blood sugar by increasing the metabolism of glucose and increasing glycogen synthesis in the liver, and inhibits platelet aggregation [44, 124].

Decrease liver Yang

Gastrodia elat Blume (天麻, Tian Ma)

The rhizome is used to subdue "exuberant *Yang*" in *liver*, to calm internal *wind* and relieve convulsions and fainting [44]. Dosage: 3–9 g/day/adult. Nontoxic; LD_{50} is not available. Its active principles are gastrodin, vanillyl alcohol, and vanillin. This herb has analgesic, anticonvulsive and sedative effects, increases coronary and cerebral blood flow, and lowers peripheral blood pressure [44, 46]. It relieves convulsion, treats hypertension, dizziness, and headache. Recent studies found it protects neurons in brain ischemia [171, 172].

Enhance Yin in liver and kidney

Lycium barbarum (枸杞子, Gou Qi Zi)

The red color fruit of *Lycium barbarum* is the medical part. Dosage: 9–15 g/day/adult. Nontoxic; LD_{50} is not available. Its water extract significantly increases nonspecific immunity, lowers blood pressure, plasma cholesterol and glucose, improves visual acuity, protects liver function, encourages generation of liver cell. It increases blood 17-ketosteroids in old men [42, 44, 169]. Lycium polysaccharides reduce the fragmentation of DNA and inhibit apoptosis [44].

Tonics for kidney Yang

Epimedium brevicorum Maxim (淫羊藿, Yin Yang Huo)

The whole plant is used for the medicine. Dosage: 10–15 g/day/adult. Nontoxic; LD_{50} is not available. The active principles are 28 flavonoids, including icariin, noricariin, and Vitamin E [42]. Extract of *Epimedium brevicorum* increases the sperm production and 17-ketosteroids excretion [44], lowers blood pressure and decreases blood sugar [42], increases the activity of immune system [44, 169] and enhances the synthesis of DNA and protein [169]. Icariin protect neurons in cerebral ischemia [173].

Ophiopogon japonicus (麦冬, Mai Dong)

The root is the medical part. Dosage: 6–15 g/day/adult. Nontoxic; LD_{50} is not available. The principles include β-sitosterol, stigmasterol, and ophiopogonin B. *Ophiopogon* increases coronary blood flow, myocardial contractility, and slowly elevates blood pressure [44].

Fructus Schisandra chinesis (五味子, Wu Wei Zi)

The fruit of *Schisandra chinesis* (*Wu Wei Zi*) is the medical part. Dosage: 3–9 g/day/adult. Nontoxic; LD_{50}: 5 g/kg in mice does not induce mortality. *Fructus Schisandra chinesis* can improve mental function, and the aqueous extract increases myocardial contractility [44].

Phytochemicals which protect plants against dangers and illness may save humans' lives; antioxidants in plants function as antioxidants in humans [174]. All of the herbal dosages are small. However, small amounts of phytochemicals also have a protective effect when they are combined [174]. All of the 19 herbs are safe and have been used of centuries, as well as documented in *Pharmacopoeia of P. R. China*.

ACKNOWLEDGMENT

In memory of Drs. Xiao, Zhenxiang (肖镇祥) and Meng, Jiamei (孟家眉), the late chairmen of Department of Neurology, Xuan-Wu Hospital, Capital University of Medical Science, Beijing, China, the pioneers in integrating Chinese Medicine and Western Medicine to combat stroke.

The assistance of Susan B. Peterson, B.A., M.A. in English for the chapter is gratefully acknowledged.

REFERENCES

1. Hachinski, V. (2007). Stroke and vascular cognitive impairment. *Stroke* **38**, 1396–1403.
2. Ginsberg, M. D. (2003). Adventures in the pathophysiology of brain ischemia: Penumbra, gene expression, neuroprotection: The 2002 Thomas Willis Lecture. *Stroke* **34**, 214–223.
3. Lo, E. H., Dalkara, T. & Moskowitz, M. A. (2003). Mechanisms, challenges and opportunities in stroke. *Nature Rev Neurosci* **4**, 399–414.
4. Cheng, Y. D., Al-Khoury, L. & Zivin, J. A. (2004). Neuroprotection for ischemic stroke: Two decades of success and failure. *Neuro Rx* **1**, 36–45.
5. Moskowitz, M. A. & Lo, E. H. (2003). Neurogenesis and apoptotic cell death. *Stroke* **34**, 324–326.

6. Jin, K., Peel, A. L., Mao, X. O., Xie, L., Cottrell, B. A., Henshall, D. C. & Greenberg, D. A. (2004). Increased hippocampal neurogenesis in Alzheimer's disease. *PNAS* **101**, 343–347.

7. Gong, X. & Sucher, N. J. (2002). Stroke therapy in traditional Chinese medicine (TCM): Prospects for drug discovery and development. *Phytomedicine* **9**, 478–484.

8. Kim, H. (2005). Neuroprotective herbs for stroke therapy in traditional eastern medicine. *Neurological Res* **27**, 287–301.

9. Shi, F. L., Hart, R. G., Sherman, D. G. *et al.* (1989). Stroke in the people's republic of China. *Stroke* **20**, 1581–1585.

10. Mena, H., Cadavid, D. & Rushing, E. J. (2004). Human cerebral infarct: A proposed histopathologic classification based on 137 cases. *Acta Neuropathol* **108**, 524–530.

11. Schiemanck, S. K., Post, M. W., Witkamp, T. D., Kappelle, L. J. & Prevo, A. J. (2005). Relationship between ischemic lesion volume and functional status in the 2nd week after middle cerebral artery stroke. *Neurorehabil Neural Repair* **19**, 133–138.

12. Tatemichi, T. K., Paik, M., Bagiella, E., Desmond, D. W., Pirro, M. & Hanzawa, L. K. (1994). Dementia after stroke is a predictor of long-term survival. *Stroke* **25**, 1915–1919.

13. Tatemichi, T. K., Paik, M., Bagiella, E., Desmond, D. W., Stern, Y., Sano, M., Hauser, W. A. & Mayeux, R. (1994). Risk of dementia after stroke in a hospitalized cohort: Results of a longitudinal study. *Neurology* **44**, 1885–1891.

14. Jendroska, K., Poewe, W., Daniel, S. E., Pluess, J., Iwerssen-Schmidt, H., Paulsen, J., Barthel, S., Schelosky, L., Cervos-Navarro, J. & DeArmond, S. J. (1995). Ischemic stress induces deposition of amyloid beta immunoreactivity in human brain. *Acta Neuropathol.* **90**, 461–466.

15. Garcia, J. H., Liu, K. F., Ye, Z. R. & Gutierrez, J. A. (1997). Incomplete infarct and delayed neuronal death after transient middle cerebral artery occlusion in rats. *Stroke* **28**, 2303–2310.

16. Butler, T. L., Kassed, C. A., Sanberg, P. R., Willing, A. E. & Pennypacker, K. R. (2002). Neurodegeneration in the rat hippocampus and striatum after middle cerebral artery occlusion. *Brain Res.* **929**, 252–260.

17. Dihne, M., Grommes, C., Lutzenburg, M., Witte, O. W. & Block, F. (2002). Different mechanisms of secondary neuronal damage in thalamic nuclei after focal cerebral ischemia in rats. *Stroke* **33**, 3006–3011.

18. Lin, B. & Ginsberg, M. D. (2000). Quantitative assessment of the normal microvasculature by endothelial barrier antigen (EBA) immunohistochemistry: Application to focal cerebral ischemia. *Brain Res* **865**, 237–244.

19. Nishigaya, K., Yagi, S., Sato, T., Kanemaru, K. & Nukui, H. (2000). Impairment and restoration of the endothelial blood–brain barrier in the rat cerebral infarction model assessed by expression of endothelial barrier antigen immunoreactivity. *Acta Neuropathol* **99**, 231–237.

20. Garcia, J. H., Liu, K. F., Yoshida, Y., Chen, S. & Lian, J. (1994). Brain microvessel: Factors altering their patency after the occlusion of a middle cerebral artery (Wistar rat). *Am J Pathol* **145**, 728–740.

21. Garcia, J. H., Liu, K. F., Yoshida, Y., Lian, J., Chen, S. & del Zoppo, G. J. (1994). Influx of leukocytes and platelets in an evolving brain infarct (Wistar rat). *Am J Pathol* **144**, 188–199.

22. Heye, N., Paetzold, C. & Cerbos-Navarro, J. (1991). The role of microthrombi and microcirculatory factors in localization and evolution of focal cerebral ischemia. *Neurosurg Rev* **14**, 7–16.

23. Zhang, Z. G., Zhang, L., Tsang, W., Goussev, A., Powers, C., Ho, K. L., Morris, D., Smyth, S. S., Coller, B. S. & Chopp, M. (2001). Dynamic platelet accumulation at the site of the occluded middle cerebral artery and in downstream microvessel is associated with loss of microvascular integrity after embolic middle cerebral artery occlusion. *Brain Res* **912**, 181–194.

24. Ritter, L. S., Stempel, K. M., Coull, B. M. & McDonagh, P. F. (2005). Leukocyte-platelet aggregates in rat peripheral blood after ischemic stroke and reperfusion. *Biol Res Nurs* **6**, 281–288.

25. Lo, A. C., Chen, A. Y., Hung, V. K., Yaw, L. P., Fung, M. K., Ho, M. C., Chung, S. S. & Chung, S. K. (2005). Endothelin-1 overexpression leads to further water accumulation and brain edema after middle cerebral artery occlusion via aquaporin 4 expression in astrocytic end-feet. *J Cereb Blood Flow Metab* **25**, 998–1011.

26. Lindvall, O. & Kokaia, Z. (2004). Recovery and rehabilitation in stroke. Stem cells. *Stroke* **35**(Suppl 1), 2691–2694.

27. Harrison, M. J. (1995). Neurologic complications of coronary artery bypass grafting: Diffuse or focal ischemia? *Ann Thorac Surg* **59**, 1356–1358.

28. Fujioka, M., Okuchi, K., Sakaki, T., Hiranatsu, K. I., Miyamoto, S. & Iwasaki, S. (1994). Specific changes in human brain following reperfusion after cardiac arrest. *Stroke* **25**, 2091–2095.

29. Furlan, A. J., Sila, C. A., Chimowitz, M. I. & Jones, S. C. (1992). Neurological complications related to cardiac surgery. *Neurol Clin* **10**, 145–166.

30. Hamill, R. J. (1995). Resuscitation: When is enough, enough? *Respir Care* **40**, 515–524.

31. Taraszewska, A., Zelman, I. B., Ogonowska, W. & Chrzanowska, H. (2002). The pattern of irreversible brain changes after cardiac arrest in humans. *Folia Neuropathol* **40**, 133–141.

32. Takahashi, S., Higano, S., Ishii, K., Matsumoto, K., Sakamoto, K., Iwasaki, Y. & Suzuki, M. (1993). Hypoxic brain damage: Cortical laminar necrosis and delayed changes in white matter at sequential MR imaging. *Radiology* **189**, 449–456.

33. Wisniewski, H. M. & Maslinska, D. (1996). Beta-protein immunoreactivity in the human brain after cardiac arrest. *Folia Neuropathol* **34**, 65–71.

34. Skovronsky, D. M., Lee, V. M.-Y. & Pratico, D. (2001). Amyloid precursor protein and amyloid β peptide in human platelets. *J Bio Chem* **276**, 17036–17043.

35. Di Luca, M., Colciaghi, F., Pastorino, L., Borroni, B., Padovani, A. & Cattabeni, F. (2000). Platelets as a peripheral district where to study pathogenetic mechanisms of Alzheimer disease: The case of amyloid precursor protein. *Eur J Pharmacol* **405**, 277–283.

36. Lin, B., Ginsberg, M. D., Busto, R. & Dietrich, W. D. (1998). Sequential analysis of subacute and chronic neuronal, astrocytic and microglial alterations after transient global ischemia in rats. *Acta Neuropathol* **95**, 511–523.

37. Lin, B., Schmidt-Kastner, R., Busto, R. & Ginsberg, M. D. (1999). Progressive parenchymal deposition of β-amyloid precursor protein in rat brain following global cerebral ischemia. *Acta Neuropathol* **97**, 359–368.

38. Dietrich, W. D., Lin, B., Globus, M. Y.-T., Green, E. J., Ginsberg, M. D. & Busto, R. (1995). Effect of delayed MK-801 [Dizocilpine] treatment with or without immediate postischemic hypothermia on chronic neuronal survival after global forebrain ischemia in rats. *J Cereb Blood Flow Meteb* **15**, 960–968.

39. Colborne, F., Sutherland, G. R. & Auer, R. N. (1999). Electron microscopic evidence against apoptosis as the mechanism of neuronal death in global ischemia. *J Neuroscience* **19**, 4200–4210.

40. Lin, B. & Ginsberg, M. D. (2000). The roles of β-amyloid precursor protein and amyloid β peptide in ischemic brain injury. *In* Pharmacology of Cerebral Ischemia 2000 (J. Krieglstein & S. Klumpp, Eds.), pp. 37–52, Medpharm Scientific Publishers, Stuttgart.

41. Pluta, R., Lossinsky, A. S., Walski, M., Wisniewski, H. M. & Mossakowski, M. J. (1994). Platelet occlusion phenomenon after short- and long-term survival following complete cerebral ischemia in rats produced by cardiac arrest. *J Hirnforsch* **35**, 463–471.

42. Hue, Z. (1994). *Traditional Chinese Medicine, the TCM Textbook for Medical School*, (3rd ed.), People's Health Publisher, Beijing, (in Chinese).

43. Phillipson, J. D. (1995). A matter of some sensitivity. *Phytochemistry* **38**, 1319–1343.

44. Huang, K. C. (1999). *Pharmacology of Chinese Herbs*, (2nd ed.), CRC Press LLC, Boca Raton.

45. Li, X., Bai, X., Qin, L., Huang, H., Xiao, Z. & Gao, T. (2003). Neuroprotective effects of Buyang huanwu decoction on neuronal injury in hippocampus after transient forebrain ischemia in rats. *Neurosci Lett* **346**, 29–32.

46. Li, Y. (1993). Medicines to improve circulation and clean out blood stasis. *In* Chinese Medicine Pharmacology (Y. K. Li & M. Y. Jiang, Eds.), 2nd ed., pp. 129–146, Chinese Medicine of China, Beijing, (in Chinese).

47. Akao, T., Kawabata, K., Yanagisawa, E., Ishihara, K., Mizuhar, Y., Wakui, Y., Sakashita, Y. & Kobashi, K. (2000). Baicalin, the predominant flavone glucuronide of scutellariae radix, is absorbed from the rat gastrointestinal tract as the aglycone and restored to its original form. *J Pharm Pharmacol* **52**, 1563–1568.

48. Zuo, F., Zhou, Z. M. & Liu, M. L. (2001). Determination of 14 chemical constituents in the traditional Chinese medicinal preparation Huangqin-Tang by high performance liquid chromatography. *Biol Pharm Bull* **24**, 693–697.

49. Lai, M. Y., Hsiu, S. L., Chen, C. C., Hou, Y. C. & Chao, P. D. (2003). Urinary pharmacokinetics of baicalein, wogonin and their glycosides after oral administration of scutellariae radix in human. *Biol Pharm Bull* **26**, 79–83.

50. Chen, L. C., Lee, M. H., Chou, M. H., Lin, M. F. & Yang, L. L. (1999). Pharmacokinetic study of paeoniflorin in mice after oral administration of paeoniae radix extract. *J Chromatogr B Biomed Sci Appl* **735**, 33–40.

51. Chen, L. C., Chou, M. H., Lin, M. F. & Yang, L. L. (2002). Pharmacokinetics of paeoniflorin after oral administration of Shao-yao-Gan-chao Tang in mice. *Jpn J Pharmacol* **88**, 250–255.

52. Chen, Y.-C., Shen, S.-C., Chen, L.-G., Lee, T. J. & Yang, L. (2001). Wogonin, baicalin, and baicalein inhibition of inducible nitric oxide synthase and cyclooxygenase-2 gene expressions induced by nitric oxide synthase inhibitors and lipopolysaccharide. *Biochem Pharmacol* **61**, 1417–1427.

53. Zhu, H., Wang, Z., Ma, C., Tian, J., Fu, F., Li, C., Guo, D., Roeder, E. & Liu, K. (2003). Neuroprotective effects of hydroxyl safflower yellow: A *in vivo* and *in vitro* studies. *Plant Med* **69**, 429–433.

54. Tsai, T. H., Liu, S. C., Tsai, P. L., Ho, L. K., Shum, A. Y. C. & Chen, C. F. (2002). The effects of the cyclosporin A, a P-glycoprotein inhibitor, on the pharmacokinetics of baicalein in the rat: A microdialysis study. *Br J Pharmacol* **137**, 1314–1320.

55. Tsai, T. & Liang, C. (2001). Pharmacokinetics of tetramethylpyrazine in rat blood and brain using microdialysis. *Int J Pharm* **216**, 61–66.

56. Liang, C., Hong, C., Chen, C. & Tsai, T. (1999). Measurement and pharmacokinetic study of tetramethylpyrazine in rat blood and its regional brain tissue by high-performance liquid chromatography. *J Chromotogr B Biomed Sci Appl* **724**, 303–309.

57. Lai, M. Y., Chen, C. C., Hsiu, S. L. & Chao, P. D. (2001). Analysis and comparison of baicalin, baicalein and wogonin contents in traditional decoctions and commercial extracts of Scutellariae Radix. *J Food Drug Analy* **3**, 145–149.

58. Morris, S. M. (1991). The genetic toxicology of 5-bromodeoxyuridine in mammalian cells. *Mutat Res* **258**, 161–188.

59. Taupin, P. (2007). BrdU immunohistochemistry for studying adult neurogenesis: Paradigms, pitfalls, limitations, and validation. *Brain Res Rev* **53**, 198–214.

60. Ley, J. J., Vigdorchik, A., Belayev, L., Zhao, W., Busto, R., Khoutorova, L., Becker, D. A. & Ginsberg, M. D. (2005). Stilbazulenyl nitrone, a second-generation azulenyl nitrone antioxidant, confers enduring neuroprotection in experimental focal cerebral ischemia in the rat: Neurobehavior, histopathology, and pharmacokinetics. *J Pharmacol* **313**, 1090–1100.

61. Arvidsson, A., Collin, T., Kirik, D., Kokaia, Z. & Lindvall, O. (2002). Neuronal replacement from endogenous precursors in the adult brain after stroke. *Nature Medicine* **8**, 963–970.

62. Braun, H., Schäfer, K. & Höllt, V. (2002). βIII Tubulin-expressing neurons reveal enhanced neurogenesis in hippocampal and cortical structures after a contusion trauma in rats. *J. Neurotrauma* **19**, 975–983.

63. Zhang, R., Zhang, Z., Wang, L., Wang, Y., Gousev, A., Zhang, L., Ho, K. L., Morshead, C. & Chopp, M. (2004). Activated neural stem cells contribute to stroke-induced neurogenesis and neuroblast migration toward the infarct boundary in adult rats. *J Cereb Blood Flow Metab* **24**, 441–448.

64. Nogawa, S., Forster, C., Zhang, F., Nagayama, M., Ross, M. E. & Iadecola, C. (1998). Interaction between inducible nitric oxide synthase and cyclooxygenase-2 after cerebral ischemia. *Proc Natl Acad Sci U S A* **95**, 10966–10971.

65. Zhao, W., Ginsberg, M. D., Prado, R. & Belayev, L. (1996). Depiction of infarct frequency distribution by computer-assisted image mapping in rat brains with middle cerebral artery occlusion. Comparison of photothrombotic and intraluminal suture models. *Stroke* **27**, 1112–1117.

66. Yamashita, T., Ninomiya, M., Acosta, P. H., Garcia-Verdugo, J. M., Sunabori, T., Sakaguchi, M., Adachi, K., Kojima, T., Hirota, Y., Kawase, T., Araki, N., Abe, K., Okano, H. & Sawamoto, K. (2006). Subventricular zone-derived neuroblasts migrate and differentiate into mature neurons in the post-stroke adult striatum. *J Neruoscience* **26**, 6627–6636.

67. Rosenstein, J. M., Krum, J. M., Sternbergerrr, L. A., Pulley, M. T. & Sternberger, N. H. (1992). Immunocytochemical expression of the endothelial barrier antigen (EBA) during brain angiogenesis. *Brain Res Dev Brain Res* **66**, 47–54.

68. Sternberger, N., Sternberger, L., Kies, M. W. & Shear, C. R. (1989). Cell surface endothelial proteins altered in experimental allergic encephalomyelitis. *J Neuroimmunol* **21**, 241–248.

69. Chan, P. H. (2005). Mitochondrial dysfunction and oxidative stress as determinants of cell death/survival in stroke. *Ann NY Acad Sci* **1042**, 203–209.

70. Iadecola, C. & Alexander, M. (2001). Cerebral ischemia and inflammation. *Curr Opin Neurol* **14**, 89–94.

71. Hamada, H., Hiramatsu, M., Edamatsu, R. & Mori, A. (1993). Free radical scavenging action of baicalein. *Arch Biochem Biophys* **306**, 261–266.

72. Okuda, S., Saito, H. & Katsuki, H. (1994). Arachidonic acid: Toxic and trophic effects on cultured hippocampal neurons. *Neuroscience* **63**, 691–696.

73. Gao, D., Sakkurai, K., Katoh, M., Chen, J. & Ogiso, T. (1996). Inhibition of microsomal lipid peroxidation by baicalein: A possible formation of an iron-baicalein complex. *Biochem Mol Biol Int* **39**, 21–25.

74. Shieh, D. E., Liu, L. T. & Lin, C. C. (2000). Antioxidant and free radical scavenging effects of baicalein, baicalin and wogonin. *Anticancer Res* **20**, 2861–2865.

75. Hsiao, G., Chen, Y. C., Lin, J., Lin, K., Chou, D., Lin, C. & Sheu, J. (2006). Inhibitory mechanisms of tetramethylpyrazine in middle cerebral artery occlusion (MCAO)-induced focal cerebral ischemia in rats. *Planta Med* **72**, 411–417.

76. Choi, B. M., Kim, H. J., Oh, G. S., Pae, H. O., Oh, H., Jeong, S., Kwon, T. O., Kim, Y. M. & Chung, H. T. (2002). 1,2,3,4,6-Penta-*O*-galloyl-beta-D-glucose protects rat neuronal cells (Neuro 2 A) from hydrogen peroxide-mediated cell death via the induction of heme oxygenase-1. *Neurosci Lett* **328**, 185–189.

77. Zhang, Z., Li, P., Wang, Z., Li, P., Zhang, W., Sun, Z., Zhang, X. & Wang, Y. (2006). A comparative study on the individual and combined effects of baicalin and jasminoidin of focal cerebral ischemia-reperfusion injury. *Brain Res* **1123**, 188–195.

78. Cho, J. & Lee, H. K. (2004). Wogonin inhibits ischemic brain injury in a rat model of permanent middle cerebral artery occlusion. *Biol Pharm Bull* **27**, 1561–1564.

79. Hsieh, C. L., Cheng, C. Y., Tsai, T. H., Lin, I. H., Liu, C. H., Chiang, S. Y., Lin, J. G., Lao, C. J. & Tang, N. Y. (2006). Paeonol reduced cerebral infarction involving the superoxide anion and microglia activation in ischemia-reperfusion injured rats. *J Ethnopharmacol* **106**, 208–215.

80. Yang, J. W., Ouyang, J. P., Liao, W. J., Tian, J., Liu, Y. M., Wei, L., Wang, B. H. & Li, K. (2005). The effects of Chinese herb angelica in focal cerebral ischemia injury in the rat. *Clin Hemorheol Microcirc* **32**, 209–215.

81. Leung, A. W., Mo, Z. X. & Zheng, Y. S. (1991). Reduction of cellular damage induced by cerebral ischemia in rats. *Neurochem Res* **16**, 687–692.

82. Romano, C., Price, M., Bai, H. Y. & Olney, J. W. (1993). Neuroprotectants in Honghua: Glucose attenuates retinal ischemic damage. *Invest Ophthalmol Vis Sci* **34**, 72–80.

83. Lee, V. M. & Pixley, S. K. (1994). Age and differentiation-related differences in neuron-specific Tubulin immunostaining of olfactory sensory neurons. *Brain Res Dev Brain Res* **83**, 209–215.

84. Kimura, Y., Matsushita, N., Yokoi-Hayashi, K. & Okuda, H. (2001). Effects of baicalein isolated from *Scutellaria baicalensis* Radix on adhesion molecule expression induced by thrombi and thrombin receptor agonist peptide in cultured human umbilical vein endothelial cells. *Planta Med* **67**, 331–334.

85. Kang, D. G., Moon, M. K., Choi, D. H., Lee, J. K., Kwon, T. O. & Lee, H. S. (2005). Vasodilatory and anti-inflammatory effects of the 1,2,3,4,6-penta-*O*-galloyl-beta-D-glucose (PGG) via a nitric oxide-cGMP pathway. *Eur J Pharmacol* **524**, 111–119.

86. Gao, D., Song, J., Hu, J., Lin, J., Zheng, L., Cai, J., Du, J. & Chen, K. (2005). Angiogenesis promoting effects of Chinese herbal medicine for activating blood circulation to remove stasis on chick embryo chorio-allantoic membrane. *Zhong Xi Jie He Za Zhi* **25**, 912–915.

87. Lei, Y., Wang, J. H. & Chen, K. J. (2003). Comparative study on angiogenesis effect of *Astragalus membranaceus* and *Angelica sinensis* in chick embryo choriollantoic membrane. *Zhongguo Zhong Yao Za Zhi* **28**, 876–878.

88. Krupinski, J., Kaluza, J., Kumar, P., Kumar, S. & Wang, J. M. (1994). Role of angiogenesis in patients with cerebral ischemic stroke. *Stroke* **25**, 1794–1798.

89. Damjanov, I. (1996). Inflammation. *In* The Pathology for the Health-related Professions (I. Damjanov, Ed.), pp. 24–43, W.B. Saunders Co., Philadelphia.

90. O'Banion, M. K. (1999). Cyclooxygenase-2: Molecular biology, pharmacology, and neurobiology. *Crit Rev Neurobiol* **13**, 45–82.

91. Hara, K., Kong, D. L., Sharp, F. R. & Weinstein, P. R. (1998). Effect of selective inhibition of cyclooxygenase 2 on temporary focal cerebral ischemia in rats. *Neurosci Lett* **256**, 53–56.

92. Shon, Y. & Nam, K. (2003). Protective effect of astragali radix extract on interleukin 1 beta induced inflammation in human amnion. *Phytother Res* **17**, 1016–1020.

93. Gui, S., Wei, W., Wang, H., Wu, L., Sun, W. & Chen, W. (2006). Effects and mechanisms of crude astragalosides fraction on liver fibrosis in rats. *J Ethnopharmacol* **103**, 154–159.

94. Li, B. Q., Fu, T., Gong, W., Dunlop, N., Kung, H., Yan, Y., Kang, J. & Wang, J. M. (2000). The flavonoid baicalin exhibits anti-inflammatory activity by binding to chemokines. *Immunopharmacology* **49**, 295–306.

95. Li, F. Q., Wang, Z., Liu, P. B. & Hong, J. S. (2005). Inhibition of microglial activation by the herbal flavonoid baicalein attenuates inflammation-mediated degeneration of dopaminergic neurons. *J Neural Transm* **112**, 331–347.

96. Nakayama, M., Uchimura, K., Zhu, R. L., Magayama, T., Rose, M., Stetler, R. A., Isakson, P. C., Chen, J. & Graham, S. H. (1998). Cyclooxygenase-2 inhibition prevents delayed death of CA1 hippocampal neurons following global ischemia. *Proc Natl Acad Sci USA* **95**, 10954–10959.

97. Koistinaho, J., Koponen, S. & Chan, P. H. (1994). Expression of cyclooxygenase-2 mRNA after global ischemia is regulated by AMPA receptors and glucocorticoids. *Stroke* **30**, 1900–1905.

98. Zhang, G. Q., Hao, X. M., Chen, S. Z., Zhou, P. A., Cheng, H. P. & Wu, C. H. (2003). Blockade of paeoniflorin on sodium current in mouse hippocampal CA1 neurons. *Acta Pharmacol Sinica* **24**, 1248–1252.

99. Petito, C. K., Feldmann, E., Pulsinelli, W. A. & Plum, F. (1987). Delayed hippocampal damage in humans following cardiorespiratory arrest. *Neurology* **37**, 1281–1286.

100. Lin, B., Ginsberg, M. D. & Busto, R. (1998). Hyperglycemic exacerbation of neuronal damage following forebrain ischemia: Microglial, astrocytic and endothelial alteration. *Acta Neuropathol* **96**, 610–620.
101. Nogawa, S., Zhang, F., Ross, M. E. & Iadecola, C. (1997). Cyclooxygenase-2 gene expression in neurons contributes to ischemic brain damage. *J Neurosci* **17**, 2746–2755.
102. Iadecola, C., Forster, C., Nogawa, S., Clark, H. B. & Ross, M. E. (1999). Cyclooxygenase-2 immunoreactivity in the human brain following cerebral ischemia. *Acta Neuropathol* **98**, 9–14.
103. Madrigal, J. L., Garcia-Bueno, B., Caso, J. R., Perez-Nievas, B. G. & Leza, J. C. (2006). Stress-induced oxidative changes in brain. *CNS Neurol Disord Drug Targets* **5**, 561–568.
104. Pepicelli, O., Fedele, E., Bonanno, G., Raiteri, M., Ajmone-Cat, M. A., Greco, A., Levi, G. & Minghetti, L. (2002). *In vivo* activation of *N*-methyl-D-aspartate receptors in the rat hippocampus increases prostaglandin E (2) extracellular levels and triggers lipid peroxidation through cyclooxygenase-mediated mechanisms. *J Neurochem* **81**, 1028–1034.
105. Kim, Y. O., Leem, K., Park, J., Lee, P., Ahn, D. K., Lee, B. C., Park, H. K., Suk, K., Kim, S. Y. & Kim, H. (2001). Cytoprotective effect of *Scutellaria baicalensis* in CA1 hippocampal neurons of rats after global cerebral ischemia. *J Ethnopharmacol* **77**, 183–188.
106. Chen, Y., Yang, L. & Lee, T. J. (2000). Oroxylin A inhibition of lipopolysaccharide-induced iNOS and COX-2 gene expression via suppression of nuclear factor-kappaB activation. *Biochem Pharmacol* **59**, 1445–1457.
107. Piao, H. Z., Jin, S. A., Chun, H. S., Lee, J. C. & Kim, W. K. (2004). Neuroprotective effect of wogonin: Potential roles of inflammatory cytokines. *Arch Pharm Res* **27**, 930–936.
108. Lee, H., Kim, Y. O., Kim, H., Kim, S. Y., Noh, H. S., Kang, S. S., Cho, G. J., Choi, W. S. & Suk, K. (2003). Flavonoid wogonin from medicinal herb is neuroprotective by inhibiting inflammatory activation of microglia. *FASEB J* **17**, 1943–1944.
109. Prieto, J. M., Recio, M. C., Giner, R. M., Manez, S., Giner-Larza, E. M. & Rios, J. L. (2003). Influence of traditional Chinese anti-inflammatory medicinal plants on leukocyte and platelet functions. *J Pharm Pharmacol* **55**, 1275–1282.
110. Sheu, J. R., Hsiao, G., Lee, Y. M. & Yen, M. H. (2001). Antithrombotic effects of tetramethylpyrazine *in vivo* experiments. *Int J Hematol* **73**, 393–398.
111. Sheu, J., Kan, Y., Hung, W., Ko, W. & Yen, M. (1997). Mechanisms involved in the antiplatelet activity of tetramethlpyrazine in human platelets. *Thromb Res* **88**, 259–270.
112. Chen, W. & Lu, Y. P. (1993). Shengmai San. *In* Formulae of Chinese Medicine (W. Chen & Y. P. Lu, Eds.), 2nd ed., pp. 200–204, School of Traditional Chinese Medicine of Shanghai, Shanghai.
113. Athanasuleas, C. L., Buckberg, G. D., Allen, B. S., Beyersdorf, F. & Kirsh, M. M. (2006). Sudden cardiac death: Directing the scope of resuscitation towards the heart and brain. *Resuscitation* **70**, 44–51.
114. Ichikawa, H. & Konishi, T. (2002). *In vitro* antioxidant potentials of traditional Chinese Medicine, Shengmai San and their relation to *in vivo* protective effect on cerebral oxidative damage in rats. *Biol Pharm Bull* **25**, 898–903.

115. Ichikawa, H., Wang, L. & Konishi, T. (2003). Role of component herbs in antioxidant activity of Shengmai San – a traditional Chinese medicine formula preventing cerebral oxidative damage in rat. *Am J Chin Med* **31**, 509–521.
116. Ichikawa, H., Wang, L. & Konishi, T. (2006). Prevention of cerebral oxidative injury by post-ischemic intravenous administration of Shengmai San. *Am J Chin Med* **4**, 591–600.
117. Watanabe, H. (1997). Candidates for cognitive enhancer extracted from medicinal plants: Paeoniflorin and tetramethylpyrazine. *Behav Brain Res* **83**, 135–141.
118. Wu, W. & Qiu, F. (1994). Experimental study on ischemia and reperfusion injury of rat liver and effects of ligustrazine and salvia compound. *Chin Med Sci J* **9**, 162–166.
119. Hua, J. & En-tan, G. (1996). Effect of postoperative treatment with a combination of Chuan Xiong and electrete on functional recovery of muscle grafts: An experimental study in the dog. *Plast Reconstr Surg* **98**, 851–855.
120. Cao, W., Zeng, Z., Zhu, Y., Luo, W., Demura, H., Naruse, M. & Shi, Y. (1998). Effects of tetramethylpyrazine, a Chinese medicine, on plasma endothelin-1 levels during acute pulmonary hypoxia in anesthetized dogs. *J Cardiovasc Pharmacol* **31**(Suppl 1), S456–S459.
121. Zheng, Z., Zhu, W., Zhou, X., Jin, Z., Liu, H., Chen, X., Pan, J., Demura, H., Naruse, M. & Shi, Y. (1998). Tetramethylpyrazine, a Chinese drug, blocks coronary vasoconstriction by endothelin-1 and decreases plasma endothelin-1 levels in experimental animals. *J Cardiovasc Pharmacol.* **31**(Suppl 1), S313–S316.
122. Feng, J., Liu, R., Wu, G. & Tang, S. (1997). Effects of tetramethylpyrazine on the release of PGI2 and TXA2 in the hypoxic isolated rat heart. *Mol Cell Biochem* **167**, 153–158.
123. Peng, W., Hucks, D., Priest, R. M., Kan, Y. M. & Ward, J. P. (1996). Ligustrazine-induced endothelium-dependent relaxation in pulmonary arteries via a NO-mediated and exogenous L-arginine-dependent mechanism. *Br J Pharmacol* **119**, 1063–1071.
124. Liu, C. & Hu, Y. (1993). Anti-inflammatory herbs. *In* Chinese Medicine Pharmacology (Y. K. Li & M. Y. Jiang, Eds.), 2nd ed., pp. 48–78, Chinese Medicine of China, Beijing, (in Chinese).
125. Sheu, J., Kan, Y., Hung, W., Lin, C. & Yen, M. (2000). The antiplatelet activity of tetramethylpyrazine is mediated through activation of NO synthase. *Life Sci* **67**, 937–947.
126. Zhang, Z., Wei, T., Hou, J., Li, G., Yu, S. & Xin, W. (2003). Iron-induced oxidative damage and apoptosis in cerebellar granule cells: Attenuation by tetramethylpyrazine and ferulic acid. *Eur J Pharmacol* **467**, 41–47.
127. Pang, P., Shan, J. & Chiu, K. (1996). Tetramethylpyrazine, a calcium antagonist. *Planta Med* **62**, 431–435.
128. Ozaki, Y. (1992). Anti-inflammatory effect of tetramethylpyrazine and ferulic acid. *Chem Pharm Bull (Tokyo)* **40**, 954–956.
129. Xiaohong, Y., Jing-Ping, O. Y. & Shuzheng, T. (2000). Angelica protects the human vascular endothelial cell from the effects of oxidized low-density lipoprotein *in vitro*. *Clin Hemorheol Microcire* **22**, 317–323.
130. Rhyu, M., Kim, J. & Kim, E. (2005). Radix angelica elicits both nitric oxide-dependent and calcium influx-mediated relaxation in rat aorta. *J Cardiovasc Pharmacol* **46**, 99–104.

131. Farooqui, A. A., Litsky, M. L., Farooqui, T. & Horrocks, L. A. (1999). Inhibitors of intracellular phospholipase A2 activity: Their neurochemical effects and therapeutical importance for neurological disorders. *Brain Res Bull* **49**, 139–153.

132. Clemens, J. A., Stephenson, D. T., Smalstig, E. B., Roberts, E. F., Johnstone, E. M., Sharp, J. D., Little, S. P. & Kramer, R. M. (1996). Reactive glia express cytosolic phospholipase A2 after transient global forebrain ischemia in rat. *Stroke* **27**, 527–535.

133. Kramer, R. M., Stephenson, D. T., Roberts, E. F. & Clemens, J. A. (1996). Cytosolic phospholipase A2 and lipid mediator release in brain. *J Lipid Mediat Cell Signal* **14**, 3–7.

134. Xue, J., Ichikawa, H. & Konishi, T. (2001). Antioxidant potential of qizhu tang, a Chinese herbal medicine, and the effect on cerebral oxidative damage after ischemia reperfusion rats. *Biol Pharm Bull* **24**, 558–563.

135. He, X., Li, C. & Yu, S. (2000). Protective effects of radix astragali against anoxic damages to *in vitro* cultured neurons. *J Tongji Med Univ* **20**, 126–127.

136. Song, Z., Ji, Z., Lo, C., Dong, T., Zhao, K., Li, O., Haines, C., Kung, S. & Tsim, K. (2004). Chemical and biological assessment of a traditional Chinese herbal decoction prepared from Radix *Astragali* and Radix *Angelicae sinensis*: Orthogonal array design to optimize the extraction of chemical constituents. *Planta Med* **70**, 1222–1227.

137. Zhang, H., Nagatsu, A., Watanabe, T., Sakakibara, J. & Okuyama, H. (1997). Antioxidative compounds isolated from safflower (*Carthamus tinctorius* L.) oil cake. *Chem Pharm Bull (Tokyo)* **45**, 1910–1914.

138. Cai, Q., Li, X. & Wang, H. (2001). Astragali and angelica protect the kidney against ischemia and reperfusion injury and accelerate recovery. *Chin Med J* **114**, 119–123.

139. Yim, T., Wu, W., Pak, W., Mak, D., Liang, S. & Ko, K. (2000). Myocardial protection against ischemia-reperfusion injury by a *Polygonum multiflrum* extract supplemented "Dang-Gui decoction for enriching blood," a compound formulation, *ex vivo*. *Phytotherapy Res* **14**, 195–199.

140. Lee, S. E., Hwang, H. J., Ha, J. S., Jeong, H. S. & Kim, J. H. (2003). Screening of medicinal plant extracts for antioxidant activity. *Life Sci* **73**, 167–179.

141. Lim, B. O., Yu, B. P., Kim, S. C. & Park, D. K. (1999). The antioxidative effect of ganhuangenin against lipid peroxidation. *Phytother Res* **13**, 479–483.

142. You, K. M., Jong, H. G. & Kim, H. P. (1999). Inhibition of cyclooxygenase/ lipoxygenase from human platelets by polyhydroxylated/methoxylated flavonoids isolated from medicinal plants. *Arch Pharm Res* **22**, 18–24.

143. Hanasaki, Y., Ogawa, S. & Fukui, S. (1994). The correlation between active oxygen scavenging and antioxidative effects of flavonoids. *Free Radic Biol Med* **16**, 845–850.

144. Gao, D., Tawa, R., Masaki, H., Okano, Y. & Sakurai, H. (1998). Protective effects of baicalein against cell damage by reactive oxygen species. *Chem Pharm Bull (Tokyo)* **46**, 1383–1387.

145. Gao, Z., Huang, K., Yang, X. & Xu, H. (2001). Protective effects of flavonoids in the roots of *Scutellaria baicalensis Georgi* against hydrogen peroxide-induced oxidative stress in HS-SY5Y cells. *Pharmacol Res* **43**, 173–178.

146. Morimoto, S., Tateishi, N., Matsuda, T., Tanaka, H., Taura, F., Furuya, N., Matsuyama, N. & Shoyama, Y. (1998). Novel hydrogen peroxide metabolism in suspension cells of *Scutellaria baicalensis Georgi*. *J Biol Chem* **273**, 12601–12611.

147. Gao, Z., Huang, K., Yang, X. & Xu, H. (1999). Free radical scavenging and antioxidant activities of flavonoids extracted from the radix of *Scutellaria baicalensis* Georgi. *Biochim Biophys Acta.* **1472**, 643–650.

148. Gabrielska, J., Oszmianski, J., Zylka, R. & Komorowska, M. (1997). Antioxidant activity of flavones from *Scutellaria baicalensis* in lecithin liposomes. *Z Naturgorsch [C]* **52**, 817–823.

149. Yokozawa, T., Dong, E., Kawai, Y., Gemba, M. & Shimizu, M. (1999). Protective effects of some flavonoids on the renal cellular membrane. *Exp Toxicol Pathol* **51**, 9–14.

150. Chen, X., Nishida, H. & Konishi, T. (2003). Baicalin promoted the repair of DNA single strand breakage caused by H_2O_2 in cultured fibroblasts. *Biol Pharm Bull* **26**, 282–284.

151. Kyo, R., Nakahata, N., Sakakibara, I., Kubo, M. & Ohizumi, Y. (1998). Baicalin and baicalein, constituents of an important medicinal plant, inhibit intracellular Ca^{2+} elevation by reducing phospholipase C activity in C6 rat glioma cell. *J Pharm Pharmacol* **50**, 1179–1182.

152. Lee, H. H., Yang, L. L., Wang, C. C., Hu, S. Y., Chang, S. F. & Lee, Y. H. (2003). Differential effects of natural polyphenols on neuronal survival in primary cultured central neurons against glutamate- and glucose deprivation-induced neuronal death. *Brain Res* **986**, 103–113.

153. Son, D., Le, P., Lee, J., Kim, H. & Kim, S. Y. (2004). Neuroprotective effect of wogonin in hippocampal slice culture exposed to oxygen and glucose deprivation. *Eur J Pharmacol* **493**, 99–102.

154. Lin, C. C. & Shieh, D. E. (1996). The anti-inflammatory activity of *Scutellaria rivularis* xtracts and its active components, baicalin, baicalein and wogonin. *Am J Chin Med* **24**, 31–36.

155. Nakamura, N., Hayasaka, S., Zhang, X. Y., Nagaki, Y., Matsumoto, M., Hayasaka, Y. & Terasawa, K. (2003). Effects of baicalin, baicalein, and wogonin on interkeukin-6 and interleukin-8 expression and nuclear factor-kappa B binding activities induced by interleukin-1 β in human retinal pigment epithelial cell line. *Exp Eye Res* **77**, 195–202.

156. Zhu, M., Rajamani, S., Kaylor, J., Han, S., Zhou, F. & Fink, A. (2004). The flavonoid baicalein inhibits fibrillation of α-synuclein and disaggregates existing fibrils. *J Bio Chem* **279**, 26846–26857.

157. Stanke-Labesque, F., Devillier, P., Bedouch, P., Cracowski, J. L., Chavanon, O. & Bessard, G. (2000). Angiotensin II-induced contractions in human internal mammary artery: Effects of cyclooxygenase and lipoxygenase inhibition. *Cardiovasc Res* **47**, 376–383.

158. Nakahata, N., Kutsuwa, M., Kyo, R., Kubo, M., Hayashi, K. & Ohizumi, Y. (1998). Analysis of inhibitory effects of scutellariae radix and baicalein on prostaglandin E2 production in rat C6 glioma cells. *Am J Chin Med* **26**, 311–323.

159. Kimura, Y., Matsushita, N. & Okuda, H. (1997). Effects of baicalein isolated from *Scutellaria baicalensis* on interleukin 1 beta- and tumor necrosis factor alpha-induced adhesion molecule expression in cultured human umbilical vein endothelial cells. *J Ethnopharmacol* **57**, 63–67.

160. Kimura, Y., Okuda, H. & Ogita, Z. (1997). Effects of flavonoids isolated from scutellariae radix on fibrinolytic system induced by trypsin in human umbilical vein endothelial cells. *J Nat Prod* **60**, 598–601.

161. Kimura, Y., Yokoi, K., Matsushita, N. & Okuda, H. (1997). Effects of flavonoids isolated from scutellariae radix on the production of tissue-type plasminogen activator and plasminogen activator inhibitor-1 induced by thrombin and thrombin receptor agonist peptide in cultured human umbilical vein endothelial cells. *J Pharm Pharmacol* **49**, 816–822.

162. Lebeau, A., Esclaire, F., Rostene, W. & Pelaprat, D. (2001). Baicalein protects cortical neurons from β amyloid (25–35) induced toxicity. *Neuroreport* **12**, 2199–2202.

163. Heo, H. J., Kim, D. O., Choi, S. J., Shin, D. H. & Lee, C. Y. (2004). Potent inhibitory effect of flavonoids in *Scutellaria baicalensis* on amyloid beta proteins-induced neurotoxicity. *J Agric Food Chem* **52**, 4128–4132.

164. Homma, M., Oka, K., Taniguchi, C., Nitsuma, T. & Hayashi, T. (1997). Systematic analysis of post-administrative Saiboku-To urine by liquid chromatography to determine pharmacokinetics of traditional Chinese Medicine. *Biomed Chromatogr* **11**, 125–131.

165. Zhang, L., Xing, D., Wang, W., Wang, R. & Du, L. (2006). Kinetic difference of baicalin in rat blood and cerebral nuclei after intravenous administration of scutellariae radix extract. *J Ethnopharmacol* **103**, 120–125.

166. Goto, H., Shimada, Y., Tanaka, N., Tanigawa, K., Itoh, T. & Terasawa, K. (1999). Effect of extract prepared from the roots of *Paeonia lactiflora* on endothelium-dependent relaxation and antioxidant enzyme activity in rats administered high-fat diet. *Phytother Res* **13**, 526–528.

167. Yasuda, T., Kon, R., Nakazawa, T. & Ohsawa, K. (1999). Metabolism of paeonol in rats. *J Nat Prod* **62**, 1142–1144.

168. Yan, D., Saito, K., Ohmi, Y., Fujie, N. & Ohtsuka, K. (2004). Paeoniflorin, a novel heat shock protein-inducing compound. *Cell Stress Chaperones* **9**, 378–389.

169. Huang, M. & Tchue, Z. (1993). Tonics. *In* Chinese Medicine Pharmacology (Y. K. Li & M. Y. Jiang, Eds.), 2nd ed., pp. 177–205, Chinese Medicine of China Press, Beijing, (in Chinese)..

170. Oh, J. K., Hyun, S. Y., Oh, H. R., Jung, J. W., Park, C., Lee, S., Park, J. H., Kim, S. Y., Kim, Y. K. & Ryu, J. H. (2007). Effects of *Anemarrhena asphodeloides* on focal ischemic brain injury induced by middle cerebral artery occlusion in rats. *Biol Pharm Bull* **30**, 38–43.

171. Yu, S. J., Kim, J. R., Lee, C. K., Han, J. E. & Lee, J. H. (2005). *Gastrodia elata* Blume and an active component, *p*-hydroxybenzyl alcohol, reduce focal ischemic brain injury through antioxidant related gene expressions. *Biol Pharm Bull* **28**, 1016–1020.

172. Kim, H., Lee, S. & Moon, K. (2003). Ether fraction of methanol extracts of *Gastrodia elata*, medicinal herb protects against neuronal cell damage after transient global ischemia in gerbils. *Phytother Res* **17**, 909–912.

173. Li, L., Zhou, Q. & Shi, J. (2005). Protective effects of icariin on neurons injured by cerebral ischemia/reperfusion. *Chin Med J* **118**, 1637–1643.

174. Joseph, J. A., Nadeau, D. A. & Underwood, A. (2002). *In* The Color Code, a Revolutionary Eating Plan for Optimum Health (J. A. Joseph, D. A. Nadeau & A. Underwood, Eds.), Hyperion, New York.

Chapter 13

Socioeconomic Aspects of the Use of Complementary and Alternative Medicine

K. Tom Xu

Department of Family and Community Medicine, School of Medicine, Texas Tech University Health Sciences Center, Lubbock, TX, USA

Abstract

This chapter discusses the socioeconomic determinants of complimentary and alternative medicine (CAM) use in the US based on empirical evidence found in the literature. The first section provides an overview of CAM use patterns in the US. The second section introduces theories from two disciplines in social sciences, sociology and economics, to establish the frameworks for further discussions. The third section discusses sociodemographic characteristics of CAM users, age, gender, race, ethnicity, culture, acculturation, health beliefs and education, and their roles in predicting CAM use. The fourth section examines factors emphasized in the microeconomic theory, price, insurance, income, and the relationship and choices between CAM and mainstream medicine. Because federal and state policies and legislations directly affect market conditions, they are analyzed along with the economic factors. The fifth section addresses barriers to CAM use. In particular, this section shows that mainstream medical providers' negative attitudes toward CAM may greatly deter patients' use of CAM. The last section concludes.

Keywords: *Economics, sociology, demographics, utilization and policy*

INTRODUCTION

More and more consumers used complementary and alternative medicine (CAM) in the past two decades. Between 1990 and 1997, the proportion of the US population who used CAM increased from 34% to 42% and the expenditure increased from $427 million to $629 million [1]. The 2002 National Health Interview Survey data, collected by the Center for Disease Control (CDC) and National Center for Health Statistics, showed that about 36% of adults used some type of CAM, excluding prayer. The fastest growing CAM types at the turn of the century were herbal medicine and yoga [2].

Many factors have contributed to the trend of CAM utilization. At the national level, increasing numbers of Americans have realized or experienced the limitations of conventional medical care that is based on Abraham Flexner's medical education model in the US. The pace of development in modern biomedical sciences seems to lag behind the prevalence of life-threatening diseases such as HIV and cancer, and chronic diseases such as diabetes and chronic pain. Consequently, patients with these conditions have incentives to seek out alternative treatments that are not based on conventional western bio-medical theories. For example, researchers have shown that the use of chiro-practic services doubled in the last two decades of the last century [3].

In response to the demand for CAM research, the Congress passed a leg-islation (P.L. 102–170) that provided $2 million to establish an office under National Institutes of Health (NIH) to investigate various CAM practices. In February 1999, this office became the National Center for Complementary and Alternative Medicine (NCCAM). The current budget for NCCAM is over $100 million. In March 2000, the White House Commission on Complementary and Alternative Medicine Policy was authorized by the President to conduct, deliver and disseminate research on CAM practices, products, access and edu-cation. The importance of CAM as part of integrated medicine is also recog-nized by several state governments. Many states' public insurance plans cover some CAM types, particularly chiropractors' visits.

It is evident that the nation's push towards the integration of CAM and mainstream medicine has yielded positive results. The current macro environ-ment has certainly improved access to CAM services as compared to 20 years ago. It is very likely to observe a higher utilization rate of CAM in the near future. Further basic, clinical and social science research on CAM are essential to ensure optimal and efficient CAM use. An important topic in CAM research is how and why consumers seek CAM care. Given a disease or health level, a host of consumers' characteristics ultimately determine whether they seek CAM care or not. As in seeking conventional medical care, whether a patient has insurance, his or her knowledge of the services, education, culture and most importantly, price and disposable income, play crucial roles in the CAM care-seeking behavior. This chapter focuses on the socioeconomic aspects of the utilization of CAM. Sociological and economic theories that can be used to explain CAM utilization are briefly reviewed. Empirical evidence from the literature is then reviewed and summarized.

THE THEORIES

Researchers have long been interested in why certain individuals seek medical care, mainstream or CAM, whereas others do not, given the same disease or health condition. From the perspective of psychology, one can argue that there are various degrees of perceived urgency. Individuals take the action of seek-ing care when the perceived urgency exceeds a critical threshold. Clearly, the threshold differs by individuals. Naturally, the next question is: what factors determine this threshold?

All behaviors in the social setting, including care-seeking, are subject to influences of factors that may not be biological. How receptive an individual is to medical treatments, whether he or she can afford the treatments, whether he or she has time for the treatments, and the availability of the treatments all play a role in defining the threshold of urgency. It is clear that there are numerous determinants; some are as "trivial" as the ability to get a babysitter, whereas others are significant, such as having health insurance or a medical care provider in the area. In order to summarize and categorize these factors and to understand the mechanisms by which the factors interact and act upon the decision to seek care, conceptual and mathematical models are built to better describe and predict individuals' care-seeking behavior.

The Behavioral Model

The behavioral model developed by Ronald Andersen in the late 1960s and early 1970s is essentially a sociological model [4]. A revised version of this model was published in 1995 [5]. The early version intends to explain why and how families use health care and to define various concepts of access to care.

The behavioral model categorizes factors that influence the utilization of health services into predisposing characteristics, enabling resources and need. Included in the predisposing characteristics are demographics, social structure, and health beliefs. Examples of the demographic characteristics are age, race, and gender. These characteristics are indicators of biological imperatives. Social structure is measured by education, occupation, ethnicity, culture and social networking. Health beliefs encompass knowledge, attitudes and values that predict the use of health care.

Enabling resources can be defined at both the personal/family and the community levels. Examples of personal/family enabling resources are income, having health insurance, having a usual source of care and having a means to reach a medical provider. At the community level, the enabling resources are mainly the availability of providers. In contrast to predisposing characteristics, most of which are exogenous or have very low mutability, enabling resources are more mutable and serve as necessary but not sufficient conditions of care-seeking.

The third category, need, can be perceived or evaluated. In most empirical studies using the behavioral model as the conceptual framework, need is often measured by either general health status or specific diseases. However, perceived health need is probably more pertinent to influencing the ultimate use of health services, at least for the first attempt to access the health care system at the beginning of an illness episode. In the behavioral model, need is dependent on certain predisposing characteristics. For example, the old and females are more likely to have the need for health services. There have been numerous studies showing genetic and epidemiological differences between races. In addition, education level may influence the formation of perceived needs.

The early version does not emphasize on how system, organization and other macro level factors affect the utilization of health services. In addition, individuals' health practices are not taken into consideration. More importantly, the interactions between factors and possible feedback loops between the determinants and outcomes are left out. The causal relationships in the early version are mostly linear. The revised behavioral model includes four components: environment, population characteristics, health behavior and outcomes. Environment includes health care system and external environment. Population characteristics include the original predisposing, enabling and need factors. Examples of health behavior are personal health practices and use of health services. Outcomes include perceived health status, evaluated health status and consumer satisfaction.

In the revised model, the use of health services is only a component of a larger concept, health behavior in general. The predisposing characteristics, enabling resources and need are retained. Different from the early version, outcomes and health behaviors can feedback to some of the mutable factors. In addition, the utilization of health services is not the ultimate outcome. Instead, it serves as a means to obtain better health outcomes and higher satisfaction.

The behavioral model constructs a concise framework that illustrates the mechanism by which the determinants of health service use and outcome interact. It conceptualizes some causal relationships. For example, environment affects population characteristics and outcomes. Population characteristics affect health behavior, which in turn determines outcomes. Many empirical researchers adopt this model and form their hypotheses. Because of the model's generalizability, extensions of the model to focus on a specific aspect, for example, patient–physician relationship as an enabling factor, can be easily achieved.

The Economic Model

The behavioral model is constructed specific to the care-seeking behavior in a social context. In contrast, the health economic model to explain the utilization of medical care is derived from microeconomics that describes individuals' general behaviors not specific to health. Microeconomics, a discipline that studies decision-making under constraints, describes an individual's social obtained under a very general premise: everyone wants to be happy and as happy as possible. Happiness is measured by the utility level.[1] Utility is obtained via consumption of goods and services that can be purchased in the market or produced by the individual using the materials purchased. However,

---

[1] Not all economists would agree that utility can be approximated by happiness. After all, utility is an economic concept whereas happiness is a psychological one. Well-being is perhaps another good proxy for utility.

consumption is constrained by the disposable income he or she possesses. His or her goal, then, is to maximize the utility by strategically and optimally allocating income to purchase goods, services and materials.[2]

One year before Ronald Andersen and John Newman published the *Societal and Individual Determinants of Medical Care Utilization in the United States*, Michael Grossman published his work that extended the conventional microeconomic model of individual behavior to health-related behaviors [6]. The Grossman model uses a human capital approach. That is, an individual invests in himself or herself through education, training and health to increase their earnings. The ultimate resource the individual has is his or her time that is fixed. His or her financial budget is determined by how he or she allocates time to work and leisure. His or her goal is to maximize utility subject to both budget and time constraints. There are several assumptions. Individuals desire health rather than medical care itself. Health cannot be purchased; instead, it can only be produced by the individual putting together input factors, for example, medical care and healthy diet, which can be purchased from the market. In addition, because health lasts more than one period of time, it depreciates. Lastly, health is both a consumption good and a investment good with a return.

The simplified Grossman model can be represented by the following:

$$\text{Max} \quad U = U[I(M,T_H), B(X,T_B);E] \qquad \text{Eq. (13.1)}$$

$$\text{s.t.} \quad T = T_H + T_B + T_L + T_W \qquad \text{Eq. (13.2)}$$

$$Y = wT_W = p_M M + p_X X \qquad \text{Eq. (13.3)}$$

Equation 13.1 states that an individual's utility (U) is a function of health (I) and all other home goods produced (B), for example, dinners and watching TV. In order to produce health, the individual needs market health input factors (M), for example, medical care, and time spent producing health (T_H). Similarly, other home goods B has to be produced by using market goods (X) as input and time (T_B). Letter E stands for technical efficiency, that is, how the individual puts health and other goods together to achieve a utility level. Equation 13.2 shows the time constraint. A given period of time, 24 hours, or a week, can be spent on producing health (T_H), producing home goods (T_B), being sick (T_L) and work (T_W). Equation 13.3 is the budget constraint. All income comes from T_W hours of work at a wage rate (w). Earned income (Y) can be spent either on health input factors at a price of p_M or home good input

---

[2] The conventional microeconomic model may leave the impression that there are no social interactions, except for market transactions. Altruism can be incorporated in the model. That is, an individual can derive utility from other individuals' high utility levels, which explains the gift-giving behaviors and donations.

factors at the price of p_X. The individual tries to maximize the utility subject to the two constraints. He or she is left to choose the levels of M, X, T_H, and T_B.[3]

Theoretically, if the functional forms of U, I and B can be established, one can mathematically solve this maximization. Many useful conclusions can be derived from this model, for example, the labor-leisure tradeoff and the effect of market wage changes, even when the model is not fully parameterized. More pertinent to our discussion is the choice of health input factors, including medical care. Without solving the equations formally, it can be seen that the choice of using medical care and how much to use are ultimately determined by production efficiency, market prices for input materials, market wage rate, consumer preferences, and technical efficiency in the production of utility.

One interesting implication of this model is the effect of aging. Intuitively, as in other non-economic models, older people tend to have more health problems, thus need more medical care, because of the biological process. The economic model implies that the reason older people use more health services is that they have a higher depreciation rate of their health stock. It reasons that a higher depreciation rate means increased cost of holding a certain level of health capital stock. Consequently, a higher level of medical care utilization is needed to reach this desired level of health capital stock.

THE CONVERGENCE OF THE BEHAVIORAL AND THE ECONOMIC MODELS

Although the behavioral and the microeconomic models have different premises, structures and mechanisms, the derived empirical model and conclusions are surprisingly similar. Many of the predisposing characteristics in the behavioral model such as age, gender, race, and culture are considered consumer preference parameters in the economic model to construct the production function and the utility function. The enabling factors such as having health insurance, waiting time, and usual source of care enter the budget and time constraint.[4] In the behavioral model, outcomes are determined by health behaviors that are predicted by population characteristics. The model also allows outcomes to feed back into mutable factors in population characteristics and health behaviors. These interactions can also been seen in the economic model in health production and the relationship between a health-state dependent utility function and the feedback of health status to the time constraint. More importantly, both models recognize that the utilization of medical care in any form is not the ultimate goal of an individual. It is health that individuals desire.

The role of education is worth further discussion in both models. In the behavioral model, education is mainly considered part of social structure in

---

[3] In theory, T_L can be determined by T_H and M.

[4] It can be argued that with a usual source of care in place, the provision of health services is more efficient because of the decreased amount of time spent in physicians' offices and a lower cost of information exchange.

predisposing characteristics. It is likely that education also influences individuals' health beliefs because persons with a higher education level are likely to have different attitudes, values and knowledge about health, conventional medical care, and CAM. More educated individuals are more likely to be employed, hence sufficient income, to enable them to seek care. According to the economic model, education has a dual role. First, it is an input factor for health production. Second, it influences production efficiency, that is, an individual with more education are more efficient in producing health using the same input factors than one with less education. Empirically, the latter role translates into the interactions between education and other input factors.

SOCIODEMOGRAPHIC DETERMINANTS OF CAM USE

Many sociodemographic characteristics of consumers predispose them to CAM use and form their preferences for various CAM treatments. Some of the predisposing characteristics and consumer preferences are determined genetically, for example, gender and race, whereas others are shaped by the environment and the social context an individual lives, for example, culture and education. To complicate the mechanism even more, genetic factors often interact with the environment to influence an individual's behavior of care-seeking. Keeping these interactions in mind, we now turn to specific sociodemographic characteristics and discuss empirical evidence of how they affect individuals' use of CAM.

Age

In studying health and health behavior, aging is often thought as only a biological concept, defined by chromosomal degradation, cellular deterioration, or progressive free radical damage, leading to the decline of heath and ultimately death. Aging is also a sociological concept, a process of gaining experience and knowledge. Health economists often consider death endogenous. That is, an individual can determine, to certain extent, of course, when he or she dies, by making choices related to health over his or her lifetime. In this regard, aging is behavioral. Consequently, many empirical studies of CAM include age as a predictor of CAM care-seeking.

Several studies have found that younger age is associated with a greater likelihood of using CAM among patients undergoing general surgeries [7], surgical patients using CAM modalities to treat anxiety [8], patients with colorectal cancer [9], patients visiting emergency departments [10], and patients with glaucoma [11]. On the other hand, among diabetic patients in a nationally representative sample, older age predicts a higher likelihood of CAM use [12]. In a review of 52 articles, the general pattern is that a younger age is associated with a higher likelihood of CAM use [13].

Interestingly, some studies have demonstrated that middle-aged (35–64) individuals are more likely to use CAM than their older and younger counterparts in various types of CAM [2, 14–17]. Among adolescents and children, being older has been found to increase the likelihood of CAM use [18, 19]. Because researchers often dichotomize age in various ways and the samples have different age groups, it is difficult to reach a simple conclusion in regard to whether older or younger individuals are more likely to seek CAM care and use more CAM services. However, based on age ranges of the samples in the empirical studies discussed here, it seems reasonable to conclude that the middle-aged are most likely to use CAM.

Health apparently is not the reason for this conclusion, for the older individuals (65 years of age or older) have more health problems. One can argue that CAM may be an idea too novel for elderly persons to adopt even when they have poor health. As compared to elderly persons and adolescents, the middle-aged not only are used to changes and new concepts yet with more life experience, but also have more exposure to diversified information because of their employment status, financial resources, social circles and knowledge of new technology. Consequently, the effect of age on CAM use is probably more socioeconomic than based on health needs.

Gender

The effect of gender on CAM use is the least ambiguous among all sociodemographic characteristics. In examining the use of various types of CAM, females are more likely than males to use CAM and tend to have to a higher utilization level. This pattern is observed among patients with cancers [9, 20–22], diabetes [23], HIV [24], multiple sclerosis [25], inflammatory eye disease [26], and smoking cessation [27]. The gender difference is also observed across all age groups, children and adolescents [19, 28], young adults [18], adults [2, 10, 14, 15, 17, 29], and elderly persons [30].

It is not surprising that females are more likely than males to use CAM. However, this pattern may have nothing to do with CAM or specific CAM types. Females are more likely to seek medical care in general. They tend to have more health needs than males. Also, females have a longer life expectancy than males. Chronic diseases and conditions are often associated with older ages. Aside from the explanation related to physical health, the gender difference is probably, in part, due to different attitudes towards mainstream medicine and CAM between females and males [31].

Race, Ethnicity, Culture and Acculturation

The influence of race and ethnicity on CAM is probably through cultural differences. For example, among Native American Indians, spirituality is a significant part of their daily lives. Consequently, spiritual healing is commonly used by this group. Chinese descendents tend to be more predisposed towards Chinese herbs and acupuncture. A higher level of religiosity among African-Americans predicts more use of prayers. It is argued that minorities may in fact be the heaviest users of alternative care due to their "long standing cultural and traditional significance" and the fact that they may face more barriers in accessing the mainstream healthcare system than their Caucasian counterparts [32].

Interestingly, several studies have indicated that "typical" CAM users are usually Caucasian [1, 15, 33, 34]. This is generally the case in studies of overall CAM use. One problem with investigations of racial and ethnic differences in CAM use is that minorities are usually under-represented in the data collection of the general population. Data on CAM use by minority populations are especially difficult to obtain because utilization of certain CAM forms, such as the use of the curanderos by Hispanics, are not well documented [32]. This may explain the observed minimal differences in CAM use by ethnicity [29, 35, 36]. In addition, what constitute complimentary and alternative therapies differ by studies, which makes the validation and comparison of these racial and ethnic differences difficult.

Non-Hispanic Whites: The most frequent users of CAM among non-Hispanic whites have been described as being employed, female, highly educated, of higher socioeconomic status, and covered by private health care insurance [1, 15, 33, 34, 37]. They tend to be heavier users of chiropractic and massage therapies [38, 39]. In a study on CAM use among women with breast cancer, white women report use of dietary methods, massage and acupuncture more often than minority groups [39].

Hispanics: Hispanics utilize herbal remedies more than non-Hispanic whites [40]. Among a sample of women with breast cancer, Latino women most often use dietary therapies and spiritual healing as a means of CAM [39]. In addition, older Hispanics are most likely to use dietary supplements, home remedies and curanderos when compared to Asians and non-Hispanic whites [38]. Moreover, Hispanics from El Paso, Texas, were found to utilize CAM to a much greater extent than national trends suggest, with massage therapists and herbalists being the CAM practitioners most often consulted [41].

African-Americans: African Americans have been found to be frequent users of orally ingested alternative therapies [39]. Relaxation techniques and spiritual healing have been cited by another study as being more frequently used by African-Americans than other minority groups [42]. One study showed that African-Americans were less likely to utilize biologically based therapies and manipulative or body-based methods than non-Hispanic whites [15].

Asian and Pacific Islanders: Oriental medicine and acupuncture are the CAM modalities most often employed by Asians [38]. In a study of ethnic differences in CAM use among individuals with cancer living in Hawaii, it was found that one in four respondents had utilized CAM at least once since diagnosis [43]. This study also found that CAM use was the heaviest among whites and Filipinos, intermediate for Native Hawaiians and Chinese and lowest for Japanese. Religious healing and prayer were the preferred methods of CAM among Filipinos, herbal medicines among Chinese and Hawaiian healing among Native Hawaiians.

Native American Indians: Alternative medicines and therapies employed by Native Americans seek to find "wholeness, balance, harmony, beauty, and meaning" among the individuals who use them [44]. A study found that 38% of the subjects who attended an urban Indian Health Service clinic saw a healer, and 86% of those who did not would consider seeing one in the future [45]. Furthermore, another study reported that 80% of Native American Indian patients with chronic illnesses in the sample showed significant, long-lasting benefits from a time-intensive treatment program that involved traditional medicine coupled with Native American healing philosophies [46].

Due to the variations across racial and ethnic groups in their CAM use, Hsiao and colleagues attempted to identify ethnic-specific CAM modalities using 9187 subjects in California [47]. For Asian-Americans, the ethnic-specific modalities are acupuncture, traditional Chinese medicine, green tea and soy products. For American Indians, the modalities are Native American healer and healing ritual. For African-Americans, the modalities are prayer for health by others and garlic pills. For Hispanics, the modality is curandero. For non-Hispanic white, the modalities are massage and osteopath. The authors further demonstrated that when ethnic-specific CAM modalities were used, the predictors of utilization differed from those used in models of overall CAM use. For example, they showed that gender was significant predicting ethnic-specific CAM use among only African-Americans and non-Hispanic whites.

Because of the important role of culture in determining CAM use, researchers have suspected that a person's nativity may influence utilization. Foreign born persons or descendents of foreign born persons may have unique values and attitudes about various CAM types and mainstream medicine in the US. For example, a study found that foreign born Latinas were more likely than their US born counterparts to believe that several behaviors, for example, early initiation of sexual intercourse and having sex during menstruation, were risk factors for cervical cancer and these beliefs were associated with a lower likelihood of receiving a Pap smear [48].

Acculturation is an adaptation process when an individual from one culture is in contact with a host culture [49]. During this process, the individual gradually takes up characteristics of the host culture and relinquish or retain his or her traditional culture. Past studies have investigated the relationship between acculturation and CAM use to establish whether less acculturated individuals are more likely to use CAM. Mixed empirical results have been found. Among Asians and Hispanics, individuals who were not proficient in English were found to be more likely to use ethnic-specific CAM modalities [47]. When the subgroups of Asians were analyzed separately, another study by Hsiao and colleagues found that acculturation was unrelated to CAM use for most subgroups [50]. In a study of 143 Koreans in New York metropolitan area, more acculturated individuals indicated preference for CAM [51]. Among Hispanics with osteoarthritis, less acculturated individuals were found to be more likely to use CAM therapies than their well acculturated counterparts [52]. The details regarding how acculturation should be measured are beyond the scope of our discussion. However, it should be noted that in most past studies of acculturation, it is language-based and/or approximated by the length of residence in the US.

Health Beliefs and Education

Whether an individual seeks medical care, be it CAM or mainstream, is partly dependent on his or her health beliefs. Health beliefs are a component of an individual's predisposing characteristics in the behavioral model and shape the individual's preferences in the economic model. Skepticism towards main-stream medicine, an aspect of health beliefs, has been shown to lower the utili-zation level [53], as well as mortality [54].

The sense of control, a key dimension of health beliefs, has been cited as a main reason for cancer patients to seek CAM care [22, 55–58]. As expected, believing that CAM therapies are safe has been reported to be a reason to use CAM [56, 59–62]. The perceived effectiveness is another main reason for patients to use CAM therapies [62–64]. However, the safety and effectiveness of CAM seem to be at odds with how modern sciences evaluate them and how mainstream culture in the western world perceives them. In a recent UK study of adults, evidence shows that positive attitudes towards science are associated with elevated skepticism about CAM [31]. As a result, it is not surprising to observe that health beliefs regarding mainstream medicine are intertwined with those regarding CAM. It has been shown that dissatisfaction with mainstream medicine and physicians are reasons for patients to use CAM [19, 64–67]. For some patients, however, the use of CAM is driven by the belief that CAM can enhance the beneficial effects and diminish the undesired side effects of main-stream medical treatments [55, 68].

Education, although traditionally considered a component of social struc-ture in the behavioral model, certainly interacts with and can shape an individ-ual's health beliefs. Most empirical studies of overall CAM use find that more educated individuals, as indicated by formal schooling, are more likely to use CAM for various diseases [8, 10, 11, 14–17, 20, 23–25, 27, 29, 30, 69]. One possible explanation for this observation is that more educated individuals have more exposure to CAM, either through formal learning or through the social circles that are diverse. More educated individuals tend to have better under-standing of health and health care. In addition, according to economic theories, better educated individuals are more efficient in producing health. They have better skills and means to seek out options and alternatives. On average, better educated individuals have more disposable income that enables them to use alternative forms of care. However, because education affects many mutable determinants of CAM use, it is difficult to sort out the exact mechanisms and pathways through which it affects CAM use.

ECONOMIC DETERMINANTS OF CAM USE

One aspect that distinguishes the economic model from the behavioral model in explaining CAM and mainstream medicine use is that market information and indicators are explicitly incorporated. The mechanisms through which income and price affect utilization are straightforward. In addition, in economic analyses of general commodities in a competitive market, a particular product or service does not monopolize the market. Consequently, the use of CAM is naturally linked to the utilization of mainstream medicine. That is, they are co-determined. The co-determination yields two possible outcomes, CAM as a complement of mainstream medicine and CAM as a substitute, which coincides with the name of *complementary* and *alternative* medicine. Following this logic, a non-mainstream therapy cannot be both complementary and alternative (substitutive) of mainstream medicine.

Price

The reasons for inadequate information regarding the market prices of CAM therapies in the literature are apparent: there are various types of CAM, many CAM type-specific prices are evaluated at the regional level, and disease-specific price combines all CAM types together. Using a nationally representative data set, one study estimated the effective price (out-of-pocket payment) of several CAM types [70]. The average price per visit for nutritional advice, acupuncture, massages, herbs and spiritual healing was found to be $49, 44, 33, 23 and 9, respectively. The national annual average out-of-pocket expenditure among CAM users was estimated to be $214 [71]. Between members of a traditional indemnity plan through a Preferred Provider Organization (PPO) and a Health Maintenance Organization (HMO) plan, the average annual costs on CAM were $376 and $347, respectively [72]. In a study of 2002 data from Washington, the median per-visit cost was $39 [73]. In treating breast, colon or prostate cancer, the annual expenditure on CAM was found to be $68 in western Washington [74]. In treating back pain, the average cost was found to be $50 in Washington [75]. For CAM use among children and adolescents, the average prices for visits and remedies were found to be $73.40 and $13.06, respectively [19]. As the results from these studies show, there is a high degree of variations in the CAM price estimates, depending on the region, type of CAM, diseases and insurance coverage.

Insurance

Insurance coverage enters the budget constraint in the economic model by modifying the effective price of CAM. There are growing numbers of insurers and employers that have included various CAM services in the insurance policies provided. In a survey of several managed care organizations in 2000, the companies indicated that meeting market demand was a key driving force for them to offer CAM coverage [76]. The most frequently covered CAM type is chiropractic service [77]. In a 2004 survey of employer benefits conducted by Kaiser Family Foundation and the Health Research and Educational Trust, about 87% of employers included chiropractic in the insurance plans offered. Due to the increased demand for CAM, states' insurance policies also have started to address issues related to CAM use. To date, many laws and regulations regarding CAM services and provisions have been passed at the state level. Among all states, Washington has been the most pioneering to include CAM in designing insurance coverage. In 1995, the "Every Category of Provider" (ECOP) law was passed. Under this law, the state requires that commercial insurance companies have to offer plans that cover all providers who are licensed to treat medical conditions the plans cover. At the federal level, some CAM types, such as chiropractic, are recognized and reimbursed by Medicare and Medicaid.

Several studies investigated the effect of CAM insurance on utilization. For example, using a nationally representative sample, one study showed that having CAM insurance was a strong independent predictor of frequent CAM use, controlling for other correlates [77]. Another study investigated the immediate effect of ECOP in Washington using data of a PPO and a HMO from 11/01/1996 through 10/31/1997 [72]. Only 1% of all patients covered for CAM used it. Enrollees of the PPO were found to be more likely to use CAM than those in the HMO. A later study of claims from three large insurance companies in Washington reported that among more than 600,000 enrollees, about 13.7% made CAM claims in 2002 [73]. This study found that patients enrolled in PPO and point-of-service (POS) plans were more likely than those enrolled in HMOs to use CAM. Empirical evidence also shows that state-level legislations seem to have made significant impact on the CAM insurance provision. In a study funded by Robert Wood Johnson Foundation based on data from 1997 and 1998, states with at least two CAM mandates demonstrated a significant increase in the likelihood of CAM use and CAM insurance provision [71]. It is inevitable that the trend of the inclusion of CAM in health insurance will continue in the future as market conditions and the health care system become more inclusive and integrative.

Income

Income imposes a limit on the available financial resources an individual has. In theory, individuals who have more income tend to consume more goods, provided that the goods are desirable. However, empirical evidence found by CAM researchers seems to be mixed. Previous studies have included income or poverty level in their analyses of CAM utilization. In the general US adult population, CAM use seems to be correlated with higher income [2]. When specific diseases and conditions are analyzed, higher income is found to be associated with higher utilization in breast cancer [78, 79], chronic liver diseases

[80], colon or prostate cancer [74], gynecologic cancers [81], chronic pain following spinal cord injury [82], HIV/AIDS [83], prostate carcinoma [84], head and neck cancers [85]. However, income is not found to be a significant predictor of CAM use for older patients with arthritis [86], patients with prostate cancer [87], children with cerebral palsy [88], chronic liver and gastrointestinal diseases [89].

The mixed results regarding the effect of income is not surprising, considering the relatively small amount an average individual spends on CAM per year. Because CAM services are still not mainstream in most individuals' consideration when choosing care, the spending on CAM is probably more "discretionary" than the amount spent on mainstream medicine. After all, the US' total spending on CAM is only a very small fraction of that on mainstream medicine. In addition, the strength of the correlation between income and CAM use is probably dependent on specific types of CAM, some of which may not financially cost an individual, for example, meditations and prayers. Furthermore, many individuals who report CAM use are those who "just want to try it out." In this scenario, either a non-significant or a positive correlation is possible.

CAM AS A SUBSTITUTE FOR OR A COMPLEMENT OF MAINSTREAM MEDICINE

Historically, CAM was often used as an alternative approach when mainstream medicine failed. The term "alternative medicine" was widely used in the 1980s [90, 91]. In the 1990s, several studies reported that many patients used CAM in conjunction with mainstream medicine for preventive and curative purposes [37, 92]. In 1999 when NCCAM gained its status of a center, Congress adopted the now commonly used term "complementary and alternative medicine."

A recent study showed that for 16 types of CAM, having difficulties obtaining mainstream medical care dramatically increased the likelihood of seeking CAM treatments [93], indicating a substitution effect. On the other hand, using a nationally representative sample, one study examined the association between the utilization of CAM and mainstream medicine and found that only 1.8% of the study population used CAM in the absence of using mainstream medicine [94], suggesting a complementary relationship between CAM and mainstream medicine. The tendency of patients to use CAM as a complement is also found among elderly diabetic patients [95].

One study explicitly examined 12 types of CAM to establish whether the substitutive or complementary relationship differed by race and ethnicity [96]. Although the use of many types of CAM was independent of mainstream medicine use, complementarity between CAM and mainstream medicine was found in three types of CAM among non-Hispanic whites and four among Asians. All significant relationships between CAM types and mainstream medicine among Hispanics and other races (predominantly Native American Indians) were substitution. The effect of substitution was the strongest among other races.

To ascertain whether the relationship between CAM and mainstream medicine is substitution or complementation has significant implications in designing insurance plans, health policies and regulations. If a particular CAM type is a substitute for mainstream medical treatments, then including it in the insurance coverage may encourage patients to seek CAM that is usually less expensive than mainstream medicine. Provided that the CAM type is efficacious and effective, its insurance coverage may lead to lowered total health care cost. In contrast, if the complementarity between a CAM type and mainstream medicine is in place, covering CAM would unambiguously increase the total expenditure, at least in the short run. In this case, it is imperative to establish that the combination of CAM and mainstream medicine is more cost-effective than the use of either. An exemplary study of the cost-effectiveness of the combination of the two showed that presenting guided-imagery to patient with heart problems before surgery decreased the length of hospital stay and pain level [97]. Another example is a study of fibromyalgia patients [98]. This study reported that users of both CAM and mainstream medicine (physician visits) and those who used only mainstream medicine had similar total expenditures because the cost per CAM visit was lower than the cost per physician visit. CAM users in this study had heavier overall disease burdens than the users of only physician visits.

BARRIERS TO CAM USE

Despite the increasing popularity of CAM in the US, the utilization rate is rather low if compared to that of mainstream medicine. The barriers to CAM exist at multiple levels, the patient, the health care system, health policies and the macro environment at large. Discussions in the previous sections examined factors at the patient level and some system level barriers, for example, CAM insurance. However, the key barrier to CAM use exists at a more macro level, that is, the society's acceptance of CAM as a legitimate approach for disease prevention, health promotion and therapeutic purposes.

Historically, CAM therapies were associated with the "New Age" movement in the 1960s. Consumers tended, and some still do, to consider CAM as non-scientific. From the perspective of research and science communities, the gold standard of randomized clinical trials (RCTs) was not met by CAM in the early days because these therapies were not originally developed from the European-styled scientific philosophy. For example, the points used by acupuncturists initially were not connected by meridians. They were individual points that ancient Chinese healers "accidentally" identified through trial and error. As more points accumulated over time, the meridians began to take shape. Using the modern sciences' terminology, these methods were at best experiments based on convenience samples. Recent CAM research has put more emphasis on RCTs of CAM to establish its efficacy and effectiveness. Although safety is often proven, the results on efficacy and effectiveness of various CAMs are mixed.

The influence of mainstream medical service providers on CAM use is strong because for most Americans, mainstream medicine is still the first line of defense against diseases. Physicians' unwillingness to accept CAM hence is one of the main barriers to CAM use. In 1965, the American Medical Association (AMA) formally declared that chiropractic was "quackery and cultism" and considered a physician's professional association with chiropractors unethical. The litigation between AMA and the chiropractic profession left the public with the impression that chiropractic was not an effective or legitimate treatment option [99]. The anti-CAM culture has certainly left a mark on the mentality of both physicians and the public. The impact is still visible today in physician–patient communications regarding CAM use. In several recent studies, researchers found that from one-third to over half of patients did not talk about CAM with their physicians [10, 38, 69, 100–103]. The consequences of no discussion of CAM with physicians can be severe, including adverse drug interactions, non-compliance, distrust and dissatisfaction with care.

Fortunately, the misperception of CAM on the part of mainstream medical care providers has diminished. In the 1990s, physicians' support and referrals for CAM grew rapidly [104]. In a study of medical care providers in New Mexico and Alaska, over 97% of surveyed providers suggested CAM to their patients [105]. About 70% of primary care clinicians in the Kentucky Ambulatory Network expressed their interest in continuing education about CAM [106]. Future medical care providers may be better prepared for patients' CAM use because many schools have included CAM education in their curricula. Studies have shown that most current students of health sciences have positive attitudes towards CAM [107, 108].

CONCLUSION

This chapter examined empirical evidence of socioeconomic predictors of CAM use based on sociological and economic theories. The utilization of CAM is influenced by factors at multiple levels, the patients, the mainstream medicine providers, the health care system, and government health policies and regulations. In general, the factors at the physician, system and policy levels are mutable. Consequently, interventions at these levels would be expected to have immediate impact for all patients. These interventions have greater impact on the trend of CAM use in the US than those targeting only patients.

To improve access to CAM services and the eventual integration of CAM and mainstream medicine, two crucial tasks must be accomplished. The first one is to establish the efficacy and effectiveness of various CAM types. This is essential in changing the perception of CAM as non-scientific. Collaboration between CAM and mainstream medicine providers would help to bridge the gap between the providers, to promote mutual respect, and to gain a deeper understanding of the nature of medicine from different perspectives. The second task is to establish the cost-effectiveness of CAM, either as a stand-alone alternative or a complement to mainstream medical treatments. The cost-effectiveness of CAM, once established, would serve as the most convincing evidence in pursuing insurance coverage of CAM in both private and public insurance plans by demonstrating CAM's financial viability.

The outlook of access to CAM services is promising. Clinics in many parts of the country are offering integrative medicine or have a network inclusion of CAM providers. Patients are more open to the idea of using CAM. If the research about the effectiveness and cost-effectiveness of CAM is successful in the near future, Americans will soon have a true integrative health care system, a system that benefits from both the East and the West, and the past and the future.

REFERENCES

1. Eisenberg, D. M., Davis, R. B., Ettner, S. L., Appel, S., Wilkey, S., Van Rompay, M. & Kessler, R. C. (1998). Trends in alternative medicine use in the United States, 1990–1997: Results of a follow-up national survey. *JAMA* **280**, 1569–1575.
2. Tindle, H. A., Davis, R. B., Phillips, R. S. & Eisenberg, D. M. (2005). Trends in use of complementary and alternative medicine by US adults: 1997–2002. *Altern Ther Health Med* **11**, 42–49.
3. Hurwitz, E. L., Coulter, I. D., Adams, A. H., Genovese, B. J. & Shekelle, P. G. (1998). Use of chiropractic services from 1985 through 1991 in the United States and Canada. *Am J Public Health* **88**, 771–776.
4. Andersen, R. & Newman, J. F. (1973). Societal and individual determinants of medical care utilization in the United States. *Milbank Mem Fund Q Health Soc* **51**, 95–124.
5. Andersen, R. M. (1995). Revisiting the behavioral model and access to medical care: Does it matter? *J Health Soc Behav* **36**, 1–10.
6. Grossman, M. (1972). On the concept of health capital and the demand for health. *J Political Economy* **80**, 223–256.
7. Velanovich, V., Hallal, N. & Shah, M. (2006). Patterns of usage of complementary and alternative medicine in general surgical patients. *Int J Surg* **4**, 206–211.
8. Wang, S. M., Peloquin, C. & Kain, Z. N. (2002). Attitudes of patients undergoing surgery toward alternative medical treatment. *J Altern Complement Med* **8**, 351–356.
9. Lawsin, C., DuHamel, K., Itzkowitz, S. H., Brown, K., Lim, H., Thelemaque, L. & Jandorf, L. (2007). Demographic, medical, and psychosocial correlates to CAM use among survivors of colorectal cancer. *Support Care Cancer* **15**, 557–564.
10. Kim, S., Hohrmann, J. L., Clark, S., Munoz, K. N., Braun, J. E., Doshi, A., Radeos, M. S. & Camargo, C. A., Jr. (2005). A multicenter study of complementary and alternative medicine usage among ED patients. *Acad Emerg Med* **12**, 377–380.
11. Rhee, D. J., Spaeth, G. L., Myers, J. S., Steinmann, W. C., Augsburger, J. J., Shatz, L. J., Terebuh, A. K., Ritner, J. A. & Katz, L. J. (2002). Prevalence of the use of complementary and alternative medicine for glaucoma. *Ophthalmology* **109**, 438–443.

12. Egede, L. E., Ye, X., Zheng, D. & Silverstein, M. D. (2002). The prevalence and pattern of complementary and alternative medicine use in individuals with diabetes. *Diabetes Care* **25**, 324–329.

13. Verhoef, M. J., Balneaves, L. G., Boon, H. S. & Vroegindewey, A. (2005). Reasons for and characteristics associated with complementary and alternative medicine use among adult cancer patients: A systematic review. *Integr Cancer Ther* **4**, 274–286.

14. Saper, R. B., Eisenberg, D. M., Davis, R. B., Culpepper, L. & Phillips, R. S. (2004). Prevalence and patterns of adult yoga use in the United States: Results of a national survey. *Altern Ther Health Med* **10**, 44–49.

15. Ni, H., Simile, C. & Hardy, A. M. (2002). Utilization of complementary and alternative medicine by United States adults: Results from the 1999 national health interview survey. *Med Care* **40**, 353–358.

16. Dessio, W., Wade, C., Chao, M., Kronenberg, F., Cushman, L. E. & Kalmuss, D. (2004). Religion, spirituality, and healthcare choices of African-American women: Results of a national survey. *Ethn Dis* **14**, 189–197.

17. Kennedy, J. (2005). Herb and supplement use in the US adult population. *Clin Ther* **27**, 1847–1858.

18. Johnson, S. K. & Blanchard, A. (2006). Alternative medicine and herbal use among university students. *J Am Coll Health* **55**, 163–168.

19. Yussman, S. M., Ryan, S. A., Auinger, P. & Weitzman, M. (2004). Visits to complementary and alternative medicine providers by children and adolescents in the United States. *Ambul Pediatr* **4**, 429–435.

20. Goldstein, M. S., Brown, E. R., Ballard-Barbash, R., Morgenstern, H., Bastani, R., Lee, J., Gatto, N. & Ambs, A. (2005). The use of complementary and alternative medicine among california adults with and without cancer. *Evid Based Complement Alternat Med* **2**, 557–565.

21. Lafferty, W. E., Bellas, A., Corage Baden, A., Tyree, P. T., Standish, L. J. & Patterson, R. (2004). The use of complementary and alternative medical providers by insured cancer patients in Washington State. *Cancer* **100**, 1522–1530.

22. Hedderson, M. M., Patterson, R. E., Neuhouser, M. L., Schwartz, S. M., Bowen, D. J., Standish, L. J. & Marshall, L. M. (2004). Sex differences in motives for use of complementary and alternative medicine among cancer patients. *Altern Ther Health Med* **10**, 58–64.

23. Bell, R. A., Suerken, C. K., Grzywacz, J. G., Lang, W., Quandt, S. A. & Arcury, T. A. (2006). Complementary and alternative medicine use among adults with diabetes in the United States. *Altern Ther Health Med* **12**, 16–22.

24. Agnoletto, V., Chiaffarino, F., Nasta, P., Rossi, R. & Parazzini, F. (2006). Use of complementary and alternative medicine in HIV-infected subjects. *Complement Ther Med* **14**, 193–199.

25. Shinto, L., Yadav, V., Morris, C., Lapidus, J. A., Senders, A. & Bourdette, D. (2006). Demographic and health-related factors associated with complementary and alternative medicine (CAM) use in multiple sclerosis. *Mult Scler* **12**, 94–100.

26. Smith, J. R., Spurrier, N. J., Martin, J. T. & Rosenbaum, J. T. (2004). Prevalent use of complementary and alternative medicine by patients with inflammatory eye disease. *Ocul Immunol Inflamm* **12**, 203–214.

27. Sood, A., Ebbert, J. O., Sood, R. & Stevens, S. R. (2006). Complementary treatments for tobacco cessation: A survey. *Nicotine Tob Res* **8**, 767–771.

28. Wilson, K. M., Klein, J. D., Sesselberg, T. S., Yussman, S. M., Markow, D. B., Green, A. E., West, J. C. & Gray, N. J. (2006). Use of complementary medicine and dietary supplements among U.S. adolescents. *J Adolesc Health* **38**, 385–394.

29. Mackenzie, E. R., Taylor, L., Bloom, B. S., Hufford, D. J. & Johnson, J. C. (2003). Ethnic minority use of complementary and alternative medicine (CAM): A national probability survey of CAM utilizers. *Altern Ther Health Med* **9**, 50–56.

30. Cherniack, E. P., Senzel, R. S. & Pan, C. X. (2001). Correlates of use of alternative medicine by the elderly in an urban population. *J Altern Complement Med* **7**, 277–280.

31. Furnham, A. (2007). Are modern health worries, personality and attitudes to science associated with the use of complementary and alternative medicine? *Br J Health Psychol* **12**, 229–243.

32. Chen, M. S. (1999). Informal care and the empowerment of minority communities: Comparisons between the USA and the UK. *Ethn Health* **4**, 139–151.

33. Bausell, R. B., Lee, W. L. & Berman, B. M. (2001). Demographic and health-related correlates to visits to complementary and alternative medical providers. *Med Care* **39**, 190–196.

34. Shumay, D. M., Maskarinec, G., Gotay, C. C., Heiby, E. M. & Kakai, H. (2002). Determinants of the degree of complementary and alternative medicine use among patients with cancer. *J Altern Complement Med* **8**, 661–671.

35. Factor-Litvak, P., Cushman, L. F., Kronenberg, F., Wade, C. & Kalmuss, D. (2001). Use of complementary and alternative medicine among women in New York City: A pilot study. *J Altern Complement Med* **7**, 659–666.

36. King, M. O. & Pettigrew, A. C. (2004). Complementary and alternative therapy use by older adults in three ethnically diverse populations: A pilot study. *Geriatr Nurs* **25**, 30–37.

37. Eisenberg, D. M., Kessler, R. C., Foster, C., Norlock, F. E., Calkins, D. R. & Delbanco, T. L. (1993). Unconventional medicine in the United States. Prevalence, costs, and patterns of use. *N Engl J Med* **328**, 246–252.

38. Najm, W., Reinsch, S., Hoehler, F. & Tobis, J. (2003). Use of complementary and alternative medicine among the ethnic elderly. *Altern Ther Health Med* **9**, 50–57.

39. Lee, M. M., Lin, S. S., Wrensch, M. R., Adler, S. R. & Eisenberg, D. (2000). Alternative therapies used by women with breast cancer in four ethnic populations. *J Natl Cancer Inst* **92**, 42–47.

40. Dole, E. J., Rhyne, R. L., Zeilmann, C. A., Skipper, B. J., McCabe, M. L. & Dog, T. L. (2000). The influence of ethnicity on use of herbal remedies in elderly Hispanics and non-Hispanic whites. *J Am Pharm Assoc (Wash)* **40**, 359–365.

41. Rivera, J. O., Ortiz, M., Lawson, M. E. & Verma, K. M. (2002). Evaluation of the use of complementary and alternative medicine in the largest United States-Mexico border city. *Pharmacotherapy* **22**, 256–264.

42. Flaherty, J. H., Takahashi, R., Teoh, J., Kim, J. I., Habib, S., Ito, M. & Matsushita, S. (2001). Use of alternative therapies in older outpatients in the United States and Japan: Prevalence, reporting patterns, and perceived effectiveness. *J Gerontol A Biol Sci Med Sci* **56**, M650–M655.

43. Maskarinec, G., Shumay, D. M., Kakai, H. & Gotay, C. C. (2000). Ethnic differences in complementary and alternative medicine use among cancer patients. *J Altern Complement Med* **6**, 531–538.

44. Cohen, K. (1998). Native American medicine. *Altern Ther Health Med* **4**, 45–57.

45. Marbella, A. M., Harris, M. C., Diehr, S. & Ignace, G. (1998). Use of Native American healers among Native American patients in an urban Native American health center. *Arch Fam Med* **7**, 182–185.

46. Mehl-Madrona, L. E. (1999). Native American medicine in the treatment of chronic illness: Developing an integrated program and evaluating its effectiveness. *Altern Ther Health Med* **5**, 36–44.

47. Hsiao, A. F., Wong, M. D., Goldstein, M. S., Yu, H. J., Andersen, R. M., Brown, E. R., Becerra, L. M. & Wenger, N. S. (2006). Variation in complementary and alternative medicine (CAM) use across racial/ethnic groups and the development of ethnic-specific measures of CAM use. *J Altern Complement Med* **12**, 281–290.

48. Hubbell, F. A., Chavez, L. R., Mishra, S. I. & Valdez, R. B. (1996). Beliefs about sexual behavior and other predictors of Papanicolaou smear screening among Latinas and Anglo women. *Arch Intern Med* **156**, 2353–2358.

49. Salabarria-Pena, Y., Trout, P. T., Gill, J. K., Morisky, D. E., Muralles, A. A. & Ebin, V. J. (2001). Effects of acculturation and psychosocial factors in Latino adolescents' TB-related behaviors. *Ethn Dis* **11**, 661–675.

50. Hsiao, A. F., Wong, M. D., Goldstein, M. S., Becerra, L. S., Cheng, E. M. & Wenger, N. S. (2006). Complementary and alternative medicine use among Asian-American subgroups: Prevalence, predictors, and lack of relationship to acculturation and access to conventional health care. *J Altern Complement Med* **12**, 1003–1010.

51. Kim, J. & Chan, M. M. (2004). Factors influencing preferences for alternative medicine by Korean Americans. *Am J Chin Med* **32**, 321–329.

52. Herman, C. J., Dente, J. M., Allen, P. & Hunt, W. C. (2006). Ethnic differences in the use of complementary and alternative therapies among adults with osteoarthritis. *Prev Chronic Dis* **3**, A80.

53. Fiscella, K., Franks, P. & Clancy, C. M. (1998). Skepticism toward medical care and health care utilization. *Med Care* **36**, 180–189.

54. Fiscella, K., Franks, P., Clancy, C. M., Doescher, M. P. & Banthin, J. S. (1999). Does skepticism towards medical care predict mortality? *Med Care* **37**, 409–414.

55. Boon, H., Stewart, M., Kennard, M. A., Gray, R., Sawka, C., Brown, J. B., McWilliam, C., Gavin, A., Baron, R. A., Aaron, D. & Haines-Kamka, T. (2000). Use of complementary/alternative medicine by breast cancer survivors in Ontario: Prevalence and perceptions. *J Clin Oncol* **18**, 2515–2521.

56. Richardson, M. A., Sanders, T., Palmer, J. L., Greisinger, A. & Singletary, S. E. (2000). Complementary/alternative medicine use in a comprehensive cancer center and the implications for oncology. *J Clin Oncol* **18**, 2505–2514.

57. Moschen, R., Kemmler, G., Schweigkofler, H., Holzner, B., Dunser, M., Richter, R., Fleischhacker, W. W. & Sperner-Unterweger, B. (2001). Use of alternative/complementary therapy in breast cancer patients: A psychological perspective. *Support Care Cancer* **9**, 267–274.

58. Eng, J., Ramsum, D., Verhoef, M., Guns, E., Davison, J. & Gallagher, R. (2003). A population-based survey of complementary and alternative medicine use in men recently diagnosed with prostate cancer. *Integr Cancer Ther* **2**, 212–216.

59. Mc, D. T. D., Walsham, N., Taylor, S. E. & Wong, L. F. (2006). Complementary and alternative medicines versus prescription drugs: Perceptions of emergency department patients. *Emerg Med J* **23**, 266–268.

60. Downer, S. M., Cody, M. M., McCluskey, P., Wilson, P. D., Arnott, S. J., Lister, T. A. & Slevin, M. L. (1994). Pursuit and practice of complementary therapies by cancer patients receiving conventional treatment. *BMJ* **309**, 86–89.

61. Begbie, S. D., Kerestes, Z. L. & Bell, D. R. (1996). Patterns of alternative medicine use by cancer patients. *Med J Aust* **165**, 545–548.

62. Tough, S. C., Johnston, D. W., Verhoef, M. J., Arthur, K. & Bryant, H. (2002). Complementary and alternative medicine use among colorectal cancer patients in Alberta, Canada. *Altern Ther Health Med* **8**, 54–56, 58–60, 62–64..

63. Risberg, T., Kaasa, S., Wist, E. & Melsom, H. (1997). Why are cancer patients using non-proven complementary therapies? A cross-sectional multicentre study in Norway. *Eur J Cancer* **33**, 575–580.

64. Ceylan, S., Hamzaoglu, O., Komurcu, S., Beyan, C. & Yalcin, A. (2002). Survey of the use of complementary and alternative medicine among Turkish cancer patients. *Complement Ther Med* **10**, 94–99.

65. Lengacher, C. A., Bennett, M. P., Kip, K. E., Keller, R., LaVance, M. S., Smith, L. S. & Cox, C. E. (2002). Frequency of use of complementary and alternative medicine in women with breast cancer. *Oncol Nurs Forum* **29**, 1445–1452.

66. Shmueli, A. & Shuval, J. (2006). Satisfaction with family physicians and specialists and the use of complementary and alternative medicine in Israel. *Evid Based Complement Alternat Med* **3**, 273–278.

67. Verhoef, M. J., Hagen, N., Pelletier, G. & Forsyth, P. (1999). Alternative therapy use in neurologic diseases: Use in brain tumor patients. *Neurology* **52**, 617–622.

68. Alferi, S. M., Antoni, M. H., Ironson, G., Kilbourn, K. M. & Carver, C. S. (2001). Factors predicting the use of complementary therapies in a multi-ethnic sample of early-stage breast cancer patients. *J Am Med Womens Assoc* **56**, 120–123, 126.

69. Navo, M. A., Phan, J., Vaughan, C., Palmer, J. L., Michaud, L., Jones, K. L., Bodurka, D. C., Basen-Engquist, K., Hortobagyi, G. N., Kavanagh, J. J. & Smith, J. A. (2004). An assessment of the utilization of complementary and alternative medication in women with gynecologic or breast malignancies. *J Clin Oncol* **22**, 671–677.

70. Bridevaux, I. P. (2004). A survey of patients' out-of-pocket payments for complementary and alternative medicine therapies. *Complement Ther Med* **12**, 48–50.

71. Sturm, R. & Unutzer, J. (2000). State legislation and the use of complementary and alternative medicine. *Inquiry* **37**, 423–429.

72. Stewart, D., Weeks, J. & Bent, S. (2001). Utilization, patient satisfaction, and cost implications of acupuncture, massage, and naturopathic medicine offered as covered health benefits: A comparison of two delivery models. *Altern Ther Health Med* **7**, 66–70.

73. Lafferty, W. E., Tyree, P. T., Bellas, A. S., Watts, C. A., Lind, B. K., Sherman, K. J., Cherkin, D. C. & Grembowski, D. E. (2006). Insurance coverage and subsequent utilization of complementary and alternative medicine providers. *Am J Manag Care* **12**, 397–404.

74. Patterson, R. E., Neuhouser, M. L., Hedderson, M. M., Schwartz, S. M., Standish, L. J., Bowen, D. J. & Marshall, L. M. (2002). Types of alternative medicine used by patients with breast, colon, or prostate cancer: Predictors, motives, and costs. *J Altern Complement Med* **8**, 477–485.
75. Lind, B. K., Lafferty, W. E., Tyree, P. T., Sherman, K. J., Deyo, R. A. & Cherkin, D. C. (2005). The role of alternative medical providers for the outpatient treatment of insured patients with back pain. *Spine* **30**, 1454–1459.
76. Pelletier, K. R. & Astin, J. A. (2002). Integration and reimbursement of complementary and alternative medicine by managed care and insurance providers: 2000 update and cohort analysis. *Altern Ther Health Med* **8**, 38–39, 42, 44 passim.
77. Wolsko, P. M., Eisenberg, D. M., Davis, R. B., Ettner, S. L. & Phillips, R. S. (2002). Insurance coverage medical conditions, and visits to alternative medicine providers: Results of a national survey. *Arch Intern Med* **162**, 281–287.
78. Gray, R. E., Fitch, M., Goel, V., Franssen, E. & Labrecque, M. (2003). Utilization of complementary/alternative services by women with breast cancer. *J Health Soc Policy* **16**, 75–84.
79. Cui, Y., Shu, X. O., Gao, Y., Wen, W., Ruan, Z. X., Jin, F. & Zheng, W. (2004). Use of complementary and alternative medicine by chinese women with breast cancer. *Breast Cancer Res Treat* **85**, 263–270.
80. Strader, D. B., Bacon, B. R., Lindsay, K. L., La, D., Brecque, R., Morgan, T., Wright, E. C., Allen, J., Khokar, M. F., Hoofnagle, J. H. & Seeff, L. B. (2002). Use of complementary and alternative medicine in patients with liver disease. *Am J Gastroenterol* **97**, 2391–2397.
81. Swisher, E. M., Cohn, D. E., Goff, B. A., Parham, J., Herzog, T. J., Rader, J. S. & Mutch, D. G. (2002). Use of complementary and alternative medicine among women with gynecologic cancers. *Gynecol Oncol* **84**, 363–367.
82. Nayak, S., Matheis, R. J., Agostinelli, S. & Shifleft, S. C. (2001). The use of complementary and alternative therapies for chronic pain following spinal cord injury: A pilot survey. *J Spinal Cord Med* **24**, 54–62.
83. Duggan, J., Peterson, W. S., Schutz, M., Khuder, S. & Charkraborty, J. (2001). Use of complementary and alternative therapies in HIV-infected patients. *AIDS Patient Care STDS* **15**, 159–167.
84. Kao, G. D. & Devine, P. (2000). Use of complementary health practices by prostate carcinoma patients undergoing radiation therapy. *Cancer* **88**, 615–619.
85. Warrick, P. D., Irish, J. C., Morningstar, M., Gilbert, R., Brown, D. & Gullane, P. (1999). Use of alternative medicine among patients with head and neck cancer. *Arch Otolaryngol Head Neck Surg* **125**, 573–579.
86. Kaboli, P. J., Doebbeling, B. N., Saag, K. G. & Rosenthal, G. E. (2001). Use of complementary and alternative medicine by older patients with arthritis: A population-based study. *Arthritis Rheum* **45**, 398–403.
87. Boon, H., Westlake, K., Stewart, M., Gray, R., Fleshner, N., Gavin, A., Brown, J. B. & Goel, V. (2003). Use of complementary/alternative medicine by men diagnosed with prostate cancer: Prevalence and characteristics. *Urology* **62**, 849–853.

88. Hurvitz, E. A., Leonard, C., Ayyangar, R. & Nelson, V. S. (2003). Complementary and alternative medicine use in families of children with cerebral palsy. *Dev Med Child Neurol* **45**, 364–370.

89. Yang, Z. C., Yang, S. H., Yang, S. S. & Chen, D. S. (2002). A hospital-based study on the use of alternative medicine in patients with chronic liver and gastrointestinal diseases. *Am J Chin Med* **30**, 637–643.

90. Furnham, A. & Smith, C. (1988). Choosing alternative medicine: a comparison of the beliefs of patients visiting a general practitioner and a homoeopath. *Soc Sci Med* **26**, 685–689.

91. Murray, J. & Shepherd, S. (1988). Alternative or additional medicine? A new dilemma for the doctor. *J R Coll Gen Pract* **38**, 511–514.

92. Lerner, I. J. & Kennedy, B. J. (1992). The prevalence of questionable methods of cancer treatment in the United States. *CA Cancer J Clin* **42**, 181–191.

93. Pagan, J. A. & Pauly, M. V. (2005). Access to conventional medical care and the use of complementary and alternative medicine. *Health Aff (Millwood)* **24**, 255–262.

94. Druss, B. G. & Rosenheck, R. A. (1999). Association between use of unconventional therapies and conventional medical services. *JAMA* **282**, 651–656.

95. Schoenberg, N. E., Stoller, E. P., Kart, C. S., Perzynski, A. & Chapleski, E. E. (2004). Complementary and alternative medicine use among a multiethnic sample of older adults with diabetes. *J Altern Complement Med* **10**, 1061–1066.

96. Xu, K. T. & Farrell, T. W. (2007). The complementarity and substitution between unconventional and mainstream medicine among racial and ethnic groups in the United States. *Health Serv Res* **42**, 811–826.

97. Tusek, D. L., Cwynar, R. & Cosgrove, D. M. (1999). Effect of guided imagery on length of stay, pain and anxiety in cardiac surgery patients. *J Cardiovasc Manag* **10**, 22–28.

98. Lind, B. K., Lafferty, W. E., Tyree, P. T., Diehr, P. K. & Grembowski, D. E. (2007). Use of complementary and alternative medicine providers by fibromyalgia patients under insurance coverage. *Arthritis Rheum* **57**, 71–76.

99. Weil, A. (1983). *Health and Healing*, Houghton Mifflin, Boston.

100. Barraco, D., Valencia, G., Riba, A. L., Nareddy, S., Draus, C. B. & Schwartz, S. M. (2005). Complementary and alternative medicine (CAM) use patterns and disclosure to physicians in acute coronary syndromes patients. *Complement Ther Med* **13**, 34–40.

101. Weiss, S. J., Takakuwa, K. M. & Ernst, A. A. (2001). Use, understanding, and beliefs about complementary and alternative medicines among emergency department patients. *Acad Emerg Med* **8**, 41–47.

102. Yates, J. S., Mustian, K. M., Morrow, G. R., Gillies, L. J., Padmanaban, D., Atkins, J. N., Issell, B., Kirshner, J. J. & Colman, L. K. (2005). Prevalence of complementary and alternative medicine use in cancer patients during treatment. *Support Care Cancer* **13**, 806–811.

103. Astin, J. A., Pelletier, K. R., Marie, A. & Haskell, W. L. (2000). Complementary and alternative medicine use among elderly persons: One-year analysis of a Blue Shield Medicare suppl ement. *J Gerontol A Biol Sci Med Sci* **55**, M4–M9.

104. Blumberg, D. L., Grant, W. D., Hendricks, S. R., Kamps, C. A. & Dewan, M. J. (1995). The physician and unconventional medicine. *Altern Ther Health Med* **1**, 31–35.

105. Brems, C., Johnson, M. E., Warner, T. D. & Roberts, L. W. (2006). Patient requests and provider suggestions for alternative treatments as reported by rural and urban care providers. *Complement Ther Med* **14**, 10–19.

106. Flannery, M. A., Love, M. M., Pearce, K. A., Luan, J. J. & Elder, W. G. (2006). Communication about complementary and alternative medicine: Perspectives of primary care clinicians. *Altern Ther Health Med* **12**, 56–63.

107. Pettersen, S. & Olsen, R. V. (2007). Exploring predictors of health sciences students' attitudes towards complementary-alternative medicine. *Adv Health Sci Educ Theory Pract* **12**, 35–53.

108. Harris, I. M., Kingston, R. L., Rodriguez, R. & Choudary, V. (2006). Attitudes towards complementary and alternative medicine among pharmacy faculty and students. *Am J Pharm Educ* **70**, 129.

Chapter 14

Noni (*Morinda citrifolia*) Fruit as a Functional Food and Dietary Supplement for an Aging Population

Amy C. Brown and Noelani Apau-Ludlum

Department of Complementary and Alternative Medicine, John A. Burns School of Medicine,
University of Hawaii at Manoa, Honolulu, HI, USA

Abstract

Background: *Morinda citrifolia* (noni) is a tree widely found throughout Asia and the Pacific Basin. Noni fruit products include its juice serving as a functional food, and dietary supplements in the form of freeze dried pills, concentrated extracts, powders, tinctures, and fruit leather. These products are claimed in the lay press as complementary treatments for a variety of medical conditions common to the aging population. Numerous questions arise from consumers and researchers seeking to separate the science from the sensationalism, but no independent review of the scientific literature has been conducted.

Purpose: To provide an independent review of PubMed articles related to the noni's potential medicinal uses in order to provide (1) a list of health conditions possibly treated in a complementary manner with noni products, and (2) an evidence-based response for health practitioners.

Methods: We conducted a literature review utilizing Medline on PubMed to summarize any research relating noni to health conditions using the key words "noni," "*Morinda citrifolia*" and "*Morinda citrifolia* and cancer."

Results: An online search of the literature, dated from inception to November 2007, resulted in a total of 125 articles. Nine of these articles were related to cancer (summarized in a review article by Brown). Other studies reviewed here investigated the use of noni for health conditions such as high blood pressure, anti-inflammation, osteoporosis related to hearing loss, tuberculosis, and HIV.

Conclusion: No conclusions can be made at this time regarding the effectiveness of noni products on various health conditions due to the limited number of research studies. Of interest, is some anti-cancer activity *in vitro* and in laboratory animals utilizing a noni precipitate and not the juice itself, anti-inflammatory action of noni and its possible benefit in arthritis, and apparent decreased bone loss in the middle ear bones that may delay hearing loss. While some interesting preliminary results have been reported, most of these studies were singular in nature, or only three to five in number for each category. As a result more research is needed in these areas to elucidate a beneficial effect, if any, of noni on these and other health conditions.

Keywords: *Noni, Morinda citrifolia, cancer, high blood pressure, osteoporosis*

INTRODUCTION

Noni juice, an extract of the *Morinda citrifolia* tree's fruit, is widely found throughout Asia and the Pacific Basin, especially in Tahiti and Hawaii. Products derived from noni fruit include its juice as a functional food, and dietary supplements in the form of freeze-dried pills, concentrated extracts, powders, tinctures, and fruit leather. Noni products are touted in the lay press as an excellent complementary treatment for a variety of medical conditions common to the aging population. However, no independent review of the literature has been conducted to determine the strength of the science behind the sensationalism surrounding noni products.

According to the Commission of Dietary Supplement Labels, it is important for health and nutrition professionals to become more knowledgeable about dietary supplements in order to help consumers make appropriate choices [1]. Part of the concern is that prescriptions and over-the-counter medications are utilized more frequently in seniors creating an increased risk for possible drug–dietary supplement interactions [2].

This is coupled with the concern that seniors are purchasing more non-vitamin, nonmineral (NVNM) dietary supplements defined as a class of dietary supplements including herbals, botanicals, proteins and amino acids [3]. The percentage of people over 65 years of age utilizing herbal/botantical dietary supplements daily varies depending on the survey conducted. Kirkpatrick [4] reported 40% of rural older adults in Idaho consumed NVNM supplements, while Gordon and Schaffer reported that among female seniors enrolled in a Kaiser-Permanente Medical Care Program, 32% had taken a NVNM in the past year, while 25% had consumed a herbal [2].

How a NVNM dietary supplement is defined influences these survey outcomes. Herbs are technically "non-woody seed-producing plants that die at the end of the vine after growing season ends." Botanicals are more broadly described as "substances derived from plants" [1]. Interpreting research using the NVNM, herbal and botanical terms becomes difficult because researchers often use them interchangeably.

As a result, data regarding the most common NVNM supplements consumed differ depending on the agency conducting the survey, the type of instrument used, and the demographics of the population surveyed. Reported use for NVNM supplements in the third National Health and Nutrition Survey was highest for lecithin, garlic, amino acids, oils (primarily fish), alfalfa, and ginseng [1].

The main reasons for NVNM supplementation in the elderly population reported by Wold [5] are arthritis, memory improvement, and generally health and well being. Cheung *et al.* found that maintaining health and treating a health condition were the primary reasons that 21% of older adults ($\geq$65 years of age) used herbal supplements. Wold's [6] survey in a healthy elderly population found glucosamine as the most frequently used NVNM followed

TABLE 14.1 Common Dietary Supplements Claimed in the Popular Press to Benefit Certain Age-Related Health Conditions

Age-Related Health Area	Selected Dietary Supplements
Aging	Antioxidants
Arthritis	Glucosamine/chondroitin, bromelain, cat's claw
Brain function	*Ginkgo biloba*, phytochemicals, alpha-lipoic acid
Cancer	Potassium, omega-3 fatty acids, antioxidants, selenium, saw palmetto for prostate cancer, probiotics
Depression (mild)	St. John's Wort, MSM, SAMe, B-vitamins
Digestive problems	Probiotics, prebiotics, digestive enzymes, fiber
Energy	Ginseng, maca
Eye health	Vitamin A (beta-carotene), E, C, zinc, lutein, lycopene
Heart	
Hypercholesterolemia	Omega-3 fatty acids, plant sterols, garlic, flaxseed oil
Hypertension	Omega-3 fatty acids, calcium, magnesium, coenzyme Q10
Immune function	Zinc, protein, vitamin C, maca
Insomnia	Certain homeopathic remedies, magnesium, chamomile tea, melatonin
Liver function	Milk thistle
Menopause	Evening primrose oil, black current oil, black cohosh, soy products, dehydorepiandrosterone (DHEA)
Osteoporosis	Calcium, vitamin D

by ginkgo biloba, chondroitin, and garlic. Women tended to consume black cohosh, borage, evening primrose, flaxseed oil, chondroitin, dehydroepiandrosterone, garlic, ginkgo biloba, glucosamine, grapeseed extract, hawthorn, and St. John's wort, while men tended to focus on alpha lipoic acid, ginkgo biloba, and grape-seed extract. Results of the surveys reporting the most common NVNM consumed would also differ if focusing on the "top-selling herbs" that are often conducted by the dietary supplement industry.

Overall, Table 14.1 lists some common dietary supplements claimed in the popular press to be useful for a variety of age-related health conditions. Despite evidence-based research supporting the use of certain NVNM dietary supplements in an elderly population, a lack of controlled, double-blind clinical studies for some of the lesser well known NVNM dietary supplements remains a problem. Noni products fall into this category and the purpose of this chapter is to provide a description of the *M. citrifolia* plant, its common uses as a functional food, a PubMed review revealing potential medicinal uses, suggested future research, and an evidence-based response for practitioners to give to seniors interested in consuming noni juice.

NATURAL HISTORY

Morinda citrifolia, is a small evergreen tree that belongs to the family Rubiaceae and its genus has 80 species. It grows mainly in the coastal areas, but can also grow up to 1300 feet [7]. It is thought to have originated in Southeast Asia before spreading throughout the Pacific via either seeds floating in the ocean or distributed by birds. Alternatively, the noni plant may have been one of the most important medicinal plants brought to Hawaii and other Pacific Basin islands by early Polynesians approximately 1500 years ago.

The migration of the tree through various countries resulted in its fruit being known by a variety of common names such as Indian Mulberry in India, Ba ji tian in China, cheesefruit in Australia, Nono in Tahiti, and noni in Hawaii [8]. The lumpy-surfaced noni fruit is produced by the plant all year. It is the size and shape of a "grenade." Initially, the unripe fruit is green, turns yellow as it ripens, and softens into a translucent sheen as it becomes over ripe (Fig. 14.1). The odor and taste of the translucent fruit is not pleasant which makes it unpalatable for many consumers unless it is first mixed with juice or some other beverage to mask the flavor [9].

Very few instances of recorded history depict the use of noni fruit or other parts of the tree among Hawaiian healers. Hawaiian history along with its medicine was passed down through generations through oral tradition. Bishop Museum records reveal that the leaf was most commonly used as a poultice over wounds, after first being held briefly over fire, to release the contents. The unripe green noni fruit was primarily used for external remedies such as mouth sores, gingivitis, toothache, and abscesses. Interviews with Hawaiian healers do not support the use of ripe fruit for other medical conditions, including

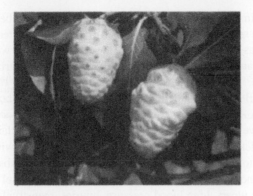

FIGURE 14.1 Noni (*Morinda citrifolia*) fruit that has ripened from a solid dark green to a cream-yellow color.

cancer. As a result, it was suggested that Chinese immigrants may have introduced their medicinal herbal techniques to the use of noni, a method of juice extraction that later grew in popularity [10].

NONI AS A FUNCTIONAL FOOD

The most common form of noni is juice derived from *M. citrifolia* fruit. Commercial concentrations range from 10% to 100% of the pure juice. Manufacturers incorporate other juices to reduce the cost and/or cover the unpalatable flavor. Noni juice can be extracted either through homemade or commercial methods. The homemade version method provides 100% noni juice. Fully ripened fruits are placed into a glass jar; some cover the fruit with a small amount of water. It is then tightly sealed so the contents naturally decompose and ferment over 1 week to 3 months depending in the quality of the fruit. The juice is then strained through cheesecloth and stored in the refrigerator.

Commercially, noni juice is manufactured in large vats and sold as juice or used to create freeze-dried pills, concentrated extracts, powders, tinctures, and even fruit leather.

Popular Uses of Noni

Noni was used in Asia and the Pacific Basin for many years before being popularized in the United States. Although the utilization of noni was prevalent in the Far East, this article only focuses on the use of noni within the United States. Its use by the Hawaiian's as a poultice (noni leaves) over external wounds or mouth sores shifted to the fruit juice as an internal remedy primarily for the treatment for cancer, diabetes, and hypertension. How this change in using noni juice occurred remains elusive, because not even the early popular uses of noni juice were purported for cancer.

The first claims within the United States of noni juice being helpful for a cornucopia of medical ailments appears to have been started by Dr. Ralph Heinicke who was a biochemist living in Hawaii (1950–1986) working for Dole Pineapple Company. Many of these broad claims were popularized through his published article, "The Pharmacologically Active Ingredient of Noni," in the Pacific Tropical Botanical Garden bulletin [11], and his 2001 book entitled *The Xeronine System. A New Biological System* [12]. It should be noted that he was the first to receive a patent on the use of noni in which he claimed one of its uses was "complete cures of hard core drug addicts with no withdrawal symptoms" (www.uspto.gov). His garden bulletin article list of unsubstantiated health claims for noni included, "arthritis, atherosclerosis, blood vessel problems, drug addiction, gastric ulcers, high blood pressure, injuries, menstrual cramps, mental depression, poor digestion, relief of pain, senility, sprains, and many others" [11].

Dr. Heinicke proposed that the active substance in noni was similar to the unknown ingredient in bromelain (pineapple enzyme) that he called "xeronine." Although no chemical structure of xeronine was ever provided, various chemical constituents in noni juice have been reported by a number of researchers who continue to decipher potential bioactive components in noni fruit juice [13–33].

Dr. Heinicke's research came to the attention of John Wadsworth, a food scientist, who according to Tahitian Noni® Juice's website, traveled to Tahiti from the United States in 1993 to find a commercial noni source. Apparently, his partner, Stephen Story, had heard a story from a neighbor returning from Tahiti about a "miracle fruit" [34]. A company was formed that was later became Tahitian Noni International, Orem, UT. This multi-level marketing (MLM) company self-reported $33 million in sales during their first year. Six years later they claimed $33 million in sales in 1 month with annual sales totaling $300 million. In 2004, the government of French Polynesia gave an award to Tahitian Noni International for "the nation's economic growth and overall positive impact (www.tahitiannoni.com)."

MEDICINAL USES OF NONI

The popularization of noni linked to commercial interests overshadowed the search for evidenced-based research revealing what, if any, medicinal value is obtained from noni juice. Numerous questions from consumers and researchers sought to separate the science from the sensationalism, but no independent review of the scientific literature had been done. As a result, Brown [9] conducted a literature review utilizing Medline on PubMed to summarize any research relating noni to health conditions. Key search words were "noni," "*Morinda citrifolia*", and "*Morinda citrifolia* and cancer." Results from the literature dated 1964 to November 2007 resulting in a total of 125 articles. Most of these articles related to health were written on the topic of cancer, and these are summarized in a review article by Brown [9]. However, other conditions were reported and include high blood pressure, inflammation, osteoporosis, tuberculosis, and HIV. The literature on these heath conditions and cancer possibly being treated by noni juice and/or its extract(s) is now briefly reviewed.

Noni and Blood Pressure

The earliest research conducted on noni relating it to a health condition was reported in French by Dang-Van-Ho from Vietnam [35, 36]. He reported that a "total root extract" was used in 58 patients and resulted in an 81% effective treatment with no side-effects [37]. In a follow-up, Youngken studied *M. citrifolia* from Thailand and India and in elegant detail delineated the root and stem structures [38]. Then, using the water-soluble part of the root administered intravenously to anesthetized dogs, they found a 26-minute marked lowering of blood pressure.

A more recent study by Ettarh [39] noted that *Morinda lucida* (L.) is widely used in Africa to treat malaria and diabetes. This sister species of *M. citrifolia* is not noni, but rather an African tree generating red fruit that grows in Nigeria and the Congo basin. He studied the effect of these leaves on the aortic rings of rats and reported a vaso-relaxing effect on aortic smooth muscle with and without endothelium. The endothelium effect is due to the endothelium release of nitric oxide, prostacyclin and endothelium-derived hyperpolarizing factor (EDHF. In aortas without endothelium, the leaf solution acted directly on smooth muscle cells by lowering intracellular calcium, however, this effect was not derived from noni (*M. citrifolia*) [39].

Noni and Anti-inflammation

Inflammation is involved in many diseases of the aging population. A small group of noni and anti-inflammation studies reveal mixed findings. Inflammation's complex pathways involve several mediators including the nitric oxide radical. In 2007, Berg *et al.* [40] studied the antioxidant and superoxide-mediated lung injury, tumor necrosis factor (TNF) and interleukin 1 (IL-1) in rats.They found that noni and noni precipitate did not protect rats against pulmonary oxygen toxicity induced by hyperoxia.

Another study by Batsu *et al.* [41] also failed to show nitric oxide scavenger activity by noni in either an *in vitro* spectrophotometric tests or in murine macrophages (*ex vitro*). However, in another *in vitro* study of the reducing and antioxidant capability of noni, strong oxygen superoxide scavenger action and potassium ferricyanide reduction was demonstrated by chromatography and UV spectrophotometry [42]. They suggested that *M. citrifolia* is a complex mixture of iridoid glycosides and flavonolglycoside antioxidant compounds.

Since noni is used to treat rheumatoid arthritis in traditional oriental medicine, a group of researchers [43] determined that noni might have anti-inflammatory properties. They injected (ip) aqueous extracts of noni derived from a slurry of ripe fruits (10 mg and 200 mg) into rats and reported a dose-dependent reduction in paw inflammation triggered by an injected pro-inflammatory.

Although not studying *M. citrifolia*, Choi *et al*. [44] researched the sister species of *Morinda officinalis* and separated its root chromatographically into monotropein and deacetylasperulosidic acid. They then studied the antinociceptive and anti-inflammatory action of the monotropein and found significant reduction in acute paw edema in hot plate exposed rats and mice. Another study on the same sister species by Kim *et al*. [45] on the methanol extraction of *M. officinalis*, demonstrated strong inhibition of nitric oxide, prostaglandin E2, TNF-alpha, nuclear factor kappa B or anti-inflammatory and antinociceptive activity.

Su *et al*. [27] purified noni and identified two new iridoid glucosides: 6-alpha-hydroxyadoxoside and 6-beta-7-beta-epoxy-8-epi-splendoside, 17 known compounds, half of which were identified for the first time in noni. All components were tested for antioxidant activity. Neolignan and Americanin A were strong antioxidants.

Noni and Osteoporosis

Anecdotally, elderly oriental people have reported hearing again after drinking noni juice. Osteoporosis might be linked to conductive hearing loss caused by diminishing middle ear bones due to osteoporosis-related changes of structure and function that naturally occur with age in postmenopausal women. A study by Langford *et al*. [46] suggested that noni juice (Tahitian Noni Juice) may increase bone remodeling and made a difference in hearing at the 8000 hz, sensorineural range. The researchers indicated that their small pilot study of eight subjects (five in the treatment group; three in the control group) needs to be repeated on a larger scale over a longer time period with pure noni juice rather than a commercial product containing lesser percentages or other potential influencing ingredients.

It is interesting to note that Seo *et al*. [47] examined the effect of providing a noni sister species, *Morindae radix* extracts, to sciatic neurectomized mice. They reported that the extract showed significant and dose-dependent suppression of decrease in hind limb thickness, tibia failure load, bone mineral density of the tibia and tibia phosphorus and calcium contents as well as increased serum osteoclacin levels. This non-noni extract was both a suppressor of bone resorption and increased bone formation *in vivo* in mice.

Noni and Tuberculosis

In 2002, Saludes *et al*. [48] studied noni leaves from the Philippines. Using *Mycobacterium tuberculosis* cultures they identified antitubercular lipids in the hexane fraction of ethanol extracted noni leaves.

Noni and HIV

In an effort to address the fast replication problem of the HIV-1 virus and persistent low level viral production in latent T cell infections which leads to drug resistant viral strains, Kamata *et al.* searched 504 bioactive compounds to identify those with inhibitory effects. They identified a component of noni root (not fruit), damnacanthal, which inhibits viral protein inducted cell death [49].

Cancer

An aging population faces an increased risk of cancer morbidity and mortality. As a result, complementary and alternative medicine (CAM) use is common among cancer patients. Mathews *et al.* [50] reported 69% of their surveyed breast cancer survivors used some form of CAM treatment. However, the percent of CAM users reported among other studies can vary depending on the definition of CAM and the type of cancer patient being surveyed. Since claims abound in the popular press about the use of noni juice against cancer, a literature review using PubMed (terms "noni", "*Morinda citrifolia*" and "*Morinda citrifolia* and cancer.") was conducted by Brown [9] to determine if any anti-cancer activity related to noni was reported in the scientific literature.

Fifteen studies (12%) of 125 articles found on noni relate to cancer studies:

- Nine of the 15 were *in vitro* studies [51–59];
- Six were *in vivo* animal studies (some data overlapped with *in vitro* studies) [51–53, 55, 60]; and
- Two were *in vivo* human studies [61, 62].

In addition, not only did noni juice concentration range from 10% to 100% in these studies, but it was tested in more than one form (extract, powder, or more commonly in a concentrated precipitate. This limited number of studies on various forms of noni is now briefly detailed to summarize the science of noni's relationship, if any, to *in vitro* or *in vivo* anti-cancer activity.

Summary of In Vitro Studies on Noni and Cancer

The majority of studies (nine total) evaluating the anti-cancer activity of noni juice or extract were conducted *in vitro* [51–59]. The first study was a brief report in 1996 by Hirazumi, a pharmacology graduate student at the University of Hawaii who studied under Dr. Furusawa in the John A. Burns School of Medicine. Most of the studies conducted by Hirazumi and Furusawa utilized a polysaccharide ethanol-precipitate and not pure noni juice. They suggested this substance stimulated the immune system through macrophages reported to release cytokines, nitric oxide (NO), interleukin-1 and interleukin-12 (IL-1, IL-12), and TNF. Other immune related factors increased were natural killer (NK) cells and cytotoxic T cells. Unrelated to the immune system was a study by Hornick *et al.* [58] showing that noni juice (5% v/v) inhibited initiation of new vessel sprouts, but other ingredients of greater concentration may have been responsible. Only a few anti-proliferation studies have been reported and these report some moderate, but not complete, inhibition on selected cancer cell lines. In 2006, Arpornsuwan [59] tested a crude extract of noni (0.1 mg/ml) against various cancer cell lines with a percent cytotoxicity ranging from 0% to 36% depending on the type of cancer cell line. There appears to be some unidentified ingredient stimulating the immune system biomarkers.

Summary of In Vivo Animal Studies

Only six studies utilizing animals have been conducted testing noni extract or fruit juice [51–53, 55, 60], however, their results suggest a bioactive in noni juice extract may slightly increase the number of mice surviving against cancer up to approximately 30% (about 1/3; 25–45%) of the time [9]. These interesting results warrant further investigation.

Summary of In Vitro Human Clinical Studies

Despite the numerous claims promoted to consumers about noni products being "effective" against cancer, only two gastric cancer case studies of limited data and one NIH clinical trial have been conducted [61–62]. The NIH Phase I human clinical trial (dose finding study) investigated the effect of noni fruit extract, in the form of freeze-dried pills and not fruit juice, given to 29 advanced cancer patients [62]. The results reported in abstract form indicated no measured tumor regression, no decrease in Brief Fatigue Inventory (BFI), and no reduction in the Center for Epidemiologic Studies Depression Scale (CES-D). However, there was a significant decrease in pain interference. No adverse events were reported on daily dosages of 4 capsules (500 mg each; 2 g total dose) with subsequent dose levels increased to 10 g (20 capsules) daily.

As with many cancers, the dietary or herbal treatment may be most effective in the early stages, as few drugs work to bring advanced cancer patients into remission for 5 or more years. Early treatment rather than advanced stage intervention is imperative for cancer treatment especially if the substance is thought to be effective through enhancing the immune system. In summary of the human research, clinical data is currently lacking to either support or refute the use of noni juice, and/or its concentrated extract, as a complementary cancer treatment [9].

SAFETY OF NONI

Potential toxicity is a common concern with many herbal and/or dietary supplements and Potterat and Hamburger [63] published an extensive review on the phytochemistry, pharmacology, and safety of *M. citrifolia* (Noni). Regarding human cases of potential toxicity, five cases to date have been reported in PubMed relating noni juice ingestion to possible harmful effects [64–67]. These case studies are explained in detail by Brown's review [9], so only a brief summary follows.

The first case in 2000 reported by Mueller [64] consisted of a 45-year-old male patient with hyperkalemia that was on a low potassium diet because of renal insufficiency. He was unaware that noni juice was a high source of potassium [68]. Although small amounts of noni juice are usually consumed on a daily basis, a cup (237 ml) has approximately the same amount of potassium (500 mg) as a cup of orange or tomato juice, or a medium banana. The other four cases involved liver hepatitis and/or jaundice. Confounding these case studies were pre-existing medical conditions and possibly prescribed drugs: Mueller's patient had renal insufficiency, Stadlbauer's [66] patients were afflicted with toxic hepatitis and chronic B-cell leukemia, and Yuce's [67] patient had multiple sclerosis. The only patient without a pre-existing condition was Millonig's [65] 45-year-old male with acute hepatitis [9].

As a result of these pre-existing medical conditions, West et al. [69, 70] (employed in the Research and Development Department of Tahitian Noni Juice, Provo, UT) reported that the causality within each of the five case studies cannot be firmly established. He also reported that four of the five case studies appeared in Europe around the time that noni fruit juice was approved as a Novel Food by the European Commission in 2003 [71] based on a 2002 report by the Scientific Committee on Food [72].

Drug–Supplement Interaction

Another possible side-effect arising from the consumption of noni products was a potential drug–supplement interaction. Carr et al. [73] suggested that noni juice interferes with the coumadin or warfarin drug, however, both Carr [73] and West [68] reported that this brand of noni juice had added vitamin K at the time. Warfarin is one of the most widely used oral anticoagulants and the degree of anticoagulation in patients is significantly affected by their vitamin K dietary intake [74]. Wittkowsky [75] reported that "patients taking warfarin are at particular risk of interactions with dietary supplements, yet approximately 30% use herbal or natural product supplements." Anticoagulant interactions with dietary supplements is currently being developed through the Clotcare Online Resource (www.clotcare.com). It is important to monitor noni products, as with all dietary supplements, to determine if they interfere with warfarin or any other drug.

LIMITATION

Only Medline articles on PubMed were utilized for the compilation of summaries found in this article. While limiting the literature review to this source ensures some degree of standardization, it also did not broaden the search to other valuable indexes such as those in botany, agriculture, anthropology, and other fields as well as other sources including, but not limited to, NapAlert and/or FDA Poison control reports. Information from the Pacific Basin (especially Tahiti) and Asia regarding indications and usage of M. citrifolia botanical use was not obtained. As a result, this review is strictly Medline-based, and while comprehensive with regard to this resource, is not entirely inclusive of all the literature or anecdotal reports, nor should it be viewed as such [9].

EVIDENCED-BASED CLINICAL RESPONSE FOR SENIORS

Medical Care

The first take-home message to clients is to maintain their medical treatments under the care of a health provider, to inform this person of any functional food and/or dietary supplement consumption, and to understand that complementary medicine is "complementary" to mainstream medicine, and preferably for healthy adults that are neither pregnant nor lactating.

Body of Evidence

Approximately 125 journal articles (as of November, 2007) exist using the key words "*Morinda citrifolia*" which is very limited in the realm of scientific studies. Since the studies conducted on noni and various health conditions are very limited in number, no conclusions can be made at this time to the effectiveness of noni products on various health conditions.

Health Conditions

The earliest research studies were conducted on high blood pressure, followed by anti-inflammation, osteoporosis related to hearing loss, tuberculosis, and HIV. While some interesting preliminary results have been reported, most of these studies were singular in nature, or only three to five in number for each category. As a result much more research is needed in these areas to elucidate a beneficial effect, if any, of noni on these and other health conditions. Of interest, is the anti-inflammatory action of noni and its possible benefit to arthritis, and the decreased bone loss in the middle ear bones that may delay hearing loss.

Cancer

Again, questions regarding noni juice and cancer can be answered with the reply that too few studies exist to make any conclusions at this time other than freeze-dried noni capsules might reduce pain perception in advanced cancer patients. In fact, only 14 studies exist on the subject of which the majority (9) were "in-the-test-tube" studies. These studies also suggest that it was the "concentrated component" in noni juice or pure noni juice that may:

1. Stimulate the immune system to "possibly" assist the body fight the cancer from within;
2. Kill a small percentage (0–36% and not 100%) of cancer cells *in vitro* depending on the type of cancer.

About 6 of the 14 studies were "animal studies" suggesting that a concentrated component in noni juice or pure noni juice may:

1. Boost the animals' immune systems; but only;
2. Slightly increases the number (about 1/3; 25–45%) of mice surviving.

Only one human clinical study exists to date. An NIH study determined that freeze-dried noni (not noni juice) may have reduced pain perception, but that it did not reverse cancer in patients with advanced cancer. However, very few conventional treatments can reverse advanced cancer either so the real question is whether or not noni juice, or its concentrated component, can influence cancer in its early stages when it might be influenced by the immune system [9].

Although a few *in vitro* and *in vivo* animals studies suggest an unidentified anti-cancer activity present to a small degree, the practicality and/or isolation of the active component warrants further research [9]. More studies are necessary to determine the potential, if any, of the specific bioactives in fermented, non-pasteurized noni juice (or if it exists in the pasteurized form) to affect early stage cancer in humans.

Potassium-Restricted Diets

Patients on low-potassium diets due to kidney, liver, or heart problems should avoid noni products. If such patients continue to consume noni products despite their healthcare providers' warning, then their potassium and liver enzyme levels should be routinely monitored.

Research Limitations

The extrapolation of these and future studies are all limited by the fact that commercial noni juice concentrations range from 10% to 100% noni juice. Perhaps, the bioactive plant component in concentrated form is more potent, or produced in the fermented noni juice product? Another question is whether or not pasteurization, common to most commercialized fruit juices, destroys the bioactive(s)?

ACKNOWLEDGMENTS/DISCLOSURES

The authors wish to thank Dr. Scot Nelson and Dr. Craig R. Elevitch, authors of *Noni: The Complete Guide for Consumers and Growers*, for their technical assistance with this manuscript and/or permission to use their noni photographs. The author, Amy C. Brown, is CEO of Natural Remedy Labs, LLC, her own biotechnology corporation located in Honolulu, Hawaii. The authors have no commercial connection with any noni product(s).

REFERENCES

1. Radimer, K. L., Subar, A. F. & Thompson, F. E. (2000). Nonvitamin, nonmineral dietary supplements: Issues and findings from NHANES III. *J Am Diet Assoc* **100**(4), 447–454.
2. Gordon, N. P. & Schaffer, D. M. (2005). Use of dietary supplements by female seniors in a large Northern California health plan. *BMC Geriatr* **9**(5), 4.
3. Archer, S. L. (2005). Nonvitamin and nonmineral supplement use among elderly people. *J Am Diet Assoc* **105**(1), 63–64.
4. Kirkpatrick, C. F., Page, R. M. & Hayward, K. S. (2006). Nonvitamin, nonmineral supplement use and beliefs about safety and efficacy among rural older adults in southeast and south central Idaho. *J Nutr Elder* **26**(1–2), 59–82.
5. Wold, R. S., Wayne, S. J., Waters, D. L. & Baumgartner, R. N. (2007). Behaviors underlying the use of nonvitamin nonmineral dietary supplements in a healthy elderly cohort. *J Nutr Health Aging* **11**(1), 3–7.
6. Wold, R. S., Lopez, S. T., Yau, C. L., Butler, L. M., Pareo-Tubbeh, S. L., Waters, D. L., Garry, P. J. & Baumgartner, R. N. (2005). Increasing trends in elderly persons' use of nonvitamin, nonmineral dietary supplements and concurrent use of medications. *J Am Diet Assoc* **105**(1), 54–63.
7. Morton, J. F. (1992). The ocean-going Noni, or Indian mulberry (*Morinda citrifolia*, Rubiaceae) and some of its "colourful" relatives. *Econ Bot* **46**, 241–256.
8. Wang, M. Y., West, B. J., Jensen, C. J., Nowicki, D., Su, C., Palu, A. K. & Anderson, G. (2002). *Morinda citrifolia* (noni): A literature review and recent advances in noni research. *Acta Pharmacol Sin* **23**(12), 1127–1141.
9. Brown, A. B. Noni (*Morinda citrifolia)* fruit as a complementary treatment for cancer: A review (in press).
10. McClatchey, W. (2002). From Polynesian healers to health food stores: Changing perspectives of *Morinda citrifolia* (Rubiaceae). *Integr Cancer Ther* **1**(2), 110–120.
11. Heinicke, R. M. (1885). The pharmacologically active ingredient of noni. *Bulletin – Pacific Tropical Botanical Garden* **15**, 10–14.
12. Heinicke, R. M. (2001). *The Xeronine System. A New Biological System*, Direct Source Publishing.
13. Akihisa, T., Matsumoto, K., Tokuda, H., Yasukawa, K., Seino, K., Nakamoto, K., Kuninaga, H., Suzuki, T. & Kimura, Y. (2007). Anti-inflammatory and potential cancer chemopreventive constituents of the fruits of *Morinda citrifolia* (Noni). *J Nat Prod* **70**(5), 754–757.
14. Bui, A. K., Bacic, A. & Pettolino, F. (2006). Polysaccharide composition of the fruit juice of *Morinda citrifolia* (noni). *Phytochemistry* **67**(12), 1271–1275.
15. Cimanga, K., Hermans, N., Apers, S., Van Miert, S., Van den Heuvel, H., Claeys, M., Pieters, L. & Vlietinck, A. (2003). Complement-inhibiting iridoids from *Morinda morindoides*. *J Nat Prod* **66**(1), 97–102.
16. Chungieng, T., Hay, L. & Montet, D. (2004). Detailed study of the juice composition of noni (*Morinda citrifolia*) fruits from Cambodia. *Fruits* **60**, 13–24.
17. Hemwimol, S., Pavasant, P. & Shotipruk, A. (2006). Ultrasound-assisted extraction of anthraquinones from roots of *Morinda citrifolia*. *Ultrason Sonochem Ultrason Sonochem* **13**(6), 543–548.

18. Kamiya, K., Tanaka, Y., Endang, H., Umar, M. & Satake, T. (2005). New anthraquinone and iridoid from the fruits of *Morinda citrifolia. Chem Pharm Bull (Tokyo)* **53**(12), 1597–1599.

19. Pawlus, A. D., Su, B. N., Keller, W. J. & Kinghorn, A. D. (2005). An anthraquinone with potent quinone reductase-inducing activity and other constituents of the fruits of *Morinda citrifolia* (noni). *J Nat Prod* **68**(12), 1720–1722.

20. Samoylenko, V., Zhao, J., Dunbar, D. C., Khan, I. A., Rushing, J. W. & Muhammad, I. (2006). New constituents from noni (*Morinda citrifolia*) fruit juice. *J Agric Food Chem* **54**(17), 6398–6402.

21. Lin, C. F., Ni, C. L., Huang, Y. L., Sheu, S. J. & Chen, C. C. (2007). Lignans and anthraquinones from the fruits of *Morinda citrifolia. Nat Prod Res* **21**(13), 1199–1204.

22. Chairungsi, N., Jumpatong, K., Suebsakwong, P., Sengpracha, W., Phutdhawong, W. & Buddhasukh, D. (2006). Electrocoagulation of quinone pigments. *Molecules* **11**(7), 514–522.

23. Sang, S., Liu, G., He, K., Zhu, N., Dong, Z., Zheng, Q., Rosen, R. T. & Ho, C. T. (2003). New unusual iridoids from the leaves of noni (*Morinda citrifolia* L.) show inhibitory effect on ultraviolet B-induced transcriptional activator protein-1 (AP-1) activity. *Bioorg Med Chem* **11**(12), 2499–2502.

24. Shotipruk, A., Kiatsongscrm, J., Pavasant, P., Goto, M. & Sasaki, M. (2004). Pressurized hot water extraction of anthraquinones from the roots of *Morinda citrifolia. Biotechnol Prog* **20**(6), 1872–1875.

25. Siddiqui, B. S., Sattar, F. A., Begum, S., Gulzar, T. & Ahmad, F. (2006). New anthraquinones from the stem of *Morinda citrifolia* Linn. *Nat Prod Res* **20**(12), 1136–1144.

26. Stalman, M., Koskamp, A. M., Luderer, R., Vernooy, J. H., Wind, J. C., Wullems, G. J. & Croes, A. F. (2003). Regulation of anthraquinone biosynthesis in cell cultures of *Morinda citrifolia. J Plant Physiol* **160**(6), 607–614.

27. Su, B. N., Pawlus, A. D., Jung, H. A., Keller, W. J., McLaughlin, J. L. & Kinghorn, A. D. (2005). Chemical constituents of the fruits of *Morinda citrifolia* (noni) and their antioxidant activity. *J Nat Prod* **68**(4), 592–595.

28. Vickers, A. (2002). Botanical medicines for the treatment of cancer: Rationale, overview of current data, and methodological considerations for phase I and II trials. *Cancer Invest* **20**(7–8), 1069–1079.

29. Wang, M., Kikuzaki, H., Csiszar, K., Boyd, C. D., Maunakea, A., Fong, S. F., Ghai, G., Rosen, R. T., Nakatani, N. & Ho, C. T. (1999). Novel trisaccharide fatty acid ester identified from the fruits of *Morinda citrifolia* (noni). *J Agric Food Chem* **47**(12), 4880–4882.

30. Wang, M., Kikuzaki, H., Jin, Y., Nakatani, N., Zhu, N., Csiszar, K., Boyd, C., Rosen, R. T., Ghai, G. & Ho, C. T. (2000). Novel glycosides from noni (*Morinda citrifolia*). *J Nat Prod* **63**(8), 1182–1183.

31. Westendorf, J., Effenberger, K., Iznaguen, H. & Basa, S. (2007). Toxicological and analytical investigations of noni (*Morinda citrifolia*) fruit juice. *J Agric Food Chem* **55**(2), 529–537.

32. Wu, Y. J., Liu, J., Wu, Y. M., Liu, L. E. & Zhang, H. Q. (2005). [Determination of polysaccharide from Chinese medicine *Morinda officinalis* how and its trace elements analysis]. *Guang Pu Xue Yu Guang Pu Fen Xi* **25**(12), 2076–2078.

33. Yao, H., Wu, H., Feng, C. H., Zhao, S. & Liang, S. J. (2004). [Relation between root structure and accumulation of anthraquinones of *Morinda officinalis*]. *Shi Yan Sheng Wu Xue Bao* **37**(2), 96–102.

34. Smillie, D. Entrepreneurs: Tales of the South Pacific. May 24, 2004. Online at http://www.forbes.com/forbes/2004/0524/178_print.html.

35. Dang-Van-Ho (1954). [A basic treatment for arterial hypertension with extracts of the roots of *Morinda citrifolia* (Cay-Nhau)]. *Presse Med* **62**(48), 1020–1021.

36. Dang-Van-Ho (1955). [Treatment and prevention of hypertension and its cerebral complications by total root extracts of *Morinda citrifolia*]. *Presse Med* **63**(72), 1478.

37. Youngken, H. W., Sr. (1958). A study of the root of *Morinda citrifolia* Linné I. *J Am Pharm Assoc Am Pharm Assoc (Baltim)*, **47**(3 Part 1), 162–165.

38. Youngken, H. W., Sr. Jenkins, H. J. & Butler, C. L. (1960). Studies on Morinda citrifolia L. II. *J Am Pharm Assoc Am Pharm Assoc* **49**, 271–273.

39. Ettarh, R. R. & Emeka, P. (2004). *Morinda lucida* extract induces endothelium-dependent and -independent relaxation of rat aorta. *Fitoterapia* **75**(3–4), 332–336.

40. Berg, J. T. & Furusawa, E. (2007). Failure of juice or juice extract from the noni plant (*Morinda citrifolia*) to protect rats against oxygen toxicity. *Hawaii Med J* **66**(2), 41–44.

41. Batsu, S. & Hazra, B. (2006). Evaluation of nitric oxide scavenging activity, *in vitro* and *ex vivo*, of selected medicinal plants traditionally used in inflammatory diseases. *Phytother Res* **20**(10), 896–900.

42. Calzuola, I., Gianfranceschi, G. L. & Marsili, V. (2006). Comparative activity of antioxidants from wheat sprouts, *Morinda citrifolia*, fermented papaya and white tea. *Int J Food Sci Nutr* **57**(3–4), 168–177.

43. McKoy, M. L., Thomas, E. A. & Simon, O. R. (2002). Preliminary investigation of the anti-inflammatory properties of an aqueous extract from *Morinda citrifolia* (noni). *Proc West Pharmacol Soc* **45**, 76–78.

44. Choi, J., Lee, K. T., Choi, M. Y., Nam, J. H., Jung, H. J., Park, S. K. & Park, H. J. (2005). Antinociceptive anti-inflammatory effect of monotropein isolated from the root of *Morinda officinalis*. *Biol Pharm Bull* **28**(10), 1915–1918.

45. Kim, I. T., Park, H. J., Nam, J. H., Park, Y. M., Won, J. H., Choi, J., Choe, B. K. & Lee, K. T. (2005). *In-vitro* and *in-vivo* anti-inflammatory and antinociceptive effects of the methanol extract of the roots of *Morinda officinalis*. *J Pharm Pharmacol* **57**(5), 607–615.

46. Langford, J., Doughty, A., Wang, M., Clayton, L. & Babich, M. (2004). Effects of *Morinda citrifolia* on quality of life and auditory function in postmenopausal women. *J Altern Complement Med* **10**(5), 737–739.

47. Seo, B. I., Ku, S. K., Cha, E. M., Park, J. H., Kim, J. D., Choi, H. Y. & Lee, H. S. (2005). Effect of *Mornidae radix* extracts on experimental osteoporosis in sciatic neurectomized mice. *Phytother Res* **19**(3), 231–238.

48. Saludes, J. P., Garson, M. J., Franzblau, S. G. & Aguinaldo, A. M. (2002). Antitubercular constituents from the hexane fraction of *Morinda citrifolia* Linn. Rubiaceae. *Phytother Res* **16**(7), 683–685.

49. Kamata, M., Wu, R. P., An, D. S., Saxe, J. P., Damoiseaux, R., Phelps, M. E., Huang, J. & Chen, I. S. (2006). Cell-based chemical genetic screen identifies damnacanthal as an inhibitor of HIV-1 Vpr induced cell death. *Biochem Biophys Res Commun* **348**(3), 1101–1106.

50. Matthews, A. K., Sellergren, S. A., Huo, D., List, M. & Fleming, G. (2007). Complementary and alternative medicine use among breast cancer survivors. *J Altern Complement Med* **13**(5), 555–562.

51. Hirazumi, A., Furusawa, E., Chou, S. C. & Hokama, Y. (1996). Immunomodulation contributes to the anticancer activity of *Morinda citrifolia* (noni) fruit juice. *Proc West Pharmacol Soc* **39**, 7–9.

52. Hirazumi, A. & Furusawa, E. (1999). An immunomodulatory polysaccharide-rich substance from the fruit juice of *Morinda citrifolia* (noni) with antitumour activity. *Phytother Res* **13**(5), 380–387.

53. Hirazumi, A., Furusawa, E., Chou, S. C. & Hokama, Y. (1994). Anticancer activity of *Morinda citrifolia* (noni) on intraperitoneally implanted Lewis lung carcinoma in syngeneic mice. *Proc West Pharmacol Soc* **37**, 145–146.

54. Furusawa, E., 2003. Anti-cancer Activity of Noni Fruit Juice Against Tumors in Mice. *Proceedings of the 2002 Hawaii Noni Conference.* University of Hawaii at Manoa, College of Tropical Agriculture and Human Resources.

55. Furusawa, E., Hirazumi, A., Story, S. & Jensen, J. (2003). Antitumour potential of a polysaccharide-rich substance from the fruit juice of *Morinda citrifolia* (noni) on sarcoma 180 ascites tumour in mice. *Phytother Res* **17**(10), 1158–1164.

56. Takashima, J., Ikeda, Y., Komiyama, K., Hayashi, M., Kishida, A. & Ohsaki, A. (2007). New constituents from the leaves of *Morinda citrifolia*. *Chem Pharm Bull (Tokyo)* **55**(2), 343–345.

57. Liu, G., Bode, A., Ma, W. Y., Sang, S., Ho, C. T. & Dong, Z. (2001). Two novel glycosides from the fruits of *Morinda citrifolia* (noni) inhibit AP-1 transactivation and cell transformation in the mouse epidermal JB6 cell line. *Cancer Res* **61**(15), 5749–5756.

58. Hornick, C. A., Myers, A., Sadowska-Krowicka, H., Anthony, C. T. & Woltering, E. A. (2003). Inhibition of angiogenic initiation and disruption of newly established human vascular networks by juice from *Morinda citrifolia* (noni). *Angiogenesis* **6**(2), 143–149.

59. Arpornsuwan, T. & Punjanon, T. (2006). Tumor cell-selective antiproliferative effect of the extract from *Morinda citrifolia* fruits. *Phytother Res* **20**(6), 515–517.

60. Wang, M. Y. & Su, C. (2001). Cancer preventive effect of *Morinda citrifolia* (noni). *Ann N Y Acad Sci* **952**, 161–168.

61. Wong, D. K. (2004). Are immune responses pivotal to cancer patient's long term survival? Two clinical case-study reports on the effects of *Morinda citrifolia* (Noni). *Hawaii Med J* **63**(6), 182–184.

62. Issell, B. F., Gotay, C., Pagano, I. & Franke, A. (2005). Quality of life measures in a phase I trial of noni. *J Clin Oncol. ASCO Annual Meeting Proceedings* **23**(16S), 8217.

63. Potterat, O. & Hamburger, M. (2007). *Morinda citrifolia* (Noni) fruit – phytochemistry, pharmacology, safety. *Planta Medica* **73**(3), 191–199.

64. Mueller, B. A., Scott, M. K., Sowinski, K. M. & Prag, K. A. (2000). Noni juice (*Morinda citrifolia*): Hidden potential for hyperkalemia? *Am J Kidney Dis* **35**(2), 310–312.

65. Millonig, G., Stadlmann, S. & Vogel, W. (2005). Herbal hepatotoxicity: Acute hepatitis caused by a noni preparation (*Morinda citrifolia*). *Eur J Gastroenterol Hepatol* **17**(4), 445–447.

66. Stadlbauer, V., Fickert, P., Lackner, C., Schmerlaib, J., Krisper, P., Trauner, M. & Stauber, R. E. (2005). Hepatotoxicity of NONI juice: Report of two cases. *World J Gastroenterol* **11**(30), 4758–4760.

67. Yuce, B., Gulberg, V., Diebold, J. & Gerbes, A. L. (2006). Hepatitis induced by Noni juice from *Morinda citrifolia*: A rare cause of hepatotoxicity or the tip of the iceberg? *Digestion* **73**(2–3), 167–170.

68. West, B. J., Tolson, C. B., Vest, R. G., Jensen, S. & Lundell, T. G. (2006). Mineral variability among 177 commercial noni juices. *Int J Food Sci* **57**(7/8), 556–558.

69. West, B. J., Jensen, C. J., Westendorf, J. & White, L. D. (2007). A safety review of noni fruit juice. *J Food Sci* **71**(8), R100–R106.

70. West, B. J., Jensen, C. J. & Westendorf, J. (2006). Noni juice is not hepatotoxic. *World J Gastroenterol* **12**(22), 3616–3619.

71. European Commission, Commission Decisions of 5 June 2003 authorizing the placing on the market of "noni juice" (juice of the fruit of *Morinda citrifolia* L.) as a novel food ingredient under Regulation (EC) Nr. 258/97 of the European Parliament and of the Council. *Official Journal of the European Union,* 2003; L 144/12:12.6.2003.

72. European Commission on Health and Consumer Protection Directorate-General. Opinion of the Scientific Committee on Food on Tahitian Noni Juice. Available at http://europa.eu.int/comm/food/fs/sc/scf/index_en.html.

73. Carr, M. E., Klotz, J. & Bergeron, M. (2004). Coumadin resistance and the vitamin supplement "Noni". *Am J Hematol* **77**(1), 103.

74. Nutescu, E. A., Shapiro, N. L., Ibrahim, S. & West, P. (2006). Warfarin and its interactions with foods, herbs and other dietary supplements. *Expert Opin Drug Saf* **5**(3), 433–451.

75. Wittkowsky, A. K. (2008). Dietary supplements, herbs and oral anticoagulants: The nature of the evidence. *J Thromb Thrombolysis* **25**(1), 72–77.

Chapter 15

Botanical Treatment for Polycystic Ovary Syndrome

Sidika E. Kasim-Karakas[1] and Susmita Mishra[2]

[1]*Division of Endocrinology, Clinical Nutrition and Vascular Medicine, Sacramento, CA, USA*
[2]*Diplomate: American Board of Internal Medicine, Women's Health Fellow, University of California, Davis Department of Obstetrics and Gynecology, CA, USA*

Keywords: *Botanicals, PCOS, insulin resistance, hirsutism, infertility*

CLINICAL CHARACTERISTICS OF THE PCOS PATIENTS

Polycystic ovary syndrome (PCOS) affects one out of 16 women. It is the most common endocrine disease affecting young women and the most common cause of anovulatory infertility [1, 2]. Approximately 6.8 million women in the USA have PCOS. The clinical abnormalities related to PCOS can be divided to two main categories: reproductive and metabolic. The reproductive abnormalities include anovulation which lead to oligomenorrhea, amenorrhea and infertility, and androgen excess which leads to hirsutism. The metabolic abnormalities include insulin resistance, obesity, dyslipidemia and hypertension [3]. In fact, 46% of the PCOS patients exhibit several of these disorders, thus fulfill the criteria for metabolic syndrome [4, 5]; 20% of the PCOS patients develop impaired glucose tolerance or type 2 diabetes before the age of 40 [6]. PCOS patients also have increased risk of premature cardiovascular disease [7, 8]. The natural course of PCOS is summarized in Fig. 15.1.

Since PCOS is a multi-faceted disease, at any given time, PCOS patients receive several medications to treat different aspects of the disease. The conventional medical approach is symptom oriented [9]. For example, oral contraceptives are used to regulate menstrual cycles and decrease hirsutism. The pharmaceuticals that block androgen receptors such as sprinolactone, or prevent the production of active forms of testosterone such as Finasteride, are also used to treat hirsutism. The insulin sensitizers, such as metformin, are prescribed to improve insulin sensitivity, help weight loss and improve lipid levels. A fascinating aspect of PCOS is that insulin sensitizers also increase

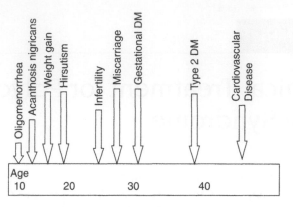

FIGURE 15.1   The natural course of PCOS.

TABLE 15.1 Potential Use of Botanicals in PCOS

PCOS				
Ovarian Dysfunction		**Metabolic Abnormalities**		
Anovulation	Androgen Excess	Insulin Resistance	Dyslipidemia	Inflammation
N-acetyl cysteine	Saw Palmetto	D Chiro-inositol	Fish oil	Fish oil
D Chiro-inositol	*Urtica diocia*	N-acetyl cysteine	Red rice yeast	Flax seed oil
Chaste berry-Vytex	N-acetyl cysteine	Chromium	D Chiro-inositol	
Flax seed	Quercetin	Magnesium	Curcumin	
White peony	*Pygeum africanum*	Fish oil		
Indole-3-carbinol	Curcumin	Cinnamon		
	Flax seed	Gymnema		
		Quercetin		
		White peony		
		Silybum marianum		

ovulation and fertility, and improve the success rate of ovulation inducers (i.e., clomiphene). Finally, hyperlipidemias may require specific treatment.

A similar goal-oriented approach can be applied to the use of botanicals as well. A number of botanicals that can improve ovarian function, androgen excess, obesity, insulin resistance, blood lipids and inflammation can exert beneficial effects in PCOS. Table 15.1 summarizes the botanicals that can potentially benefit PCOS patients.

Although the list of botanicals which can be used for PCOS is extensive, only a few of these have been directly tested in PCOS patients. Potential benefit has been extrapolated from other patient populations with similar reproductive or metabolic abnormalities. The botanicals and supplements reviewed in this chapter are those that are commonly recommended by complementary medicine providers and natural medicine websites. However it cannot be overemphasized that more prospective mechanistic and safety related data are necessary to refine the use of botanicals for PCOS.

TARGETED USE OF BOTANICALS FOR PCOS

Ovarian dysfunction

Anovulation

Polycystic ovary syndrome is the most common cause of anovulatory infertility. These patients fail to ovulate because normal ovulation requires the maturation of multiple follicles, followed by selection of the dominant follicle. In PCOS, multiple follicles start to maturate but there is a failure in the selection of the dominant follicle. This arrest in the ovulatory cycle results in the formation of multiple small cysts – giving the disease its name. Anovulation is usually associated with the decreased number of menses (oligomenorrhea) or no menses (amenorrhea). In addition, the stroma of the ovary is enlarged and the number of theca cells that produce the male hormone testosterone is increased. This leads to androgen excess and contributes to anovulation.

The incomplete follicular maturation and increased testosterone secretion are partly caused by the abnormalities in hypothalamic pituitary axis which result in excess production of luteinizing hormone (LH) and deficient production of follicle-stimulating hormone (FSH) [9]. Secretion of LH vs. FSH from the pituitary is regulated by the pulse frequency of the hypothalamic gonadotropin-releasing hormone (GnRH). Increased pulse frequency favors secretion of LH-β subunit. In contrast, decreased pulse frequency favors transcription of FSH-β subunit. PCOS patients exhibit increased GnRH pulse frequency leading to preferential LH synthesis. The cause of this abnormality is unknown.

In the ovaries, FSH stimulates the maturation of the follicles and estrogen production in the granulosa cell while LH stimulates the secretion of androgens from the ovarian theca cells. Consequently, increased LH to FSH ratio promotes the androgen synthesis and interferes with normal follicle maturation and ovulation.

Importantly, insulin acts synergistically with LH to enhance the androgen production of theca cells. In addition, insulin inhibits hepatic synthesis of sex hormone-binding globulin (SHBG), the key circulating protein that binds to testosterone. Thus, the unbound bioavailable fraction of testosterone increases. Reducing circulating insulin levels by various means improves ovarian function, increase ovulation and fertility [10–15].

The traditional treatments for inducing ovulation and increasing fertility include clomiphene (a selective estrogen receptor modulator) and insulin sensitizers (such as metformin or thiozalidinediones).

Botanical treatments can be used either by themselves or in combination with the traditional treatments. They increase ovulation either by regulating the hypothalamic pituitary function or by reducing insulin resistance. The botanicals that have been used for this purpose are as follows:

i. *N-acetyl cysteine* (NAC): It is a derivative of the amino acid cysteine and is a well recognized antioxidant. A recent study demonstrated that NAC effectively augmented ovulation in PCOS patients when given in conjunction with clomiphene, as compared to clomiphene alone [16]. Patients were given clomiphene citrate 50 mg tablets twice daily alone or with NAC 1200 mg/day orally for 5 days starting on day 3 of the menstrual cycle. The ovulation rate significantly improved with the addition of NAC (17.9% vs. 52%) as well as serum progesterone levels and endometrial thickness. The success of NAC may depend upon the severity of the disease: In a clomiphene-resistant PCOS population, addition of NAC did not increase ovulation while metformin increased ovulation significantly [17].

ii. **d Chiro-inositol**: It is a relative of inositol which is manufactured through the breakdown of phytic acids found in vegetables, fruits, legumes, whole grains (especially buckwheat) and nuts. It is a phosphoglycan mediator of the insulin action. A study reported that insulin resistant PCOS patients had low inositol levels; and d chiro-inositol supplementation reduced insulin resistance and plasma testosterone levels [18]. A prospective study randomized 44 PCOS patients to 1200 mg of d chiro-inositol or placebo daily for 6 or 8 weeks. Nineteen of the 22 (86%) patients in the d chiro-inositol group ovulated during treatment as compared with 6 of the 22 (27%) patients in the placebo group [19]. Presently d chiro-inositol is unavailable in a drug or supplement form. Inositol and Pinitol are available; and both have been reported to reduce blood glucose at doses of 200 mg and 600 mg twice daily, respectively. In another placebo controlled study, 136 PCOS women who took inositol had significantly higher ovulation frequency [20]. Although these supplements are generally considered safe, inositol can signal activation of serotonin receptors and could theoretically worsen manic or bipolar disorder and should not be used in conjunction with selective serotonin reuptake inhibitors (SSRI drugs) and 5-hydroxytryptamine receptor agonists.

iii. **Chaste berry**: Vitex is a standardized supplement containing the extract and pure dried powder of the whole fruit of the chaste tree plant (*Vitex agnus-castus*). It is considered to be a hormone modulator and widely used in correcting irregular menses and improving premenstrual syndrome. Vitex can increase progesterone by regulating LH release and inhibit the release of prolactin by acting as a dopaminergic agent. In a study, 93 women who had tried to conceive for 6–36 months were given a supplement containing chaste berry, L arginine, vitamins and minerals; progesterone level, menstrual cycle length, pregnancy rate and side effects were documented. After 3 months, the supplementation group demonstrated increased mid-luteal progesterone and normalized menstrual cycles compared to no significant changes in the placebo group [21]. Fourteen out of the 53 women who received the supplementation became pregnant as compared to 4 of the 40 women who received the placebo. Three other women in the supplement group conceived after 6 months. The recommended dose is 1–4 ml of a 1:2 dried plant tincture of 500–1000 mg of dried berries daily.

iv. **Flaxseed**: Flax and soy products contain significant amounts of phytoestrogens [22]. They are particularly good sources of isoflavones and lignans (the main classes of phytoestrogens found in the human diet). The structure of phytoestrogens is similar to the estrogen/antiestrogen tamoxifen. Asian women have been found to have menstrual cycle length 2–3 days longer than Western women which may be due to the larger consumption of phytoestrogens in their diet [23]. However studies directly comparing flaxseed intake and menstrual cycle length have not been statistically significant. Based on these observations, 1–2 tablespoons of ground flax seed or 1–2 capsule of flax lignan 78 mg/day have been recommended.

v. **White peony**: Paeoniliflorin is derived from the dried root of *Paenoia lactiflora Pall.* A number of effects have been attributed to Paeonia including elevating progesterone and lowering androgens. *In vitro* studies demonstrated an increase in the aromatase enzyme activity, which is responsible for converting testosterone to estrogen, and consequently decreased testosterone levels. A study from Japan found that Unkei-to, which contains paeonia, stimulates both estrogen and progesterone secretion in human granulosa cells suggesting stimulatory effects on both steroideogenesis and the ovulatory process within the ovary [24]. In a Japanese clinical trial involving 34 PCOS women, a formula containing *Glycyrrhiza glabra* and *Paeonia lactiflora* (Shakuyaku-Kanzo-To™) was added to the regular diet for 12 weeks. In those women who became pregnant, the mean serum testosterone levels were decreased by 35% from the baseline, whereas those who did not become pregnant testosterone did not change [25]. In a clinical trial in China, the same formula was given to 20 PCOS women; testosterone levels decreased in 90% of the subjects; and 25% them conceived. The daily dose for Paeonia used ranged between 4.5 and 9 ml of a 1:2 dried plant extract.

vi. **Indole-3-carbinol (I-3-C)**: It is isolated from cruciferous vegetables increases the 2-hydroxylation of estrogens. Although I-3-C exhibits both estrogenic and anti-estrogenic properties in animal models, its effects on ovulation and fertility have not been studied in humans [26].

Androgen Excess/Hirsutism

In PCOS, ovaries produce excess testosterone. In addition, SHBG which binds the testosterone in the circulation is decreased [27]. Consequently, a larger fraction of testosterone is biologically available. Blood levels of SHBG correlates inversely with insulin sensitivity; thus insulin resistant individuals have low SHBG levels [27]. At the hair follicles, testosterone binds to the androgen receptor and then it is converted to the more active form dihydro testosterone (DHT). The androgen excess causes male pattern hair distribution: excess facial and body hair along with scalp hair loss.

The conventional treatment for androgen excess comprise oral contraceptives which suppress ovarian testosterone production and increase SHBG; spironolactone which blocks the binding of testosterone to the androgen receptor; and Finastride which inhibits the conversion of testosterone to DHT [28]. There are botanical treatments with similar actions. These include:

i. **Saw Palmetto**: Saw Palmetto is a berry found on the palm tree (*Serenoa repens*). It is widely used for the treatment of benign prostatic hypertrophy because it inhibits 5 reductase enzyme which converts testosterone to DHT [29–31]. Thus, saw palmetto can reduce the clinical consequences of testosterone excess such as hirsutism, male pattern balding and acne. Despite the lack of controlled studies of saw palmetto in PCOS patients, it is widely used with anecdotal good results and without side effects. A common starting dose is 320 mg one capsule a day with the option of increasing to two capsules later on.

ii. **Urtica dioica**: It is more commonly known as stinging nettle. The roots of the nettle contain a mixture of compounds including lectins, phenols, sterols and lignans. *Uritica dioica* has been used in the treatment of benign prostate hypertrophy because it inhibits the binding of SHBG to its receptor and thereby increases the availability of SHBG to bind testosterone [32–34]. Dosages of 50–200 mg are given daily. Although *Urtica dioica* has not been clinically tested in PCOS patients, it is conceivable that increased SHBG activity can increase the binding of the excess androgen and help to alleviate hirsutism, acne and male pattern baldness.

iii. **N-acetyl-cysteine**: which has been outlined in the previous section, has been shown to decrease total testosterone levels and free androgen index at the doses between 1.8 and 3 g/day, over a 6-week period [35].

iv. **Quercetin**: It is a flavonoid found in onions, grapes and green vegetables and exerts anti-proliferative effects against various malignant cells by decreasing insulin like growth factor (IGF)1. A study investigating the secretion of IGF1 and IGF-binding protein in human prostate cells showed that quercetin treatment decreased IGF and increased IGF-binding protein levels [36]. IGF1 also stimulates testosterone production in the ovarian stroma [37]. Thus it is conceivable that quercetin may inhibit secretion of testosterone by interfering with the effect of IGF1 on the ovarian stroma.

v. *Pygeum africanum*: It is extracted from the bark of the African plum tree. In Europe it has been used for prevention and treatment of benign prostate hypertrophy. The dosage used in trials is 25 mg daily. It is thought to act by reducing prolactin levels and by acting on the sex steroid hormone receptors [38]. As with many of the botanicals, more prospective studies are needed to assess its benefits.

vi. **Curcumin**: It is a polyphenolic compound found in the spice turmeric. In the human prostate cancer cell lines, curcumin has exhibited potent anti-androgen activity [39]. The mechanism of action was novel because curcumin behaved like 17α-substituted DTH. Thus it is speculated that curcumin may have a role in alleviating the androgen excess in PCOS.

vii. **Flax seed**: As stated previously, flaxseed is a good source of phytoestrogens, specifically lignans and isoflavones, which may stimulate the synthesis of SHBG. It has been reported that urinary lignan concentrations correlate directly with serum SHBG levels [23]. However, small intervention trials failed to show any significant increase in SHBG or consistent changes in sex steroids with flax seed supplementation [22, 40]. Effects of flax lignans on PCOS have not been tested.

Metabolic Abnormalities

Obesity

In the USA the majority of PCOS patients are obese. Relatively modest weight loss, approximately 6% of the original weight, improves fertility in PCOS [41, 42]. Thus, the botanicals that facilitate weight loss can be extremely useful in PCOS. These botanicals are discussed in another chapter in this book.

Insulin Resistance

Recognition of insulin resistance as a common characteristic of PCOS has revolutionized the management of PCOS. It is now well accepted that the insulin sensitizers used for treating diabetic patients, such as metformin or thiozalidinediones, can be prescribed to reduce insulin resistance in PCOS [43–45]. Nondiabetic PCOS patients can also use these agents because insulin sensitizers do not cause hypoglycemia. Furthermore, insulin sensitizers improve the ovarian function; regulate menstrual cycles and increase ovulation and fertility. In addition, metformin can facilitate weight loss whereas thiozalidinediones can cause weight gain [46]. Metformin can also prevent miscarriages and is safe during pregnancy [47–50].

The success of insulin sensitizers in PCOS lead to the use of the botanicals with similar effects. These agents are as follows:

i. **d Chiro-inositol**: The action and potential benefits of d chiro-inositol has been outlined earlier in the section under anovulation/Infertility.

ii. *N*-acetyl–cysteine: In a study including 6 lean and 31 obese PCOS subjects, supplementation with 1.8–3g/day of NAC was associated with no change in glucose area under the curve (AUC). However, the insulin AUC was decreased in hyperinsulinemic patients, indicating increased insulin sensitivity in this population [35]. Thus, NAC can be used to reduce insulin resistance in PCOS.

iii. **Chromium**: It has been widely studied in the treatment of hyperglycemia. The results have been variable depending on the type of chromium and the dose: In hyperglycemic subjects on a low chromium diet, supplementation with 200 mcg chromium improved glucose tolerance and circulating insulin levels, whereas normoglycemic subjects did not benefit from chromium supplementation [51]. A recent study which investigated the effects of 1000 mcg of chromium piconilate supplementation on insulin sensitivity in obese PCOS women reported a significant improvement in the glucose disposal rate [52].

iv. **Magnesium**: Low serum magnesium (Mg) as well as high ionized calcium (Ca) to magnesium ratio has been associated with insulin resistance and diabetes mellitus. A study assessing the cation profile of PCOS patients compared with control women found significantly lower serum Mg and higher Ca/Mg ratio in PCOS patients [53]. However there was no correlation between these minerals and the steroid hormones (estrogen, progesterone and testosterone) in the PCOS women or controls.

v. **Fish oils**: These comprise omega-3 (*n*-3) polyunsaturated fatty acids (PUFAs), specifically eicosapentanoic acid (EPA) and docosahexanoic acid (DHA). These PUFAs are used preferentially for energy production and increase glycogen storage. A large body of evidence indicates that fish oils reverse insulin resistance caused by high-fat or sucrose feeding by reducing adipocyte cell size and the release of fatty acids from the adipose tissue. The decrease in circulating fatty acid levels facilitates the glucose utilization in the muscle and improves whole-body insulin sensitivity [54–56]. Effects of fish oils on insulin resistance in PCOS patients are currently under investigation.

vi. **Cinnamon**: This spice has traditionally been recommended for type 2 diabetes mellitus. Patient with type 1 diabetes do not benefit from cinnamon [57]. According to a recent literature search, three prospective, placebo controlled, peer reviewed clinical trials evaluated the effect of cinnamon supplementation in type 2 diabetes: Two studies reported modest decrease in blood glucose, while one study showed no significant change [58]. Although there is no established effective dose, the doses commonly used range between 1 and 4 g of cinnamon powder or 200 and 300 mg of cinnamon extract. Effects of cinnamon were also studied in a small number of PCOS patients. Daily ingestion of 1000 mg of cinnamon for 8 weeks improved glucose response during oral glucose tolerance test (OGTT) and the insulin resistance parameters in PCOS [59].

vii. **Gymnema**: It is an ayurvedic herb used as antidiabetic, hypoglycemic, and lipid lowering agent. Gymnemic acid, isolated from the leaves of the herb, alters the perception of taste buds for sweets. It also inhibits the glycosidase enzyme in the intestine and reduces the absorption of glucose [60]. The daily dose of Gymnema used is 3.5–11 ml of the extract.

viii. **Quercetin**: Although quercetin has been studied for the treatment of neuropathy in diabetes, there has been no evidence to suggest beneficial effects on either blood glucose or insulin resistance. Its effects on IGF1 have been outlined under the Androgen excess section of this chapter.

ix. **White peony**: There is limited evidence suggesting that Paeonia may lower glucose in the setting of insulin resistance. This may be the mechanism underlying its beneficial effects on ovulation – as discussed earlier.

x. *Silybum marianum*: More commonly known as milk thistle, has numerous therapeutic properties. A randomized double-blinded study which compared silybum (200 mg 3 times daily) to placebo in 51 type 2 diabetic patients showed significant decreases in glycosylated hemoglobin (HbA1c), fasting blood glucose, total cholesterol, LDL-cholesterol, triglyceride and the liver enzymes [61]. The more common use of this botanical has been in liver disorders. Due to its antioxidant properties, silybum exerts anti-proliferative effects on the liver cells, suggesting a potential hepato-protective effect [62]. Since fatty liver is common in PCOS [63–66], this botanical may be beneficial in this population.

Dyslipidemia

Approximately 50% of the PCOS patients fulfill the criteria for the Metabolic Syndrome and are at risk for cardiovascular disease [4, 5, 8, 67, 68]. Thus, management of PCOS goes beyond addressing the ovulatory function and infertility, and involves management of long-term health risks. The most common lipoprotein abnormality seen in PCOS is dyslipidemia which is characterized by high plasma triglyceride and low HDL-cholesterol. Some patients have mixed hyperlipidemia characterized by elevations of triglyceride and cholesterol. The following botanicals can be used to treat these disorders:

i. **Fish oils**: Fish oils have potent triglyceride lowering effects. They act through a dual mechanism: Fish oils decrease lipogenesis by decreasing sterol regulatory element binding protein (SREBP) production by the liver X receptor (LXR). They also increase peroxisomal β-oxidation of the fatty acids by regulating peroxisome proliferator-activated receptor (PPAR) α [69]. Although the traditional lipid risk factor for atherogenesis is the LDL-cholesterol, recent research has underlined the importance of elevated triglyceride concentrations in cardiovascular disease. Omega-3 fatty acids in doses of 2–4 g/day can lower serum triglyceride by approximately 25–30% within 4 weeks of treatment [70–72]. It should be mentioned however that fish oils also cause a small increase in LDL-cholesterol [70, 72]. So far, there is no evidence to suggest that the increase in LDL-cholesterol caused by fish oils leads to an increase in cardiac events. In addition, when added to the statins, fish oils cause further reduction in triglyceride, suggesting a complementary mechanism of action [73].

ii. **Red rice yeast**: It is produced by cultivating the fungus *Monascus purpureus* on polished rice. It contains several substances including sterols, monounsaturated fats, isoflavones and mevinolin. Mevinolin is a potent inhibitor of the HMG CoA reductase, and in fact, it is marketed as the prescription medication Lovastatin. A recent meta analysis including 93 randomized controlled trials reported significant decreases in total cholesterol with red rice yeast. [74]. Notably, there was no statistically significant differences in total cholesterol lowering, LDL lowering and HDL increasing effects of the two red rice yeast preparations (*Xuezhikang* 1.2 g/day or *Zhibituo* 3.15 g/day) vs. 10–20 mg/day doses of simvastatin, pravastatin, atorvastatin or fluvastatin. As compared to fibrates, red rice yeast preparations were more effective in lowering in LDL, less effective in lowering triglyceride and equally effective in increasing HDL. Across the trials red rice yeast was more potent in improving all lipid parameters as compared to inositol, fish oil, and conjugated estrogen. Seventy-seven trials reported adverse effects outcomes, the most common being dizziness, decreased appetite, back ache, abdominal distention and diarrhea. A small number of patients had elevated in serum blood urea nitrogen and liver enzymes. Since the active component of red rice yeast is identical to a prescription medicine, the Food and Drug Administration has recently issued a warning regarding the use of red rice yeast [75].

iii. **d Chiro-inositol**: As discussed above this compound improves several metabolic abnormalities and ovulatory function in PCOS women. The report in the New England Journal of Medicine (NEJM) indicated that PCOS women supplemented with d chiro-inositol had a significant decrease in the plasma triglyceride as compared to the placebo [19]. Although total cholesterol also decreased from the baseline level, this decrease was similar to that seen with the placebo group. High density lipoprotein- and LDL-cholesterol concentrations did not change.

iv. **Curcumin**: which was described under the androgen excess section has also been studied for its potential benefits on the lipid profile. The are conflicting data showing both a modest increase and a decrease in total-cholesterol without any change in HDL-cholesterol [76].

Inflammation

The circulating inflammatory markers such as C-reactive protein (CRP), interleukin (IL)-6, tumor necrosis factor (TNF) α are considered non-traditional risk factors for cardiovascular disease. Women with PCOS have increased inflammatory markers in the circulation [77, 78]. It is not clear however whether this increase is related directly to PCOS or a consequence of obesity which commonly accompanies PCOS [79].

Fish and flax seed oils may be used to reduce inflammation in PCOS because the prostaglandins and leukotrienes produced from omega-3 polyunsaturated fatty acids have anti-inflammatory effects [80]. However, there is evidence to suggest that these oils may not be very effective *in vivo* for reducing inflammation [81].

In summary, several botanicals and supplements listed above are used as complementary and alternative treatments for PCOS. The use of some these agents is supported by well designed trials. On the other hand, several products are being used based on the speculated benefits. At the present there is little information regarding the safety profile of these treatments and their interactions with conventional treatments. These limitations should not cast a shadow over these agents but rather emphasize the need for continued research to understand the mechanistic reasons for the apparent benefits of these agents in the treatment of PCOS.

REFERENCES

1. Dunaif, A. & Thomas, A. (2001). Current concepts in the polycystic ovary syndrome. *Annu Rev Med* **52**, 401–419.
2. Legro, R. S. (2001). Polycystic ovary syndrome: The new millenium. *Mol Cell Endocrinol* **184**, 87–93.
3. Legro, R. S., Kunselman, A. R. & Dunaif, A. (2001). Prevalence and predictors of dyslipidemia in women with polycystic ovary syndrome. *Am J Med* **111**, 607–613.
4. Ehrmann, D. A., Liljenquist, D. R., Kasza, K., Azziz, R., Legro, R. S. & Ghazzi, M. N. (2006). Prevalence and predictors of the metabolic syndrome in women with polycystic ovary syndrome. *J Clin Endocrinol Metab* **91**, 48–53.
5. Glueck, C. J., Papanna, R., Wang, P., Goldenberg, N. & Sieve-Smith, L. (2003). Incidence and treatment of metabolic syndrome in newly referred women with confirmed polycystic ovarian syndrome. *Metabolism* **52**, 908–915.
6. Legro, R. S., Kunselman, A. R., Dodson, W. C. & Dunaif, A. (1999). Prevalence and predictors of risk for type 2 diabetes mellitus and impaired glucose tolerance in polycystic ovary syndrome: A prospective, controlled study in 254 affected women. *J Clin Endocrinol Metab* **84**, 165–169.
7. Talbott, E. O., Zborowskii, J. V. & Boudraux, M. Y. (2004). Do women with polycystic ovary syndrome have an increased risk of cardiovascular disease? Review of the evidence. *Minerva Ginecol* **56**, 27–39.
8. Shroff, R., Kerchner, A., Maifeld, M., Van Beek, E. J., Jagasia, D. & Dokras, A. (2007). Young obese women with polycystic ovary syndrome have evidence of early coronary atherosclerosis. *J Clin Endocrinol Metab* **92**, 4609–4614.
9. Ehrmann, D. (2005). Polycystic ovary syndrome. *N Engl J Med*, 1223–1236.
10. Park, K. H., Kim, J. Y., Ahn, C. W., Song, Y. D., Lim, S. K. & Lee, H. C. (2001). Polycystic ovarian syndrome (PCOS) and insulin resistance. *Int J Gynaecol Obstet* **74**, 261–267.

11. Nestler, J. E., Stovall, D., Akhter, N., Iuorno, M. J. & Jakubowicz, D. J. (2002). Strategies for the use of insulin-sensitizing drugs to treat infertility in women with polycystic ovary syndrome. *Fertil Steril* **77**, 209–215.

12. Dunaif, A., Scott, D., Finegood, D., Quintana, B. & Whitcomb, R. (1996). The insulin-sensitizing agent troglitazone improves metabolic and reproductive abnormalities in the polycystic ovary syndrome. *J Clin Endocrinol Metab* **81**, 3299–3306.

13. Azziz, R., Ehrmann, D., Legro, R. S. *et al.* (2001). Troglitazone improves ovulation and hirsutism in the polycystic ovary syndrome: A multicenter, double blind, placebo-controlled trial. *J Clin Endocrinol Metab* **86**, 1626–1632.

14. Majuri, A., Santaniemi, M. & Rautio, K. *et al.* (2007). Rosiglitazone treatment increases plasma levels of adiponectin and decreases levels of resistin in overweight women with PCOS: A randomized placebo-controlled study. *Eur J Endocrinol* **156**, 263–269.

15. Cheang, K. I., Sharma, S. T. & Nestler, J. E. (2006). Is metformin a primary ovulatory agent in patients with polycystic ovary syndrome? *Gynecol Endocrinol* **22**, 595–604.

16. Badawy, A., State, O. & Abdelgawad, S. (2007). N-Acetyl cysteine and clomiphene citrate for induction of ovulation in polycystic ovary syndrome: A cross-over trial. *Acta Obstet Gynecol Scand* **86**, 218–222.

17. Elnashar, A., Fahmy, M., Mansour, A. & Ibrahim, K. (2007). N-acetyl cysteine vs. metformin in treatment of clomiphene citrate-resistant polycystic ovary syndrome: A prospective randomized controlled study. *Fertil Steril* **88**, 406–409.

18. Kennington, A. S., Hill, C. R., Craig, J. et al. (1990). Low urinary chiro-inositol excretion in non-insulin-dependent diabetes mellitus. *N Engl J Med* **323**, 373–378.

19. Nestler, J. E., Jakubowicz, D. J., Reamer, P., Gunn, R. D. & Allan, G. (1999). Ovulatory and metabolic effects of D-chiro-inositol in the polycystic ovary syndrome. *N Engl J Med* **340**, 1314–1320.

20. Gerli, S., Mignosa, M. & Di Renzo, G. C. (2003). Effects of inositol on ovarian function and metabolic factors in women with PCOS: A randomized double blind placebo-controlled trial. *Eur Rev Med Pharmacol Sci* **7**, 151–159.

21. Westphal, L. M., Polan, M. L. & Trant, A. S. (2006). Double-blind, placebo-controlled study of Fertilityblend: A nutritional supplement for improving fertility in women. *Clin Exp Obstet Gynecol* **33**, 205–208.

22. Phipps, W. R., Martini, M. C., Lampe, J. W., Slavin, J. L. & Kurzer, M. S. (1993). Effect of flax seed ingestion on the menstrual cycle. *J Clin Endocrinol Metab* **77**, 1215–1219.

23. Tham, D. M., Gardner, C. D. & Haskell, W. L. (1998). Clinical review 97: Potential health benefits of dietary phytoestrogens: A review of the clinical, epidemiological, and mechanistic evidence. *J Clin Endocrinol Metab* **83**, 2223–2235.

24. Sun, W. S., Imai, A., Tagami, K., Sugiyama, M., Furui, T. & Tamaya, T. (2004). *In vitro* stimulation of granulosa cells by a combination of different active ingredients of unkei-to. *Am J Chin Med* **32**, 569–578.

25. Takahashi, K. & Kitao, M. (1994). Effect of TJ-68 (shakuyaku-kanzo-to) on polycystic ovarian disease. *Int J Fertil Menopausal Stud* **39**, 69–76.

26. Rogan, E. G. (2006). The natural chemopreventive compound indole-3-carbinol: State of the science. *In Vivo* **20**, 221–228.

27. Jayagopal, V., Kilpatrick, E. S., Jennings, P. E., Hepburn, D. A. & Atkin, S. L. (2003). The biological variation of testosterone and sex hormone-binding globulin (SHBG) in polycystic ovarian syndrome: Implications for SHBG as a surrogate marker of insulin resistance. *J Clin Endocrinol Metab* **88**, 1528–1533.

28. Koulouri, O. & Conway, G. S. (2007). A systematic review of commonly used medical treatments for hirsutism in women. *Clin Endocrinol (Oxf).*

29. Dimitrakov, J. D. (2006). Saw palmetto for benign prostatic hyperplasia. *N Engl J Med* **354**, 1950–1951.

30. Casner, P. R. (2006). Saw palmetto for benign prostatic hyperplasia. *N Engl J Med* **354**, 1950–1951.

31. Yang, J. & Te, A. E. (2005). Saw palmetto and finasteride in the treatment of category-III prostatitis/chronic pelvic pain syndrome. *Curr Urol Rep* **6**, 290–295.

32. Hryb, D. J., Khan, M. S., Romas, N. A. & Rosner, W. (1995). The effect of extracts of the roots of the stinging nettle (Urtica dioica) on the interaction of SHBG with its receptor on human prostatic membranes. *Planta Med* **61**, 31–32.

33. Schottner, M., Gansser, D. & Spiteller, G. (1997). Interaction of lignans with human sex hormone binding globulin (SHBG). *Z Naturforsch [C]* **52**, 834–843.

34. Schottner, M., Gansser, D. & Spiteller, G. (1997). Lignans from the roots of Urtica dioica and their metabolites bind to human sex hormone binding globulin (SHBG). *Planta Med* **63**, 529–532.

35. Fulghesu, A. M., Ciampelli, M. & Muzj, G.etal. (2002). N-acetyl-cysteine treatment improves insulin sensitivity in women with polycystic ovary syndrome. *Fertil Steril* **77**, 1128–1135.

36. Vijayababu, M. R., Arunkumar, A., Kanagaraj, P. & Arunakaran, J. (2006). Effects of quercetin on insulin-like growth factors (IGFs) and their binding protein-3 (IGFBP-3) secretion and induction of apoptosis in human prostate cancer cells. *J Carcinog* **5**, 10.

37. Qin, K. N. & Rosenfield, R. L. (1998). Role of cytochrome P450c17 in polycystic ovary syndrome. *Mol Cell Endocrinol* **145**, 111–121.

38. Melo, E. A., Bertero, E. B., Rios, L. A. & Mattos, D., Jr. (2002). Evaluating the efficiency of a combination of Pygeum africanum and stinging nettle (Urtica dioica) extracts in treating benign prostatic hyperplasia (BPH): Double-blind, randomized, placebo controlled trial. *Int Braz J Urol* **28**, 418–425.

39. Ohtsu, H., Xiao, Z., Ishida, J. *et al.* (2002). Antitumor agents. 217. Curcumin analogues as novel androgen receptor antagonists with potential as anti-prostate cancer agents. *J Med Chem* **45**, 5037–5042.

40. Hutchins, A. M., Martini, M. C., Olson, B. A., Thomas, W. & Slavin, J. L. (2001). Flaxseed consumption influences endogenous hormone concentrations in postmenopausal women. *Nutr Cancer* **39**, 58–65.

41. Norman, R. J., Davies, M. J., Lord, J. & Moran, L. J. (2002). The role of lifestyle modification in polycystic ovary syndrome. *Trends Endocrinol Metab* **13**, 251–257.

42. Norman, R. J., Homan, G., Moran, L. & Noakes, M. (2006). Lifestyle choices, diet, and insulin sensitizers in polycystic ovary syndrome. *Endocrine* **30**, 35–43.

43. Conway, G. S. (2000). Hyperinsulinaemia and polycystic ovary syndrome. *Hum Fertil (Camb)* **3**, 93–95.

44. Dunaif, A., Xia, J., Book, C. B., Schenker, E. & Tang, Z. (1995). Excessive insulin receptor serine phosphorylation in cultured fibroblasts and in skeletal muscle.

A potential mechanism for insulin resistance in the polycystic ovary syndrome. *J Clin Invest* **96**, 801–810.

45. Dunaif, A. (1997). Insulin resistance and the polycystic ovary syndrome: mechanism and implications for pathogenesis. *Endocr Rev* **18**, 774–800.

46. Mitkov, M., Pehlivanov, B. & Terzieva, D. (2006). Metformin versus rosiglitazone in the treatment of polycystic ovary syndrome. *Eur J Obstet Gynecol Reprod Biol* **126**, 93–98.

47. Vandermolen, D. T., Ratts, V. S., Evans, W. S., Stovall, D. W., Kauma, S. W. & Nestler, J. E. (2001). Metformin increases the ovulatory rate and pregnancy rate from clomiphene citrate in patients with polycystic ovary syndrome who are resistant to clomiphene citrate alone. *Fertil Steril* **75**, 310–315.

48. Nestler, J. E. (2006). Is metformin or clomiphene citrate more effective for ovulation induction in polycystic ovary syndrome? *Nat Clin Pract Endocrinol Metab* **2**, 128–129.

49. Jakubowicz, D. J., Iuorno, M. J., Jakubowicz, S., Roberts, K. A. & Nestler, J. E. (2002). Effects of metformin on early pregnancy loss in the polycystic ovary syndrome. *J Clin Endocrinol Metab* **87**, 524–529.

50. Glueck, C. J., Wang, P., Kobayashi, S., Phillips, H. & Sieve-Smith, L. (2002). Metformin therapy throughout pregnancy reduces the development of gestational diabetes in women with polycystic ovary syndrome. *Fertil Steril* **77**, 520–525.

51. Anderson, R. A., Polansky, M. M., Bryden, N. A. & Canary, J. J. (1991). Supplemental-chromium effects on glucose, insulin, glucagon, and urinary chromium losses in subjects consuming controlled low-chromium diets. *Am J Clin Nutr* **54**, 909–916.

52. Lydic, M. L., McNurlan, M., Bembo, S., Mitchell, L., Komaroff, E. & Gelato, M. (2006). Chromium picolinate improves insulin sensitivity in obese subjects with polycystic ovary syndrome. *Fertil Steril* **86**, 243–246.

53. Muneyyirci-Delale, O., Nacharaju, V. L., Dalloul, M. *et al.* (2001). Divalent cations in women with PCOS: Implications for cardiovascular disease. *Gynecol Endocrinol* **15**, 198–201.

54. Kasim-Karakas, S. (2007). *Omega-3 Fatty Acids and Insulin Resistance*, CRC Press LLC, Boca Raton, FL.

55. Lombardo, Y. B., Hein, G. & Chicco, A. (2007). Metabolic syndrome: Effects of n-3 PUFAs on a model of dyslipidemia, insulin resistance and adiposity. *Lipids* **42**, 427–437.

56. Storlien, L. H., Higgins, J. A., Thomas, T. C. et al. (2000). Diet composition and insulin action in animal models. *Br J Nutr* **83**(Suppl 1), S85–S90.

57. Altschuler, J. A., Casella, S. J., MacKenzie, T. A. & Curtis, K. M. (2007). The effect of cinnamon on A1C among adolescents with type 1 diabetes. *Diabetes Care* **30**, 813–816.

58. Pham, A. Q., Kourlas, H. & Pham, D. Q. (2007). Cinnamon supplementation in patients with type 2 diabetes mellitus. *Pharmacotherapy* **27**, 595–599.

59. Wang, J. G., Anderson, R. A., Graham, G. M., 3rd. et al. (2007). The effect of cinnamon extract on insulin resistance parameters in polycystic ovary syndrome: A pilot study. *Fertil Steril* **88**, 240–243.

60. Kimura, I. (2006). Medical benefits of using natural compounds and their derivatives having multiple pharmacological actions. *Yakugaku Zasshi* **126**, 133–143.

61. Huseini, H. F., Larijani, B., Heshmat, R. *et al.* (2006). The efficacy of Silybum marianum (L,) Gaertn. (silymarin) in the treatment of type II diabetes: A randomized, double-blind, placebo-controlled, clinical trial. *Phytother Res* **20**, 1036–1039.

62. Gebhardt, R. (2003). Antioxidative, antiproliferative and biochemical effects in HepG2 cells of a homeopathic remedy and its constituent plant tinctures tested separately or in combination. *Arzneimittelforschung* **53**, 823–830.

63. Brown, A. J., Tendler, D. A., McMurray, R. G. & Setji, T. L. (2005). Polycystic ovary syndrome and severe nonalcoholic steatohepatitis: Beneficial effect of modest weight loss and exercise on liver biopsy findings. *Endocr Pract* **11**, 319–324.

64. Cerda, C., Perez-Ayuso, R. M., Riquelme, A. *et al.* (2007). Nonalcoholic fatty liver disease in women with polycystic ovary syndrome. *J Hepatol* **47**, 412–417.

65. Gambarin-Gelwan, M., Kinkhabwala, S. V., Schiano, T. D., Bodian, C., Yeh, H. C. & Futterweit, W. (2007). Prevalence of nonalcoholic fatty liver disease in women with polycystic ovary syndrome. *Clin Gastroenterol Hepatol* **5**, 496–501.

66. Setji, T. L., Holland, N. D., Sanders, L. L., Pereira, K. C., Diehl, A. M. & Brown, A. J. (2006). Nonalcoholic steatohepatitis and nonalcoholic Fatty liver disease in young women with polycystic ovary syndrome. *J Clin Endocrinol Metab* **91**, 1741–1747.

67. Essah, P. A. & Nestler, J. E. (2006). Metabolic syndrome in women with polycystic ovary syndrome. *Fertil Steril* **86**(Suppl 1), S18–S19.

68. Shroff, R., Syrop, C. H., Davis, W., Van Voorhis, B. J. & Dokras, A. (2007). Risk of metabolic complications in the new PCOS phenotypes based on the Rotterdam criteria. *Fertil Steril* **88**, 1389–1395.

69. Kasim-Karakas, S. (2007). *Omega-3 Fatty Acids and Lipoprotein Metabolism*, CRC Press LLC, Boca Raton, FL.

70. Kasim, S. E., Stern, B., Khilnani, S., McLin, P., Baciorowski, S. & Jen, K. L. (1988). Effects of omega-3 fish oils on lipid metabolism, glycemic control, and blood pressure in type II diabetic patients. *J Clin Endocrinol Metab* **67**, 1–5.

71. Kasim-Karakas, S. E. (1995). Impact of n-3 fatty acids on lipoprotein metabolism. *Curr Opin Lipidol* **6**, 167–171.

72. Kasim-Karakas, S. E., Herrmann, R. & Almario, R. (1995). Effects of omega-3 fatty acids on intravascular lipolysis of very-low-density lipoproteins in humans. *Metabolism* **44**, 1223–1230.

73. Aligeti, V. R., Gandhi, M., Braden, R., Rezk, A. & Elam, M. B. (2007). Effect of combination lipid-modifying therapy on the triglyceride lowering effect of fish oil. *Am J Med Sci* **333**, 168–172.

74. Liu, J., Zhang, J., Shi, Y., Grimsgaard, S., Alraek, T. & Fonnebo, V. (2006). Chinese red yeast rice (Monascus purpureus) for primary hyperlipidemia: A meta-analysis of randomized controlled trials. *Chin Med* **1**, 4.

75. SoRelle, R. (2000). Appeals Court says Food and Drug Administration can regulate cholestin. *Circulation* **102**, E9012–E9013.

76. Baum, L., Cheung, S. K., Mok, V. C. *et al.* (2007). Curcumin effects on blood lipid profile in a 6-month human study. *Pharmacol Res* **56**, 509–514.

77. Diamanti-Kandarakis, E., Alexandraki, K., Piperi, C. *et al.* (2006). Inflammatory and endothelial markers in women with polycystic ovary syndrome. *Eur J Clin Invest* **36**, 691–697.

78. Diamanti-Kandarakis, E., Paterakis, T. & Kandarakis, H. A. (2006). Indices of low-grade inflammation in polycystic ovary syndrome. *Ann N Y Acad Sci* **1092**, 175–186.
79. Mohlig, M., Spranger, J., Osterhoff, M. *et al.* (2004). The polycystic ovary syndrome per se is not associated with increased chronic inflammation. *Eur J Endocrinol* **150**, 525–532.
80. Calder, P. C. (2001). Polyunsaturated fatty acids, inflammation, and immunity. *Lipids* **36**, 1007–1024.
81. Murphy, K. J., Galvin, K., Kiely, M., Morrissey, P. A., Mann, N. J. & Sinclair, A. J. (2006). Low dose supplementation with two different marine oils does not reduce pro-inflammatory eicosanoids and cytokines in vivo. *Asia Pac J Clin Nutr* **15**, 418–424.

Chapter 16

Eggs and Health: Nutrient Sources and Supplement Carriers

Gita Cherian

Department of Animal Sciences, Oregon State University, Corvallis, OR, USA

Abstract

The chicken egg is a storehouse of several biologically active nutrients such as polyunsaturated fatty acids, cholines, sialic acid, sphingolipids, and antioxidants. However, concern over the possible risks of high saturated fat and cholesterol has led to the reduction in per capita consumption of eggs. Incorporation of functional nutrients into eggs could lead to alternate and novel health-promoting nutrients for humans. In this regard, several functional nutrients such as omega-3 fatty acids, conjugated linoleic acids, vitamin E, vitamin D, selenium, folic acid, lutein, zeaxanthin, and iodine have been incorporated into eggs, making eggs an excellent choice as a functional food. Particular emphasis is given in this chapter to research conducted during the past two decades on enrichment of chicken eggs with functional nutrients, their health effects in humans and the role of eggs as an alternate route to provide those nutrients that are in short supply or lacking in the current human diet.

Key words: *Eggs, bioactive nutrients, omega-3 fatty acids, functional food*

INTRODUCTION

The chicken egg has been an important part of the human diet since the dawn of civilization. It is the only food from the animal kingdom that can provide nutrients to humans as well as sustain a new life (when fertile) upon incubation. Thus the egg contains several nutrients that are essential for life. In a typical American diet, eggs supplied <10% of total calories, 2.0% fat and 3.9% proteins in addition to many biologically active nutrients that are essential for maintaining human health [1]. This chapter describes the chicken egg's composition, nutrient content of the edible portion and the eggs' role as a carrier in providing health-promoting nutrients to humans. Particular emphasis is given to research conducted during the past two decades on enrichment of chicken eggs with functional nutrients, their health effects in humans and the role of eggs as an alternate route to provide those nutrients that are in short supply or lacking in the current human diet.

TABLE 16.1 Nutrient Content of a Large Raw Egg (adapted from http://www.aeb.org/food/nutrient.html)

Nutrient	Whole egg	White	Yolk
Water (g)	37.7	29.3	8.1
Food energy (calories)	72.0	17.0	55.0
Protein (g)	6.29	3.60	2.70
Total lipid (g)	5.00	0.0	5.0
Total carbohydrates (g)	0.39	0.21	0.61
Ash (g)	0.47	0.21	0.29
Minerals (mg)	412.4	225.0	187.4
Vitamin A (IU)	244.0	—	244.0
Vitamin D (IU)	18.0		18.0
Vitamin E (mg)	0.48		0.48
B vitamins (mg)	221.5	2.03	220.7

EGG COMPOSITION

The egg is comprised of four main parts: yolk, egg white or albumen, shell membranes, and shell. In general, the shell contributes 9–11%, the yolk 25–33% and the egg white 56–64% [2]. The total edible portion of the egg is 89–91%. The egg yolk is a homogeneously emulsified fluid and is the first part of the egg to develop. Egg yolk is comprised of 51–52% water, 16–17% protein, 31–33% fat including cholesterol, fat soluble vitamins and pigments, 0.2–1.0% carbohydrates and some minerals (1%) [3]. Egg white is composed of mainly water (80%), and proteins (11%), with the remaining made up of carbohydrates (<0.4%) and water soluble vitamins and pigments. Other inorganic components include phosphorus, magnesium and trace amounts of iron and sulfur comprise less than 0.05%. The nutrient content of a large egg is shown in Table 16.1. As can be seen from Table 16.1, protein and fat constitute the major macro nutrients in the egg.

Lipids

Among the macronutrients, lipids are one of the main components of the egg comprising 5.0–5.5 g in an average 60-g egg. Almost all lipids are present in the yolk as lipoprotein complexes. Trace levels of lipids have been observed in the white. Yolk lipids include neutral lipids or triacylglycerol, phospholipids, and free cholesterol. Triacylglycerol and phospholipids are the major components of yolk lipids comprising up to 65 and 32%, respectively [4] (Table 16.2).

TABLE 16.2 Major Lipid Classes and their Proportions in Chicken Eggs (adapted from references [3, 5])

Major lipid and fatty acid fractions	Proportion (%)
Triglyceride	63–65
Cholesterol	4.9–5.0
Cholesterol ester	1.0
Phospholipids	30–31
Phosphatidylcholine	21.0
Phosphatidyl ethanolamine	7.3
Phosphatidyl serine	0.9
Sphingolipids	0.9

Egg phospholipids are made up of phosphatidyl choline (lecithin), phosphatidyl ethanolamine, phosphatidyl serine, and sphingolipids. Minor levels of lysophosphatidyl choline and phosphatidyl ethanolamine are also present. Egg phospholipids are also rich in long-chain polyunsaturated fatty acids (PUFA) such as docosahexaenoic acid (DHA; C22:6 n-3) and arachidonic acid (C20:4–6). Egg phospholipids, due to their amphipathic nature, are widely used as emulsifiers in the baking, pharmaceutical, animal feed, and cosmetic industries. In addition, several fat soluble vitamins and pigments are present in egg lipids making egg a multifunctional and multinutritional food. However, egg lipids are not fully exploited in the food industry to its full potential in comparison to plant-derived lipids.

Egg Fatty Acids

Fatty acids are the most prevalent components of triglycerides and phospholipids and may constitute over 4 g in an average egg. Egg fatty acids are of different chain lengths varying from 14 to 22 carbons and of different degrees of saturation as well as different configurations. Egg fatty acids include saturated fatty acids, monounsaturated fatty acids and omega-6 and omega-3 polyunsaturated fatty acids (PUFA). A list of some of the common fatty acids in egg yolk with their systemic names, shorthand notations and concentrations is shown in Table 16.3. Several factors influence the fatty acid composition of egg including the hen's ration, strain, age and the storage and cooking methods employed. However, diet is the major determinant of yolk fatty acid composition [5].

Saturated Fatty Acids

The predominant saturated fatty acids in eggs are palmitic (C16:0) and stearic (C18:0). The content of these two fatty acids in chicken eggs may range from 22% to 26% and 8% to 10%, respectively. There are also minor amounts of

TABLE 16.3 Systemic Names and Shorthand Notations of Some of the Common Fatty Acids and their Content in Chicken Eggs*

Common or systemic names	Shorthand notation	Concentration
Myristic acid	C14:0	0.50
Palmitic acid	C16:0	26.0
Palmitoleic acid	C16:1	3.2
Stearic acid	C18:0	9.4
Oleic acid	C18:1 n-9	43.0
Linoleic acid	C18:2 n-6	15.0
α-Linolenic acid	C18:3 n-3	0.5
Arachidonic acid	C20:4 n-6	1.7
Eicosapentaenoic acid (EPA)	C20:5 n-3	0.1
Docosatetraenoic acid	C22:4 n-6	0.1
Docosapentaenoic acid (DPA)	C22:5 n-3	0.2
Docosahexaenoic acid (DHA)	C22:6 n-3	1.2

*Values reported as fatty acids (%) and may vary due to hen's diet, strain, or age.

other saturated fatty acids such as C14 and C20. Total saturated fatty acids in eggs may constitute 30–35%.

Monounsaturated Fatty Acids

The monounsaturated fatty acids in eggs are mainly palmitoleic (C16:1), oleic (C18:1), constituting to 42–46%. Other minor monounsaturated fatty acids such as 20:1 and 22:1 are present in trace amounts. Oleic acid (C18:1) is the major monounsaturated fatty acid in chicken eggs. The monounsaturated fatty acid content is affected by diet composition. Feeding PUFA-rich oils (e.g., sunflower oil, canola, flax) and conjugated linoleic acid (CLA) alters the content of yolk monounsaturated fatty acids [6].

Omega-6 (n-6) and Omega-3 (n-3) Polyunsaturated Fatty Acids

Eggs contain both omega-6 and omega-3 fatty acids. The predominant omega-6 fatty acid in egg lipids is linoleic acid (C18:2 n-6). Other omega-6 fatty acids may include arachidonic (C20:4 n-6), C22:4 n-6, and C22:5 n-6. The content of long-chain omega-6 PUFA (>20-carbon) may vary from 1% to 2% and is reflected by the type of the diet [4]. The content of omega-3 fatty acids in eggs is contributed by α-linoleic (C18:3 n-3), eicosapentaenoic acid (C20:5 n-3), docosapentaenoic (C22:5 n-3), and DHA. Among these, DHA is the major omega-3 fatty acid in the egg. The α-linolenic content in regular eggs is under 1% of total lipids. DHA may constitute between 1% and 3%. The content of omega-3 and omega-6 PUFA is a reflection of the hen's dietary fat. Addition of flax, chia, marine oil or other products such as marine algae into the diet leads to significant increases in α-linolenic, eicosapentaenoic, docosapentaenoic, and DHA in eggs [4].

Sterols

The major sterol in yolk lipids is cholesterol, which is found in the free form. Cholesterol content may vary from 11 mg/g to 14 mg/g yolk or 200 mg to 220 mg/average egg. Although diet has very little effect on egg cholesterol [4] other factors such as egg weight, yolk size and strain of bird may affect the content of egg cholesterol [7, 8].

EGG PROTEINS

Proteins constitute another macronutrient in eggs and a typical egg would provide approximately 6 g of protein. Adding two eggs into the diet will meet about 30% of the recommended dietary allowance (RDA) for protein in the United States. Egg proteins distributed in the yolk and white are complete proteins with a good balance of essential amino acids and high digestibility (>90%). The protein value of whole egg protein is considered to be 100 and is used as a standard for measuring nutritional quality of other food proteins. Egg white contains about 11% proteins. The major egg white proteins are ovalbumin (54%), ovotransferrin (14%), ovomucoid (11%), ovomucin (3.5%), lysozyme (3.5%), and globulins (8%). Lysozyme is widely used in the food industry due to its antibacterial properties. Most yolk proteins exist as lipoproteins. Low-density lipoprotein is the major protein, accounting up to 65% of total yolk proteins. The high-density lipoprotein exists as a complex with phosphoprotein as "phosvitin." Other yolk proteins include livetin and a riboflavin-binding protein. Egg yolk also contains other immune proteins such as immunoglobulins. In eggs immunoglobulin Y (IgY) is present predominantly in the yolk, whereas IgA and IgM are present in the white. Efforts have been made to separate IgY to be used for pharmaceutical and food industry purposes. Due to the multifunctional (gelling, emulsifying, foaming, binding) and pharmacological properties, egg proteins are highly desirable ingredients in baking and the food and drug industries.

EGG MICRONUTRIENTS

Egg micronutrients include fat soluble and water soluble vitamins, minerals and pigments (Table 16.1). Most fat soluble vitamins are concentrated in the yolk and water soluble vitamins in yolk and white. In addition, there are minor nutrients and pigments in the egg constituting up to 0.02%. The yolk pigments include xanthophylls and carotenes which contribute to the yellow color. The avian egg contains several kinds of free sugars and glycoconjugates. Glucose is the most common of the free sugars and constituting up to 0.7, 0.8, and 0.7% in the whole egg, albumen, and yolk, respectively. Total carbohydrate in the whole egg, white, and yolk constitutes to 0.61, 0.34, and 0.30 g, respectively. Most of the carbohydrates in egg are oligosaccharides bound to protein. Sialic acid is a functional carbohydrate in egg with pharmacological potential due to its involvement in cell adhesion, receptor functions, and defense mechanisms. The inorganic components of egg white are sulfur, potassium, sodium, and chlorine. Many of the micro nutrients in the egg can be manipulated by dietary means. However, vitamin E, selenium and pigments are the nutrients that are highly researched for diet-modification purposes.

DIET AND HEALTH

Major advancement has been made in the past two decades in our understanding of the mechanisms whereby diet can influence health. As a result, functional foods have been introduced as a new concept for foods that provide health benefits beyond basic nutrition. Consumer interest in functional foods is evidenced by the wide range of health-promoting specialty foods available and supplements in the marketplace. Annual sales of functional foods in the United States is estimated to be over $50 billion. Among the different nutrients, omega-3 fatty acids have captured world-wide attention due to their several positive effects on human heath [9]. Beneficial effects of omega-3 fatty acids in the prevention and management of coronary heart disease, hypertension, renal diseases, thrombosis, depression, type-2 diabetes, Crohn's disease, and rheumatoid arthritis, in addition to the role of these fatty acids in brain and visual development in infants have been reported [9].

CHICKEN EGGS AS FUNCTIONAL FOODS AND SUPPLEMENT CARRIERS

Claims of beneficial health effects of certain fatty acids such as omega-3 led to extensive research on manipulating the fatty acid composition of chicken eggs [3]. This has led to the creation of several brands of specialty eggs with labels such as designer, super, or modified (to name a few) in super markets world-wide. At present, specialty eggs in US markets comprise about 5% and are growing by 1% a year. A national retail study conducted in US cities in 2001 indicated an average price of $2.18 for specialty eggs (range from $0.88 to $4.38) vs. $1.23 for regular white eggs with no special claims [10]. The success of creating and marketing eggs enriched with omega-3 led to attempts by several researchers in modifying other nutrients in eggs. Some of these nutrients include fatty acids (CLA), antioxidant vitamins (vitamin E, vitamin A), B vitamins and minerals (selenium, iodine, vitamin B12, manganese) [3]. A list of some of these nutrients, their concentrations in eggs and their potential benefit to humans is shown in Table 16.4.

TABLE 16.4 A List of Some of the Bioactive Nutrients Reported in Eggs and their Functional Roles[a]

Components	Content/egg*	Potential benefits[b]
Carotenoids		
Carotenes	100–209 µg	Neutralizes free radicals, which may damage cells; bolster cellular antioxidant defense; can be made into vitamin A in the body
Lutein + Zeaxanthin	1.33–1.91 mg	May contribute to maintenance of healthy vision
Lycopene	.08–8.5 mg	May contribute to maintenance of prostate health
Fatty Acids		
Monounsaturated fatty acids	1.7–3.3 mg	May reduce risk of CHD
Omega-3 fatty acids (α-linolenic, EPA, DPA, DHA)	100–650 mg	May contribute to maintenance of heart health and maintenance of mental and visual function, may reduce risk of CHD, may contribute to maintenance of mental and visual function
Conjugated linoleic acid (CLA)	0.15–0.9 g	Maintains desirable body composition and healthy immune function
Minerals		
Phosphorus	110 mg	May reduce the risk of osteoporosis
Selenium	7.1–43.4 µg	Neutralizes free radicals, which may damage cells; may contribute to healthy immune function
Vitamins		
Vitamin A	100 µg	May contribute to maintenance of healthy vision, immune function, and bone health; may contribute to cell integrity
Vitamin B2 (Riboflavin)	0.16–0.24 mg	Helps support cell growth; helps regulate metabolism
Niacin	0.05–1.94 mg	Helps support cell growth; helps regulate metabolism
Vitamin B12	0.84–3.35 µg	May contribute to maintenance of mental function; helps regulate metabolism and supports blood cell formation
Folic Acid	20–50 µg	Maintains healthy pregnancy
Biotin	10–18 µg	Helps regulate metabolism and hormone synthesis
Vitamin D	18–90 IU	Helps regulate calcium and phosphorus; helps contribute to bone health; may contribute to healthy immune function; helps support cell growth
Vitamin E (Tocopherols + tocotrienols)	0.70–6.7 mg	Neutralizes free radicals, may contribute to healthy immune function and maintenance of heart health
Sphingolipids	2250 µmol/kg	Maintain membrane structure, modulate cholesterol metabolism
Choline	300 mg	Involved in brain function, memory and learning ability

CHD = *coronary heart disease.*
[a]*Values reported are a range of those nutrients reported in conventional eggs or those from hens fed modified diets.*
[b]*FDA approved health claim established for component.*

Why Omega-3 Fatty Acids?

Current consumption of omega-3 fatty acids in the United States is 1.4 g/day α-linolenic acid (C18:3 *n*-3) and 0.2 g/day of long chain (>20-carbon omega-3) [11]. Although no official dietary recommendations have been made in the US, nutritional scientists suggest including α-linolenic acid at 2.2 g/day and long-chain omega-3 (C20:5 *n*-3 + C22:6 *n*-3) at 0.65 g/day [11]. Therefore an additional 0.8 and 0.45 g/day of α-linolenic acid and long-chain omega-3 is needed in the current US diet. Although marine foods are the major source of omega-3, cost, consumer preference, and seasonal availability limit the US percapita consumption of marine-based omega-3 fatty acids. To accommodate for the 57% (α-linolenic acid) and 225% (long-chain omega-3) increase in omega-3, alternate dietary sources of omega-3 fatty acids need to be provided.

Flax seeds and marine oil have been added to the layer diet to increase omega-3 in eggs. Eggs from flax-fed hens are high in 18-carbon omega-3 (C18:3 *n*-3) and those from fish-oil based diets are rich in long-chain >20-carbon omega-3 PUFA (e.g., eicosapentaenoic, DHA). A detailed review of omega-3 studies in avians is written elsewhere [4]. Addition of two eggs from hens fed 10% flax to the daily diet could provide up to 440 mg α-linolenic acid and 100 mg of DHA. Similarly, addition of two eggs from hens fed diets with 3.0% fish oil could provide 20 mg α-linolenic acid and 340 mg DHA. Several authors have reported beneficial effects of omega-3 enriched eggs in humans including infants and seniors (Table 16.5). Most studies report significant increases in serum α-linolenic, and DHA with omega-3 eggs. The effect of consumption of omega-3 eggs on total blood cholesterol has been controversial. Interestingly, several researchers have reported higher levels of high density lipoprotein cholesterol with the consumption of omega-3 eggs. Thus, including two eggs (flax-fed) will meet over 55% of the extra α-linolenic needed in the US diet. Similarly, including two eggs (fish oil-fed) will meet over 75% of the extra DHA needed in the US diet. Although feeding flax and fish oil over 10 and 3%, irrespectively to hens has been reported to increase the α-linolenic and DHA content in eggs, additions exceeding these levels may lead to off-flavors and reduced sensory appeal of omega-3 enriched eggs. Table 16.6 shows the contribution of eggs in meeting the recommended daily allowance of several nutrients including omega-3 fatty acids.

Conjugated Linoleic Acids (CLA)

Recently, another fatty acid namely CLA, has received considerable attention for its anticarcinogenic, antiatherogenic, hypocholesterolemic, immunomodulatory, and body fat reduction properties [12]. CLA is the generic name for a group of positional and geometric conjugated dienomic isomers of linoleic acid. Current intake of CLA is estimated to be several hundred milligrams/day [13]. Based on animal data, it is estimated that approximately 3 g/day of CLA would be required to produce beneficial effects in humans [14]. Several researchers

TABLE 16.5 Omega-3 Fatty Acid-Rich Egg Consumption and Reported Health Effects in Adults and Infants (adapted from reference [25])

No. of Egg	Week/days fed	Reported responses
4 eggs/day	4 weeks	No change in plasma total cholesterol, reduction in serum triglycerides, and systolic and diastolic blood pressure
4 eggs/day	2 weeks	Reduction in serum triglycerides. No change in total or HDL cholesterol, increase in omega-3 PUFA, DHA of platelet phospholipids
2 eggs/day	18 days	Increase in plasma HDL cholesterol, reduction in plasma triglycerides. No change in total cholesterol or and LDL cholesterol
2 eggs/day	4 weeks	Reduction in plasma triglycerides, total cholesterol, systolic blood pressure in adults
4 eggs/day	14 weeks	Increased DHA, omega-3 PUFA in platelet phospholipids, no change in plasma triglycerides, total cholesterol or HDL cholesterol in adults
2 eggs/day	18 days	Increase in plasma HDL cholesterol, reduction in plasma triglycerides. No change in total cholesterol or LDL cholesterol
7 eggs/week	24 weeks	Increase in HDL cholesterol, EPA, DHA, and total omega-3 PUFA
2 eggs/week	6 weeks	Increase in linolenic and docosahexaenoic acids of breast milk in nursing women
1 egg/day	8 weeks	Increased blood levels of docosahexaenoic acid, vitamin E, and lutein in adults
12 eggs/week	6 weeks	Reduction in serum triglyceride in adults
4 eggs/week	6 months	Increase in erythrocyte docosahexaenoic acids of formula-fed infants
4 eggs/week	6 weeks	Decrease in platelet aggregation in adults
4 eggs/week	6 months	Increase plasma omega-3 fatty acids, docosahexaenoic acids and blood content of iron in infants
6 eggs/week	4 weeks	No effect on serum total, LDL or HDL cholesterol. Increase in serum α-linolenic and triglycerides
DHA- enriched egg powder (150 mg/day)	9 months	Increased DHA and arachidonic acid in elderly patients

PUFA = *polyunsaturated fatty acids*, HDL = *high density lipoprotein*, LDL = *low density lipoprotein*.

TABLE 16.6 Eggs as Supplement Carriers: Reported Values of Nutrients and Percent of Recommended Dietary Allowance Provided[a]

Nutrient	Level reported in one serving[b]	Percent RDA Supplied
α-Linolenic acid (18:3 n-3)	400–800 mg	>40
Docosahexaenoic Acid	400 mg	>100
Total omega-3 fatty acids	500–1600 mg	>50
Conjugated linoleic acid	150–900 mg	RDA not established
Vitamin A	150 ug	16.6
Vitamin D	1.2–10 ug	23–30
Vitamin E	8–38 mg	>150
Vitamin K	260 ug	>200
Thiamin	134 ug	11.2
Riboflavin	490 ug	37.6
Pyridoxine	66 ug	5.0
Biotin	36 ug	>100
Folic Acid	20 ug	5.0
Niacin	154 ug	1.0
Pantothenic acid	2410 ug	48
Vitamin B12	6.7 ug	>250
Lutein	1.91 mg	RDA not established
Selenium	64–87 ug	>130
Choline	300 mg	1/3 of the RDA

[a] *Range of nutrient values reported in regular or eggs obtained from hens fed modified diets. Adapted from references [4, 17, 20].*
[b] *One serving = 2 average size eggs.*

have reported incorporating CLA into chicken eggs through diet. The CLA content varied from 0.21 to 0.9 g per average egg. The CLA supplied per serving (two eggs) could meet 14–58% of the suggested requirements for humans [6].

Choline

Chicken eggs are a rich source of choline (associated with phosphatidyl choline in phospholipids). Choline is responsible for the structural integrity and signaling function of phopholipid-rich cell membranes. One large egg contains about 300 mg of choline which provides 60% of the recommended daily intake of choline for adults, including pregnant and lactating women [15].

Sphingolipids

The sphingolipid content of eggs has been reported to be the highest of any food at 2250 umol/kg [16]. Sphingolipids are critical for the maintenance of membrane structure and modulate the behavior of extracellular matrix proteins.

Vitamins and Minerals

The egg content of several minor nutrients and the percent RDA supplied upon consumption of one serving (two eggs) is shown in Table 16.6. A recent survey in the US indicated that eggs contributed ~10% of vitamin B6, 10–20% of folate, and >20% of vitamin A, E, and B12 [1]. Several researchers have focused on producing eggs with higher levels of vitamins than regular eggs [17, 18, 19]. However, the efficiency of hens in transferring dietary vitamin to eggs is varied for different vitamins, with efficiency ranging from 5% to 80%. With the objective of producing eggs that can meet >50% of the daily recommended intake of vitamins, Leeson and Caston [17] fed vitamin-enriched diets to hens. For the 12 vitamins explored (A, D3, E, K, B1, B2, B6, biotin, folic acid, niacin, pantothenic acid, and vitamin B12), meaningful enrichment (meeting >20% of RDA) was noted only for vitamin D3, Vitamin E, pantothenic acid, and vitamin B12. In another study, House et al. [19] reported that by adding folic acid to the diet of laying hens, it was possible to increase the folate concentration of egg yolk two to fourfold. A folate enriched egg can potentially contain 12.5% of the RDA for this vitamin. These authors stated that the form of folate present in eggs is highly bioavailable since it is already in its metabolically active form (5-methyltetrahydrofolate) [19].

Due to the popularity of omega-3 specialty eggs, vitamin E enrichment of eggs has been most documented. This is because, incorporation of vitamin E has provided added antioxidant protection and product stability especially in specialty eggs rich in omega-3. The successful enrichment of chicken eggs with selenium has also been documented [20, 21]. Consumption of one serving of eggs enriched with selenium can meet ~100% of the RDA [21] (Table 16.6). Since selenium consumption in many countries falls below the RDA, such eggs may provide an alternate route to provide selenium to the human diet [20].

Egg Pigments

Several pigments are present in all parts of the egg. The yolk has the highest pigment content, constituting to 0.02%. The lipid matrix of the egg yolk provides a readily bioavailable dietary source of fat-soluble pigments. Carotenoid pigments constitute a group of lipid-soluble compounds. Carotenoids are of biological importance for their light-absorbing properties, antioxidant functions and immunomodulatory functions. The yolk carotenes are classified as xanthophylls and carotenes. Leutin, zeaxanthin, and cryptoxanthin belong to the xanthophyll group and β-carotene belongs to the carotene group. Lutein and zeaxanthin are two carotenoid pigments that accumulate in the retina of the eye [22]. These pigments protect the retina by absorbing blue light which damages the retina [23], leading to age-related macular degeneration. Humans cannot synthesize lutein and zeaxanthin; therefore these pigments should be provided in the diet. Hens accumulate xanthophylls (lutein, zeaxanthin, and capsanthin) in the egg mainly from their diet. The yolks of chicken eggs produced commercially contain large amounts of the carotenoids lutein and zeaxanthin (~292 ug/yolk and ~213 ug/yolk, respectively) as compared to other dietary carotenoids. β-carotene is present in small amounts (~3.6 ug/yolk) and lycopene is undetectable. It has been reported that the bioavailability of egg yolk lutein is higher than that in supplements and green vegetables [24, 25].

CHICKEN EGGS AS FUNCTIONAL FOODS AND SUPPLEMENT CARRIERS – FUTURE

Increased consumer awareness that certain nutrients may have beneficial effects on health and disease prevention has led to seeking these nutrients from food or supplements. In eggs, these health-promoting nutrients include omega-3 fatty acids, fat soluble vitamins, carotenoid pigments such as lutein and zeaxanthin, choline, B vitamins, and minerals. There is opportunity to enhance these nutrients in eggs through diet manipulation as reported in Table 16.4. However, feeding strategies should not increase the cost of egg production or be detrimental to the health of birds. Therefore, use of feed ingredients that are not usually consumed by humans should be investigated. Chicken eggs, due to their high content of nutrients, low cost and versatility in food preparation are a popular food item for all cultures and all ages. Although consumers are willing to pay extra for nutrient-modified eggs [9], the real value for humans from nutrient-enriched eggs comes only if those nutrients are in short supply in the diet and if consumption of such eggs contributes significantly to the daily recommended intake of the nutrient, without side effects on human health. Therefore, in order to be accepted by consumers, the health effects of nutrient-modified eggs need to be investigated clinically in different age and ethnic groups. This will enhance the nutritional potential of chicken eggs as supplement carriers to humans. Such research will generate new knowledge in using functional food strategies to prevent or alleviate the progression of chronic disease and to defend human health.

ACKNOWLEDGMENTS

The Ott Professorship awarded to G. Cherian, and financial support from the Linus Pauling Institute and Oregon State University Experiment Station Hatch Project are acknowledged.

REFERENCES

1. Song, W. O. & Kerver, J. M. (2001). Nutritional contribution of eggs to American diets. *J Am Coll Nutr* **19**, 556S–562S.
2. Cherian, G., Holsonbake, Y. B. & Goeger, M. P. (2002). Fatty acid composition and egg components of specialty eggs. *Poultry Sci* **81**, 30–33.
3. Stadelman, W. J. & Coterill, O. J. (1977). *Egg Science and Technology*, pp. 1–38, AVI, Westport.
4. Cherian, G. (2008). Omega-3 fatty acids: Studies in Avians, Chapter 13. *In* Wild-Type Food in Health Promotion and Disease Prevention: The Columbus® Concept (F. De Meester & R. R. Watson, Eds.), pp. 169–178, Humana Press.
5. Cherian, G. (2005). Eggs: Biology and nutrition, Chapter 153. *In* Handbook of Food Science, Technology and Engineering (Y. H. Hui, Ed.), Vol. IV, CRC Press, Taylor and Francis Group, Boca Raton, FL, USA.
6. Cherian, G. (2006). Conjugated linoleic acid (CLA) for health: chicken eggs as alternative sources of CLA, Chapter 3. *In* The Amazing Egg: Nature's Perfect Functional Food for Health Promotion (J. S. Sim & H. H. Sunwoo, Eds.), pp. 49–64, University of Alberta.
7. Naber, E. C. (1983). Nutrient and drug effects on cholesterol metabolism in the hen. *Fed Proc* **42**, 2486–2493.
8. Jiang, Z. & Sim, J. S. (1991). Egg cholesterol values in relation to the age of laying hens and to egg size and yolk weights. *Poultry Sci* **70**, 1838–1841.
9. Simopoulos, A. P. (2000). Human requirement for *n*-3 polyunsaturated fatty acids. *Poultry Sci* **79**, 91–970.
10. Patterson, P. H., Koelkebeck, K. W., Bell, D. D., Carey, J. B., Anderson, K. E. & Darre, M. J. (2001). Egg marketing in national supermarkets: Specialty eggs-Part 2. *Poultry Sci* **80**, 390–395.
11. Kris-Etherton, P. M., Taylor, D. S., Yu-Poth, S., Huth, P., Moriarty, K., Fishell, V. & Hargrove, R. L. (2000). The polyunsaturated fatty acids in the food chain in the United States. *Am J Clin Nutr.* **71**, 179S–188S.
12. Belury, M. A. (2002). Dietary conjugated linoleic acid in health: Physiological effects and mechanisms of action. *Ann Rev Nutr* **22**, 505–531.
13. Fritsche, J., Rickert, H., Steinhart, M. P., Yurawecz, M. M., Mossaba, N., Sehat, J. A., Roach, G., Kramer, J. K. G. & Ku, Y. (1999). Conjugated linoleic acid (CLA) isomers: Formation, analysis, amounts in foods and dietary intake. *Fett Lipid* **101**, 272–276.
14. Ha, Y. L., Grimm, N. K. & Pariza, M. W. (1989). Newly recognized anticarcinogenic fatty acids: Identification and quantification in natural and processed cheeses. *J Agric Food Chem* **37**, 75–81.
15. Zeisel, S. H. (2000). Choline: Needed for normal development of memory. *J Am Coll Nutr* **19**, 528S–531S.
16. Vesper, H. V., Schmeiz, E. M., Nikolava-Karakashan, M. N., Dillehay, D. V. & Merrill, A. H. (1999). Sphingolipids in food and the emerging importance of sphingolipids to nutrition. *J Nutr* **129**, 1239–1250.
17. Leeson, S. & Caston, L. J. (2003). Vitamin enrichment of Eggs. *J Appl Poult Res* **12**, 24–26.

18. Mattila, P., Valaja, J., Rossow, L., Venäläinen, E. & Tupasela, T. (2004). Effect of vitamin D_2- and D_3-enriched diets on egg vitamin D content, production, and bird condition during an entire production period. *Poultry Sci* **83**, 433–440.

19. House, J. D., Braun, K., Ballance, D. M., O'Connor, C. P. & Guenter, W. (2002). The enrichment of eggs with folic acid through supplementation of the laying hen diet. *Poultry Sci* **81**, 1332–1337.

20. Surai, P. F. & Sparks, N. H. C. (2001). Designer eggs: From improvement of egg composition to functional food. *Trends in Food Sci Technol* **12**, 7–16.

21. Sparks, N. H. C. (2006). The hen's egg – its role in human nutrition changing? *World Poultry Sci* **62**, 308–315.

22. Ribaya-Mercado, J. D. & Blumberg, J. B. (2004). Lutein and zeaxanthin and their potential roles in disease prevention. *J Am Coll Nutr* **23**, 567S–587S.

23. Krinsky, N. I., Landrum, J. T. & Bone, R. A. (2003). Biologic mechanisms of the protective role of lutein and zeaxanthin in the eye. *Annu Rev Nutr* **23**, 171–201.

24. Chung, H. Y., Rasmussen, H. M. & Johnson, E. J. (2004). Lutein bioavailability is higher from lutein-enriched eggs than from supplements and spinach in men. *J Nutr* **134**, 1887–1893.

25. Cherian, G. (2003). Functional food attributes of *n*-3 polyunsaturated and conjugated linoleic acid enriched chicken eggs. *Nutritional Genomics and Functional Foods* **1**, 47–53.

Chapter 17

Berries and Cancer

Paul E. Milbury

Antioxidants Research Laboratory, Jean Mayer USDA Human Nutrition Research Center on Aging at Tufts University, Boston, MA

Abstract

The sum of epidemiologic evidence showing a protective effect of diets rich in fruits and vegetables against cancer is not as strong as originally thought. Nevertheless there is *in vitro* evidence suggesting that the biologically active phytochemicals from berries have anti-carcinogenic activity. Many of these compounds also show anti-carcinogenic effects in animal cancer models. *In vitro* experiments have contributed much to the knowledge base regarding probable mechanisms of action that support chemoprotective activities of berry phytochemicals at the molecular level. These chemopreventive mechanisms include prevention of radical damage, DNA stabilization, detoxification, inhibition of inflammatory processes such as cyclooxygenase-2 expression, and induction of apoptosis. However, much of the *in vitro* research on the anti-cancer effects of berries and their components has been conducted at concentrations that are not relative to the *in vivo* bioavailability and metabolism of the compounds studied. Many phytochemicals present in berries are poorly absorbed by animals or humans and those that are absorbed are rapidly metabolized and excreted by xenobiotic metabolism. Indeed, this activation of phase II metabolism is a putative chemoprotective mechanism. Much of the anti-cancer bioactivity observed *in vitro* still requires additional research with animals and humans to verify these effects *in vivo*. Additional necessary research includes concerted efforts to identify the bioavailability, metabolism, and tissue distribution of berry phytochemicals and their metabolites not only to the circulation but also to the target tissues. Research is also needed to determine whether berry phytochemicals augment or interfere with current day chemotherapeutic protocols.

Keywords: *Berries, cancer, phenolics, phytochemicals, in vitro, in vivo*

INTRODUCTION

Plants are the consummate chemist and, via evolution over the millennia, have diversified their genome and biosynthetic pathways to produce an enormous number of distinct phytochemicals. Unlike animals, plants are not proficient at "cleaning up" their genomes or disposing of genes no longer unnecessary to present functional needs. As a result classes of phytochemicals within a single plant often include many structurally similar but subtly different members. These phytochemicals either function in plants presently or have functioned in the past to attract mutual partners or repelling predators. In many cases phytochemicals that were once harmful to organisms are still present in fruits and berries and in other cases mutualism results in delivery of beneficial phytochemicals to animal partners in the mutuality beneficial relationship. For example vitamin C is a beneficial phytochemical to fruit eating animals that have lost the capacity to synthesize it. In contrast, amygdalin remains in stones of bitter almonds, peaches, and apricots although it is toxic to animals. Yet humans have used it as a natural and traditional anti-cancer drug [1]. As is the case for many phytochemicals, laboratory evidence suggests bioefficacy for amygdalin while clinical trials fail to support its anti-cancer efficacy. Such may be the case for many phytochemicals from berries.

The body of *in vitro* evidence suggesting chemoprotective and anti-cancer effects for many berry phytochemicals continues to grow and there are promising animal studies; however, the small number of intervention studies conducted to date have produced mixed results even for the ability of antioxidant rich berries in reducing radical induced DNA damage. Data from *in vivo* studies that show anti-cancer effects of berry phytochemicals suggests that these chemoprotective effects may depend upon multiple mechanistic pathways, synergy of action by phytochemicals, and may be cancer specific for particular berries. This chapter contains a review of many of the recent studies of the anti-cancer effects of berries, berry extracts, and a small number of the myriad individual phytochemicals contained within berries.

WHAT IS A BERRY?

Before any discussion of the health benefits of berries can proceed, a problem of terminology must be addressed. In the culinary arts and in the common language usage, the term berry is a generic term describing any small, edible fruit with multiple seeds. Botanist, however, have a more restrictive definition of the term that technically excludes aggregate fruits, including the raspberry the blackberry, and the boysenberry. The definition of a berry in botanical terms refers to an indehiscent fruit derived from a single ovary having one or many seeds within a fleshy wall or pericarp. Indehiscent fruit do not open spontaneously at maturity to release seeds. This definition includes fruits such as the cranberry, grape, and tomato. If asked, the vast majority of people would not recognize a tomato as a berry but would readily identify small, sweet, juicy, and brightly colored fruits as berries regardless of its botanical structure.

For the purposes of this chapter, we will consider the term berry to be the common term and as such will refer to the small, edible, colored fruits with multiple seeds and include plants of the species *Vaccinium*, *Sambucus*, *Fragaria*, and *Rubus*. A non-exhaustive list of commonly known berries is listed in Table 17.1,

TABLE 17.1 Names of Berries with Synonyms and Latin Names

Popular botanical and common berries		
Common name	Synonyms	Latin name
Highbush blueberry		*Vaccinium corymbosum*
Lowbush blueberry		*Vaccinium angustifolium*
Bilberry	European blueberry, whortleberry	*Vaccinium myrtillus*
Cranberry		*Vaccinium macrocarpon*
Lowbush cranberry	Mountain cranberry, cowberry lingonberry	*Vaccinium oxycoccus*
Huckleberry		*Vaccinium ovatum*
Boxberry	Checkerberry, spiceberry, teaberry or wintergreen	*Gaultheria procumbens*
Pomegranate		*Punica granatum*
Kiwifruit		*Actinidia chinensis*
Banana		*Musa sapientum*
Blackcurrant		*Ribes nigrum*
Redcurrant		*Ribes triste*
Dewberry		*Rubus idaeus*
Loganberry		*Rubus loganobaccus*
Shadberry	Juneberry, Saskatoon, serviceberry	*Amelanchier laevis*
Hackberry	Sugarberry	*Celtis reticulata*
Persimmon		*Diospyros virginiana*
Acerola	Barbados or West Indian cherry, surinam cherry	*Maldighia glabra*
Mulberry		*Morus rubra*
Wolfberry	Snowberry	*Lycium barbarum*
Elderberry		*Sambucus nigra*
Açai	Palmberry, goji	*Euterpe oleracea*
Grapes		*Vitis vinifera*
Chili pepper		*Capsicum sp*
Blackberry		*Rubus villosus*
Raspberry		*Rubus idaeus*
Boysenberry		*Rubus sp*
Strawberry		*Fragaria sp*

TABLE 17.2 Public and Scientific Perception of Berries

		Botanical designation	
		Berry	Not a berry
Common usage	Berry	Blackcurrant, redcurrant, cranberry, blueberry, and gooseberrya	Strawberry. blackberry, raspberry, and boysenberry
	Not a berry	Tomato, persimmon, eggplant, guava, chili pepper, pomegranate, avocado, kiwifruit, grape, and banana	Apple, peach, and cherry

and Table 17.2 contains illustrations of common misconceptions between the botanical and common perception of what a berry is.

Although evolution is responsible for the fact that we have such a diversity of fruits, it is humans that engage in taxonomy and comparative anatomy. Most frugivores (fruit eaters) recognize berry fruits primarily by color and size; for it is the color that plants use to attract animals to such small fruits in a scheme to disperse their seeds, much like the process used to attract birds and insects during fertilization. By eating the fruit, animals unwittingly participate in the biological process termed mutualism. Upon eating the berries, we obtain nutrients and the plants that bore them obtain mobility for their seeds. Any animal could serve the role of seed carrier, but in the case of berries, this role has been reserved primarily for animals with vision capable of distinguishing color change in the fruit that indicates the point in time when the seeds are mature. When seeds are immature and not ready for dispersal the fruits carry bitter tasting flavonoids to discourage herbivores. As berries ripen, they undergo a shift in flavonoid ratios favouring the colored anthocyanins while also increasing in sugar content [2]. The cranberry may be an exception to this generalization by evolving away from increased levels of sugar, perhaps driven by adaptation to a water seed dispersal scheme that has little need to attract animals with reward of sugar.

Is a little sugar all humans have derive from co-evolution and mutualism? Perhaps, in consuming berries there are more benefits for the animal than just a few calories. For humans, and some bats and birds, evolution as frugivores may have lead to the permitted loss of specific metabolic pathways and a form of obligatory mutualism [3, 4]. Without vitamin C from fruits, humans are subject to scurvy, and without another source of vitamin C long term existence is not possible. Throughout evolution humans did not see berries and think, "Ah, vitamin C." Rather, humans saw berries as a sweet tasty food source and their shamans even saw them as medicine. Do additional evolutionary benefits arise from mutualism, conferred by the berry producing plant to the berry consuming animal?

A SHORT HISTORY OF FRUIT AND VEGETABLE INTAKE AND CANCERS

By the early 1990s roughly 200 studies had examined the relationship between fruit and vegetable intake and cancers of the breast, cervix, ovary, esophagus, oral cavity, lung, stomach, colon, bladder, and pancreas. This evidence was reviewed in 1992 and the weight of evidence suggested that individuals in the lowest quartile for fruit and vegetable intake have twice the risk of developing cancer compared with those in the highest quartile [5]. In 1997 the American Institute for Cancer Research published a report from the World Cancer Research Fund that concluded the evidence for protective effects of fruits and vegetables against cancers of the esophagus, stomach, and lung was "convincing" but the evidence for protection of fruits (as opposed to vegetables) against cancers of the colon and rectum was not strong [6]. By the time The International Agency for Research on Cancer (IARC), which is part of the World Health Organization, published its 387-page review in 2003 of research on the relationship between fruits, vegetables, and cancer [7], inclusion of data from cohort studies had weekend the strong evidence proffered by earlier case-control studies. The IARC concluded that data from studies in humans show "There is limited evidence for a cancer-preventive effect of consumption of fruit and of vegetables for cancers of the mouth and pharynx, esophagus, stomach, colon-rectum, larynx, lung, ovary (vegetables only), bladder (fruit only), and kidney. There is inadequate evidence for a cancer-preventive effect of consumption of fruit and of vegetables for all other sites." The IARC went on to examine the combined data from human epidemiological, animal, and other types of studies, and concluded that that eating more fruit "probably lowers the risk of cancers of the esophagus, stomach and lung" and "possibly reduces the risk of cancers of the mouth, pharynx, colon-rectum, larynx, kidney, and urinary bladder." These reports dealt largely with the relationship between total fruit and total vegetable consumption and cancers. The IARC itself pointed out that these summaries may overlook the possibility that specific fruits (or vegetable) may be protective against particular cancers.

The early epidemiological conclusions had already fostered interest in identifying which fruits and vegetables provide the best protection against the development of cancer and what bioactive constituents may be responsible for the chemopreventive qualities of those fruits and vegetables. The identification of protective substances in fruits and vegetables and the mechanisms by which they protect against cancer is inextricably linked to understanding the etiologic pathways leading to cancer. By the turn of the century investigators were realizing the common denominator in pathogenesis of most chronic diseases, including cancer, is the involvement of oxidative stress, via the actions of reactive oxygen and nitrogen species and biological damage inflicted by uncontrolled radical [8–10]. Indeed there was molecular evidence that cancer was associated with radical induced DNA damage and that, in isocaloric diets, individuals consuming fruits and vegetables had lower levels of excreted markers of DNA damage [11]. Dietary plants contain hundreds of electron donating antioxidants. Among edible vegetables, berries of the family of Rosaceae (*Rubus* and *Fragaria*) and those of the family of Ericaceae (*Vaccinium*) are particularly rich in antioxidant compounds when compared to other fruit species [12, 13]. In tests of potential to quench radicals, berries prove to be the fruits highest in total antioxidant capacity [14–16]. Berries and fruits have also been shown to increase postprandial antioxidant capacity of human plasma [17]. Yet, with the exception of evidence for prevention of digestive tract cancers, evidence for an anti-carcinogenic effect of berries in human studies is weak. *In vitro* and animal studies show that extracts from some berries can decrease biomarkers of DNA damage and carcinogenesis. The mechanisms of action are being defined but it is clear they are manifold and complex and will probably represent many synergistic interactions.

PHYTOCHEMICALS IN BERRIES

The major nutrient and non-nutrient bioactive antioxidant components of berry fruits are comprised predominantly of the phenolics and polyphenolics compounds and ascorbic acid. While berry plants can synthesize ascorbic acid via multiple pathways, present concentrations vary significantly among berries and contents data is not complete for all berries.

Phenolics and polyphenolics are a large and chemically diverse class of antioxidant compounds found in most fruits [18]. They include the anthocyanins, the flavonols (e.g., quercetin), flavanols, ellagic acid derivatives such as ellagitannins and ellagic acid itself, and stilbenes (e.g., resveratrol). The phenolic content of berries depends not only on the species and variety of berry, but also on environmental factors and the stage of fruit. While most berries experience their highest concentrations of anthocyanins at ripeness, certain berries, such as the strawberry experience declining levels of ellagic acid as they ripen [12].

Gallotannins and ellagitannins are hydrolysable tannins that represent the most abundant phenols in berries [20]. Hydrolysable tannins are rich in hydroxyl groups and are thus strong antioxidants and they can be hydrolyzed to ellagic acid. Tannins also have anti-cancer activities [21] however the relevance of anti-cancer potential must also be tempered by an understanding of what is bioavailable to *in vivo* tumors. Proanthocyanidins are condensed tannins, large branched molecules that result from the polymerization of flavan-3-ols. Flavan-3-ols are reduction of anthocyanidins and leucoanthocyanidins. Berry proanthocyanidins have been linked to prevention of urinary tract infections, cataracts, diabetes, and colon cancer [22–26]; however, much of this research has been conducted *in vitro* and in animal studies where it is not clear that proanthocyanidin or their metabolites are responsible for observed effects.

Another group of phenolic flavonoids abundant in berries belonging to the class termed anthocyanins and are the components of berries responsible for their color. In plants anthocyanin pigments are glycosylated forms of aglycone base structures defined as anthocyanidins. Anthocyanidins structures confer particular colors: cyanidins are red, delphinidins are blue, pelargonidins are red-purple. The glycosylated forms exist in various ratios in berry fruits resulting in the endless hues observable in various berries. Blueberries and bilberries are rich in cyanidins and delphinidins and are blue [27] while other berries such as the strawberry, rich in pelargonidins, are red in color [28]. Other flavonoids found in berries include catechin, quercetin, and kaempferol.

Another phenolic in the stilbene class, resveratrol, has received notoriety lately for its ability to mimic caloric restriction in mice on high caloric diets and its presence in wine. Resveratrol is not only present in grape berry, but is also present in other berries and a growing body of evidence points to its potential as an anti-cancer agent.

As with any living organism, many phenolic acids have been identified in berries. Berries also contain high levels of other compounds believed to reduce malignant transformation, including the B vitamins, such as folic acid, essential minerals such as calcium and selenium.

CURRENT THEORIES REGARDING CHEMOPROTECTION AND ANTI-TUMORIGENIC PHYTOCHEMICAL COMPOUNDS

The concept of chemoprevention was first forwarded by Sporn in 1979 [29] and has since blossomed into a field of molecular research examining the ability of natural and pharmacologic chemicals to not only to prevent, but also to cure cancer. In the current era of molecular drug development, the National Cancer Institute (NCI) has encouraged development of highly specific, targeted therapies for the treatment of cancer. Recent advances in our understanding of the genetic and molecular changes involved in the progression of malignant cells have accelerated development of targeted drugs to treat specific tumors. However, to date only a modest clinical benefit, limited to subsets of patients, has been demonstrated. Furthermore, despite a high degree of target selectivity, the use of targeted therapies often is associated with systemic toxicity [30]. Meanwhile, although funded to a lower level, research has proceeded on the anti anti-cancer activity of naturally occurring molecules [31]. In most cases, when an epidemiologic association is observed between a food and reduction in incidence of cancer, the next steps in the research effort generally involve separation of putative bioactive components and investigation of the effects of these components in cell culture and animal model. To some degree this effort to determine chemopreventive effects depends heavily on what markers or measures of anti-cancer mechanism is chosen. To qualify as a chemopreventive compound a phytochemical must either prevent cancer initiation by enhancing genomic stability, preventing carcinogens from reaching and activating their cellular targets, or suppress cancer cell growth.

Cancer initiation can be prevented via antioxidant mechanisms that scavenging reactive oxygen and nitrogen species and limiting the extent of oxidative damage to DNA and other critical cellular mechanisms or by enhancing repair of damaged DNA. Initiation can also be prevented by altering the uptake, metabolism and clearance of carcinogen by enhancing detoxification. Once initiation has occurred, cancer promotion and progression can be inhibited by disrupting pre-neoplastic signal transduction, transcriptional regulation, and cell cycle regulation and/or by establishing (or re-establishing) apoptotic cell death [32]. Cancer cells show increased reactive oxygen species (ROS) production and this trait has been linked to genomic instability and cancer initiation and progression [33]. The theory of ROS induced cancer raises the question of the corollary. Dietary antioxidants may present a means of chemoprevention by lowering ROS and protecting cells from cancer [34]. While the oxidative stress theory first brought investigators to investigate berry phytochemicals as anti-cancer agents, the evidence demonstrating that consumption of berries can reduce oxidative stress *in vivo* is mixed with null and positive effects [35–37].

Most of the literature supporting the efficacy of any oxidants against cancer is based on *in vitro* studies and from chemical carcinogen induced tumor animal models [38]. Much of this literature has been recently reviewed in light of the potential for berry phytochemicals to act as cancer chemotherapeutic agents by protecting against genomic instability [39]. Unfortunately, much of the research on phytochemicals conducted *in vitro* was done without consideration of the bioavailability and metabolism of the phytochemicals examined. Many plant phytochemicals are not absorbed by animal or human subjects at levels that have been studied *in vitro*. The compounds that do exert anti-carcinogenic effects at realistic doses may be responsible for the effects seen by berries and other phenolic rich foods; however, much more research is required to verify the *in vivo* effects of individual compounds. It should be highlighted that synergistic effects between multiple compounds may be responsible for effects observed by whole berries or extracts where effects are not observed (or below observable limits) for individual berry components.

In light of the fact that berries possess predominently water soluble antioxidants or polyphenolic antioxidants with relatively low bioavailability, the question has been raised about how effectively dietary antioxidants compete with endogenous antioxidants *in vivo* as direct radical quenchers.

Plant polyphenolic, and especially flavonoids such as anthocyanins, are excellent antioxidant *in vitro*; however, *in vivo*, their more important chemoprotective role may be as modulators of signal transduction pathways, gene regulation, and regulators detoxifying enzymes (e.g., glutathione *S*-transferase (GST), NADPH (nicotinamide adenine dinucleotide phosphate): quinone oxidoreductase and heme oxygenase) [40]. An excellent review of the effects of flavonoids on mammalian cells is presented by Middleton *et al.* [41] including chemoprotective effects citing studies of mutagenicity, anti-carcinogenic and apoptotic effects, anti-proliferative activity, effects on differentiation, adhesion, metastasis, heat shock proteins, multidrug resistance, and xenobiotic metabolism. Middleton *et al.* also extensively review studies of flavonoid effects on enzyme systems, many directly relevant to carcinogenesis and inflammation.

An example of the effects phytochemicals can have is found in the modulation of the antioxidant response element or electrophile responsive element (ARE/EpRE). Detailed studies of the detoxification enzymes revealed the existence of the ARE, a DNA sequence regulating the cellular response to many chemopreventive agents as well as the response of cells to changes in redox status [42]. Many of the phytochemicals in berries, especially the flavonoids, activate different pathways resulting in ARE modulation of numerous chemoprotective genes, including the pro-inflammatory cyclooxygenase 2 (COX2) gene. The PKC (protein kinase C), PI3K, MAPK (mitogen-activated protein kinase), JNK (c-Jun NH_2-terminal kinases) pathways can all be affected by berry phytochemicals [43] and all these pathways can modify the relationship between the transcription factor Nrf2 and Keap1, its negative regulator initiating translocation of Nrf2 to the nucleus activating the ARE [44]. Other pathways affected in phytochemicals chemoprotection are reviewed elsewhere [45].

IN VITRO EVIDENCE OF BERRY CHEMOPREVENTION

Carcinogenesis begins with alteration of the genomic stability in the process of initiation leading to mutagenesis. Damage to DNA induced by carcinogenic compounds, their reactive metabolites, or reactive oxygen and nitrogen species results in mutations of critical genes regulating proliferation, cell death, or apoptosis. These mutations are exacerbated by damage to the DNA repair mechanisms themselves. The inevitable result of un-repairable damage to these genes is loss of cell death capability and cancer proliferation. Strong evidence exists from *in vitro* studies that berries can intervene in many of the mechanisms of cancer at multiple stages in cancer development and there are several reviews of these effects for individual berries [46–48].

Strawberry, blueberry, and raspberry extracts induce cell death in breast and cervical cancer cell lines [49] and their juices are more potent inhibitors of chemically induced mutagenesis than are juices of many other berries [50]. Blackberry juice and purees have also been shown to inhibit mutagenesis [51] via the *in vitro* Ames test, a relatively reliable *in vitro* indicator of *in vivo* chemoprotective potential. Further tests of blackberries however have shown that there is a high degree of variability in anti-mutagenic potency even within varieties or cultivars within a species [52]. These differences are linked to phytochemical content and may vary with soils, microclimate, cultivation practices, and stage of ripeness. For example, a difference in the *in vitro* ability to inhibit proliferation has been suggested between organically and conventionally cultivated strawberries that was attributed to their antioxidant levels [53].

Both extracts and individual berry phytochemicals have been examined for their anti-mutagenic qualities. Some of these in vitro experiments clearly point to the existence of synergistic effects between berry components in chemoprotection. Cranberry phenolics, ellagic acid, and rosmarinic acid have synergistic interactions in inhibiting chemically induced (sodium azide and

N-methyl-N′-nitro-N-nitrosoguanidine) mitogenesis in a Salmonella typhimurium tester system against the mutagens whereas ellagic acid and rosmarinic acid were equally effective in protecting the DNA from oxidative damage [54]. Ellagic acid and rosmarinic acid enhanced the anti-mutagen activity of cranberry phenolics suggesting that these compounds may protect cells from mutations by modulating DNA repair systems.

A few *in vitro* and *in vivo* studies have demonstrated anthocyanins ability to reduce cancer cell proliferation and to inhibit tumor formation [55–57]. Berry anthocyanins anti-carcinogenic properties appear to stem from their ability to affect multiple mechanisms, including inhibition of cyclooxygenase enzymes (such as COX2) and blocking activation of a MAPK pathway [58]. Anthocyanins are phytochemical components that are present in all berries and although the individual components, concentrations, and ratios may vary between berries, their presence may contribute to the overall potential of any berry's anti-carcinogenic properties.

Strawberry extracts containing high antioxidant activity levels of the enzymes glutathione peroxidase, superoxide dismutase, guaiacol peroxidase, ascorbate peroxidase, and glutathione reductase have been shown to inhibit proliferation of a human lung epithelial cancer cell line and inhibit tetradecanoylphorbol-13-acetate (TPA) or ultraviolet-B (UVB) induced activator protein-1 (AP-1) and nuclear factor-kappaB (NF-κB) when applied to JB6 P$^+$ mouse epidermal cells *in vitro* [59]. The implication of down-regulation of AP-1 and NF-κB activities is the blockade of MAPK signaling, and suppressing cancer cell proliferation and transformation.

Organic extracts of black raspberries have also been shown to inhibit benzo(a)pyrene (BaP)-induced cell transformation *in vitro* via inhibiting AP-1 and NF-κB transactivation in mouse epidermal JB6 Cl 41 cells mediated via inhibition of MAPK activation and inhibitory subunit B phosphorylation, respectively [60]. None of the fractions was found to affect p53-dependent transcription activity. In view of the important roles of AP-1 and NFB in tumor promotion/progression, these results suggest that the ability of black raspberries to inhibit tumor development may be mediated by impairing signal transduction pathways leading to activation of AP-1 and NFB. The methanolic fraction appears to be the major fraction responsible for the inhibitory activity of black raspberries. Experiments with components of black raspberries, ellagic acid, ferulic acid, and β-sitosterol, as well as with ethanolic extracts of black raspberries have demonstrated that components within black raspberries can inhibited the growth of premalignant and malignant oral cells [61]. Evidence was presented suggesting that these effects on cell proliferation of premalignant and malignant human oral cells may involve specific berry components that interfere with aberrant signaling pathways regulating cell cycle progression.

Similarly, blackberry extracts inhibit 12-O-tetradecanoylphorbol-13-acetate (TPA) induced proliferation of cancer cells and neoplastic transformation of a human lung cancer cell line, A549 and blackberry extract pretreatment of these cells inhibits 8-hydroxy-2'-deoxyguanosine (8-OHdG) formation induced by UVB irradiation [62]. Furthermore, blackberry extract blocked UVB- or TPA-induced phosphorylation of extracellular signal-regulated protein kinases and (JNK), but not p38 kinase. These results indicated that an extract from fresh blackberry may inhibit tumor promoter-induced carcinogenesis and associated cell signaling. The chemopreventive effects of blackberry may be via blockade of ROS-mediated AP-1 and MAPK activation.

In experiments using human breast cancer MCF-7 cells, cranberry extracts possessed the ability to suppress proliferation and evidence has been presented that partly attribute this effect to both the initiation of apoptosis and the G1 phase arrest [63]. Observation that cranberry presscake (the material remaining after squeezing juice from the berries) fed to mice bearing human breast tumor MDA-MB-435 cells decrease the growth and metastasis of tumors led to examination of cranberry anti-tumor activity in other tumor types. *In vitro* experiments showed varying degrees of inhibition of proliferation by a cranberry flavonoid extract fraction in the androgen-dependent prostate cell line LNCaP and DU145, the estrogen-independent breast line MDA-MB-435, the breast (MCF-7), skin (SK-MEL-5), colon (HT-29), lung (DMS114), and brain (U87) cell lines [64]. Experiments in MDA-MB-435 cells demonstrated blockade of cell cycle progression and induction of apoptosis as the likely mechanisms responsible for these effects. The dried extracts and flavonoid fractions of blueberries show anti-proliferation and apoptotic activities toward HT-29 and Caco-2 cells. Flavonol, tannin, and anthocyanin fractions inhibited cell proliferation better than did the phenolic acid fraction; however, the anthocyanin fraction also increased DNA fragmentation, indicating the induction of apoptosis. These findings suggest that blueberry intake may reduce colon cancer risk [65].

Different fractions of phenolic compounds in blueberries and muscadine grapes have been investigated for their effects on HepG2 liver cancer cell viability and apoptosis [66]. Polyphenols were extracted from four cultivars of each berry species and further separated into phenolic acids, tannins, flavonols, and anthocyanins fractions. The phenolic acid fractions both muscadine grapes and blueberries inhibited HepG2 cell proliferation. Once again, however, the greatest inhibitory effects were observed from the anthocyanin fractions. Flavonol and tannin fractions did show anti-proliferative activities. Anthocyanin fractions of both berries increased DNA fragmentation compared to control suggesting that both blueberries and grapes may contribute to reduction in liver cancer risk. Another group found a different active anti-cancer ingredient in muscadine grapes effective against a different human cancer cell line. Four polyphenolics fractions of the muscadine grape extracts, (1) an ellagitannin-rich fraction, (2) a free ellagic acid and flavonoids fraction, (3) an anthocyanin, and (4) an ellagic acid glycosides fraction had inhibitory effects on vital cell parameters. These effects correlated with the ellagic acid glycosides and flavonoids and also to the antioxidant capacity. The investigators concluded that the anti-cancer properties of red muscadine juice were related to ellagic acid components within the grapes [67].

Extracts of six commercial berries, blackberry, black raspberry, blueberry, cranberry, red raspberry, and strawberry, have been evaluated for their ability to inhibit the growth of human oral (KB, CAL-27), breast (MCF-7), colon (HT-29, HCT116), and prostate (LNCaP) tumor cell lines at concentrations ranging from 25 µg/ml to 200 µg/ml [68]. A dose-dependent inhibition of cell proliferation in all of the cell lines was observed. The berry extracts were also shown to induce apoptosis in Ht-29 colon cancer cells with black raspberry and strawberry extracts showing the most potency.

Fractionated extracts of four *Vaccinium* species (lowbush blueberry, bilberry, cranberry, and lingonberry) show anti-carcinogenic properties *in vitro* by inducing the phase II xenobiotic detoxification enzyme quinone reductase and inhibiting tumor promoter phorbol 12-myristate 13-acetate induction of ornithine decarboxylase [69]. In these *in vitro* experiments components of the hexane/chloroform fraction of bilberry and of the proanthocyanidin fraction of lowbush blueberry, cranberry, and lingonberry exhibit potential anti-carcinogenic activity as evaluated by *in vitro* screening tests.

High molecular weight tannins of proanthocyanidin-rich fractions from both wild and cultivated blueberries have inhibitory effects *in vitro* on the proliferation of prostate cancer cells. While different proanthocyanin fractions from wild and cultivated blueberries showed different activities, in general proanthocyanins suppressed proliferation of the androgen-sensitive prostate cancer cell line, LNCaP, but are even more effective at inhibiting the androgen insensitive prostate cancer cell line, DU145 [70]. Questions remain regarding the bioavailability of tannins and proanthocyanins to tissue tumor sites. While the amount day intake of proanthocyanidins from berries and other plant sources generally represents an amount twice that of other flavonoids, the bioavailability of proanthocyanidins above the dimer level is improbable. *In vitro* effects of proanthocyanidins must be tempered by the realization that they are unlikely to have effects in tissues where delivery to an active site in interstitial space is required.

Another important anti-cancer therapeutic property of berries and berry components derives from their ability to inhibit angiogenesis. Angiogenesis, while essential during growth, development and normal wound healing, is also necessary to the process of tumor growth and malignancy. Cancer cells secrete growth factors such as vascular endothelial growth factor. Tumors cannot grow without a blood supply and stimulation of new capillaries is essential to their growth and to formation of additional tumors resulting in the process of malignancy. Berry extracts of strawberry, bilberry, wild blueberry, cranberry, elderberry, and raspberry seeds inhibit angiogenesis by inhibiting tumor necrosis factor-alpha (TNF-α) induced VEGF expression in human HaCaT keratinocytes [71]. Using a matrigel assay this study also showed that edible berries impair angiogenesis in human dermal microvascular endothelial cells. Black raspberry extracts are also anti-angiogenic in a human tissue-based *in vitro* fibrin clot angiogenesis assay. Assay-guided fractionation of a crude black raspberry extract identified one of the active compounds as gallic acid.

However, individual subfractions were not as potent as the original extract implying multiple active ingredients that may be additive or synergistic in their anti-angiogenic effects [72].

Lately, interest is growing in the effects of microflora on phytochemical constituents of foods and the consequent health implications. Interestingly, the bacteria Serratia vaccinii, isolated from blueberry microflora, is capable of increasing the antioxidant capacity of berry juices by increasing its phenolic content. Saskatoon berry, cranberry, strawberry, and grape wines co-fermented with Serratia and wine yeast in anaerobic fermentations were high in antioxidant activity and strongly inhibited activated-macrophage NO (nitric oxide) production and induced tumor necrosis factor-alpha production [73]. It remains to be determined if this effect extends to other cell types, and its implication for cancer is unclear. This data does bring forward the concept that berry phytochemicals that are consumed, are also available to gastrointestinal (GI) microflora that can alter and metabolize them, generating bioavailable compounds that have not been thoroughly investigated.

PHYTOCHEMICALS IN VITRO AND IN VIVO

In vitro studies have generally employed berry extracts or individual berry chemical components used at µg/ml concentrations. These concentrations are far higher than the concentrations either expected or found *in vivo*. Nevertheless, some of the activities observed *in vitro* have been observed in animal studies. As cited above, the potential chemopreventive activities include reduced proliferation, increased apoptosis, and cell cycle arrest in tumor cells, down-regulation of expression and activity of inflammatory enzymes and signaling pathways and enhancement of carcinogen detoxification pathways. Strawberry and saw palmetto berry extract have been shown to inhibit COX enzymes *in vitro* in prostate cancer cells suggesting berry components could modulate the inflammatory process [74] yet there is insufficient research conducted to date to verify that these effects exist *in vivo*. In many cases there is disconnect between the concentrations required to produce these effects *in vitro* and the levels of compounds reaching tissues *in vivo*. There are, however, several points that must be kept in mind. Bioavailability of all berry phytochemicals to the various tissues has not yet been thoroughly investigated [75] and when phytochemicals are absorbed they are metabolized. Many of the *in vitro* anti-cancer studies were conducted using compounds that are not physiologically relevant. For example, no study to date has identified the aglycone anthocyanidins in plasma much less tissues. Studies have identified the original plant anthocyanins and the animal produced glucuronide and/or methylated metabolites in circulation [76–80]; however, currently there is little direct evidence of anthocyanin aglycones existing in the circulation or urine of humans [78]. The absorption, metabolism and pharmacokinetics of anthocyanins have been recently reviewed [81] and as is the case for many berry phytochemicals, basic aspects of their absorption and metabolism need to be more fully investigated. Furthermore, little or nothing is known about the biological activity of individual metabolites. Another point to keep in mind involves the concept of biological synergy of pho-tochemical compounds [82]. The concept has been forwarded to explain why combinations of natural phytochemicals acquired through whole-food consump-tion in fruits and vegetables show health benefits not seen in the individual com-ponents at physiologically relevant concentrations.

IN VIVO EVIDENCE OF BERRY CHEMOPREVENTION

Nitric oxide is now recognized as playing important roles in cancer etiology and progression and it can influence the outcome of cancer treatment. It is synthe-sized by the action of nitric oxide synthases on the amino acid arginine. Nitric oxide plays a role in production of nitrite and important signal regulator in mam-malian cells [83]; however, it can also react with other oxygen radicals produc-ing peroxynitrite, nitrogen dioxide, and dinitrogen trioxide, highly damaging reactive nitrogen species. These are potent inducers of apoptosis and necrosis. However, they can also inhibit DNA repair mechanisms, leading to mutation and carcinogenesis. There is clear evidence that administration of competitive inhibi-tors of nitric oxide synthetase can significantly slow the growth of solid tumors in rodent models. Both inhibition and over-production of nitric oxide can pro-vide strategies for cancer therapy and these have been reviewed [84].

In vitro and *in vivo* experiments have been conducted to investigate berry inhibition of nitrosation. When whole strawberries were provided immediately after an amine-rich diet with a nitrate, *N*-nitrosodimethylamine (NDMA) excre-tion in humans was decreased by 70% compared to ingestion of an amine-rich diet with a nitrate [85]. These results suggest that consumption of whole straw-berries can reduce endogenous NDMA formation. *In vivo*, dietary freeze-dried strawberries have been shown to possess the ability to inhibit NMBA-induced tumorigenesis in the rat esophagus [86]. Rats consuming diets containing 5 and 10% freeze-dried strawberries experienced reductions in esophageal tumor mul-tiplicity of over 50% with the higher dose compared to control diet fed animals. In further studies of arylalkyl isothiocyanates inhibition of NMBA-induced tumorigenicity and DNA methylation, freeze-dried strawberry preparation were not as effective as phenylpropyl isothiocyanate or phenylethyl isothiocyanate in inhibiting NMBA-induced esophageal carcinogenesis in the F344 rat esophagus [87]. The chemopreventive activity of the strawberries could not be attributed solely to the ellagic acid content of the berries.

Reduced glutathione (L-gamma-glutamyl-L-cysteinyl-glycine, GSH) is the prevalent low-molecular weight thiol in mammalian cells and the primary endog-enous defence molecule against oxidative radical damage, and plays critical roles in detoxification and cell signaling (involved in the regulation of gene expression, apoptosis, and cell proliferation). Two enzymes are responsible for GSH synthe-sis, γ-glutamylcysteine synthetase and glutathione synthetase. Alterations in GSH concentrations been demonstrated to be a common feature of many pathological diseases, including cancer. GSH modulation has been recently to modulate redox-sensitive components of signal transduction cascades [88].

Transgenic mice expressing luciferase controlled by the γ-glutamylcysteine synthetase heavy subunit promoter were used to investigate the effects of berry juices or extracts on γ-glutamylcysteine synthetase. Transgenic mice fed berry juices or extracts or ellagic acid showed upregulation of γ-glutamylcysteine synthetase via change in GCSh promoter activity [89]. The experiments showed that there were responders or nonresponders among the animals. Thus berry consumption can lead to *in vivo* induction of γ-glutamylcysteine synthetase, a protective enzyme that is chemopreventive.

As previously mentioned, activation of MAPK pathways has been implicated in cell migration, proteinase induction, apoptosis, and angiogenesis, that is events involved in tumorigenesis and metastasis [90]. Different kinases in the MAPK family including JNK, p38, and ERK regulate cell migration via distinct mechanisms. Inhibition of MAPK pathways and pro-carcinogenic mechanisms mediated by AP-1, NF-κB, and COX2 by berry extracts and berry phytochemical components may contribute to the suppression of tumor cell proliferation and metastasis *in vivo*. In a combination of *in vitro* and *in vivo* experiments in rodents, the berry anthocyanin cyanidin-3-glucoside (C3G) has been shown to exhibits chemoprevention and chemotherapeutic activities by interfering with signal transduction via AP-1, MAPK, NF-κB, COX2, and TNF-α [91].

The ability of berry extracts and phytochemicals to modulate TNF-α and other signal transduction pathway components *in vitro* and *in vivo* suggest strongly that they may also inhibit angiogenesis in animals. Hemangiomas represent a powerful model to study *in vivo* angiogenesis. Mouse endothelioma cells injected into compatible host animals proliferate to form blood vessel conduits that fuse with the systemic circulation, drawing blood into the hemangioma. Monocyte chemotactic protein 1 recruits macrophages to sites of infection or inflammation and facilitate angiogenesis. Wild blueberry and the berry mix (OptiBerry) significantly inhibit inducible monocyte chemotactic protein 1 transcription and inducible NF-κB transcription in endothelioma cells [92] diminishing their ability to form hemangioma. These data provide *in vivo* evidence substantiating the anti-angiogenic property of edible berries.

Lyophilized black raspberries are also effective against NMBA-induced esophageal tumorigenesis in the F344 rat during both the initiation and post-initiation phases of carcinogenesis showing similar potency as strawberries [93]. Lyophilized black raspberries inhibited formation of the promutagenic adduct O^6-methylguanine and significantly reduced tumor incidence and multiplicity, proliferation indices and preneoplastic lesion formation.

Blueberries, un-like strawberries and black raspberries, are not able to inhibit NMBA-induced tumorigenesis in the rat esophagus [94]. They differ from strawberries and black raspberries, however, in that they contain only small amounts of the chemopreventive agent ellagic acid. Blueberries did not reduce the formation of NMBA-induced O^6-methylguanine adducts in esophageal DNA when fed at 10% of the diet.

Of the alimentary tract cancers, therapeutic protocols against oral cavity cancers are perhaps the most ineffective. Using a hamster cheek pouch model, black raspberries have been shown to inhibit 7,12-dimethylbenz(a) anthracene (DMBA)-induced oral cavity tumors [95]. The mechanisms for the observed effects of black raspberries on chemically induced oral and esophageal cancer appear to be mediated by down-regulation of COX2, inducible nitric oxide synthase, and c-Jun [96].

Further down the alimentary tract, lyophilized black raspberries had effects on azoxymethane (AOM)-induced aberrant crypt foci, colon tumors, and urinary 8-hydroxy-2'-deoxyguanosine (8-OHdG) levels in male Fischer 344 rats [97]. Aberrant crypt foci multiplicity decreased in berry fed animals relative to the AOM only group. Total tumor multiplicity and adenocarcinoma multiplicity declined and, although not significant, a tumor burden was observed in all berry fed groups. Urinary 8-OHdG levels, a marker of DNA damage, were reduced in the berry fed animals. The research concerning berry effects on esophageal and colon cancer has recently been reviewed [98].

Research began in humans in autumn of 2006 to examine the potential benefits of dietary black raspberries on Barrett's esophageal cancer. This is the first human clinical trial of dietary berries as a preventative dietary agent against cancer. Interim findings from 10 patients suggest that daily consumption of lyophilized black raspberries decreases urinary excretion of two markers of oxidative stress, 8-epi-prostaglandin F2 (8-Iso-PGF2) and, to a lesser extent, 8-hydroxy-2'-deoxyguanosine (8-OHdG), among patients with Barrett's esophageal cancer [99].

A Chinese study showed that wolfberries reduce DNA strand breakage via a buccal cell comet assay in a limited number of healthy humans compared with controls [100]. Other studies of berry consumption in humans have shown that Aronia, blueberry and boysenberry juice decreases in oxidative DNA damage in blood cells [101]. However, all berries do not appear to prevent DNA damage in humans. Human consumption of blackcurrant juice for 3 weeks resulted in an increase in oxidative DNA damage when compared to control subjects [102]. While controversial, it has been suggested that the high vitamin C content of blackcurrant juice (210 mg/l) was acting as a pro-oxidant as blackcurrant anthocyanins alone was neither protective nor did it cause increased DNA damage. Other berry supplementation studies using cranberries [103] or blueberries [104] at nutritionally relevant levels also showed no reductions in DNA damage. The ability of berries or their extracts to prevent genomic instability by diminishing DNA damage has not been unequivocally proved in humans.

To date relatively few of the bioactive compounds identified in berries have proceeded to clinical trials for cancer prevention [105–107]. Indeed there are currently only half a dozen trials of any phase listed at http://www.cancer. gov/clinicaltrials [108] being conducted in the United States using either fruit extracts or components identified as active components from them. In addition to that of dried raspberries mentioned above, trials are currently underway using mistletoe, resveratrol, grape pro-anthocyanins, and strawberries. These studies include phase II, phase I trial for "Resveratrol for Patients With Colon Cancer," a phase I "Study of Resveratrol in Patients With Resectable Colorectal Cancer," a phase I "Biomarker Study of Dietary Grape-Derived Low Dose Resveratrol for Colon Cancer Prevention," a phase II "Randomized Study of Fruit and Vegetable Extracts in Patients With Stage I-IVB Head and Neck Cancer," a phase I "Pilot Chemoprevention Study of IH636 Grape Seed Proanthocyanidin Extract in Healthy Postmenopausal Women at High Risk of Developing Breast Cancer," and a phase II randomized study of "Mistletoe as Complementary Treatment in Patients With Advanced Non-Small-Cell Lung Cancer (NSCLC), Treated With Carboplatin/Gemcitabine Chemotherapy Combination."

CONCLUSIONS

In vitro and *in vivo* evidence suggests that lyophilized berries, berry extracts, and berry phytochemicals including proanthocyanins (or their metabolites), anthocyanins, other flavonoids such as quercetin, ellagic acid, and stilbenes have efficacy in preventing some cancers. Very little is known regarding the effects of berries on metastasis. Much more research is necessary to understand the bioavailability, tissue distributions, and metabolism of berry phytochemicals. Research to date suggests that different berries may possess different efficacies against different cancers. A high degree of synergy exists between berry phytochemicals in their chemoprotective activities and this is likely driven by actions that modulate a variety of pathways affecting carcinogenesis and pro-carcinogenic mechanisms such as inflammation and angiogenesis.

There is a deficit of animal studies examining the effects of dietary berries on breast and colon cancer. No studies have yet investigated the degree to which berry phytochemicals will complement or interfere with current chemotherapy protocols.

REFERENCES

1. Milazzo, S., Ernst, E., Lejeune, S. & Schmidt, K. (2006). Laetrile treatment for cancer. *Cochrane Database of Systematic Reviews* (Issue 2), Art. No.: CD005476. DOI: 10.1002/14651858.CD005476.pub2.
2. Cipollini, M. L. & Levey, D. J. (1997). Secondary metabolites of fleshy vertebrate-dispersed fruits: Adaptive hypotheses and implications for seed dispersal. *The American Naturalist* **150**, 346–372.
3. Challem, J. J. (1997). Did the loss of endogenous ascorbate propel the evolution of Anthropoidea and Homo sapiens? *Med-Hypotheses* **48**, 387–392.
4. Blomme, T., Vandepoele, K., De Bodt, S., Simillion, C., Maere, S. & Van de Peer, Y. (2006). The gain and loss of genes during 600 million years of vertebrate evolution. *Genome Biol* **7**, R43.

5. Block, G., Patterson, B. & Subar, A. (1992). Fruit, vegetables, and cancer prevention: A review of the epidemiological evidence. *Nutr Cancer* **18**, 1–29.

6. World Cancer Research Fund (1997). *Food, Nutrition and the Prevention of Cancer: A Global Perspective*, pp. 216–251, American Institute for Cancer Research, Washington, DC.

7. International Agency for Research on Cancer (2003). Fruit and Vegetables, IARC Press, Lyon, France.

8. Beckman, K. B. & Ames, B. N. (1998). The free radical theory of aging matures. *Physiol Rev* **78**, 547–581.

9. Halliwell, B. (1996). Antioxidants in human health and disease. *Annu Rev Nutr* **16**, 33–50.

10. Sies, H. (1997). Oxidative stress: Oxidants and antioxidants. *Exp Physiol* **82**, 291–295.

11. Simic, M. G. & Bergtold, D. S. (1991). Dietary modulation of DNA damage in human. *Mutation Research/Fundamental and Molecular Mechanisms of Mutagenesis* **250**, 17–24.

12. Proteggente, A. R., Pannala, A. S., Paganga, G., Van Buren, L., Wagner, E., Wiseman, S., Van De Put, F., Dacombe, C. & Rice-Evans, C. A. (2002). The antioxidant activity of regularly consumed fruit and vegetables reflects their phenolic and vitamin C composition. *Free Radical Res* **36**, 217–233.

13. Sun, J. S., Chu, Y. F., Wu, X. & Liu, R. H. (2002). Antioxidant and antiproliferative activities of common fruits. *J Agric Food Chem* **50**, 7449–7454.

14. Halvorsen, B. L., Holte, K., Myhrstad, M. C., Barikmo, I., Hvattum, E., Remberg, S. F., Wold, A. B., Haffner, K., Baugerød, H., Andersen, L. F., Moskaug, Ø., Jacobs, D. R., Jr. & Blomhoff, R. (2002). A systematic screening of total antioxidants in dietary plants. *J Nutr* **132**, 461–471.

15. du Toit, R., Volsteedt, Y. & Apostolides, Z. (2001). Comparison of the antioxidant content of fruits, vegetables and teas measured as vitamin C equivalents. *Toxicology* **14**, 63–69.

16. Wu, X., Beecher, G. R., Holden, J. M., Haytowitz, D. B., Gebhardt, S. E. & Prior, R. L. (2004). Lipophilic and hydrophilic antioxidant capacities of common foods in the United States. *J Agric Food Chem* **52**, 4026–4037.

17. Prior, R. L., Gu, L., Wu, X., Jacob, R. A., Sotoudeh, G., Kader, A. A. & Cook, R. A. (2007). Plasma antioxidant capacity changes following a meal as a measure of the ability of a food to alter *in vivo* antioxidant status. *J Am Coll Nutr* **26**, 170–181.

18. Macheix, J.-J., Fleuriet, A. & Billot, J. (1990). *Fruit Phenolics*, CRC Press, Boca Raton, FL.

19. Williner, M. R., Pirovani, M. E. & Güemes, D. R. (2003). Ellagic acid content in strawberries of different cultivars and ripening stages. *J SciFood Agric* **83**, 842–845.

20. Kahkonen, M. P., Hopia, A. I. & Heinonen, M. (2001). Berry phenolics and their antioxidant activity. *J Agric Food Chem* **49**, 4076–4082.

21. Castonguay, H. U., Gali, E. M., Perchellet, X. M., Gao, M., Boukharta, G., Jalbert, T., Okuda, T., Yoshida, T., Hatano, & Perchellet, J. P. (1997). Antitumorigenic and antipromoting activities of ellagic acid, ellagitannins and oligomeric anthocyanin and procyanidin. *Int J Oncol* **10**, 367–373.

22. Ariga, T. (2004). The antioxidative function, preventive action on disease and utilization of proanthocyanidins. *Biofactors* **21**, 197–201.
23. Williamson, G. & Manach, C. (2005). Bioavailability and bioefficacy of polyphenols in humans. II. Review of 93 intervention studies. *Am J Clin Nutr* **81**, 243S–255S.
24. Ahuja, S., Kaak, B. & Roberts, J. (1998). Loss of fimbrial adhesion with the addition of *Vaccinium macrocarpon* to the growth medium of P-fimbriated *Escherichia coli*. *J Urol* **159**, 559–562.
25. Ofek, I., Goldhar, J., Zafriri, D., Lis, H., Adar, R. & Sharon, N. (1991). Anti-*Escherichia coli* adhesin activity of cranberry and blueberry juices. *N Engl J Med* **324**, 1599.
26. Durukan, A. H., Evereklioglu, C., Hurmeric, V., Kerimoglu, H., Erdurman, C., Bayraktar, M. Z. & Mumcuoglu, T. (2006). Ingestion of IH636 grape seed proanthocyanidin extract to prevent selenite-induced oxidative stress in experimental cataract. *J Cataract Refract Surg* **32**, 1041–1045.
27. Jaakola, L., Määttä, K., Pirttila, A. M., Törrönen, R., Kärenlampi, S. & Hohtola, A. (2002). Expression of genes involved in anthocyanin biosynthesis in relation to anthocyanin, proanthocyanidin, and flavonol levels during bilberry fruit development. *Plant Physiol* **130**, 729–739.
28. da Silva, F. L., Escribano-Bailón, M. T., Alonso, J. J. P. & Santos-Buelga, C. (2007). Anthocyanin pigments in strawberry. *Food Sci Technol* **40**, 374–382.
29. Sporn, M. B. (1976). Approaches to prevention of epithelial cancer during the preneoplastic period. *Cancer Res* **36**, 2699–2702.
30. Penas-Prado, M. & Gilbert, M. R. (2007). Molecularly targeted therapies for malignant gliomas: Advances and challenges. *Expert Rev Anticancer Ther* **7**, 641–661.
31. Johnson, I. T. (2007). Phytochemicals and cancer. *Proc Nutr Soc* **66**, 207–215.
32. Liu, R. H. (2004). Potential synergy of phytochemicals in cancer prevention: Mechanism of action. *J Nutr* **134**, 3479S–3485S.
33. Burhans, W. C. & Weinberger, M. (2007). DNA replication stress, genome instability and aging. *Nucleic Acids Res* **35**, 7545–7556.
34. Visioli, F., Grande, S., Bogani, P. & Galli, C. (2004). The role of antioxidants in the mediterranean diets: Focus on cancer. *Eur J Canc Prev* **13**, 337–343.
35. Barnett, L. E., Broomfield, A. M., Hendriks, W. H., Hunt, M. B. & McGhie, T. K. (2007). The *in vivo* antioxidant action and the reduction of oxidative stress by boysenberry extract is dependent on base diet constituents in rats. *J Med Food* **10**, 281–289.
36. Harris, G. K., Gupta, A., Nines, R. G., Kresty, L. A., Habib, S. G., Frankel, W. L., LaPerle, K., Gallaher, D. D., Schwartz, S. J. & Stoner, G. D. (2001). Effects of lyophilized black raspberries on azoxymethane-induced colon cancer and 8-hydroxy-2'-deoxyguanosine levels in the Fischer 344 rat. *Nutr Cancer* **40**, 125–133.
37. Wood, L. G., Gibson, P. G. & Garg, M. L. (2006). A review of the methodology for assessing *in vivo* antioxidant capacity. *J Sci Food Agric* **86**, 2057–2066.
38. Chen, C. & Kong, A. N. (2005). Dietary cancer-chemopreventive compounds: From signaling and gene expression to pharmacological effects. *Trends Pharmacol Sci* **26**, 318–326.

39. Duthie, S. J. (2007). Berry phytochemicals, genomic stability and cancer: Evidence for chemoprotection at several stages in the carcinogenic process. *Mol Nutr Food Res* **51**, 665–674.

40. Milbury, P. E., Graf, B., Curran-Celentano, J. M. & Blumberg, J. B. (2007). Bilberry (*Vaccinium myrtillus*) anthocyanins modulate heme oxygenase-1 and glutathione *S*-transferase-pi expression in ARPE-19 cells. *Invest Ophthalmol Vis Sci* **48**, 2343–2349.

41. Middleton, E., Jr., Kandaswami, C. & Theoharides, T. C. (2000). The effects of plant flavonoids on mammalian cells: Implications for inflammation, heart disease, and cancer. *Pharmacol Rev* **52**(4), 673–751.

42. Hayes, J. D. & McMahon, M. (2001). Molecular basis for the contribution of the antioxidant responsive element to cancer chemoprevention. *Cancer Lett* **28**, 103–113.

43. Chen, C. & Kong, A. N. (2004). Dietary chemopreventive compounds and ARE/EpRE signaling. *Free Radic Biol Med* **36**, 1505–1516.

44. Nguyen, T., Sherratt, P. J. & Pickett, C. B. (2003). Regulatory mechanisms controlling gene expression mediated by the antioxidant response element. *Annu Rev Pharmacol Toxicol* **43**, 233–260.

45. Bode, A. M. & Dong, Z. (2005). Signal transduction pathways in cancer development and as targets for cancer prevention. *Prog Nucleic Acid Res Mol Biol* **79**, 237–297.

46. Juranić, Z. & Zizak, Z. (2005). Biological activities of berries: From antioxidant capacity to anti-cancer effects. *Biofactors* **23**, 207–211.

47. Neto, C. C. (2007). Cranberry and blueberry: Evidence for protective effects against cancer and vascular diseases. *Mol Nutr Food Res* **51**, 652–664.

48. Neto, C. C. (2007). Cranberry and its phytochemicals: A review of *in vitro* anticancer studies. *J Nutr* **137**(1 Suppl), 186S–193S.

49. Wedge, D. E., Meepagala, K. M., Magee, J. B., Smith, S. H., Huang, G. & Larcom, L. L. (2001). Anticarcinogenic activity of strawberry, blueberry, and raspberry extracts to breast and cervical cancer cells. *J Med Food* **4**, 49–52.

50. Smith, S., Tate, P. L., Huang, G., Magee, J. B., Meepagala, K. M., Wedge, D. E. & Larcom, L. L. (2004). Antimutagenic activity of berry extracts. *J Med Food* **7**, 450–455.

51. Tate, P., Kuzmar, A., Smith, S. W., Wedge, D. E. & Larcom, L. L. (2003). Comparative effects of eight varieties of blackberry on mutagenesis. *Nutr Res* **23**, 971–979.

52. Tate, P., Stanner, A., Shields, K., Smith, S. & Larcom, L. (2006). Blackberry extracts inhibit UV-induced mutagenesis in *Salmonella typhimurium* TA100. *Nutr Res* **26**, 100–104.

53. Olsson, M. E., Andersson, C. S., Oredsson, S., Berglund, R. H. & Gustavsson, K. E. (2006). Antioxidant levels and inhibition of cancer cell proliferation *in vitro* by extracts from organically and conventionally cultivated strawberries. *J Agric Food Chem* **54**, 1248–1255.

54. Vattem, D. A., Jang, H.-D., Levin, R. & Shetty, K. (2006). Synergism of cranberry phenolics with ellagic acid and rosmarinic acid for antimutagenic and DNA protection functions. *J Food Biochem* **30**, 98–116.

55. Hou, D. X. (2003). Potential mechanisms of cancer chemoprevention by anthocyanins. *Curr Mol Med* **3**, 149–159.

56. Kang, S., Seeram, N., Nair, M. & Bourquin, L. (2003). Tart cherry anthocyanins inhibit tumor development in Apc(Min) mice and reduce proliferation of human colon cancer cells. *Cancer Lett* **194**, 13–19.

57. Koide, T., Hashimoto, Y., Kamei, H., Kojima, T., Hasegawa, M. & Terabe, K. (1997). Antitumor effect of anthocyanin fractions extracted from red soybeans and red beans *in vitro* and *in vivo*. *Cancer Biother. Radiopharm* **12**, 277–280.

58. Hou, D. X., Kai, K., Li, J. J., Lin, S., Terahara, N., Wakamatsu, M., Fujii, M., Young, M. R. & Colburn, N. (2004). Anthocyanidins inhibit activator protein 1 activity and cell transformation: Structure-activity relationship and molecular mechanisms. *Carcinogenesis* **25**, 29–36.

59. Wang, S. Y., Feng, R., Lu, Y., Bowman, L. & Ding, M. (2005). Inhibitory effect on activator protein-1, nuclear factor-kappaB, and cell transformation by extracts of strawberries (Fragaria × ananassa Duch). *J Agric Food Chem* **53**, 4187–4193.

60. Huang, C., Huang, Y., Li, J., Hu, W., Aziz, R., Tang, M., Sun, N., Cassady, J. & Stoner, G. D. (2002). Inhibition of benzo(a)pyrene diol-epoxide-induced transactivation of activated protein 1 and nuclear factor kb by black raspberry extracts. *Cancer Res* **62**, 6857–6863.

61. Han, C., Ding, H., Casto, B., Stoner, G. D. & D'Ambrosio, S. M. (2005). Inhibition of the growth of premalignant and malignant human oral cell lines by extracts and components of black raspberries. *Nutr Cancer* **51**, 207–217.

62. Feng, R., Bowman, L. L., Lu, Y., Leonard, S. S., Shi, X., Jiang, B.-H., Castranova, V., Vallyathan, V. & Ding, M. (2004). Blackberry extracts inhibit activating protein 1 activation and cell transformation by perturbing the mitogenic signalling pathway. *Nutr Cancer* **50**, 80–89.

63. Sun, J. & Liu, R. H. (2006). Cranberry phytochemical extracts induce cell cycle arrest and apoptosis in human MCF-7 breast cancer cells. *Cancer Lett* **241**, 124–134.

64. Ferguson, P. J., Kurowska, E., Freeman, D. J., Chambers, A. F. & Koropatnick, D. J. (2004). A flavonoid fraction from cranberry extract inhibits proliferation of human tumor cell lines. *J Nutr* **134**, 1529–1535.

65. Yi, W. G., Fischer, J., Krewer, G. & Akoh, C. C. (2005). Phenolic compounds from blueberries can inhibit colon cancer cell proliferation and induce apoptosis. *J Agric Food Chem* **53**, 7320–7329.

66. Yi, W., Akoh, C. C., Fischer, J. & Krewer, G. (2006). Effects of phenolic compounds in blueberries and muscadine grapes on Hepg2 cell viability and apoptosis. *Food Res Int* **39**, 628–638.

67. Mertens-Talcott, S. U., Lee, J. H., Percival, S. S. & Talcott, S. T. (2006). Induction of cell death in Caco-2 human colon carcinoma cells by ellagic acid rich fractions from muscadine grapes (*Vitis rotundifolia*). *J Agric Food Chem.* **54**, 5336–5343.

68. Seeram, N. P., Adams, L. S., Zhang, Y., Lee, R., Sand, D., Scheuller, H. S. & Heber, D. (2006). Blackberry, black raspberry, blueberry, cranberry, red raspberry, and strawberry extracts inhibit growth and stimulate apoptosis of human cancer cells *in vitro*. *J Agric Food Chem* **54**, 9329–9339.

69. Bomser, J., Madhavi, D. L., Singletary, K. & Smith, M. A. L. (1996). *In vitro* anticancer activity of fruit extracts from *Vaccinium* species. *Planta Med* **62**, 212–216.

70. Schmidt, B. M., Erdman, J. W. & Lila, M. A. (2006). Differential effects of blueberry proanthocyanidins on androgen sensitive and insensitive human prostate cancer cell lines. *Cancer Lett* **231**, 240–246.

71. Roy, S., Khanna, S., Alessio, H. M., Vider, J., Bagchi, D., Bagchi, M. & Sen, C. K. (2002). Anti-angiogenic property of edible berries. *Free Radic Res* **36**, 1023–1031.

72. Liu, Z., Schwimer, J., Liu, D., Greenway, F. L., Anthony, C. T. & Woltering, E. A. (2005). Black raspberry extract and fractions contain angiogenesis inhibitors. *Agric Food Chem* **53**, 3909–3915.

73. Voung, R., Martin, J. & Matar, C. (2006). Antioxidant activity of fermented berry juices and their effects on nitric oxide and tumor necrosis factor-alpha production in macrophages 264.7 gamma NO(–) cell line. *J Food Biochem* **30**, 249–268.

74. Goldmann, W. H., Sharma, A. L., Currier, S. J., Johnston, P. D., Rana, A. & Sharma, C. P. (2001). Saw palmetto berry extract inhibits cell growth and Cox-2 expression in prostatic cancer cells. *Cell Biol Int* **25**, 1117–1124.

75. Kalt, W., Blumberg, J. B., McDonald, J. E., Vinqvist-Tymchuk, M. R., Fillmore, S. A., Graf, B. A., O'Leary, J. M. & Milbury, P. E. (2008). Identification of anthocyanins in the liver, eye, and brain of blueberry-fed pigs. *J Agric Food Chem* **56**, 705–712.

76. Milbury, P. E., Cao, G., Prior, R. L. & Blumberg, J. (2002). Bioavailablility of elderberry anthocyanins. *Mech Ageing Dev* **123**, 997–1006.

77. Kay, C. D., Mazza, G. & Holub, B. J. (2005). Anthocyanins exist in the circulation primarily as metabolites in adult men. *J Nutr* **135**, 2582–2588.

78. Felgines, C., Talavera, S., Gonthier, M. P., Texier, O., Scalbert, A., Lamaison, J. L. & Remesy, C. (2003). Strawberry anthocyanins are recovered in urine as glucuro- and sulfoconjugates in humans. *J Nutr* **133**, 1296–1301.

79. Mazza, G., Kay, C. D., Cottrell, T. & Holub, B. J. (2002). Absorption of anthocyanins from blueberries and serum antioxidant status in human subjects. *J Agric Food Chem* **50**, 7731–7737.

80. Wu, X., Pittman, H. E., 3rd. & Prior, R. L. (2004). Pelargonidin is absorbed and metabolized differently than cyanidin after marionberry consumption in pigs. *J Nutr* **134**, 2603–2610.

81. Kay, C. D. (2006). Aspects of anthocyanin absorption, metabolism and pharmacokinetics in humans. *Nutr Res Rev* **19**, 137–146.

82. Liu, R. H. (2004). Potential synergy of phytochemicals in cancer prevention: Mechanism of action. *J Nutr* **134**, 3479S–3485S.

83. Bryan, N. S., Fernandez, B. O., Bauer, S. M., Garcia-Saura, M. F., Milsom, A. B., Rassaf, T., Maloney, R. E., Bharti, A., Rodriguez, J. & Feelisch, M. (2005). Nitrite is a signaling molecule and regulator of gene expression in mammalian tissues. *Nat Chem Biol* **1**, 290–297.

84. Hirst, D. G. & Robson, T. (2007). Nitrosative stress in cancer therapy. *Front Biosci* **1**, 3406–3418.

85. Chung, M. J., Lee, S. H. & Sung, N. J. (2002). Inhibitory effect of whole strawberries, garlic juice or kale juice on endogenous formation of *N*-nitrosodimethylamine in humans. *Cancer Lett* **182**, 1–10.

86. Carlton, P. S., Kresty, L. A., Siglin, J. C., Morse, M. A., Lu, J., Morgan, C. & Stoner, G. D. (2001). Inhibition of *N*-nitrosomethylbenzylamine-induced

tumorigenesis in the rat esophagus by dietary freeze-dried strawberries. *Carcinogenesis* **22**, 441–446.

87. Stoner, G. D., Kresty, L. A., Carlton, P. S., Siglin, J. C. & Morse, M. A. (1999). Isothiocyanates and freeze-dried strawberries as inhibitors of esophageal cancer. *Toxicol Sci* **52**(Suppl), 95–100.

88. Franco, R., Schoneveld, O. J., Pappa, A. & Panayiotidis, M. I. (2007). The central role of glutathione in the pathophysiology of human diseases. *Arch Physiol Biochem* **113**, 234–258.

89. Carlsen, H., Myhrstad, M. C., Thoresen, M., Moskaug, J.Ø. & Blomhoff, R. (2003). Berry intake increases the activity of the gamma-glutamylcysteine synthetase promoter in transgenic reporter mice. *J Nutr* **133**, 2137–2140.

90. Reddy, K. B., Nabha, S. M. & Atanaskova, N. (2003). Role of MAP kinase in tumor progression and invasion. *Cancer Metastasis Rev* **4**, 395–403.

91. Ding, M., Feng, R., Wang, S. Y., Bowman, L., Lu, Y., Qian, Y., Castranova, V., Jiang, B. H. & Shi, X. (2006). Cyanidin-3-glucoside, a natural product derived from blackberry, exhibits chemopreventive and chemotherapeutic activity. *J. Biol. Chem.* **281**, 17359–17368.

92. Atalay, M., Gordillo, G., Roy, S., Rovin, B., Bagchi, D., Bagchi, M. & Sen, C. K. (2003). Anti-angiogenic property of edible berry in a model of hemangioma. *FEBS Lett* **544**, 252–257.

93. Kresty, L. A., Morse, M. A., Morgan, C., Carlton, P. S., Lu, J., Gupta, A., Blackwood, M. & Stoner, G. D. (2001). Chemoprevention of esophageal tumorigenesis by dietary administration of lyophilized black raspberries. *Cancer Res* **61**, 6112–6119.

94. Aziz, R. M., Nines, R., Rodrigo, K., Harris, K., Hudson, T., Gupta, A., Morse, M., Carlton, P. & Stoner, G. D. (2002). The effect of freeze-dried blueberries on *N*-nitrosomethylbenzylamine tumorigenesis in the rat esophagus. *Pharmaceutical Biology (Formerly International Journal of Pharmacognosy)* **40**(Suppl), 43–49.

95. Casto, B. C., Kresty, L. A., Kraly, C. L., Pearl, D. K., Knobloch, T. J., Schut, H. A., Stoner, G. D., Mallery, S. R. & Weghorst, C. M. (2002). Chemoprevention of oral cancer by black raspberries. *Anticancer Res* **22**(6C), 4005–4015.

96. Chen, T., Hwang, H., Rose, M. E., Nines, R. G. & Stoner, G. D. (2006). Chemopreventive properties of black raspberries in *N*-nitrosomethylbenzylamine-induced rat esophageal tumorigenesis: Down-regulation of cyclooxygenase-2, inducible nitric oxide synthase, and c-Jun. *Cancer Res* **66**, 2853–2859.

97. Harris, G. K., Gupta, A., Nines, R. G., Kresty, L. A., Habib, S. G., Frankel, W. L., LaPerle, K., Gallaher, D. D., Schwartz, S. J. & Stoner, G. D. (2001). Effects of lyophilized black raspberries on azoxymethane-induced colon cancer and 8-hydroxy-2'-deoxyguanosine levels in the Fischer 344 rat. *Nutr Cancer* **40**, 125–133.

98. Stoner, G. D., Wang, L. S., Zikri, N., Chen, T., Hecht, S. S., Huang, C., Sardo, C. & Lechner, J. F. (2007). Cancer prevention with freeze-dried berries and berry components. *Semin Cancer Biol Oct* **17**, 403–410.

99. Kresty, L. A., Frankel, W. L., Hammond, C. D., Baird, M. E., Mele, J. M., Stoner, G. D. & Fromkes, J. J. (2006). Transitioning from preclinical to clinical chemopreventive assessments of lyophilized black raspberries: Interim results

show berries modulate markers of oxidative stress in Barrett's esophagus patients. *Nutr Cancer* **54**, 148–156.

100. Szeto, Y. T., Benzie, I. F., Collins, A. R., Choi, S. W., Cheng, C. Y., Yow, C. M. & Tse, M. M. (2005). A buccal cell model comet assay: Development and evaluation for human biomonitoring and nutritional studies. *Mutat Res* **578**, 371–381.

101. Bub, A., Watzl, B. & Blockhaus, M. (2003). Fruit juice consumption modulates antioxidant status, immune status and DNA damage. *J Nutr Biochem* **14**, 90–98.

102. Moller, P., Loft, S., Alfthan, G. & Freese, R. (2004). Oxidative DNA damage in circulating mononuclear blood cells after ingestion of blackcurrant juice or anthocyanin-rich drink. *Mutat Res* **551**, 119–126.

103. Duthie, S. J., Jenkinson, A. M., Crozier, A., Mullen, W., Pirie, L., Kyle, J., Yap, L. S., Christen, P. & Duthie, G. G. (2006). The effects of cranberry juice consumption on antioxidant status and biomarkers relating to heart disease and cancer in healthy human volunteers. *Eur J Nutr* **45**, 113–122.

104. Wilms, L. C., Hollman, P. C. H., Boots, A. W. & Kleinjans, J. C. S. (2005). Protection by quercetin and quercetin-rich fruit juice against induction of oxidative DNA damage and formation of BPDE-DNA adducts in human lymphocytes. *Mutat Res* **582**, 155–162.

105. Graf, B. A., Milbury, P. E. & Blumberg, J. B. (2005). Flavonols, flavones, flavanones, and human health: Epidemiological evidence. *J Med Food* **8**, 281–290.

106. Tsuda, H., Ohshima, Y., Nomoto, H., Fujita, K., Matsuda, E., Iigo, M., Takasuka, N. & Moore, M. A. (2004). Cancer prevention by natural compounds. *Drug Metab Pharmacokinet* **19**, 245–263.

107. Thomasset, S. C., Berry, D. P., Garcea, G., Marczylo, T., Steward, W. P. & Gescher, A. J. (2007). Dietary polyphenolic phytochemicals: Promising cancer chemopreventive agents in humans? A review of their clinical properties. *Int J Cancer* **120**, 451–458.

108. http://www.cancer.gov/clinicaltrials, last accessed Jan, 28, 2008.

Chapter 18

Flavonoids and Cardiovascular Health

Pon Velayutham Anandh Babu and Dongmin Liu

Department of Human Nutrition, Foods and Exercise, College of Agriculture and Life Sciences, Virginia Polytechnic Institute and State University, Blacksburg, Virginia, USA

Abstract

Flavonoids are considered as health promoting, disease preventing dietary supplements and are focus of much current nutritional and therapeutic interest. They are found ubiquitously in higher plants with variable phenolic structures. Epidemiological, *in vitro* and animal studies indicate that flavonoids exert protection against cardiovascular diseases. Flavonoids possess the bioactivity to beneficially affect the cardiovascular risk factors such as lipoprotein oxidation, dyslipidemia, endothelial dysfunction and blood platelet aggregation. The cardioprotective effect of flavonoids can be attributed to its antioxidant, antithrombogenic, and lipid lowering properties and also its effect on promoting endothelial function. This chapter is to provide an overview of the recent research developments on the protective effect of flavonoids, particularly tea flavonoids on cardiovascular health. Though many experimental evidences on flavonoids are promising, substantial studies are still required to prove the effectiveness for cardiovascular disease prevention and/or treatment and further understand the mechanism underlying this action of flavonoids.

Keywords: *Flavonoids, tea, dyslipidemia, oxidative stress, platelets, endothelial dysfunction, cardiovascular disease*

INTRODUCTION

Flavonoids are a ubiquitous group of naturally occurring polyphenolic compounds characterized by the flavan nucleus and represent one of the most prevalent classes of compounds in fruits, vegetables and plant-derived beverages. More than 8000 compounds with flavonoids structure have been identified, many of which are responsible for the attractive colors of flowers, fruits and leaves. In plants, these compounds afford protection against ultraviolet radiation, pathogens, and herbivores [1, 2].

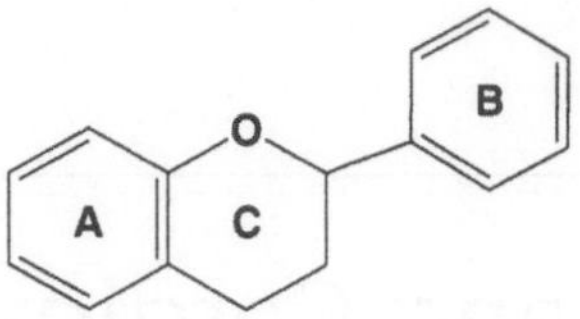

FIGURE 18.1　Basic chemical structure of flavonoids.

Flavonoids are considered as health promoting and disease preventing dietary supplements. Epidemiological, clinical and animal studies reveal that flavonoids may exert protective effects against various disease conditions including cardiovascular disease and cancer. Flavonoids also possess antibacterial, antiviral, and anti-inflammatory effects. Population studies have shown that flavonoid intake is inversely correlated with mortality from cardiovascular disease [3–6]. Flavonoids have been reported to beneficially impact parameters associated with atherosclerosis, including lipoprotein oxidation, blood platelet aggregation, and vascular reactivity. Antioxidant, antithrombotic, anti-inflammatory, and hypolipidemic properties are illustrated to play a significant role in the lower cardiovascular mortality observed with higher flavonoid intake [4, 5, 7]. Thus recently flavonoids are the focus of much current nutritional and therapeutic interest.

Continued studies of the mechanisms underlying the biological effects of plant flavonoids may provide new strategies for the prevention and treatment of cardiovascular disease. A thorough knowledge and understanding about flavonoids and their health benefits will help establish the dietary recommendations for flavonoids. This chapter provides an overview of recent developments on the biological activities responsible for the cardioprotective effect of flavonoids. Though variety of flavonoids play significant role in cardiovascular diseases, this article will specifically focus on tea flavonoids.

STRUCTURE AND CLASSIFICATION

Flavonoids are benzo-γ-pyrone derivatives consisting of phenolic and pyrane rings and are classified according to substitutions [3]. Flavonoids have a common basic chemical structure as shown in Fig. 18.1. The structural components common to most of the flavonoids include basic flavonoid skeleton and various combination of multiple hydroxyl and methoxyl group substituents. All of the major classes of flavonoids are comprised of three six-membered rings: an aromatic A-ring fused to a heterocyclic C-ring that is attached through a single carbon–carbon bond to an aromatic B-ring. Flavonoids differ in the arrangements of hydroxyl, methoxyl, and glycosidic side groups, and in the conjugation between the A- and B- rings. Based on specific structural differences, flavonoids are classified into six major classes: flavonols, flavones, flavanones, flavanols, anthocyanidins, and isoflavones [8]. The six main groups

TABLE 18.1 Flavonoid Subclasses, Representative Dietary Flavonoids, and Common Food Sources

Flavonoid subclass	Prominent dietary flavonoids	Food sources
Flavanol	Catechin, epicatechin, epicatechin gallate, epigallocatechin, epigallocatechin gallate	Tea, cocoa, red wines, chocolate, apples, hops
Flavone	Rutin, apigenin, luteolin, chrysin, diosmetin	Red wine, tomato skin, citrus, parsley, red pepper, herbs, cereals, vegetables
Flavonol	Kaempferol, quercetin, myricetin, rutin	Black tea, grape fruit, broccoli, onion, broccoli, tomato, tea, red wine, cranberry grapes, red wine
Flavanone	Naringenin, eriodictyol	Citrus fruits, peppermint, grapefruits
Isoflavone	Genistein, daidzein	Legumes (e.g., soybean)
Anthocyanidin	Apigenidin, cyanidin	Colored fruits, cherry, raspberry, strawberry

of flavonoids with the best-known members of each group and food source in which they are present are listed in Table 18.1. The molecular structure of each group of flavonoids is given in Fig. 18.2. The contents of the flavonoids in common foods have been reported in numerous publications [2–5] and are also available in the United States Department of Agriculture databases.

The hydroxyl groups found on all three rings are potential sites for links to carbohydrates. Flavonoids that are bound to one or more sugar molecules are known as flavonoid glycosides, whereas those that are not conjugated to sugar molecules are called aglycones. With the exception of flavan-3-ols, flavonoids occur in plants and most foods as glycosides. The structure complexity of flavonoids is further increased with the linking of acetyl and malonyl groups to the sugar conjugates. The combination of flavonoid structures, sugars, and acylation contribute to their complexity and the large number of individual molecules (>5000) that have been identified [8].

Tea Flavonoids

Tea, the dried leaves of the plant *Camellia sinensis*, is a popular beverage consumed worldwide. It can be categorized into three types, depending on

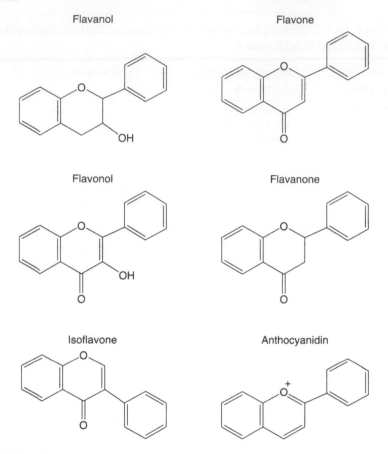

FIGURE 18.2 Molecular structure of six major flavonoids.

the level of oxidation, that is green tea (non-oxidized), oolong tea (partially oxidized), and black tea (oxidized). Green tea manufactured by inactivating the enzyme polyphenol oxidase in the fresh leaves by either firing or by steaming, to prevent the enzymatic oxidation of catechins. Green tea is an excellent source of polyphenol antioxidants, known as green tea catechins. The important catechins of green tea are (–)-epicatechin (EC), (–)-epicatechin-3-gallate (ECG), (–)-epigallocatechin (EGC), and (–)-epigallocatechin-3-gallate (EGCG). In manufacturing black tea, the leaves are crushed to allow the polyphenol oxidase to catalyze the oxidation, leading to polymerization of catechins. Theaflavins and thearubigins, are complex condensation products, called as derived polyphenols, generated during the processing of black tea. In green tea, catechins represent 80–90% and flavonols <10% of total flavonoids. The catechin content of black tea is only 20–30% whereas the theaflavins and thearubigins represent ~10 and 50–60% of total flavonoids [9].

Absorption

Though there are no long-term stores of flavonoids in the body, they do concentrate in certain tissues at concentrations that are adequate to exert biological effects. The flavonoids that are absorbed sufficiently to exert a possible effect on cardiovascular parameters *in vivo* include isoflavones, flavonols, flavanones, and the flavan-3-ols. For these flavonoids, a dose of 50 mg would give rise to a maximum plasma concentration (C_{max}) between 0.4 μM ((−)epicatechin) and 2.5 μM (genistein) [10]. Four classes of flavonoids (flavonols, flavanones, isoflavones, and flavan-3-ols) can be predicted to be absorbed in sufficient amounts to exert biological effects even as conjugated forms [11]. Studies indicate that catechins and their gut flora metabolites are well absorbed. The increase in plasma total catechin concentration is greater after ingestion of single large dose of green tea than one of black tea solids (equivalent to 3–6 cups), ranging from 0.6 μmol/l to 1.8 μmol/l and from 0.2 μmol/l to 0.34 μmol/l, respectively [12].

EPIDEMIOLOGICAL STUDIES

Many epidemiological studies have evaluated the relationship between flavonoid intake and cardiovascular disease risk [13–16]. There is considerable evidence that flavonoid consumption can reduce the risk of cardiovascular diseases and total mortality. In Zutphen study, which assessed 805 male subjects over a period of 5 years, reported that incidence of fatal and nonfatal first myocardial infarction and mortality from stroke decreased significantly with intake of flavonoids, derived mainly from tea, in a dose-dependent manner [15]. A follow-up of this study found that high intake of flavonoids significantly lowered the risk of stroke in study participants [17]. In a case-control study it was reported a 44% reduction in cardiovascular risk in the individuals drinking more than one cup of tea per day [18]. Consistently, a cohort study demonstrated a 31% and 39% reduction in cardiovascular risk in moderate and heavy tea drinkers after adjustment of other risk factors [19]. In Saudi Coronary Artery Disease Study it was found that those who drank more than six cups of tea per day (>480 ml) had significantly lower prevalence of coronary heart disease than non-tea drinkers [20]. A large Japanese population study of over 40,000 middle-aged Japanese found that those who drank just over to two cups (about 17 ounces) of green tea per day reduced their risk of death from cardiovascular disease by 22–33%, compared to those who drank less than a half-cup of green tea daily [21].

Epidemiological studies also show that flavonoids can improve the cardiovascular risk factors such as hypertension, dyslipidemia, and endothelial dysfunction and reduce the cardiovascular mortality. In a cross-sectional study, the consumption of 120–599 ml of green tea per day for at least 1 year reduced the risk of developing hypertension by 46%, compared to those subjects consuming less than 120 ml/day. Consuming more than 600 ml/day reduced the risk by 65% [22]. In Japanese subjects undergoing coronary angiography, it was observed that there is an inverse relationship between green tea consumption and coronary atherosclerosis [23]. Consumption of 8 g powdered green tea per day for 2 weeks was shown to enhance flow mediated blood vessel dilation in chronic smokers and it was suggested that green tea consumption may prevent future cardiovascular events in smokers [24]. In a randomized, double-blind, placebo-controlled, cross-over study, supplementation of 300 mg EGCG daily for 2 weeks acutely improved brachial artery flow mediated dilation in subjects with endothelia dysfunction. A Japanese study involving 1371 men older than 40 years of age reported the association between the consumption of >10 cups (1500 ml) of green tea a day with a decreased serum concentration of total cholesterol, LDL, and triglycerides, and with an increased HDL concentration [25]. In clinical study it was found that regular ingestion of tea resulted in a significant and consistent increase in endothelium-dependent and endothelium-impendent blood vessel dilation [26]. Although many studies suggest the beneficial effect of flavonoids on cardiovascular risk, few studies indicate that there is no significant inverse relationship between flavonoids intake and cardiovascular disease [16, 27]. This discrepancy could be due to the differences in flavonoid doses used, treatment duration, ages of subjects and other experimental conditions.

BIOCHEMICAL MECHANISMS

Cardiovascular disease is multifactorial involving oxidative stress, abnormalities in lipid profile, disturbances in vascular tone, and platelet aggregation. Flavonoids were reported to improve these abnormalities and improve the markers of cardiovascular health by several mechanisms.

Antioxidant Effect

The pathological mechanisms involved in cardiovascular diseases include the generation of supraphysiological levels of reactive oxygen species (ROS). ROS cause deleterious effects on cellular membrane and internal structure which alter the cardiac metabolism and contribute to the onset of cardiovascular disease. To reduce the oxidative stress and to maintain redox homeostasis humans have endogenous and exogenous mechanisms. Dietary flavonoids including tea have been largely studied for their strong antioxidant capacities and are considered as an important endogenous antioxidant. The best described property of almost every group of flavonoids is their capacity to act as antioxidants [2–5, 28]. The antioxidant effects are reported to be a primary mechanism that mediates the cardioprotective role of tea [6]. It is well documented that flavonoids can exert both direct and indirect antioxidant effects on cardiovascular system [6, 29, 30]. Flavonoids present antioxidant activity through scavenging free radicals, chelating redox active transition metal ions, inhibiting redox sensitive transcription factors, inhibiting pro-oxidant enzymes and inducing antioxidant enzymes [3–6, 29].

An increase in plasma antioxidant capacity after consumption of flavonoids especially green or black tea was reported using different assay systems [31]. Consumption of green tea and encapsulated green tea extracts for 1–4 weeks has been demonstrated to decrease biomarkers of oxidative status [32]. Green tea consumed within a balanced controlled diet was shown to improve overall the antioxidative status and to protect against oxidative damage in humans [33]. Accordingly, a significant increase in plasma antioxidant capacity was reported in humans after consumption of moderate amounts of green tea [34]. On the contrary, few studies reported that chronic green and black tea consumption had either little or no increase in plasma antioxidant activity [31]. Studies show that the rise in plasma antioxidant capacity peaks about 1–2 hours after tea ingestion and subsides shortly thereafter [32]. It was proposed that this could be due to limited absorption and rapid metabolism and excretion of tea catechins [31].

Flavonoids can be oxidized by radicals, resulting in a more stable, less-reactive radicals. This is due to the high reactivity of the hydroxyl group of the flavonoids with the reactive compound of the radicals. Therefore, flavonoids can stabilize the ROS and prevent oxidative injury by directly scavenging the free radicals. Flavonoids can directly scavenge superoxides and highly reactive oxygen-derived radical peroxynitrite. Green tea catechins can act as scavengers of free radicals and thereby prevent radical damage. Catechins isolated from green tea have been shown to scavenge (or neutralize) H_2O_2 and O_2 generated by the xanthine–xanthine oxidase system [35].

Flavonoids possess ideal structural chemistry for free radical scavenging activities. Due to the number and arrangements of their phenolic hydroxyl groups catechins are excellent electron donors and efficient scavengers of free radicals such as superoxide anions, singlet oxygen, nitric oxide, and peroxynitrite [31, 32]. The scavenging activity of different catechin molecules is related to the number of *o*-dihydroxyl and *o*-hydroxyketol groups, C2–C3 double bonds, concentration, solubility, the accessibility of the active group to the oxidant, and the stability of the reaction product [36, 37]. Several important features of the radical scavenging mechanism are delocalization of electrons, formation of intra- and intermolecular hydrogen bonds, rearrangements of molecules and chelatation of metals that may be involved in oxidation [38, 39]. The *o*-trihydroxyl group and 3-gallate esters in catechins appear to play an important role in antioxidant activity, radical scavenging, and preventing oxidative destruction of biological compounds. EGCG is the most potent tea antioxidant with four dihydroxyl groups [36] and its additional phenyl hydroxyl groups makes this gallate-containing catechin more able to donate the proton due to resonance delocalization [40].

Tea flavonoids can also chelate iron and copper to prevent their participation in Fenton and Haber-Weiss reaction in protecting cells against transition metal-catalyzed free radical formation [41, 42]. The o-3'4'-hydroxyl group of the B ring and gallate moiety of gallocatechins was reported to be the metal binding site for catechins [43, 44].

Tea catechins were shown to modulate the redox-sensitive transcription factors such as nuclear factor kappa B (NF-κB) and activator protein-1 (AP-1) in cardiovascular cells [45]. NF-κB has been shown to participate and mediate various oxidative stress-regulated vascular events. Administration of EGCG during reperfusion significantly decreased IκB kinase activity resulting in reduction of IκBα degradation and NF-κB activity. In this study, EGCG treatment also reduced the AP-1 activity by diminishing phosphorylation of c-Jun [46]. Oral administration of green tea catechins was reported to decrease the activity of NF-κB in murine cardiac transplants [47].

The two important ROS generating enzymes are inducible nitric oxide synthase (iNOS) which produce large quantities of nitric oxide upon stimulation of inflammatory cells and xanthine oxidase which oxidizes hypoxanthine and xanthine to uric acid. Different types of cells, including endothelial cells and macrophages produce nitric oxide (NO). Endothelial-derived NO through the activity of constitutive NO synthase is important for maintaining the dilation of blood vessels. However higher concentrations of NO produced by iNOS in macrophages can cause oxidative damage. The activated macrophages to a great extent increase the simultaneous production of both NO and superoxide anions. NO reacts with free radicals, thereby producing the highly damaging peroxynitrite. Peroxynitrite can directly oxidize low-density lipoprotein (LDLs), resulting in irreversible damage to the cell membrane. Flavonoids by directly scavenging the free radicals reduce the formation of peroxynitrite, resulting in less damage. Indeed, flavonoids result in a reduction in ischemia-reperfusion injury by interfering with iNOS activity and catechins were reported to suppress the expression of iNOS [48, 49]. It has been hypothesized that NO scavenging plays a role in the therapeutic effects of tea flavonoids. The xanthine oxidase metabolic pathway has been implicated as an important route in the oxidative damage to tissues, particularly after ischemia-reperfusion. During reperfusion, xanthine oxidase reacts with molecular oxygen, thereby releasing superoxide. Catechins were reported to inhibit the reaction catalyzed by xanthine oxidase and reduce the oxidative damage [50]. EGCG inhibits xanthine oxidase to produce uric acid and also acts as a scavenger of superoxide [51]. Therefore, the antioxidative activity of polyphenols may be due not only to their ability to scavenge superoxide, but also because of their ability to block xanthine oxidase and relative oxidative signal transducers [51]. Cyclooxygenase and lipoxygenase play an important role as inflammatory mediators. They are able to oxidize proteins other than their regular substrates, thereby aggravating oxidative damage and tea catechins were shown to inhibit both types of oxygenases [52]. Epicatechin inhibited 15-lipooxygenase mediated LDL oxidation more effectively than ascorbic acid or α-tocopherol at similar concentration [53].

Several studies have found that catechins are able to up-regulate and/or activates enzymes that play important roles in cellular antioxidant defense mechanisms. Hairless mice given 0.2% green tea catechins increase the activity of superoxide dismutase, catalase and glutathione peroxidase [54]. Both black and green tea induces the expression of catalase in aortas of spontaneously hypertensive rats [28]. Administration of green tea extract (containing 80% catechins) was shown to favorably modulate the activities of antioxidant enzymes such as catalase, superoxide dismutase, and glutathione peroxidase in the aorta and heart of diabetic rats [55].

Tea catechins also have the ability to participate in vitamin E recycling and thus complement some of the functions of glutathione (GSH), one of the antioxidant systems essential for cellular protection [56]. The vitamin E sparing effect of flavonoids was reported earlier and green tea was shown to increase the plasma GSH level [57]. Several animal studies state that tea administration prevented a decrease in tissue GSH concentrations [55, 58, 59]. Catechins also limit consumption of α-tocopherol and allow it to act as a scavenger within cell membranes while catechins scavenge aqueous peroxy radicals near the membrane surface [56].

Increased lipid peroxidation has important implications for vascular disease such as atherogenesis. The markers of lipid peroxidation were shown to be reduced by flavonoids in both *in vitro* and *in vivo* studies [4]. While it is not completely clear which components in tea primarily contribute to this effect, in animal studies, tea catechins administration was shown to decrease plasma levels of thiobarbituric acid reactive substances (TBARS), a widely used lipid oxidation marker [57]. The catechins in tea exhibit the most powerful antioxidant activity, 20 times more potent than vitamin C, which may essentially attributable to the observed inhibitory effect of tea on lipid peroxidation [60]. Consistently, a diet containing 1% tea catechins inhibited dietary polyunsaturated fatty acid-induced lipid peroxidation as determined by measuring plasma TBARS in Wistar rats [61]. Plasma TBARS were also lower in hamsters given green or black tea in their drinking water [62]. Green tea was shown to inhibit lipid peroxidation in the plasma and lens of diabetic rats [63]. It was report that treatment with green tea for 4 weeks can reduce the lipid peroxidation in the aorta and heart of diabetic rats [55].

While increasing evidence provides such a beneficial effect of green tea extract on lipid peroxidation, adequate dosage intake and treatment duration may be important to achieve this effect in humans. Recent studies showed that a significant 22% decrease in plasma TBARS after consumption of 3 g/day of green tea extract (equivalent to 10 cups/day of green tea) for 4 weeks compared with a placebo [64]. However no significant changes in plasma TBARS were found in studies where volunteers consumed green tea extract equivalent to two cups of tea acutely or three cups of tea daily for 7 days [65, 66].

LDL is by far the most studied risk factor for cardiovascular disease. At the first stage, LDL deposits at lesion sites of the arterial wall and is subjected to oxidation when protector such as tocopherols are depleted. Oxidation of LDL then induces modifications in lipoproteins, stimulates inflammatory reactions, causes monocytes and monocyte-derived macrophages to uptake oxidized LDL, and ultimately leads to the formation of lipid-loaden foam cells and atherosclerotic plaques. These plaques protrude from the inner surface of the arteries, narrow the lumen, and reduce blood flow which leads to coronary heart disease. Flavonoids including tea catechins were reported to inhibit the oxidation of LDL both *in vitro* and in animal studies [2–5]. EGCG was reported to be very effective among the tea catechins in reducing the LDL oxidation and has a lipoprotein bound antioxidant activity greater than tocopherol. Peroxynitrite, a potent oxidant generated by the reaction of NO with superoxide in the vascular endothelium, induces LDL oxidation and pro-inflammatory cytokine mediated myocardial dysfunction [67, 68]. Catechins could also decrease the peroxynitrite-induced nitration of tyrosine and protect the apolipoprotein B-100 of LDL from peroxynitrite induced modification of critical amino acids, which contribute to it surface charge [69]. The addition of flavonoids to the macrophages conserved the α-tocopherol content of the LDL and delayed the onset of lipid peroxidation [4].

Effect on Lipid Profile

Hyperlipidemia, an elevation of lipids in the blood stream, is one of the major risk factors for the development of cardiovascular disease. A casual relationship between the elevated plasma lipids and the development of atherosclerotic plaques has been well established [70]. Evidence suggests that drugs with the ability to lower LDL-cholesterol also reduce the probability of cardiovascular death. Flavonoids especially green tea catechins affect lipid metabolism by various mechanisms and prevent the appearance of atherosclerotic plaque. Catechins influence intestinal lipid absorption, luminal lipid hydrolysis and intestinal uptake and intracellular processing of lipids. It is well documented that tea is associated with beneficial effects on lipid profile and with reductions of atherosclerotic lesions in various models of hyperlipidemia.

In hypercholesterolemic rats, green tea considerably reduces serum and liver cholesterol, the atherogenic index, and liver weight by lowering the deposition of lipids [71]. In a cholesterol-fed hamster model, black and green tea consumption was reported to reduce the plasma cholesterol levels by 20 and 28%, respectively [62]. Green tea extract (300 mg/kg body weight) treatment for 4 weeks was shown to reduce the accumulation of cholesterol in the heart of diabetic rats [72]. Rats fed a cholesterol-rich diet and given Chinese green tea or jasmine tea for 8 weeks had significantly lower cholesterol levels in serum and liver. It was hypothesized that due to poor absorption and greater availability of green tea catechins in the intestinal lumen, it is possible that the lipid-lowering effect of green tea and catechins is mediated, at least in part, via their influence on the intestinal lipid digestion and absorption [73]. Green tea and its catechins interfere with the luminal emulsification, hydrolysis, and micellar solubilization of lipids [73]. It was demonstrated that mixtures of catechins extracted from Japanese green tea lowered the absorption of cholesterol and triglyceride in rats with thoracic lymph-duct cannula [74]. Studies also observed that a mixture of EGCG and ECG was more effective than a mixture of EC and EGC in lowering the absorption of cholesterol, suggesting that the gallate esters of green tea catechins were more potent inhibitors of cholesterol absorption [74].

The micellar solubilization of hydrolyzed lipids is the critical step for the uptake and absorption of lipids by the enterocyte. Green tea may influence the uptake of cholesterol and other lipids by the enterocyte through interaction with transporters, particularly those exposed to the intestinal lumen [73]. Tea catechins, in particular gallate esters are shown to decrease the cholesterol absorption by forming insoluble co-precipitates of cholesterol and decreasing the bile acid induced micellar solubility [74]. However, EC, one of green tea catechins, inhibits cholesterol absorption primarily by binding to cholesterol, thereby increasing fecal excretion of cholesterol [75]. In addition, catechins may have direct inhibitory effect on cholesterol synthesis. It was recently found that green tea catechins are potent and selective inhibitors of rat squalene epoxidase, a rate limiting enzyme of cholesterol biosynthesis. The presence of galloyl moiety was suggested to be important for squalene epoxidase inhibition activity [76]. Therefore, the hypocholesterolemic effect of tea catechins may be a collective result of their inhibitory action on cholesterol absorption and biosynthesis and their action on enhanced cholesterol excretion.

In a randomized cross-over study, consumption of moderate (224 mg) and high (674 mg) amounts of catechins 3 times, along with a standardized light meal (bread and 20 g butter) was shown to reduce the postprandial triglyceride response by 15.1% and 28.7%, respectively [77]. Green tea catechins were shown to inhibit the action of digestive lipases. Tea catechins, particularly those with a galloyl moiety, dose-dependently inhibit the activity of pancreatic lipase, thereby suppressing triacylglycerol absorption and postprandial hypertriacylglycerolemia [74]. In addition, green tea catechins at the levels achievable by typical daily intake, markedly altered the physicochemical properties of a lipid emulsion by increasing its particle size and reducing the surface area [78]. These changes reduce the interaction of pancreatic lipase with fat and therefore decrease the rate of hydrolysis of fat [78]. EGCG was identified as the main catechin compound present on the lipid phase of the emulsion that is responsible for the changes in emulsion properties [79]. It was proposed that the hydroxyl moieties of EGCG interact with the hydrophilic head group of phosphatidyl choline at the exterior of a lipid emulsion by forming hydrogen bonds, and that such interaction may lead to formation of cross-links followed by coalescence of the emulsion droplets [79]. The postprandial hypertriacylglycerolemia is a risk factor for coronary heart disease and these results thus suggest that catechins with a galloyl moiety may have a beneficial effect on this disease.

EGCG also has been shown to exert a potent inhibitory effect on pancreatic phospholipase A_2, which may also be attributable to the decreased absorption of lipid because luminal phosphatidyl choline hydrolysis is critical to facilitating intestinal lipid digestion and absorption [73, 80]. Regarding this, EGCG may interact with the surface phosphatidyl choline of a lipid emulsion and hinder the access to the substrate by phospholipase A_2. Alternatively, EGCG may directly interact with the enzyme protein and subsequently alter its conformation and catalytic activity [81, 82].

It was also suggested that green tea may inhibit intestinal acyl CoA: cholesterol acyltransferase in the enterocyte [83]. Green tea catechins may influence critical steps involved in the assembly and secretion of chylomicrons from the enterocyte into the lymphatics [73]. The synthesis of fatty acid is the key step for lipogenesis. The suppression of lipogenesis by oolong, black, pu-erh, and green tea leaves has been demonstrated in the experimental animals [84]. EGCG profoundly suppress fatty acid synthase (FAS) gene transcription through the epidermal growth factor (EGF) receptor/phosphoinositide-3 kinase (PI3K)/Akt/Sp-1 signal transduction pathway [85]. In addition, EGCG and ECG were shown to inhibit the activity of acetyl CoA carboxylase, which catalyzes the carboxylation of acetyl-CoA to malonyl-CoA, the rate limiting step in fatty acid biosynthesis [86]. Green tea administered to hamster fed a high fat diet had higher fecal excretion of total fatty acids [75].

Several studies indicate that green tea flavonoids can favorably modify the lipoproteins. EGCG was reported to suppress LDL-cholesterol but promote HDL-cholesterol in rats fed with high fat and high cholesterol diet [87]. Two cross-sectional studies conducted in Japan showed that green tea consumption was associated with a lower ratio of LDL-cholesterol to HDL-cholesterol [25, 88]. Apolipoprotein B (ApoB) is the primary apolipoprotein component in LDL that comprises of 90% of total protein mass. While it is still unclear exactly what functional role ApoB plays in LDL, high levels of ApoB are related to the pathogenesis of atherosclerosis. Interestingly, green tea EC supplemented in either diet or drinking water was shown to reduce ApoB and improve the balance of apolipoproteins [75]. In addition, treatment with green tea extract for 4 weeks has been shown to reduce LDL- and VLDL-cholesterol whereas increase HDL-cholesterol in diabetic rats [72].

Effect on Vascular Homeostasis

One of the most important focuses of cardiovascular disease research is on the function of endothelial cells, which not only serve as a biological barrier separating circulating blood and peripheral tissues, but also secrete various vasoactive substances for maintaining normal vascular function. Vascular endothelial cells playing a central role in vascular homeostasis and alterations in the endothelial function contribute to the pathogenesis of cardiovascular diseases [89]. Endothelial cells regulate vascular homeostasis by producing factors that act locally in the vessel wall and lumen. Endothelium-derived vasodilator, NO, regulates important aspects of vascular tone and homeostasis [90]. NO inhibits expression of leukocyte adhesion molecules at the endothelial surface and prevents the interaction of leukocytes and endothelial cells, thereby exerting anti-inflammatory and antiatheroclerotic effects, given that it is well recognized now that inflammation is involved in all stages of the pathogenesis of atherosclerosis. In addition, NO prevents platelet adhesion, platelet aggregation, and vascular smooth muscle cell proliferation [89]. Thus the reduced production or bioavailability of NO can lead to endothelial dysfunction which is one of the initial steps in atherogenesis, even before structural changes in the vessel wall become apparent. Indeed, a growing body of literature demonstrates that endothelial dysfunction is linked to future cardiovascular events. Therefore, agents that are capable of preventing damage to endothelial cells or of restoring endothelial function may have important clinical implications. Many interventions known to reduce cardiovascular risk such as lipid lowering agents, angiotensin converting enzyme inhibitors, angiotensin receptor blockers have the ability to reverse endothelial dysfunction in patients with cardiovascular disease [91]. Furthermore, endothelial function has evolved into a clinically useful endpoint for developing efficacious strategy for the prevention and treatment of cardiovascular disease [92].

Several studies demonstrated that flavonoid containing beverages have beneficial effects on endothelial function. Data from experimental and clinical studies suggest that tea constituents significantly improved endothelial function, thereby providing a plausible mechanism for the beneficial effects of tea in patients with cardiovascular disease. Duffy et al. [93] reported that tea consumption reverses endothelial dysfunction. Both short- and long-term consumption of black tea improved endothelium-dependent flow-mediated dilation of the brachial artery in patients with coronary disease, whereas flow-mediated vessel dilation was not affected by an acute dose of caffeine, suggesting that caffeine content of tea was not responsible for the observed results [93]. Hodgson and colleagues reported that consumption of five cups of black tea per day for 4 weeks improved brachial artery flow-mediated dilation in a group of otherwise healthy subjects with modest hypercholesterolemia [26]. Administration of EGCG (200 mg/kg for 3 weeks) was shown to reduce systolic blood pressure and enhanced endothelial function [94]. These studies suggest that reversing endothelial dysfunction is one of the mechanisms to explain the beneficial effect of tea consumption on cardiovascular disease risk.

While the precise mechanism by which tea improves endothelial function is not exactly clear, recent studies demonstrating that tea consumption was also associated with an improvement in nitroglyerin-mediated vascular dilation, suggest that tea may improve the bioactivity of endothelium-derived NO and/or have a beneficial effect on the function of vascular smooth muscle. Actually, animal studies demonstrated tea catechins evoked endothelium- and NO-dependent vasorelaxation in precontracted rat aortic rings [95]. In cultured endothelial cells, EGCG rapidly activates endothelial NO synthase (eNOS) activity without altering eNOS protein content, an effect that is mediated through the PI3K/Akt-dependent pathway [96]. Interestingly, activation of PI3K/Akt and eNOS by EGCG in endothelial cells requires ROS and Fyn, a protein associates with the p85 subunit of PI3K [97]. Green tea catechins were also shown to inhibit the proliferation of aortic smooth muscle cells via activation of p53 to prevent the development of atherosclerosis [98]. EGC and ECG were reported to be an active inhibitors of H_2O_2 induced endothelial cell injury [99].

One of the earliest events in the development of atherosclerosis is the recruitment of inflammatory white blood cells from the blood to the arterial wall and is dependent on the expression of adhesion molecules by the vascular endothelial cells that line the inner walls of blood vessels [100]. Vascular smooth muscle cells (SMC) adhesion and migration are critical events in disease-related vascular remodeling such as atherosclerosis. EGCG and ECG were reported as potent inhibitors on SMC adhesion by interfering with SMC's integrin $\beta 1$ expression and binding to extracellular matrix proteins [101]. EGCG was also shown to reduce cytokine-induced VCAM-1 expression and monocyte adhesion to endothelial cells [102]. EGCG was also reported to inhibit SMC migration at low concentrations [101]. Green tea catechins suppress or inhibit the proliferation of aortic SMC which produce connective tissue leading to luminal narrowing and sclerosis of the arteries [103].

Effect on Platelet Abnormalities

Blood platelet activation and aggregation also have an integral role in the development of cardiovascular disease. Variations in the platelet sensitivity correlated directly to mortality from coronary artery disease. There is extensive evidence that antiplatelet therapy reduces cardiovascular disease risk. Dietary flavonoids can inhibit platelet activation and aggregation. Animal studies have reported the beneficial effects of tea consumption on platelet aggregation. Tea consumption reduced plasma concentrations of P-selectin, a cell adhesion molecule secreted by activated endothelial cells and platelets that mediate the interaction of activated endothelial cells or platelets with leukocytes, therefore a useful marker of *in vivo* platelet aggregation [104]. Platelet activation and subsequent thromboembolism are important pathological mechanisms of ischemic cardiovascular events.

Several flavonoids inhibited platelet adhesion, aggregation and secretion [4]. Kang *et al.* [105] reported that green tea catechins can inhibit adenosine diphosphate (ADP)- and collagen-induced rat platelet aggregation *ex vivo* in a dose-dependent manner. EGCG and other tea catechins were also shown to dose-dependently inhibit ADP-, collagen-, epinephrine- and calcium ionophore-induced human platelet aggregation *in vitro* without changing the coagulation parameters such as activated partial thromboplastin time, prothrombin time, and thrombin time [105]. It was proposed that the mode of antithrombotic action of tea may be due to antiplatelet activities rather than to anticoagulant activity. Thrombin-induced aggregation was reduced in platelets from rats that drank green tea. Another study reports that the antiplatelet activity of green tea catechins is mediated by inhibition of cytoplasmic calcium increase, which leads to the inhibition of fibrinogen-GPIIb/IIIa binding via the activation of Ca^{2+}-ATPase and inhibition of inositol 1,4,5-triphosphate formation [106]. However, Sugatani et al. proposed that catechins may reduce the production of platelet activating factor (PAF) by inhibiting acetyl-CoA: lysoPAF acetyltransferase [107]. EGCG can inhibit PAF decreasing the stickiness of platelets and decreasing the probability of platelet aggregation. EGCG was reported to block tyrosine phosphorylation and reduce gene expression of platelet-derived growth factor-β-receptor [108].

Platelet aggregation contributes to acute thrombus formation, followed by embolization of stenosed arteries. Adhesion of activated platelets to vascular endothelium generates lipid peroxidation and ROS which inhibit endothelial production of prostacyclin and NO. Tea catechins may protect against thrombosis by directly scavenging free radicals, thereby maintaining proper concentrations of endothelial prostacyclin and NO. Arachidonic acid, which release is increased in inflammatory conditions, is metabolized by platelets to form prostaglandin, endoperoxides, and thromboxane A2, leading to platelet activation and aggregation. Flavonoids are believed to exert antiaggregating effect mainly through inhibition of thromboxane A2 formation possibly as a result of suppressing arachidonic acid liberation and thromboxane A2 synthase [109].

Platelet responses can involve activation of phospholipase C and phospholipase A2, as well as hydrolytic release of arachidonic acid and its subsequent conversion through cyclooxygenase to thromboxane A2, which potentiates platelet activation. The effects of green tea catechins on phospholipase A2 activity and the antithrombotic reaction of platelets have been investigated in diabetic rats [110]. Catechin supplementation maintains normal level of platelet thromboxane A2 formation and improves platelet aggregation. The antiplatelet effect of flavonoids may be explained by both inhibition of thromboxane synthesis and thromboxane receptor antagonism.

CONCLUSION

Epidemiological, clinical and experimental studies suggest that flavonoids, particularly tea flavonoids have beneficial effects on cardiovascular system and reduce the risk of cardiovascular disease. The underlying mechanisms involve improved endothelial function, antioxidative, antithrombiotic, and lipid lowering effects. Though many experimental evidences on flavonoids are promising, substantial studies are still required to prove the effectiveness for cardiovascular disease prevention and/or treatment and further understand the mechanism underlying this action of flavonoids.

ACKNOWLEDGMENT

Supported by grants from the American Heart Association Mid-Atlantic Affiliate (to D. Liu) and the National Center for Complementary and Alternative Medicine (NIH R21AT002739 to D. Liu).

REFERENCES

1. Moon, Y. J., Wang, X. & Morris, M. E. (2006). Dietary flavonoids: Effects on xenobiotic and carcinogen metabolism. *Toxicol In Vitro* **20**, 187–210.
2. Erdman, J. W., Jr., Balentine, D., Arab, L., Beecher, G., Dwyer, J. T., Folts, J., Harnly, J., Hollman, P., Keen, C. L., Mazza, G., Messina, M., Scalbert, A., Vita, J., Williamson, G. & Burrowes, J. (2007). Flavonoids and heart health: Proceedings of the ILSI North America Flavonoids Workshop, May 31–June 1, 2005, Washington, DC. *J Nutr* **137**, 718S–737S.
3. Heim, K. E., Tagliaferro, A. R. & Bobilya, D. J. (2002). Flavonoid antioxidants: Chemistry, metabolism and structure-activity relationships. *J Nutr Biochem* **13**, 572–584.
4. Middleton, E., Kandaswami, C. & Theoharides, T. C. (2000). The effects of plant flavonoids on mammalian cells: implications for inflammation, heart disease, and cancer. *Pharmacological reviews.* **52**, 673–751.
5. Nijveldt, R. J., van Nood, E., van Hoorn, D. E., Boelens, P. G., van Norren, K. & van Leeuwen, P. A. (2001). Flavonoids: a review of probable mechanisms of action and potential applications. *Am J Clin Nutr* **74**, 418–425.
6. Stangl, V., Dreger, H., Stangl, K. & Lorenz, M. (2007). Molecular targets of tea polyphenols in the cardiovascular system. *Cardiovascular Res* **73**, 348–358.
7. Arts, I. C. & Hollman, P. C. (2005). Polyphenols and disease risk in epidemiologic studies. *Am J Clin Nutr* **81**, 317S–325S.
8. Beecher, G. R. (2003). Overview of dietary flavonoids: nomenclature, occurrence and intake. *J Nutr* **133**, 3248S–3254S.
9. Balentine, D. A., Wiseman, S. A. & Bouwens, L. C. (1997). The chemistry of tea flavonoids. *CritRev Food Sci Nutr* **37**, 693–704.
10. Manach, C., Williamson, G., Morand, C., Scalbert, A. & Remesy, C. (2005). Bioavailability and bioefficacy of polyphenols in humans. I. Review of 97 bioavailability studies. *Am J Clin Nutr* **81**, 230S–242S.
11. Williamson, G., Barron, D., Shimoi, K. & Terao, J. (2005). *In vitro* biological properties of flavonoid conjugates found *in vivo*. *Free Radic Res* **39**, 457–469.
12. Riemersma, R. A., Rice-Evans, C. A., Tyrrell, R. M., Clifford, M. N. & Lean, M. E. (2001). Tea flavonoids and cardiovascular health. *QJM* **94**, 277–282.
13. Yochum, L., Kushi, L. H., Meyer, K. & Folsom, A. R. (1999). Dietary flavonoid intake and risk of cardiovascular disease in postmenopausal women. *Am J Epidemiol* **149**, 943–949.
14. Knekt, P., Jarvinen, R., Reunanen, A. & Maatela, J. (1996). Flavonoid intake and coronary mortality in Finland: A cohort study. *BMJ (Clinical Research Ed.)* **312**, 478–481.
15. Hertog, M. G., Feskens, E. J. & Kromhout, D. (1997). Antioxidant flavonols and coronary heart disease risk. *Lancet* **349**, 699.

16. Hertog, M. G., Sweetnam, P. M., Fehily, A. M., Elwood, P. C. & Kromhout, D. (1997). Antioxidant flavonols and ischemic heart disease in a Welsh population of men: The Caerphilly Study. *Am J Clin Nutr* **65**, 1489–1494.

17. Keli, S. O., Hertog, M. G., Feskens, E. J. & Kromhout, D. (1996). Dietary flavonoids, antioxidant vitamins, and incidence of stroke: The Zutphen study. *Arch Intern Med* **156**, 637–642.

18. Sesso, H. D., Gaziano, J. M., Buring, J. E. & Hennekens, C. H. (1999). Coffee and tea intake and the risk of myocardial infarction. *Am J Epidemiol* **149**, 162–167.

19. Mukamal, K. J., Maclure, M., Muller, J. E., Sherwood, J. B. & Mittleman, M. A. (2002). Tea consumption and mortality after acute myocardial infarction. *Circulation* **105**, 2476–2481.

20. Hakim, I. A., Alsaif, M. A., Alduwaihy, M., Al-Rubeaan, K., Al-Nuaim, A. R. & Al-Attas, O. S. (2003). Tea consumption and the prevalence of coronary heart disease in Saudi adults: Results from a Saudi national study. *Preventive Med* **36**, 64–70.

21. Kuriyama, S., Shimazu, T., Ohmori, K., Kikuchi, N., Nakaya, N., Nishino, Y., Tsubono, Y. & Tsuji, I. (2006). Green tea consumption and mortality due to cardiovascular disease, cancer, and all causes in Japan: The Ohsaki study. *JAMA* **296**, 1255–1265.

22. Yang, Y. C., Lu, F. H., Wu, J. S., Wu, C. H. & Chang, C. J. (2004). The protective effect of habitual tea consumption on hypertension. *Arch Intern Med* **164**, 1534–1540.

23. Sasazuki, S., Kodama, H., Yoshimasu, K., Liu, Y., Washio, M., Tanaka, K., Tokunaga, S., Kono, S., Arai, H., Doi, Y., Kawano, T., Nakagaki, O., Takada, K., Koyanagi, S., Hiyamuta, K., Nii, T., Shirai, K., Ideishi, M., Arakawa, K., Mohri, M. & Takeshita, A. (2000). Relation between green tea consumption and the severity of coronary atherosclerosis among Japanese men and women. *Ann Epidemiol* **10**, 401–408.

24. Kim, W., Jeong, M. H., Cho, S. H., Yun, J. H., Chae, H. J., Ahn, Y. K., Lee, M. C., Cheng, X., Kondo, T., Murohara, T. & Kang, J. C. (2006). Effect of green tea consumption on endothelial function and circulating endothelial progenitor cells in chronic smokers. *Circ J* **70**, 1052–1057.

25. Imai, K. & Nakachi, K. (1995). Cross sectional study of effects of drinking green tea on cardiovascular and liver diseases. *BMJ (Clinical research ed.)* **310**, 693–696.

26. Hodgson, J. M., Puddey, I. B., Burke, V., Watts, G. F. & Beilin, L. J. (2002). Regular ingestion of black tea improves brachial artery vasodilator function. *Clin Sci (Lond)* **102**, 195–201.

27. Sesso, H. D., Paffenbarger, R. S., Jr., Oguma, Y. & Lee, I. M. (2003). Lack of association between tea and cardiovascular disease in college alumni. *Int J Epidemiol* **32**, 527–533.

28. Negishi, H., Xu, J. W., Ikeda, K., Njelekela, M., Nara, Y. & Yamori, Y. (2004). Black and green tea polyphenols attenuate blood pressure increases in stroke-prone spontaneously hypertensive rats. *J Nutr* **134**, 38–42.

29. Cabrera, C., Artacho, R. & Gimenez, R. (2006). Beneficial effects of green tea: A review. *J Am College Nutr* **25**, 79–99.

30. Basu, A. & Lucas, E. A. (2007). Mechanisms and effects of green tea on cardiovascular health. *Nutr Rev* **65**, 361–375.

31. Higdon, J. V. & Frei, B. (2003). Tea catechins and polyphenols: Health effects, metabolism, and antioxidant functions. *Crit RevFood Sci Nutr* **43**, 89–143.

32. Khan, N. & Mukhtar, H. (2007). Tea polyphenols for health promotion. *Life Sciences* **81**, 519–533.

33. Erba, D., Riso, P., Bordoni, A., Foti, P., Biagi, P. L. & Testolin, G. (2005). Effectiveness of moderate green tea consumption on antioxidative status and plasma lipid profile in humans. *J Nutr Biochem.* **16**, 144–149.

34. Leenen, R., Roodenburg, A. J., Tijburg, L. B. & Wiseman, S. A. (2000). A single dose of tea with or without milk increases plasma antioxidant activity in humans. *Eur J Clin Nutr* **54**, 87–92.

35. Ruch, R. J., Cheng, S. J. & Klaunig, J. E. (1989). Prevention of cytotoxicity and inhibition of intercellular communication by antioxidant catechins isolated from Chinese green tea. *Carcinogenesis* **10**, 1003–1008.

36. Dufresne, C. J. & Farnworth, E. R. (2001). A review of latest research findings on the health promotion properties of tea. *J Nutr Biochem* **12**, 404–421.

37. Guo, Q., Zhao, B., Shen, S., Hou, J., Hu, J. & Xin, W. (1999). ESR study on the structure–antioxidant activity relationship of tea catechins and their epimers. *Biochimica et biophysica acta* **1427**, 13–23.

38. van Acker, S. A., de Groot, M. J., van den Berg, D. J., Tromp, M. N., Donne-Op den Kelder, G., van der Vijgh, W. J. & Bast, A. (1996). A quantum chemical explanation of the antioxidant activity of flavonoids. *Chem Res Toxicol* **9**, 1305–1312.

39. Morel, I., Lescoat, G., Cogrel, P., Sergent, O., Pasdeloup, N., Brissot, P., Cillard, P. & Cillard, J. (1993). Antioxidant and iron-chelating activities of the flavonoids catechin, quercetin and diosmetin on iron-loaded rat hepatocyte cultures. *Biochem Pharmacol* **45**, 13–19.

40. Liao, S., Kao, Y. H. & Hiipakka, R. A. (2001). Green tea: Biochemical and biological basis for health benefits. *Vitamins and Hormones* **62**, 1–94.

41. Mira, L., Fernandez, M. T., Santos, M., Rocha, R., Florencio, M. H. & Jennings, K. R. (2002). Interactions of flavonoids with iron and copper ions: A mechanism for their antioxidant activity. *Free Radic Res* **36**, 1199–1208.

42. Miller, N. J., Castelluccio, C., Tijburg, L. & Rice-Evans, C. (1996). The antioxidant properties of theaflavins and their gallate esters – radical scavengers or metal chelators? *FEBS Lett* **392**, 40–44.

43. Hider, R. C., Liu, Z. D. & Khodr, H. H. (2001). Metal chelation of polyphenols. *Methods Enzymol* **335**, 190–203.

44. Kumamoto, M., Sonda, T., Nagayama, K. & Tabata, M. (2001). Effects of pH and metal ions on antioxidative activities of catechins. *Biosci Biotechnol Biochem* **65**, 126–132.

45. Khan, N., Afaq, F., Saleem, M., Ahmad, N. & Mukhtar, H. (2006). Targeting multiple signaling pathways by green tea polyphenol (–)-epigallocatechin-3-gallate. *Cancer Res* **66**, 2500–2505.

46. Aneja, R., Hake, P. W., Burroughs, T. J., Denenberg, A. G., Wong, H. R. & Zingarelli, B. (2004). Epigallocatechin, a green tea polyphenol, attenuates myocardial ischemia reperfusion injury in rats. *Molecular Medicine (Cambridge, Mass.)* **10**, 55–62.

47. Suzuki, J., Ogawa, M., Sagesaka, Y. M. & Isobe, M. (2006). Tea catechins attenuate ventricular remodeling and graft arterial diseases in murine cardiac allografts. *Cardiovasc Res* **69**, 272–279.

48. Lin, Y. L. & Lin, J. K. (1997). (–)-Epigallocatechin-3-gallate blocks the induction of nitric oxide synthase by down-regulating lipopolysaccharide-induced activity of transcription factor nuclear factor-kappaB. *Mol Pharmacol* **52**, 465–472.

49. Chan, M. M., Fong, D., Ho, C. T. & Huang, H. I. (1997). Inhibition of inducible nitric oxide synthase gene expression and enzyme activity by epigallocatechin gallate, a natural product from green tea. *Biochem Pharmacol* **54**, 1281–1286.

50. Aucamp, J., Gaspar, A., Hara, Y. & Apostolides, Z. (1997). Inhibition of xanthine oxidase by catechins from tea (*Camellia sinensis*). *Anticancer Res* **17**, 4381–4385.
51. Lin, J. K., Chen, P. C., Ho, C. T. & Lin-Shiau, S. Y. (2000). Inhibition of xanthine oxidase and suppression of intracellular reactive oxygen species in HL-60 cells by theaflavin-3,3'-digallate, (–)-epigallocatechin-3-gallate, and propyl gallate. *J Agric Food Chem* **48**, 2736–2743.
52. Hong, J., Smith, T. J., Ho, C. T., August, D. A. & Yang, C. S. (2001). Effects of purified green and black tea polyphenols on cyclooxygenase- and lipoxygenase-dependent metabolism of arachidonic acid in human colon mucosa and colon tumor tissues. *Biochem Pharmacol* **62**, 1175–1183.
53. da Silva, E. L., Abdalla, D. S. & Terao, J. (2000). Inhibitory effect of flavonoids on low-density lipoprotein peroxidation catalyzed by mammalian 15-lipoxygenase. *IUBMB Life* **49**, 289–295.
54. Khan, S. G., Katiyar, S. K., Agarwal, R. & Mukhtar, H. (1992). Enhancement of antioxidant and phase II enzymes by oral feeding of green tea polyphenols in drinking water to SKH-1 hairless mice: Possible role in cancer chemoprevention. *Cancer Res* **52**, 4050–4052.
55. Babu, P. V., Sabitha, K. E. & Shyamaladevi, C. S. (2006). Therapeutic effect of green tea extract on oxidative stress in aorta and heart of streptozotocin diabetic rats. *Chem Biol Interact* **162**, 114–120.
56. Zhu, Q. Y., Huang, Y., Tsang, D. & Chen, Z. Y. (1999). Regeneration of alpha-tocopherol in human low-density lipoprotein by green tea catechin. *J Agric Food Chem* **47**, 2020–2025.
57. Frei, B. & Higdon, J. V. (2003). Antioxidant activity of tea polyphenols *in vivo*: Evidence from animal studies. *J Nutr* **133**, 3275S–3284S.
58. Sur-Altiner, D. & Yenice, B. (2000). Effect of black tea on lipid peroxidation in carbon tetrachloride treated male rats. *Drug MetabolDrug Interac* **16**, 123–128.
59. Guleria, R. S., Jain, A., Tiwari, V. & Misra, M. K. (2002). Protective effect of green tea extract against the erythrocytic oxidative stress injury during mycobacterium tuberculosis infection in mice. *Mol Cell Biochem* **236**, 173–181.
60. Vinson, J. A., Dabbagh, Y. A., Serry, M. M. & J, J. (1995). Plant flavonoids, especially tea flavonols, are powerful antioxidants using an *in vitro* oxidation model for heart disease. *J Agric Food Chem* **43**, 2798–2799.
61. Nanjo, F., Honda, M., Okushio, K., Matsumoto, N., Ishigaki, F., Ishigami, T. & Hara, Y. (1993). Effects of dietary tea catechins on alpha-tocopherol levels, lipid peroxidation, and erythrocyte deformability in rats fed on high palm oil and perilla oil diets. *Biol Pharmaceut Bullet* **16**, 1156–1159.
62. Vinson, J. A. & Dabbagh, Y. A. (1998). Effect of green and black tea supplementation on lipids, lipid oxidation and fibrinogen in the hamster: Mechanisms for the epidemiological benefits of tea drinking. *FEBS Lett* **433**, 44–46.
63. Vinson, J. A. & Zhang, J. (2005). Black and green teas equally inhibit diabetic cataracts in a streptozotocin-induced rat model of diabetes. *J Agric Food Chem* **53**, 3710–3713.
64. Freese, R., Basu, S., Hietanen, E., Nair, J., Nakachi, K., Bartsch, H. & Mutanen, M. (1999). Green tea extract decreases plasma malondialdehyde concentration but does not affect other indicators of oxidative stress, nitric oxide production, or hemostatic factors during a high-linoleic acid diet in healthy females. *Eur J Nutr* **38**, 149–157.

65. Nakagawa, K., Ninomiya, M., Okubo, T., Aoi, N., Juneja, L. R., Kim, M., Yamanaka, K. & Miyazawa, T. (1999). Tea catechin supplementation increases antioxidant capacity and prevents phospholipid hydroperoxidation in plasma of humans. *J Agric Food Chem* **47**, 3967–3973.

66. Miura, Y., Chiba, T., Miura, S., Tomita, I., Umegaki, K., Ikeda, M. & Tomita, T. (2000). Green tea polyphenols (flavan 3-ols) prevent oxidative modification of low density lipoproteins: An *ex vivo* study in humans. *J Nutr Biochem* **11**, 216–222.

67. Leeuwenburgh, C., Hardy, M. M., Hazen, S. L., Wagner, P., Oh-ishi, S., Steinbrecher, U. P. & Heinecke, J. W. (1997). Reactive nitrogen intermediates promote low density lipoprotein oxidation in human atherosclerotic intima. *J Biol Chem* **272**, 1433–1436.

68. Moore, K. P., Darley-Usmar, V., Morrow, J. & Roberts, L. J., 2nd. (1995). Formation of F2-isoprostanes during oxidation of human low-density lipoprotein and plasma by peroxynitrite. *Circulation Res* **77**, 335–341.

69. Pannala, A. S., Rice-Evans, C. A., Halliwell, B. & Singh, S. (1997). Inhibition of peroxynitrite-mediated tyrosine nitration by catechin polyphenols. *Biochem Biophys Res Commun* **232**, 164–168.

70. Miura, Y., Chiba, T., Tomita, I., Koizumi, H., Miura, S., Umegaki, K., Hara, Y., Ikeda, M. & Tomita, T. (2001). Tea catechins prevent the development of atherosclerosis in apoprotein E-deficient mice. *J Nutr* **131**, 27–32.

71. Yang, T. T. & Koo, M. W. (1997). Hypocholesterolemic effects of Chinese tea. *Pharmacol Res* **35**, 505–512.

72. Babu, P. V. A., Sabitha, K. E. & Shyamaladevi, C. S. (2006). Green tea extract impedes dyslipidaemia and development of cardiac dysfunction in streptozotocin-diabetic rats. *Clin Exper Pharmacol Physiol* **33**, 1184–1189.

73. Koo, S. I. & Noh, S. K. (2007). Green tea as inhibitor of the intestinal absorption of lipids: Potential mechanism for its lipid-lowering effect. *J Nutr Biochem* **18**, 179–183.

74. Ikeda, I., Imasato, Y., Sasaki, E., Nakayama, M., Nagao, H., Takeo, T., Yayabe, F. & Sugano, M. (1992). Tea catechins decrease micellar solubility and intestinal absorption of cholesterol in rats. *Biochimica et Biophysica Acta* **1127**, 141–146.

75. Chan, P. T., Fong, W. P., Cheung, Y. L., Huang, Y., Ho, W. K. & Chen, Z. Y. (1999). Jasmine green tea epicatechins are hypolipidemic in hamsters (*Mesocricetus auratus*) fed a high fat diet. *J Nutr* **129**, 1094–1101.

76. Abe, I., Seki, T., Umehara, K., Miyase, T., Noguchi, H., Sakakibara, J. & Ono, T. (2000). Green tea polyphenols: Novel and potent inhibitors of squalene epoxidase. *Biochem Biophys Res Commun* **268**, 767–771.

77. Unno, T., Tago, M., Suzuki, Y., Nozawa, A., Sagesaka, Y. M., Kakuda, T., Egawa, K. & Kondo, K. (2005). Effect of tea catechins on postprandial plasma lipid responses in human subjects. *Br J Nutr* **93**, 543–547.

78. Armand, M., Pasquier, B., Andre, M., Borel, P., Senft, M., Peyrot, J., Salducci, J., Portugal, H., Jaussan, V. & Lairon, D. (1999). Digestion and absorption of 2 fat emulsions with different droplet sizes in the human digestive tract. *Am J Clin Nutr* **70**, 1096–1106.

79. Shishikura, Y., Khokhar, S. & Murray, B. S. (2006). Effects of tea polyphenols on emulsification of olive oil in a small intestine model system. *J Agric Food Chem* **54**, 1906–1913.

80. Wang, S., Noh, S. K. & Koo, S. I. (2006). Green tea catechins inhibit pancreatic phospholipase A(2) and intestinal absorption of lipids in ovariectomized rats. *J Nutr Biochem* **17**, 492–498.

81. Hollman, P. C., Tijburg, L. B. & Yang, C. S. (1997). Bioavailability of flavonoids from tea. *Crit Rev Food Sci Nutr* **37**, 719–738.
82. Guharay, J., Sengupta, B. & Sengupta, P. K. (2001). Protein–flavonol interaction: Fluorescence spectroscopic study. *Proteins* **43**, 75–81.
83. Loest, H. B., Noh, S. K. & Koo, S. I. (2002). Green tea extract inhibits the lymphatic absorption of cholesterol and alpha-tocopherol in ovariectomized rats. *J Nutr* **132**, 1282–1288.
84. Kuo, K. L., Weng, M. S., Chiang, C. T., Tsai, Y. J., Lin-Shiau, S. Y. & Lin, J. K. (2005). Comparative studies on the hypolipidemic and growth suppressive effects of oolong, black, pu-erh, and green tea leaves in rats. *J Agric Food Chem* **53**, 480–489.
85. Yeh, C. W., Chen, W. J., Chiang, C. T., Lin-Shiau, S. Y. & Lin, J. K. (2003). Suppression of fatty acid synthase in MCF-7 breast cancer cells by tea and tea polyphenols: A possible mechanism for their hypolipidemic effects. *Pharmacogenomics J* **3**, 267–276.
86. Watanabe, J., Kawabata, J. & Niki, R. (1998). Isolation and identification of acetyl-CoA carboxylase inhibitors from green tea (*Camellia sinensis*). *Biosci Biotechnol Biochem* **62**, 532–534.
87. Chisaka, T., Matsuda, H., Kubomura, Y., Mochizuki, M., Yamahara, J. & Fujimura, H. (1988). The effect of crude drugs on experimental hypercholesteremia: Mode of action of (–)-epigallocatechin gallate in tea leaves. *Chem Pharmaceut Bullet* **36**, 227–233.
88. Kono, S., Shinchi, K., Wakabayashi, K., Honjo, S., Todoroki, I., Sakurai, Y., Imanishi, K., Nishikawa, H., Ogawa, S. & Katsurada, M. (1996). Relation of green tea consumption to serum lipids and lipoproteins in Japanese men. *J Epidemiol/ Japan Epidemiological Association* **6**, 128–133.
89. Vita, J. A. (2005). Polyphenols and cardiovascular disease: Effects on endothelial and platelet function. *Am J Clin Nutr* **81**, 292S–s297S.
90. Ignarro, L. J., Buga, G. M., Wood, K. S., Byrns, R. E. & Chaudhuri, G. (1987). Endothelium-derived relaxing factor produced and released from artery and vein is nitric oxide. *Proceedings of the National Academy of Sciences of the United States of America* **84**, 9265–9269.
91. Widlansky, M. E., Gokce, N., Keaney, J. F., Jr. & Vita, J. A. (2003). The clinical implications of endothelial dysfunction. *J Am Coll Cardiol.* **42**, 1149–1160.
92. Vita, J. A. & Keaney, J. F., Jr. (2002). Endothelial function: A barometer for cardiovascular risk. *Circulation* **106**, 640–642.
93. Duffy, S. J., Keaney, J. F., Jr., Holbrook, M., Gokce, N., Swerdloff, P. L., Frei, B. & Vita, J. A. (2001). Short- and long-term black tea consumption reverses endothelial dysfunction in patients with coronary artery disease. *Circulation* **104**, 151–156.
94. Potenza, M. A., Marasciulo, F. L., Tarquinio, M., Tiravanti, E., Colantuono, G., Federici, A., Kim, J. A., Quon, M. J. & Montagnani, M. (2007). EGCG, a green tea polyphenol, improves endothelial function and insulin sensitivity, reduces blood pressure, and protects against myocardial I/R injury in SHR. *Am J Physiol* **292**, E1378–E1387.
95. Tijburg, L. B., Mattern, T., Folts, J. D., Weisgerber, U. M. & Katan, M. B. (1997). Tea flavonoids and cardiovascular disease: A review. *Critic Rev Food Sci Nutr* **37**, 771–785.
96. Lorenz, M., Wessler, S., Follmann, E., Michaelis, W., Dusterhoft, T., Baumann, G., Stangl, K. & Stangl, V. (2004). A constituent of green tea, epigallocatechin-3-gallate, activates endothelial nitric oxide synthase by a phosphatidylinositol-3-OH-kinase-, cAMP-dependent protein kinase-, and Akt-dependent pathway and leads to endothelial-dependent vasorelaxation. *J Biol Chem* **279**, 6190–6195.

97. Kim, J. A., Formoso, G., Li, Y., Potenza, M. A., Marasciulo, F. L., Montagnani, M. & Quon, M. J. (2007). Epigallocatechin gallate, a green tea polyphenol, mediates NO-dependent vasodilation using signaling pathways in vascular endothelium requiring reactive oxygen species and Fyn. *J Biol Chem* **282**, 13736–13745.

98. Hofmann, C. S. & Sonenshein, G. E. (2003). Green tea polyphenol epigallocatechin-3 gallate induces apoptosis of proliferating vascular smooth muscle cells via activation of p53. *FASEB J* **17**, 702–704.

99. Chang, W. C. & Hsu, F. L. (1991). Inhibition of platelet activation and endothelial cell injury by flavan-3-ol and saikosaponin compounds. *Prostaglandins, Leukotrienes, and Essential Fatty Acids* **44**, 51–56.

100. Stocker, R. & Keaney, J. F., Jr. (2004). Role of oxidative modifications in atherosclerosis. *Physiological Rev* **84**, 1381–1478.

101. Lo, H. M., Hung, C. F., Huang, Y. Y. & Wu, W. B. (2007). Tea polyphenols inhibit rat vascular smooth muscle cell adhesion and migration on collagen and laminin via interference with cell–ECM interaction. *J Biomed Sci* **14**, 637–645.

102. Ludwig, A., Lorenz, M., Grimbo, N., Steinle, F., Meiners, S., Bartsch, C., Stangl, K., Baumann, G. & Stangl, V. (2004). The tea flavonoid epigallocatechin-3-gallate reduces cytokine-induced VCAM-1 expression and monocyte adhesion to endothelial cells. *Biochem Biophys Res Commun* **316**, 659–665.

103. Yokozawa, T., Oura, H., Nakagawa, H., Sakanaka, S. & Kim, M. (1995). Effects of a component of green tea on the proliferation of vascular smooth muscle cells. *Biosci Biotechnol Biochem* **59**, 2134–2136.

104. Hodgson, J. M., Puddey, I. B., Mori, T. A., Burke, V., Baker, R. I. & Beilin, L. J. (2001). Effects of regular ingestion of black tea on haemostasis and cell adhesion molecules in humans. *Eur J Clin Nutr* **55**, 881–886.

105. Kang, W. S., Lim, I. H., Yuk, D. Y., Chung, K. H., Park, J. B., Yoo, H. S. & Yun, Y. P. (1999). Antithrombotic activities of green tea catechins and (–)-epigallocatechin gallate. *Thrombosis Res* **96**, 229–237.

106. Kang, W. S., Chung, K. H., Chung, J. H., Lee, J. Y., Park, J. B., Zhang, Y. H., Yoo, H. S. & Yun, Y. P. (2001). Antiplatelet activity of green tea catechins is mediated by inhibition of cytoplasmic calcium increase. *J Cardiovasc Pharmacol* **38**, 875–884.

107. Sugatani, J., Fukazawa, N., Ujihara, K., Yoshinari, K., Abe, I., Noguchi, H. & Miwa, M. (2004). Tea polyphenols inhibit acetyl-CoA:1-alkyl-sn-glycero-3-phosphocholine acetyltransferase (a key enzyme in platelet-activating factor biosynthesis) and platelet-activating factor-induced platelet aggregation. *Int Arch Allergy Immunol* **134**, 17–28.

108. Sumpio, B. E., Cordova, A. C., Berke-Schlessel, D. W., Qin, F. & Chen, Q. H. (2006). Green tea, the "Asian paradox," and cardiovascular disease. *J Am College Surg* **202**, 813–825.

109. Son, D. J., Cho, M. R., Jin, Y. R., Kim, S. Y., Park, Y. H., Lee, S. H., Akiba, S., Sato, T. & Yun, Y. P. (2004). Antiplatelet effect of green tea catechins: A possible mechanism through arachidonic acid pathway. *Prostaglandins, Leukotrienes, and Essential Fatty Acids* **71**, 25–31.

110. Yang, J. A., Choi, J. H. & Rhee, S. J. (1999). Effects of green tea catechin on phospholipase A2 activity and antithrombus in streptozotocin diabetic rats. *J Nutr Sci Vitaminol (Tokyo)* **45**, 337–346.

Chapter 19

Ibogaine and the Treatment of Opiate Addiction

Emily J. Richer, MPH

Department of Public Health Policy and Management, University of Arizona, Mel and Enid Zuckerman College of Public Health, Tucson, AZ, USA

Abstract

Ibogaine is a hallucinogen which has gained attention in the treatment of opioid addiction. Preliminary scientific studies have indicated that Ibogaine can reduce drug cravings, weaken withdrawal symptoms, and improve self-control. Due to the severe side effects, Ibogaine is not often used recreationally, and it has a low potential for addiction. Ibogaine is currently a Schedule I Controlled Substance in the United States, which means it is illegal to manufacture, buy, possess, or distribute without a DEA (drug enforcement administration) license. Ibogaine is administered in many clinics throughout the world, most prevalently in Canada, Europe, and Latin America. There are risks of fatalities with Ibogaine. Due to this fact, advocates say it should be used as a last resort. Not enough tests have been conducted to examine its safety, but its potential is promising and should be investigated.

Keywords: *Ibogaine, Iboga root, opiates, addiction, treatment*

INTRODUCTION

Ibogaine is an indole alkaloid found in the roots of an exotic rainforest shrub native to West Africa called *Tabernanthe iboga* [1]. Ibogaine is a hallucinogen which has gained attention due to its use in the treatment of opioid addiction. It is extracted from the root of the Iboga shrub and is being studied and tested for the treatment of substance abuse, in particular opioid addictions. Preliminary scientific studies in the Americas and Europe indicate that Ibogaine can create immediate reductions in drug cravings, weaken withdrawal symptoms, and improve self-control [1]. The chemical name of Ibogaine is 12-methoxyibogamine, and the chemical formula is $C_{20}H_{26}N_2O$ [2]. Currently Ibogaine is used in the form of crystalline hydrochloride salt. This process prevents decomposition during extraction from the root [2].

At low doses (5 mg/kg of body weight) Ibogaine has a mild stimulant effect, similar to that of caffeine [3]. Chewing the root of the shrub can deliver low doses of Ibogaine. When used in high doses (20–30 mg/kg of body weight) Ibogaine is a strong, long-lasting hallucinogen and is currently classified as a psychedelic [4]. There are three types of hallucinogens: psychedelics, dissociatives, and deliriants [4]. Ibogaine, like all drugs of abuse, is considered a psychoactive. Psychoactive drugs cause subjective changes in perception, thought, emotion, and consciousness. Unlike other psychoactive drugs, such as stimulants and opioids, the hallucinogens do not merely amplify familiar states of mind, but rather induce experiences that are qualitatively different from those of ordinary consciousness. These experiences are often compared to non-ordinary forms of consciousness such as trances, meditations, conversion experiences, and dreams [5]. The term *psychedelic* was coined in the 1960s and means "mind viewing." Prior to that, starting in 1931, the hallucinogens were referred to as "phantastica" meaning that they could create a world of fantasy within a person's mind [5].

Ibogaine is an indole hallucinogen. The basic structure of the neurotransmitter serotonin is referred to as an indole nucleus. Other hallucinogens, such as LSD (lysergic acid diethylamide) and psilocybin, also contain the indole structure [2]. Ibogaine is not widely used like other hallucinogens, such as LSD, Psilocybin Mushrooms, and Peyote, but it does have effects similar to ones produced by those. Due to the severe side effects, Ibogaine is not often used recreationally, and its potential for addiction is extremely low. Ibogaine lasts much longer than other psychedelics, often having an active window of 24 hours and sometimes even up to 48 hours. Ibogaine is usually ingested in the form of a powder and is taken orally, most often put into a capsule then swallowed. Once ingested it is often physically and mentally exhausting and produces ataxia for as long as 12 hours. A state of panic usually hits the user within the first 2 hours of ingestion. Excessive sweating and nausea that may lead to vomiting is not uncommon throughout the experience, especially in the first 4–6 hours. Some people who have taken Ibogaine said that once the first few hours passed, it was an interesting experience where they visualized everything from when they started using drugs, to life experiences, to intense "storms of vibrant colors and unusual textures" [2].

HISTORY OF IBOGAINE

Ibogaine has been used in some countries for many centuries. In the mid-1800s Ibogaine was used in Gabon, Africa in initiation rights of the Bwiti religion. When boys would come of age, usually around age 9–12, it was tradition to have them ingest large amounts of the root and, once they got through the day or two long "trip," they were thought to be adult men [2]. During this 24-hour period they were cared for by older members of the community who would stay awake by chewing on Ibogaine roots. It was known even then that when using Ibogaine at the hallucinogenic level, suffocation and other side effects could be risks.

In 1901 Dybowski and Landrin first isolated Ibogaine from the root of the shrub [2]. In 1966 the total synthesis was accomplished by G. Buchi, and since then several further totally synthetic routes have been developed [2]. The use of Ibogaine in treating substance use disorders in human subjects was first proposed by Howard Lotsof in US Patent 4,499,096 which was awarded in 1985 [6]. Ibogaine's ability to attenuate opioid withdrawal was first confirmed by a rat study done by Michailo Dzoljic and associates in 1988 and again in 1994 [3]. Since then there have been numerous studies, but there have not been any peer-reviewed studies demonstrating statistically significant long term improvement following Ibogaine administration to humans with drug abuse problems.

IBOGAINE AND LEGAL ISSUES

Ibogaine is denoted as a Schedule I Controlled Substance in the United States, which means it is illegal to manufacture, buy, possess, or distribute without a DEA license [7]. To be categorized as a Schedule I drug the following three statements must all be true: (1) The substance has a high potential for abuse; (2) The substance has no currently accepted medical use in treatment in the United States; (3) There is a lack of accepted safety for use of the drug under medical supervision [5].

After the Harrison Act was passed in 1914, narcotics became less freely available and more expensive [8]. Prior to this time heroin had been sold in stores and manufactured by the Bayer Company. In the early 1900s growing opiate abuse was recognized as a problem [2]. Ibogaine was regulated by the US Food and Drug Administration in 1967 pursuant to its authority to regulate stimulants, depressants, and hallucinogens granted by the 1965 Drug Abuse Control Amendments (DACA) to the Federal Food, Drug, and Cosmetic Act. In 1970, with the passage of the Controlled Substances Act, it was classified as a Schedule I Controlled Substance. Since that time, several other countries including Sweden, Denmark, Belgium, and Switzerland have also banned the sale and possession of Ibogaine [1]. Two non-profit organizations in the United States advocate Ibogaine to patients. A treatment center in Florida actually provides Ibogaine to patients, and a center in New York helps patients locate treatment facilities, which are mostly in Canada [9, 10]. Presently, only two arrests have been recorded for the use of Ibogaine. Jack Brian Hout and his wife, Karen Sue Hout, were arrested for conspiring to import Ibogaine. They had both suffered from opiate addictions and had Ibogaine shipped to them from Belize to their home in Casper, Wyoming in December of 2005 [2].

PHARMACOLOGY OF IBOGAINE

The pharmacology of Ibogaine is complex, affecting many different neurotransmitter systems simultaneously [2]. Ibogaine is metabolized in the human body by cytochrome P450 2D6; the major metabolite is noribogaine [2].

Noribogaine is most potent as a serotonin reuptake inhibitor. "Among recent proposals for Ibogaine mechanisms of action is activation of the glial cell line derived neurotrophic factor (GDNF) pathway in the ventral tegmental area (VTA) of the brain. The work has been accomplished in preclinical opiate research where 30 mg/kg of Ibogaine caused increases in RNA expression of GDNF in keeping with reduction of opiate intake in the rat, absent of neurotoxicty or cell death" [6].

STUDIES ABOUT IBOGAINE

Many studies of the effects of Ibogaine on rats have been conducted. In 1994 the journal *Behavioural Brain Research* published a study done by Susanne Cappendijk, Durk Fekkes, and Michailo Dzoljic on the effects of Ibogaine in morphine-addicted rats [6]. Male Wistar rats, weighing 290–330 g, were housed in groups and had free access to food and water. The room was kept at a constant temperature (21°C) and humidity (55%). Morphine dependence was induced by implantation of a morphine base pellet on the back of the rat under ether anesthesia. All of the morphine-addicted rats were only used once. The morphine-dependent rats were separated into two groups, some treated with Ibogaine and the others with water. The rats were not given morphine again and were studied and observed for withdrawal symptoms. Upon withdrawal, the rats treated with water had severe withdrawal symptoms including diarrhea, chewing, excess grooming, shaking, chattering, and jumping. The rats treated with Ibogaine had a few of the same symptoms, like diarrhea and shaking, but not to the same extent, and the symptoms didn't last as long. After a few days, the rats that had been given Ibogaine did not show any withdrawal symptoms, but those given water were still exhibiting withdrawal symptoms. The study was conducted by the Addiction Research Institute in Rotterdam [11].

Similar studies have been done with human subjects. Dr. Mash of the University of Miami, Department of Neurology obtained a large sample size case series study of human volunteers. Taking part in this study were 274 addicts from self-help programs (202 males and 72 females) who were dependent on opiates [2]. European and American addiction selfhelp groups provided testimonials that drug cravings and opiate withdrawal symptoms were blocked after only a single dose administration of Ibogaine [2].

Ibogaine has provided scientists with a new tool to study the brain to understand the addict's motivation for treatment. Future developments include the possibility of delivering the long-acting metabolite of Ibogaine with a system similar to that of a nicotine patch, but because of the extreme side effects, it would be a one-time-use patch. This technology might even be developed to stabilize people with other types of addictions, such as drugs and alcohol. One shortcoming of Ibogaine in its current form is that for it to be successful, the patient has to have enough substance-free time to have effects of other drugs out of the body [12].

EFFECTS OF IBOGAINE

Once ingested, Ibogaine affects the neurotransmitters and actually "resets" them by essentially clearing them. This process is thought to delete the history of opiate dependency. To use Ibogaine for the purposes of curing an opioid addiction, there must not be any opiates present in the body, which otherwise could result in fatality [1]. A period of clean time away from all substances is recommended for a minimum of a few days prior to taking Ibogaine. Once subjects ingest the Ibogaine, they usually become sick with symptoms, such as excessive sweating and vomiting. After the initial side effects subside, many users of Ibogaine report experiencing visual phenomena during a waking dream state, such as instructive replays of life events that led to their addiction. Others report therapeutic visions that help them conquer the fears and negative emotions that drive their addiction. The ensuing time is said to be both physically and mentally exhausting. After 24–48 hours, the initial hallucinations wear off. It is believed that intensive counseling and therapy following the treatment is very important. Some patients require a second or third treatment session with Ibogaine over the course of the next 12–18 months, as it provides a greater efficacy in extinguishing the opiate addiction. Only a small minority of patients relapse completely into opiate addiction within weeks of treatment [9].

IBOGAINE ADMINISTRATION

Ibogaine is being administered in many clinics throughout the world, most prevalently in Canada, Latin America, and Europe. In the United States, two drug rehabilitation centers encourage patients to seek Ibogaine therapy. The Dora Weiner Foundation in New York, founded by Howard Lotsof in 1983, and named after his grandmother, advocates Ibogaine use to its patients [9]. According to its mission statement, "the activities of the foundation are exclusively charitable, educational, and scientific with the intent to encourage and promote public knowledge of research in the study of chemical dependence and substance-related disorders and to advocate for the rights of patients being treated for dependence to drugs. In furtherance of its activities DWF will encourage the exchange of information among persons interested in such study and works through activities which include sponsoring research, conferences, seminars, and workshops" [9]. The foundation explains that "Ibogaine provides a somewhat different scenario wherein the medication's discovery as an anti-addictive agent came from the drug using counter culture" [1]. Lotsof has maintained a strong working relationship with patients and patient advocates who were incorporated into early research through the International Coalition for Addict Self-Help (ICASH).

The second United States treatment facility, the Healing Transitions Institute for Addiction, is located in Miami, Florida. For decades this facility has been researching Ibogaine's therapeutic effects. This institute was founded by Dr. Deborah Mash of the University of Miami, Department of Neurology, who is recognized worldwide as a leading neuroscientist and neuropharmacologist. Over the past 15 years, her research has been continuously supported by a variety of peer-reviewed basic science research grants. Dr. Mash has reported results of her studies on aging, neurodegenerative and neuropsychiatric disorders, and drug and alcohol abuse in more than 250 articles and presentations [1]. According to Dr. Mash, "many drug dependent clients enter treatment in a revolving door manner; from one program to the next, only to find themselves unable to break out of the vicious cycle of relapse. Ibogaine is an important first step on the road to recovery" [13].

Dr. Mash has been an advocate of Ibogaine and has found success with it in her patients. People have come from around the country to participate in her research studies on Ibogaine. In July 1996, Dr. Mash was interviewed by Pacifica Radio reporter Paul DeRienzo about her research with Ibogaine. Dr. Mash's goal was to study Ibogaine in a "credible laboratory, in a credible medical center with appropriate people looking over everyone's shoulder" to collect appropriate data [13]. To possess the Ibogaine needed to go forward with her research, Dr. Mash had to file with the Drug Enforcement Administration and be granted a Schedule I license, which she said was a time consuming process. In addition, she had to file with the University of Miami's Human Subjects Review Board to obtain permission to have people ingest Ibogaine. Dr. Mash had to present her case in front of people from various disciplines: medical ethicists, clinicians, and other scholars. Once the board accepted her proposal, Dr. Mash had to "convince the Public Health Service to garner some sort of support from the National Institute on Drug Abuse" which had funded work that Dr. Mash did earlier. Lastly, in order to work with Ibogaine and human subjects, Dr. Mash had to win approval from the Food and Drug Administration. Only then, could Dr. Mash proceed with her research on the effects of Ibogaine on human subjects [1].

In a testimonial of the positive effects of Ibogaine, a patient of Dr. Mash (C.M. from Denver) writes, "Who would have thought that over 14 months ago I'd now be clean and sober? Who could have imagined I'd be happy, joyous and free from the sickness that I've lived with each and every hour of each and every day – let alone still be alive to speak of it? I'll never forget the night that I got to Miami and met Dr. Mash and her staff. I couldn't know that this program – these wonderful people and the root Ibogaine – was to be the catalyst for change in my life, the catapult to hurl me into my recovery. I was someone who hadn't long to live and I could barely get well enough to take Ibogaine. Now I hate to even imagine missing the chance. I couldn't have dreamed a better dream. I could go on for hours about how Ibogaine changed my life. I am willing: willing to change, to live, to love and to be loved" [13].

RISKS OF IBOGAINE

Some risks of fatalities are associated with the use of Ibogaine. Due to this fact, advocates for the drug say it should be used as a last resort. As of February 2006, at least eight people had died in Europe and the United States from using Ibogaine. Dr. Mash, in referring to one fatality, stated that a patient whose heart is not strong should not receive this treatment [12]. Most of the fatalities occurred under "remarkable circumstances: some of the fatalities being several days after Ibogaine consumption. Four persons had taken less than half of the dose recommended for drug therapy. To date, there is no conclusive explanation for the fatalities" [12]. Some scientists suspect that the deceased had taken opioids concurrent with Ibogaine, which is known to cause fatalities. Fatalities were only documented at doses over 10 mg/kg. The effects of Ibogaine in small amounts on the autonomic nervous system are well known. Tablets with a total of 8 mg of Ibogaine (which is a trace amount) were sold in the 1960s in Europe as a stimulant [8].

OPIOID ADDICTION AND TREATMENT

Opiate use and abuse has been recognized as a problem for thousands of years. The opium poppy was cultivated in lower Mesopotamia as long ago as 3400 BC [5]. In Homer's *Odyssey* there is a passage that refers to the common use of opium, and that was said to be in the year 1000 BC. In the 1800s there were numerous Opium dens in England [5]. The oldest known treatment for opiate addiction was written about in 1902 in a medical guide which recommended reduced use, gradually stopping, cold showers, travel abroad, and a change of lifestyle such as going west to work on a cattle ranch or in a mine. Today many people are affected by heroin addiction. Opiates are strong central nervous system depressants, but regular users develop physiological tolerance allowing gradually increased doses. In combination with other depressants, such as alcohol, even experienced users can easily overdose. Today, three treatments are medically recognized: Methadone, LAAM, and Buprenorphine [5].

Methadone is a synthetic narcotic analgesic developed in Germany during World War II. It was found to be a substitute for the then-unavailable opium-based agent. It is said to be quite effective if taken orally, and it has a long duration, which means it needs to be taken less frequently then recreational heroin. The withdrawal symptoms are also less severe. Although long approved as a narcotic analgesic, methadone gained fame as a drug useful in treatment programs for heroin dependence [14]. When taking methadone, either by pill or injection, some patients will gradually reduce the dose to eventually be weaned off the drug. Others must remain on a high dose. Methadone use can result in abnormal drug-seeking behavior, addiction, and dependence, just like heroin use can [5]. There are many side effects associated with taking Methadone. Some common ones are nausea, vomiting, constipation, lightheadedness, dizziness, dry mouth, drowsiness, blurred vision, flushing, and increased sweating. Methadone clinics are set up to deliver the drug to patients daily. A negative stigma is associated with methadone clinics, and they are often not successful because they need to see all patients daily. Essentially, methadone is a substitute drug to opiates.

In 1993, the FDA approved another synthetic opiate, L-alpha-acetyl-methanol (LAAM) for use in treating narcotic-dependent patients. Due to the fact that LAAM is metabolized in the liver, it has longer-lasting effects than methadone. Instead of daily visits, patients are able to take the drug only 3 times a week, which is the major advantage of LAAM [14]. Otherwise, it is quite similar to Methadone.

Because a large number of opioid-dependent individuals do not respond well to the Methadone and LAAM treatments, another drug has recently been approved. It is a semi-synthetic opioid analgesic called Buprenorphine. Buprenorphine first received FDA approval in 2002 and is marketed under the name Suboxine [5]. Buprenorphine is a partial opioid antagonist. This means that it has a relatively large margin of safety and low overdose potential, which differs from both Methadone and LAAM [14]. It works by preventing with-drawal symptoms, since Buprenorphine is actually a type of narcotic (opioid) itself. The packaging for Buprenorphine states that it should be used as part of a complete narcotic dependence treatment plan [5]. It has side effects similar to Methadone, which include drowsiness, dizziness, weakness, constipation, and vomiting. A growing number of scientists have reported that intravenous her-oin self-administration is significantly reduced when heroin dependent research participants are maintained on Buprenorphine [14]. Buprenorphine, however, is very costly, so it is not an option for patients with a limited income.

CONCLUSION AND RECOMMENDATIONS

Of the three available treatments for opiate addicts (Buprenorphine, Methadone, and LAAM) none are a perfect solution, and all could be improved upon as far as actually helping substance abusers stop using opiates. The current sys-tem of delivering Methadone is fraught with problems. Methadone clinics continue to wrestle with a negative stigma, which discourages people from seeking help, and their required daily visits are problematic for many with jobs and other obligations. Use of the drug Ibogaine could be implemented into treatment that would prove more successful than the others. Not enough tests have been conducted to satisfactorily examine its safety, but its poten-tial is promising and should be investigated. Although, the main focus of this paper has been on Ibogaine and opiate addiction, newer research is testing its beneficial effects on alcohol, cocaine, and methamphetamine abuse. Some sci-entists, namely Howard Lotsof, are of the opinion that Ibogaine might help all addictions. If that proves to be the case, Ibogaine should be reconsidered for treatment and be taken off the Schedule I status, to become a prescribed medicine. The potential for abuse and recreational use is low in Ibogaine, due to the fact that it has such intense negative side effects. Hallucinogens are rarely described as addictive, so with its low potential for addiction, Ibogaine's inclusion as a Schedule I is inappropriate. Although some deaths were caused by its use, Ibogaine might prove to be a preferred alternative and, in fact, a more successful remedy in treating substance abuse.

REFERENCES

1. Healing Transitions Institute for Addiction, "Ibogaine," http://www.ibogaine.net. (accessed April 15, 2007).
2. Wikipedia Online Encyclopedia, "Ibogaine," http://.en.wikipedia.org/wiki/ibogaine. (accessed April 3, 2007).
3. Erowid Online Library, "Psychoactive Vault," http://www.erowid.org. (accessed April 3, 2007).
4. Wikipedia Online Encyclopedia, "Hallucinogens," http://en.wikipedia.org/wiki/hallucinogens. (accessed April 15, 2007).
5. Ksir, C. & Ray, O. (2004). *Drugs, Society, and Human Behavior*, 10th Edition, McGraw Hill, New York.
6. Cappendijk, S., Fekkes, D. & Dzoljic, M. (1994). The inhibitory effect of norharman on morphine withdrawal syndrome in rats: Comparison with Ibogaine. *Behav Brain Res* **65**, 117–119.
7. Wikipedia Online Encyclopedia, "Controlled Substances Act," http://en.wikipedia.org/wiki/controlled_substances_act. (accessed April 15, 2007).
8. Wikipedia Online Encyclopedia, "Heroin," http://en.wikipedia.org/wiki/heroin. (accessed April 3, 2007).
9. Dora Weiner Foundation Website, "About," http://www.doraweiner.org. (accessed April 15, 2007).
10. Lane, A. (December 9, 2005). Couple to be Held in Jail. The Casper Star-Tribune, Local News section.
11. Mash, D. C. (2005). Ibogaine therapy. *Addictions* S05–S322.
12. Maas, U. & Strubelt, S. (2006). Fatalities after taking Ibogaine in addiction treatment could be related to sudden cardiac death caused by autonomic dysfunction. *Medical Hypotheses* **67**, 960–964.
13. The Ibogaine Series, "Uncovering Ibogaine the Deborah Mash Interview with Paul DeRenzio," http://pdr.autono.net/mash.htm. (accessed December 28, 2007).
14. WebMD, "Drugs A-Z," http://www.webmd.com. (accessed April 3, 2007).

Chapter 20

The Potential of Caffeine for the Inhibition of Cognitive Decline in the Aged

Gabriel Keith Harris and Caroline R. Summers

Department of Food, Bioprocessing, and Nutrition Sciences, North Carolina State University, Raleigh, NC, USA

Abstract

The global phenomenon of a growing elderly population is likely to bring about an increase in the incidence of age-related cognitive decline and stimulate interest in the development of strategies to prevent it. Various reports have suggested that moderate to high consumption of caffeine and some other stimulants have potentially beneficial effects on several measures of cognition, including improved attention and enhanced information processing speed. Due to the widespread use of caffeine, it is unclear as to whether consumers experience additional cognitive benefits relative to nonconsumers or if the observed effects are only the result of reductions in withdrawal symptoms upon re-administration of caffeine. Although caffeine appears to be metabolized similarly in the young and old, few studies have examined the effects of caffeine on cognition in the elderly. (The majority of studies on the effects of caffeine and other stimulants have involved young adult subjects.) Thus, the purpose of this chapter is to examine the known and potential effects of caffeine on the prevention or inhibition of cognitive decline in the aged. These potential benefits are weighed against the known side effects of stimulants, such as hypertension, sleeplessness, and anxiety. The interaction of diet and other lifestyle factors with stimulants and the development of dosing regimens that may more specifically enhance cognition with fewer side effects are also discussed.

Keywords: *Caffeine, cognitive decline, stimulants, disease prevention, elderly*

INTRODUCTION

In 2007, the youngest members of the United State's "Baby Boom" generation entered their fifth decade of life [1]. Given their projected life expectancy of approximately 70 years, it is probable that the incidence of age-related conditions, including cognitive decline, will increase in the coming decades [2]. By the year 2030, nearly 20% of the US population is projected to be 65 years of age or older [3]. This trend is not restricted to Western nations as the percentage of persons over 65 years of age is expected to increase worldwide from its present 7.5–12% over the same time period [4]. Although the age distribution of developing countries is still shifted in the direction of the young, worldwide birth and death rates have declined over the past century and are projected to continue declining, resulting in an increase in the aged population [5]. Since dementia risk rises from 1.5% at age 65–30% at age 80, dementia-related diseases will be a worldwide issue in subsequent decades [6]. The aging of global populations has spurred an increased interest in diseases associated with the aging process. Although they have not been strictly defined in terms of chronological age, the terms "aged" or "elderly" will be used interchangeably in this chapter to refer to individuals 65 years of age or older.

Aside from physical limitations, one of the most obvious effects of advanced age is a decline in mental capacity, principally demonstrated by a reduced ability to acquire and retain new information (short and long-term memory), impaired attention, and decreased speed of information processing [7]. Functionally, this results in difficulty in attaining new skills and in "multi-tasking." This may partially explain the contention over the Federal Aviation Administration's proposal to raise mandatory retirement age for airline pilots from 60 to 65 years of age [8]. Age-associated cognitive decline can be grouped into two general categories: normal aging and pathological cognitive decline due to disease. Although normal aging results in all of the impairments described above, diseases such as Alzheimer's and Parkinson's, as well as conditions such as stroke result in a much more rapid decline of mental abilities.

Caffeine has been reported to improve mental function, but most of these studies have been conducted in the young or under conditions of sleep deprivation or induced fatigue. This leaves many unanswered questions with regard to the effects of caffeine and other stimulants on cognitive decline in the elderly. This chapter therefore addresses the following questions regarding caffeine:

1. Can caffeine slow the gradual cognitive decline associated with normal aging?
2. Can caffeine prevent or delay the onset of diseases associated with rapid cognitive decline?
3. Are caffeine's potential benefits outweighed by negative side effects?
4. How does diet affect caffeine's function relative to cognitive decline?

CAFFEINE CHEMISTRY AND CONSUMPTION PATTERNS

Caffeine is a methylxanthine (Fig. 20.1) that is found in a variety of plant products, most notably coffee, tea, and caffeinated soft drinks, while the structurally similar methylxanthines, theophylline, and theobromine are found primarily in tea and chocolate, respectively [9–11]. Caffeine, theophylline, and, to a lesser

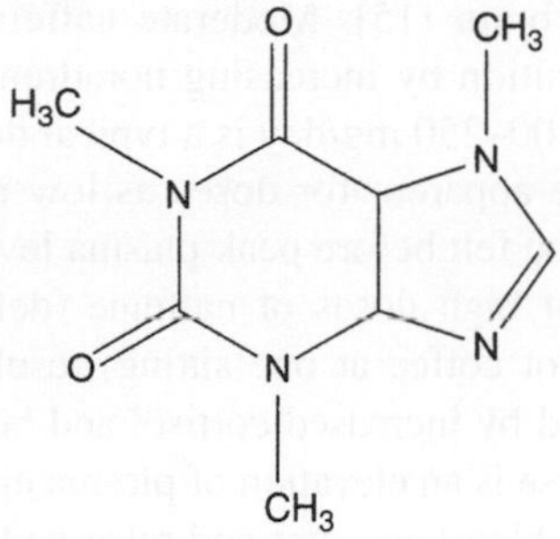

FIGURE 20.1 Caffeine structure.

degree, theobromine, function as stimulants. Caffeine is by far the most frequently consumed stimulant in the world and for that reason will be the focus of this chapter [12]. Caffeine consumption varies widely by country. According to 1998 data, the highest annual consumption per capita was observed in Finland, Sweden, and Denmark (greater than 10 kg of coffee beans were consumed per person per year). In contrast, per capita consumption in the United States was less than half that amount (4.7 kg/person/year). This translates to approximately 200 mg of caffeine or two cups of coffee per person per day [12].

CAFFEINE MECHANISMS

The known stimulant effects of caffeine and other methylxanthines at typical consumption levels (100–250 mg, or the equivalent of approximately 1–2.5 cups of coffee) are primarily due to their function as non-specific inhibitors of adenosine receptors A_1 and A_{2A}. The adenosine A_1 receptor is distributed throughout the central nervous system, with the highest concentrations in regions of the brain associated with the formation of new memories (hippocampus), language (cerebral cortex), and motor skills (cerebellum). Binding of adenosine to A_1 receptors serves to lower intracellular levels of the secondary messenger cyclic AMP (adenosine monophosphate). In contrast, adenosine A_{2A} receptors are localized to the basal ganglia, which serve numerous cognitive functions, and to areas of the brain associated with both learning and memory (nucleus caudatus and putamen), as well as with reward and addictive behavior (nucleus accumbens) and the sense of smell (tuberculum olfactarium) [13]. Unlike A_1 receptors, binding of adenosine to A_{2A} receptors raises intracellular cyclic AMP in GABAergic neurons and opposes the stimulatory effects of dopamine binding to its D_2 target receptors [14]. Regardless of receptor type, binding of adenosine to target receptors has a general depressant effect of slowing heart rate, lowering blood pressure, and reducing spontaneous activity.

Caffeine acts as a stimulant by either stabilizing (where A_1 and A_{2A} receptors are found together) or by increasing (where A_1 receptors predominate) cyclic AMP levels. Recent evidence indicates that A_1 and A_{2A} receptor proteins may form heteromers in the brain [15]. Moderate caffeine intake has also been reported to improve cognition by increasing noradrenaline turnover in human subjects [16]. Although 100–250 mg/day is a typical dose for many consumers, caffeine's effects may be apparent for doses as low as 60 mg (approximately one cup of tea) and may be felt before peak plasma levels are reached [17].

Acute consumption of high doses of caffeine (defined here as 500 mg, or approximately five cups of coffee at one sitting) results in activation of stress responses as demonstrated by increased cortisol and beta-endorphin levels. The result of this stress response is an elevation of plasma epinephrine levels. This, in turn, raises heart rate and blood pressure and releases free fatty acids from storage [18]. The mechanism by which this stress response is initiated is not entirely clear, and may involve both inhibition of adenosine receptors and of phosphodiesterase (the enzyme that converts cyclic AMP to AMP). The conversion of cyclic AMP to AMP inactivates cyclic AMP's secondary messenger function. The inhibition of phosphodiesterase was once thought to be the primary mechanism by which caffeine exerted its stimulatory effects. More recent reports have suggested that the concentration of caffeine necessary to inhibit phosphodiesterase may be as much as 10 times greater than that needed to inhibit adenosine receptors, so it appears unlikely that phosphodiesterase plays a major role at normal caffeine consumption levels [13]. This is especially true for the aged, who generally tend to consume less caffeine than younger persons [7].

Genetic factors appear to influence caffeine consumption patterns and response to caffeine intake. A study of caffeine consumption among fraternal (335 women) and identical twins (486 women) found that genetics may have an influence on the effects of caffeine consumption. Based on data from the twins study, it was estimated that between 35% and 77% of caffeine consumption patterns could be explained by genetic factors [19]. A population-based study of 2735 individuals found that the 1083TT polymorphism of the adenosine A_{2A} receptor was associated with lower caffeine dependence. The authors hypothesized that this was indicative of a greater resistance to caffeine dependency [20]. A double-blind study of 54 men and 46 women who were self-reported infrequent caffeine users found that two separate polymorphisms of the A2A receptor gene were linked to anxiety after consuming 150 mg of caffeine. These two polymorphisms have also been linked to panic disorders [21].

One of the most well-known and most frequently reported effects of caffeine is its ability to temporarily stave off fatigue and drowsiness [22]. There is disagreement among researchers, however, as to whether the reported improvements in cognition are real or are nothing more than an alleviation of withdrawal symptoms (known as the "withdrawal reversal hypothesis") [23]. In support of this hypothesis, Rogers et al. indicated that among regular caffeine consumers, no additional benefits are observed from caffeine intake until 8 hours after a morning dose [23]. In contrast, a study by Haskell et al. indicated that caffeine did appear to have some effects beyond the reversal of withdrawal symptoms. This conclusion was based on measurable improvements (reaction time, memory tasks, alterness) both in non-deprived chronic caffeine users and in non-consumers of caffeine. Caffeine was reported to improve mood in chronic consumers and to improve performance in caffeine-naive subjects to a greater degree than chronic users [25]. Other authors have logically argued that observable effects in habitual non-consumers show that caffeine's effects are not exclusively due to the reversal of withdrawal symptoms [26].

In addition to debate over the withdrawal reversal hypothesis, the effects of chronic caffeine consumption on cognitive function are largely unknown. Many studies that have examined the effects of caffeine on cognition have used either habitual caffeine consumers deprived of caffeine for varying lengths of time or individuals who do not choose to consume caffeine on a regular basis. Neither of these approaches addresses the effects of caffeine in habitual users. In rodent studies, one physiological response to caffeine consumption appeared to be an increase in the number of adenosine receptors in the brain. Marangos *et al.* reported a 20–30% increase in the number of adenosine receptors in the caffeine treated rodents versus control rodents over a period of several weeks [27]. Whether this response is indicative of caffeine tolerance in chronic users (as would seem logical) or if it suggests a change in cognition is still unknown [28]. Short-term caffeine consumption in caffeine-naive or caffeine-deprived subjects is known to have negative side effects, namely reductions in cerebral blood flow and impaired glucose tolerance [29, 30]. In contrast, chronic caffeine consumption has no effect on blood flow to the brain [31]. Although it is well known that habitual caffeine users develop a tolerance to caffeine, some authors have suggested that the tolerance is incomplete in that an intake above a certain level of caffeine would demonstrate effects similar to those observed in habitual non-users [31,32]. Based on recent animal study data, this incomplete tolerance may primarily involve A_{2A} receptor antagonism [15].

CAFFEINE AND NORMAL AGING

Can caffeine slow the gradual cognitive decline associated with normal aging? The answer(s) to this question are mixed, particularly with regard to memory. The Maastricht aging study, which included individuals ranging from 24 years to 81 years of age, has been used on two separate occasions as a source of data to examine the effects of caffeine on cognitive decline. The first report involved 1875 members of the study and found that consumption of coffee and tea, used as surrogates for caffeine intake, did not prevent cognitive decline, but did appear to improve certain aspects of cognition such as long-term memory and motor speed relative to age-matched peers [33]. In a subsequent report involving 1376 members of the Maastricht study, caffeine intake did not significantly affect memory, but did appear to slow declines in information processing speed [34]. As part of the second report, members of the Maastricht aging study were tested for choice reaction time or the time required to choose between or among a variety of options and then tested again 6 years later. The results indicated that increasing caffeine consumption was associated with improvements in this psychomotor measure of cognition only. A cross-sectional study of 9003 British adults who participated in the Health and Lifestyle Survey reported that coffee and tea consumption improved simple and choice reaction time, as well as incidental verbal memory (the ability to remember words or speech), and visuo-spatial reasoning (the ability to think about and manipulate shapes). As with other studies, coffee and tea consumption were used as surrogates for caffeine consumption. The reported effects were dose-dependent in terms of the amount of beverage consumed and were stronger for coffee than for tea. If the observed effects were due to caffeine, this would be logical since a particular volume of coffee contains approximately twice the caffeine as an equal volume of tea. The effects also appeared to be greater for the elderly than for the young [32].

Not all studies comparing the effects of tea and coffee consumption on cognition have reported coffee to be superior. The Surugaya Project, a cross-sectional Japanese study involving 1003 subjects in their seventh decade of life reported that tea, but not coffee consumption, was associated with a reduced risk of "normal" cognitive decline, as assessed by the mini-mental state examination. This examination included a questionnaire designed to be used as a rapid screening technique for dementia in clinical settings. Interestingly, green tea was more protective than oolong tea or coffee in this study [35]. Since green tea contains less caffeine per serving than coffee (approximately 50 mg in green tea versus approximately 100 mg in coffee) non-caffeine components of this beverages may merit further investigation, especially with regard to their ability to prevent cognitive decline.

If, as indicated by other authors, normal cognitive aging can be viewed as a progressive loss of alertness or arousal, stimulants may be potentially beneficial. A study by Rees *et al.* reported that the consumption of 250 mg of pure caffeine in non-withdrawn young and old subjects improved cognitive performance and reduced fatigue-associated declines in performance in older people [36]. This double-blind parallel study involved 48 men and women, with half of the study participants in the 20–25 age range and half in the 50–65 age range. Caffeine appeared to be particularly effective at inhibiting the late-day declines in cognitive performance observed in the 50–65 year age group relative to those receiving the placebo. This finding is in keeping with the increase in fatigue that occurs with aging, coupled with studies indicating that physical fatigue adversely affects mental performance. van Duinen *et al.* reported that caffeine maintained performance and accuracy during a fatiguing motor task, suggesting that the aged may benefit from this approach [37]. To summarize, caffeine does appear to have potential benefits relative to cognitive decline in normal aging, particularly with regard to improved reaction time and attention. Effects on short and long-term memory have been reported, but are less well-established.

CAFFEINE AND DISEASE PREVENTION

Can caffeine or other stimulants prevent or delay the onset of diseases associated with rapid cognitive decline? The answer to this question appears to be yes, at least with regard to Parkinson's and Alzheimer's diseases. The effects of caffeine on Parkinson's disease risk appear to be both dose and gender dependent. A 22-year prospective study of 6710 Finnish men and women, aged 50–79 at the outset of the study reported that those consuming 10 or more cups of coffee per day had a relative risk of 0.26 of developing Parkinson's disease relative to those who did not drink coffee [38]. Although these results are striking, the practical significance of this very high level of coffee consumption for those that consume 1–2 cups per day is unclear. In the Cancer Prevention Study II Cohort, a U.S.-based prospective study of greater than one million people, coffee intake was reported to be inversely associated with Parkinson's disease mortality in men and in women who did not use postmenopausal estrogen. In contrast, coffee consumption was associated with an increased relative risk of Parkinson's disease mortality in women who underwent postmenopausal estrogen therapy [39]. A previous study of 77,713 women from the nurses health study also reported that coffee consumption was only protective against Parkinson's disease in the absence of estrogen therapy [40]. Unlike the results for women, data from the health professional's follow-up study and other prospective studies indicates that caffeine from coffee and other caffeine-containing beverages appears to be consistently protective against Parkinson's disease for men [41].

Based on human, animal, and cell culture studies, caffeine and other A_{2A} receptor antagonists may play a role in preventing Alzheimer's disease. A case control study involving 54 subjects with probable diagnosis of Alzheimer's disease to 54 age and sex-matched controls found that individuals that consumed 199 mg of caffeine (approximately two cups of coffee) per day for the previous 20 years were at a significantly lower risk of developing the desease than those consuming less caffeine. This was true after controlling for other dementia risk factors including hypertension, diabetes, stroke, head trauma, and family history [42]. A meta-analysis of two case controls and two prospective studies examining the effects of coffee on Alzheimer's disease also reported that coffee was protective [43]. Since it was pointed out earlier that chronic caffeine consumption increased the number of adenosine receptors, it is interesting to note that Alzheimer's patients have been reported to lose adenosine A_1 receptors, specifically in the hippocampal region of the brain [44].

Based on animal study data, caffeine may prevent Alzheimer's disease by protecting against beta-amyloid toxicity through adenosine A_1 receptor inhibition. Although caffeine is a non-specific inhibitor of adenosine A_1 and A_{2A} receptors, only A_1 receptor antagonists appear to protect against beta-amyloid toxicity [45]. A second animal study that used transgenic mice highly susceptible to the formation of beta-amyloid plaques showed that caffeine protected against their formation via inhibition of presenilin-1 and beta-secretase, and through normalization of adenosine levels, which were reduced in animals not treated with caffeine [46]. These animal studies are of interest since the presence of beta-amyloid proteins is considered to be a major causative factor in the etiology of Alzheimer's disease. Data collected from cell culture work on a neuroblastoma cell line indicate that caffeine may protect against Alzheimer's through the induction of neutral endopeptidases that are capable of degrading beta-amyloid proteins [47]. Interestingly, green tea ingredients, such as epicatechin and epigallocatechin gallate also induced neutral endopeptidase activity in this model, raising the possibility that non-stimulant food ingredients may augment the protective effects of caffeine.

In addition to direct preventative effects against Parkinson's and Alzheimer's diseases, caffeine consumption may also indirectly inhibit cognitive decline via prevention of type II diabetes, a disease associated with accelerated rates of cognitive decline [48, 49]. Several authors who have analyzed data from the nurses health study and the health professional's follow-up study have reported that coffee, tea, and caffeine consumption are generally associated with a reduced risk of type II diabetes [30, 50, 51]. As mentioned earlier, acute caffeine intake in caffeine-naive subjects is associated with impaired glucose tolerance. However, regular caffeine users do not experience impaired glucose tolerance. This may be due to tolerance to caffeine, to non-caffeine components present in caffeinated beverages, or both. In support of this idea, a study by Battram *et al.* reported that caffeine from coffee caused glucose intolerance to a lesser degree than pure caffeine [52].

NEGATIVE SIDE EFFECTS OF CAFFEINE

Although caffeine consumption may have some benefits with regard to slowing normal cognitive decline and the prevention of diseases associated with rapid cognitive decline, it is important to consider the potentially negative effects of caffeine consumption in the elderly. Potential concerns include the hypertensive and anxiety-producing effects of caffeine, as well as withdrawal symptoms and possible drug interactions. Data from the nurses health studies I and II involving 155,594 women found that neither caffeine in general nor caffeine consumption via coffee were significantly associated with the diagnosis of hypertension, although the reasons for this observation are unclear [53]. Among men, caffeine appears to have the greatest effects on those already diagnosed with hypertension. A study of 182 men, categorized as having optimal, normal, high-normal, or stage I hypertension, were administered 250 mg of caffeine. An hour after caffeine administration, men in the stage I and high normal categories were most likely to exhibit elevated blood pressure readings consistent with hypertension [54]. Caffeine withdrawal symptoms can result from doses as low as 100 mg/day and range from lethargy to headaches to muscle and joint pain. Withdrawal symptoms peak between 24 hours and 48 hours after cessation of use and may last for up to a week. Since the elderly are more likely to undergo medical procedures more frequently than the young, it is important to consider the effects of caffeine use and withdrawal on these patients [55]. Caffeine withdrawal symptoms often result in self-medication via re-administration of caffeine. This suggests that caffeine produces significant dependency.

INTERACTIONS BETWEEN DIET AND CAFFEINE

A number of dietary and lifestyle factors appear to influence the effects of caffeine on cognitive decline. These include: the consumption of caffeine with or without meals, the timing of those meals, and the non-caffeine chemical composition of caffeine-containing beverages. Smith and co-workers examined the effects of caffeine consumed with breakfast, lunch, and dinner. Coffee consumed after either a hot or cold breakfast was reported to improve memory related to concepts, the ability to recognize items, and free recall. Improved logical reasoning was also observed in a double-blind, placebo-controlled trial involving 24 men and 24 women, all university students. In this study, caffeine was added directly to decaffeinated coffee at 4 mg/kg body weight, or approximately equivalent to the caffeine content in three cups of regular coffee. In addition to effects on cognition, caffeine also significantly increased blood pressure and pulse rate [56]. Caffeine consumed with lunch effectively eliminated the post-lunch declines in attention. The effects of caffeine were greatest on less anxious individuals, as they are also the ones that have the largest drops in attention after lunch [57]. In a double-blind, placebo-controlled trial involving 24 men and 24 women, the consumption of 3 mg/kg body weight caffeine, or approximately equal to the amount of caffeine in two cups of regular coffee after an evening meal, improved alertness compared to subjects that did not consume caffeine [58]. Little data exists regarding the interactive effects of individual macronutrients with caffeine on cognitive function. A randomized, double-blinded crossover study used to test the interaction of caffeine and glucose reported a synergistic improvement in memory and in attention when 75 mg of caffeine and 37.5 g of glucose were ingested at the same time after an overnight fast [59].

Aside from coffee, tea is the most common means of caffeine consumption. Coffee contains a wide variety of chemical compounds, but, unlike those in tea, no single compound in coffee has been reported to influence caffeine's stimulatory effects. In contrast, tea contains a number of substances that may modulate caffeine's effects, including theanine and catechins. Theanine is an amino acid found in green, oolong, and black teas and is a biochemical precursor of catechins. Catechins are flavonoid compounds. Rogers *et al.* observed that theanine effectively opposed the hypertensive effects of caffeine in a randomized, double-blind, placebo-controlled group of 48 adults between 18 years and 28 years of age [60]. Both theanine and catechins have been reported to possess neuroprotective effects in animal models in which an ischemic stroke was simulated [61, 62]. Due to its theanine content, tea may be preferable to coffee in terms of caffeinated beverage consumption for the elderly, especially for those suffering from hypertension.

SUMMARY

In this chapter, we have discussed the known and potential effects of caffeine and other stimulants on the aged. Several observations and recommendations can be made relative to the effects of caffeine on cognitive decline in the elderly. First and most obvious, the small number of studies involving elderly subjects makes firm conclusions difficult. As the elderly population grows worldwide and the expected burden of Parkinson's, Alzheimer's and other age-related forms of cognitive decline rises, the need for this information will also increase. Second, the data related to the effects of caffeine on cognition is difficult to interpret due to the myriad of assessment tools. Standardization of cognitive testing across studies is an essential step in ensuring that experimental results are comparable. Third, caffeine does appear to have potential cognitive benefits for the elderly, particularly with regard to reducing fatigue, improving reaction time and attention, and enhancing mood. Fourth, the side effects of caffeine, especially hypertension, need to be carefully considered before recommendations for its use are made for elderly persons. Further studies are needed to identify optimal caffeine dosing regimens, or more selective stimulants that can separate caffeine's apparent cognitive benefits from its known side effects.

REFERENCES

1. Martin, J. A., Hamilton, B. E., Sutton, P. D., Ventura, S. J., Menacker, F. & Kirmeyer, S. (2006). Births: Final Data for 2004. National Vital Statistics Reports 55.
2. National Center for Health Statistics (2006). Health, United States, 2006, with Chartbook on Trends in the Health of Americans (http://www.cdc.gov/nchs/data/hus/hus06.pdf#027).
3. He, W., Sengupta, M., Velkoff, V. A. & DeBarros, K. A. (2006). 65+ in the United States: 2005. (U.S. Census Bureau) http://www.census.gov/prod/2006pubs/p23-209.pdf.
4. US Census Bureau (2007). International Database (http://www.census.gov/ipc/www/idb/).
5. United Nations (2001). World Population Prospects: The 2000 Revision (http://www.unece.org/stats/trend/register.htm).
6. Ritchie, K. & Lovestone, S. (2002). The dementias. *Lancet* **360**, 1759–1766.
7. van Boxtel, M. P. J. & Schmitt, J. A. J. (2004). Age-related changes in the effects of coffee on memory and cognitive performance. *In* Coffee, Tea, Chocolate, and the Brain, (A. Nehlig, Ed.), pp. 85–94, CRC Press, Boca Raton.
8. Federal Aviation Administration (2007). Washington Headquarters Press Release: FAA to Propose Pilot Retirement Age Change (http://www.faa.gov/news/press_releases/news_story.cfm?newsId = 8027).
9. US Department of Agriculture, ARS (2007). USDA National Nutrient Database for Standard Reference, Release 20. Nutrient Data Laboratory Home Page (http://www.ars.usda.gov/ba/bhnrc/ndl).
10. Calviño, A. M., Tamasi, O. P. & Ciappini, M. C. (2005). Note. Caffeine content and dynamical bitterness of yerba mate *Ilex paraguariensis* infusions. *Food Sci Technol Int* **11**, 401–407.
11. Thomas, J. B., Yen, J. H., Schantz, M. M., Porter, B. J. & Sharpless, K. E. (2004). Determination of caffeine, theobromine, and theophylline in standard reference

material 2384, baking chocolate, using reversed-phase liquid chromatography. *J Agric Food Chem* **52**, 3259–3263.

12. Lundsberg, L. (1998). Caffeine consumption. *In* Caffeine (G. A. Spiller, Ed.), pp. 200–222, CRC Press, New York.
13. Daly, J. W. & Fredholm., B. B. (2004) Mechanisms of action of caffeine on the nervous system. In *Coffee, Tea, Chocolate, and the Brain* (A. Nehlig, Ed.), pp. 1–11, CRC Press, Boca Raton.
14. Daly, J. W. (2007). Caffeine analogs: Biomedical impact. *Cell Mol Life Sci* **64**, 2153–2169.
15. Ferre, S., Ciruela, F., Borycz, J., Solinas, M., Quarta, D., Antoniou, K., Quiroz, C., Justinova, Z., Lluis, C., Franco, R. & Goldberg, S. R. (2008). Adenosine A1-A2A receptor heteromers: New targets for caffeine in the brain. *Front Biosci* **13**, 2391–2399.
16. Smith, A., Brice, C., Nash, J., Rich, N. & Nutt, D. J. (2003). Caffeine and central noradrenaline: Effects on mood, cognitive performance, eye movements and cardiovascular function. *J Psychopharmacol* **17**, 283–292.
17. Durlach, P. J. (1998). The effects of a low dose of caffeine on cognitive performance. *Psychopharmacology (Berl)* **140**, 116–119.
18. Absi, M. & Lovallo, W. R. (2004). Caffeine's effects on the human stress axis. *In* Coffee, Tea, Chocolate, and the Brain, (A. Nehlig, Ed.), pp. 113–124, CRC Press, Boca Raton.
19. Kendler, K. S. & Prescott, C. A. (1999). Caffeine intake, tolerance, and withdrawal in women: a population-based twin study. *Am J Psychiatry* **156**, 223–228.
20. Cornelis, M. C., El-Sohemy, A. & Campos, H. (2007). Genetic polymorphism of the adenosine A2A receptor is associated with habitual caffeine consumption. *Am J Clin Nutr* **86**, 240–244.
21. Alsene, K., Deckert, J., Sand, P. & de Wit, H. (2003). Association between A2a receptor gene polymorphisms and caffeine-induced anxiety. *Neuropsychopharmacology* **28**, 1694–1702.
22. McLellan, T. M., Kamimori, G. H., Voss, D. M., Tate, C. & Smith, S. J. (2007). Caffeine effects on physical and cognitive performance during sustained operations. *Aviat Space Environ Med* **78**, 871–877.
23. Rogers, P. J., Heatherley, S. V., Hayward, R. C., Seers, H. E., Hill, J. & Kane, M. (2005). Effects of caffeine and caffeine withdrawal on mood and cognitive performance degraded by sleep restriction. *Psychopharmacology (Berl)* **179**, 742–752.
24. Heatherley, S. V., Hayward, R. C., Seers, H. E. & Rogers, P. J. (2005). Cognitive and psychomotor performance, mood, and pressor effects of caffeine after 4, 6 and 8 h caffeine abstinence. *Psychopharmacology (Berl)* **178**, 461–470.
25. Haskell, C. F., Kennedy, D. O., Wesnes, K. A. & Scholey, A. B. (2005). Cognitive and mood improvements of caffeine in habitual consumers and habitual non-consumers of caffeine. *Psychopharmacology (Berl)* **179**, 813–825.
26. Seidl, R., Peyrl, A., Nicham, R. & Hauser, E. (2000). A taurine and caffeine-containing drink stimulates cognitive performance and well-being. *Amino Acids* **19**, 635–642.
27. Marangos, P. J., Boulenger, J. P. & Patel, J. (1984). Effects of chronic caffeine on brain adenosine receptors: Regional and ontogenetic studies. *Life Sci* **34**, 899–907.

28. Holtzman, S. G., Mante, S. & Minneman, K. P. (1991). Role of adenosine receptors in caffeine tolerance. *J PharmacolExper Ther* **256**, 62–68.
29. Haase, C. G., Becka, M., Kuhlmann, J. & Wensing, G. (2005). Influences of caffeine, acetazolamide and cognitive stimulation on cerebral blood flow velocities. *Prog Neuropsychopharmacol Biol Psychiatry* **29**, 549–556.
30. Salazar-Martinez, E., Willett, W. C., Ascherio, A., Manson, J. E., Leitzmann, M. F., Stampfer, M. J. & Hu, F. B. (2004). Coffee consumption and risk for type 2 diabetes mellitus. *Ann Intern Med* **140**, 1–8.
31. Watson, J. M., Sherwin, R. S., Deary, I. J., Scott, L. & Kerr, D. (2003). Dissociation of augmented physiological, hormonal and cognitive responses to hypoglycaemia with sustained caffeine use. *Clin Sci (Lond)* **104**, 447–454.
32. Jarvis, M. J. (1993). Does caffeine intake enhance absolute levels of cognitive performance? *Psychopharmacology (Berl)* **110**, 45–52.
33. Hameleers, P. A., Van Boxtel, M. P., Hogervorst, E., Riedel, W. J., Houx, P. J., Buntinx, F. & Jolles, J. (2000). Habitual caffeine consumption and its relation to memory, attention, planning capacity and psychomotor performance across multiple age groups. *Hum Psychopharmacol* **15**, 573–581.
34. van Boxtel, M. P., Schmitt, J. A., Bosma, H. & Jolles, J. (2003). The effects of habitual caffeine use on cognitive change: A longitudinal perspective. *Pharmacol Biochem Behav* **75**, 921–927.
35. Kuriyama, S., Hozawa, A., Ohmori, K., Shimazu, T., Matsui, T., Ebihara, S., Awata, S., Nagatomi, R., Arai, H. & Tsuji, I. (2006). Green tea consumption and cognitive function: A cross-sectional study from the Tsurugaya Project 1. *Am J Clin Nutr* **83**, 355–361.
36. Rees, K., Allen, D. & Lader, M. (1999). The influences of age and caffeine on psychomotor and cognitive function. *Psychopharmacology (Berl)* **145**, 181–188.
37. van Duinen, H., Lorist, M. M. & Zijdewind, I. (2005). The effect of caffeine on cognitive task performance and motor fatigue. *Psychopharmacology (Berl)* **180**, 539–547.
38. Saaksjarvi, K., Knekt, P., Rissanen, H., Laaksonen, M. A., Reunanen, A. & Mannisto, S. (2007). Prospective study of coffee consumption and risk of Parkinson's disease. *Eur J Clin Nutr*, (epub ahead of print) (http://www.ncbi.nlm.nih.gov/entrez/query.fcgi?cmd = Retrieve&db = PubMed&dopt = Citation&list_uids = 17522612).
39. Ascherio, A., Weisskopf, M. G., O'Reilly, E. J., McCullough, M. L., Calle, E. E., Rodriguez, C. & Thun, M. J. (2004). Coffee consumption, gender, and Parkinson's disease mortality in the cancer prevention study II cohort: The modifying effects of estrogen. *Am J Epidemiol* **160**, 977–984.
40. Ascherio, A., Chen, H., Schwarzschild, M. A., Zhang, S. M., Colditz, G. A. & Speizer, F. E. (2003). Caffeine, postmenopausal estrogen, and risk of Parkinson's disease. *Neurology* **60**, 790–795.
41. Ascherio, A., Zhang, S. M., Hernan, M. A., Kawachi, I., Colditz, G. A., Speizer, F. E. & Willett, W. C. (2001). Prospective study of caffeine consumption and risk of Parkinson's disease in men and women. *Ann Neurol* **50**, 56–63.
42. Maia, L. & de Mendonca, A. (2002). Does caffeine intake protect from Alzheimer's disease? *Eur J Neurol* **9**, 377–382.
43. Barranco Quintana, J. L., Allam, M. F., Serrano Del Castillo, A. & Fernandez-Crehuet Navajas, R. (2007). Alzheimer's disease and coffee: A quantitative review. *Neurol Res* **29**, 91–95.

44. Kalaria, R. N., Sromek, S., Wilcox, B. J. & Unnerstall, J. R. (1990). Hippocampal adenosine A1 receptors are decreased in Alzheimer's disease. *Neurosci Lett* **118**, 257–260.

45. Dall'Igna, O. P., Fett, P., Gomes, M. W., Souza, D. O., Cunha, R. A. & Lara, D. R. (2007). Caffeine and adenosine A(2a) receptor antagonists prevent beta-amyloid (25-35)-induced cognitive deficits in mice. *Exp Neurol* **203**, 241–245.

46. Arendash, G. W., Schleif, W., Rezai-Zadeh, K., Jackson, E. K., Zacharia, L. C., Cracchiolo, J. R., Shippy, D. & Tan, J. (2006). Caffeine protects Alzheimer's mice against cognitive impairment and reduces brain beta-amyloid production. *Neuroscience* **142**, 941–952.

47. Ayoub, S. & Melzig, M. F. (2006). Induction of neutral endopeptidase (NEP) activity of SK-N-SH cells by natural compounds from green tea. *J Pharm Pharmacol* **58**, 495–501.

48. Cukierman, T., Gerstein, H. C. & Williamson, J. D. (2005). Cognitive decline and dementia in diabetes – systematic overview of prospective observational studies. *Diabetologia* **48**, 2460–2469.

49. Ryan, C. M. (2005). Diabetes, aging, and cognitive decline. *Neurobiol Aging* **26**(Suppl 1), 21–25.

50. Paynter, N. P., Yeh, H. C., Voutilainen, S., Schmidt, M. I., Heiss, G., Folsom, A. R., Brancati, F. L. & Kao, W. H. (2006). Coffee and sweetened beverage consumption and the risk of type 2 diabetes mellitus: The atherosclerosis risk in communities study. *Am J Epidemiol* **164**, 1075–1084.

51. Iso, H., Date, C., Wakai, K., Fukui, M. & Tamakoshi, A. (2006). The relationship between green tea and total caffeine intake and risk for self-reported type 2 diabetes among Japanese adults. *Ann Intern Med* **144**, 554–562.

52. Battram, D. S., Arthur, R., Weekes, A. & Graham, T. E. (2006). The glucose intolerance induced by caffeinated coffee ingestion is less pronounced than that due to alkaloid caffeine in men. *J Nutr* **136**, 1276–1280.

53. Winkelmayer, W. C., Stampfer, M. J., Willett, W. C. & Curhan, G. C. (2005). Habitual caffeine intake and the risk of hypertension in women. *JAMA* **294**, 2330–2335.

54. Hartley, T. R., Sung, B. H., Pincomb, G. A., Whitsett, T. L., Wilson, M. F. & Lovallo, W. R. (2000). Hypertension risk status and effect of caffeine on blood pressure. *Hypertension* **36**, 137–141.

55. Griffiths, R. R., Evans, S. M., Heishman, S. J., Preston, K. L., Sannerud, C. A., Wolf, B. & Woodson, P. P. (1990). Low-dose caffeine physical dependence in humans. *J Pharmacol Exp Ther* **255**, 1123–1132.

56. Smith, A., Kendrick, A., Maben, A. & Salmon, J. (1994). Effects of breakfast and caffeine on cognitive performance, mood and cardiovascular functioning. *Appetite* **22**, 39–55.

57. Smith, A. P., Rusted, J. M., Eaton-Williams, P., Savory, M. & Leathwood, P. (1990). Effects of caffeine given before and after lunch on sustained attention. *Neuropsychobiology* **23**, 160–163.

58. Smith, A., Maben, A. & Brockman, P. (1994). Effects of evening meals and caffeine on cognitive performance, mood and cardiovascular functioning. *Appetite* **22**, 57–65.

59. Scholey, A. B. & Kennedy, D. O. (2004). Cognitive and physiological effects of an "energy drink": An evaluation of the whole drink and of glucose, caffeine and herbal flavouring fractions. *Psychopharmacology (Berl)* **176**, 320–330.

60. Rogers, P. J., Smith, J. E., Heatherley, S. V. & Pleydell-Pearce, C. W. (2007). Time for tea: Mood, blood pressure and cognitive performance effects of caffeine and theanine administered alone and together. *Psychopharmacology (Berl)* **195**, 569–577.

61. Weinreb, O., Mandel, S., Amit, T. & Youdim, M. B. (2004). Neurological mechanisms of green tea polyphenols in Alzheimer's and Parkinson's diseases. *J Nutr Biochem* **15**, 506–516.

62. Kakuda, T. (2002). Neuroprotective effects of the green tea components theanine and catechins. *Biol Pharm Bull* **25**, 1513–1518.

Chapter 21

Five or More Servings of Fruit and Vegetables Each Day for Better Health!

Lyn M. Steffen

Division of Epidemiology and Community Health, University of Minnesota School of Public Health, Minneapolis, MN, USA

Abstract

Over 2.5 million deaths were attributable to low fruit and vegetable intake according to the World Health Organization. Epidemiologic evidence has shown low consumption of fruit and vegetables is associated with higher risk of cardiovascular disease (CVD), stroke, type 2 diabetes, high blood pressure, osteoporosis, certain cancers, and obesity, although study findings are not consistent. Paradoxically, the French population has a high intake of saturated fat, but a low rate of CVD. A recent study demonstrated that polyphenols (i.e., red wine, fruit, or vegetable intake) consumed together with high fat foods may reduce the effect of dietary fat on the development of atherosclerosis. Further, findings from two meta-analyses provide strong support for the *Dietary Guidelines for Americans* that consuming more than 5 servings of fruit and vegetables daily is beneficial for cardiovascular health. However, study results are inconsistent regarding the relation between fruit and vegetables and several other chronic diseases, including peripheral artery disease, type 2 diabetes, cancer, and obesity. Higher intake of fruit and vegetables is inversely associated with blood pressure, as shown in several studies. Moreover, recent studies of novel CVD biomarkers, including inflammation and oxidative stress, have shown lower concentrations of these biomarkers with greater amounts of fruit and vegetable intake. Fruit and vegetables are colorful packages of phytochemicals that promote health. Despite the favorable effects of fruit and vegetables, intake is not sufficient in the majority of populations nationally or internationally; only 23–26% of adults consume at least 5 servings of fruit and vegetables each day. Clearly, nutrition education interventions are necessary to promote fruit and vegetable consumption in adult and youth populations.

Keywords: *Fruit and vegetables, cardiovascular disease, stroke, blood pressure, oxidative stress*

INTRODUCTION

Over 2.5 million deaths were attributable to low fruit and vegetable intake according to the World Health Organization [1]. Epidemiologic evidence has shown low consumption of fruit and vegetables is associated with higher risk of cardiovascular disease [2–4], stroke [5], type 2 diabetes [6], high blood pressure [7,8], osteoporosis [9], certain cancers [10, 11], and obesity [12], although study findings are not consistent [11, 13, 14].

According to the *Dietary Guidelines for Americans*, children and adults should eat a sufficient number and variety of fruits and vegetables each day while staying within individual energy needs [15]. In particular, foods from all five vegetable subgroups should be eaten several times a week, including dark green, orange, legumes, starchy vegetables, and other vegetables. The *Dietary Guidelines for Americans*, first developed in 1980 and updated in 2005 by the United States Department of Agriculture (USDA) and the Department of Health and Human Services (DHHS), "provides science-based advice to promote health and reduce risk for major chronic disease through diet and physical activity" [15]. In addition, the USDA also developed a tool called the Food Guide Pyramid (found at www.myPyramid.gov) which translates the *Dietary Guidelines for Americans* into messages that may assist consumers to improve their eating habits [16].

PREVALENCE OF FRUIT AND VEGETABLE CONSUMPTION

Results from Behavioral Risk Factor Surveillance System (BRFSS), a national survey, show that the proportion of US adults consuming at least 5 servings of fruit and vegetables daily increased from 19% in 1991 to 22% in 1994 and to 23% in 1996 [17]. Findings from the National Health and Nutrition Examination Survey (NHANES) III conducted in 1988–1994 and in 1999–2002 were similar with only 24.3 and 23.6% of US adults, respectively, consuming at least 5 servings of fruit and vegetables each day [18]. Even though the "5 A Day for Better Health" nutrition education campaign was conducted in 1991, only a small proportion of adults increased their fruit and vegetable consumption [19]. However, in the 1999–2002 NHANES, 84–88% of older adults (65+ years old) and 70% of adults ages 19–64 years reported consuming some fruit each day. Most (94–96%) adults reported eating almost 2 servings of vegetables on a given day [18].

In Europe, guidelines for consumption of fruit and vegetables vary by country from 400 g/day to 750 g/day [20]. However, similar to the US, only 27% of adult women achieve the minimum intake of 400 g/day, with an average of 297 g/day [21]. According to the Australian National Nutrition Survey results, the average daily intake of fruit and vegetables for men was 138 and 285 g, respectively; while women reported 132 and 230 g, respectively [22]. Clearly, national and international interventions are necessary to promote fruit and vegetable consumption in adult and youth populations.

NUTRIENTS AND FOOD COMPOUNDS IN FRUIT AND VEGETABLES

Why are fruit and vegetables beneficial to health? Fruit and vegetables are colorful foods chock full of different combinations of nutrients and bioactive compounds interacting with one another that may subsequently lead to better health for individuals who eat plenty of them [23].

Bioactive Compounds

There are four major classes of bioactive compounds found in fruit and vegetables, including nitrogen-containing alkaloids, phenolics and polyphenolics, sulfur-containing compounds, and terpenoids. Polyphenols, "bioactive" food compounds that are found in fruits, vegetables, coffee, tea, chocolate, and soy, have been shown to protect against chronic disease, including coronary heart disease (CHD) [24]. Major polyphenol subgroups include flavonoids, flavonols, phenolic acids, anthocyanidins, and tannins. Over two-thirds of the polyphenols consumed in the diet are flavonoids [25]. The French population has been known to consume a diet high in saturated fat and also red wine; interestingly, the French have a low incidence of CHD. This phenomenon has been labeled "the French Paradox." Even though saturated fat intake is positively associated with CHD, the food compounds resveratrol and flavonoids found in red wine (grapes) are known for their antioxidant, antithrombotic, and anti-inflammatory activities [26]. Thus, if consumed together, polyphenols may reduce the effect of fatty food consumption on the development of atherosclerosis [27]. In a prospective study of women living in Iowa, dietary intake of flavanones, anthocyanidins, and fruit rich in flavonoids were associated with reduced risk of death due to all causes and CHD [28]. The polyphenolic compounds in fruit and vegetables may also be beneficial in slowing the neuronal deficits of aging [29]. The flavonoid anthocyanidin (e.g., found in blueberries) is known for potent antioxidant and anti-inflammatory activity and inhibition of lipid peroxidation. Although most nutrition intervention studies of cognitive function in aging have used rat models, recent studies have shown significantly improved cognitive and motor behavioral performance in animals supplemented with blueberries [30, 31].

Total Antioxidant Capacity

Fruits and vegetables are major sources of antioxidants, including vitamin C, folate, carotenoids (alpha carotene, beta carotene, lycopene, lutein, and zeaxanthin), and selenium, as well as the previously mentioned bioactive compounds (nitrogen-containing alkaloids, phenolics and polyphenolics, sulfur-containing compounds, and terpenoids). There are situations in which the levels of the individual antioxidant components may not be useful, but one measure of total antioxidant potency of total dietary intake or in the plasma would be beneficial to answer a research question. Total antioxidant capacity (TAC) may be measured in the extracellular fluid and is the sum of endogenous and food-derived antioxidants or it may be measured in foods and is the sum of all antioxidants in the food. TAC may be determined by Trolox equivalents antioxidant capacity assay (TEAC), total radical-trapping antioxidant parameter (TRAP), and ferric reducing-antioxidant power (FRAP) [32].

In a cross-sectional study, TAC in foods, particularly in fruits and vegetables, was evaluated relative to biomarkers and chronic disease. The average of three 1-day dietary records was used to determine the TAC of food and beverages consumed by 243 healthy adults [33]. Dietary TAC was significantly higher in adults with low plasma high-sensitivity C-reactive protein (hCRP) levels than in those with lower hCRP levels. In addition, individuals with high CRP levels also had increased levels of white blood cells, greater BMI (body mass index) and waist circumferences, less insulin sensitivity, lower levels of HDL (high-density lipoprotein) and beta-carotene, and were more likely to have hypertension than those with low CRP levels. This anti-inflammatory effect could be one of the mechanisms by which fruits, vegetables, and red wine have been shown to be protective against cardiovascular disease.

Nutrient- vs. Food-Based–Disease Relations

There are numerous studies examining the relations between single nutrients or nutrient scores, as in the example above, and chronic disease or risk factors for a disease. However, nutrients are not consumed in isolation and there likely is important synergy among the nutrients, particularly in foods. Because we eat foods, it is logical to conduct analysis of food-based–disease relationships. In the following example, we evaluate the relations of nutrient and food intakes with incident VTE (venous thromboembolism) . To examine these relations, data were analyzed from the ARIC study – the Atherosclerosis Risk in Communities – a prospective study of almost 16,000 African American and white middle-aged adults recruited from one of four field centers, including Minneapolis, MN, Jackson, MS, Forsythe County, NC, and Washington County, MD. Investigators found that consumption of 4 or more servings of fruit and vegetables per day was associated with lower incidence of VTE as shown in Table 21.1 [34]. To support the food findings, nutrient intakes of vitamin B6 and folate were also inversely related to VTE. Studying the effect of a food or diet pattern on the outcome-of-interest may be synonymous to studying the interaction among nutrients in a food [23].

FRUIT AND VEGETABLE INTAKE REDUCES THE RISK OF CHRONIC DISEASE

Consumption of 5 or more servings of fruit and vegetables each day is recommended to reduce the risk of chronic disease, including CHD [35], stroke [35],

TABLE 21.1 Hazard Ratios (HR) of Venous Thromboembolism Across Quintiles of Dietary Intake, ARIC, 1987–2001 ($n = 14,962$) (adapted from Steffen *et al.* [34])

	Quintiles of dietary intake					p_{trend}
	1	2	3	4	5	
			Folate (mcg/day)			
Range of intake	<160	160–206	206–249	249–310	>310	
No. of cases	57	34	40	32	34	
HR (95% CI)	1.0	0.58 (0.37, 0.91)	0.66 (0.41, 1.05)	0.49 (0.28, 0.86)	0.49 (0.24, 1.02)	0.06
			Vitamin B6 (mg/day)			
Range of intake	<1.25	1.25–1.57	1.57–1.86	1.86–2.26	>2.26	
No. of cases	54	40	38	33	32	
HR (95% CI)	1.0	0.66 (0.43, 1.02)	0.57 (0.35, 0.93)	0.44 (0.25, 0.78)	0.37 (0.17, 0.80)	0.007
			Fruit and vegetables (servings/day)			
Range of intake	<2.5	2.5–3.5	3.5–4.5	4.5–5.8	>5.8	
No. of cases	56	41	35	28	37	
HR (95% CI)	1.0	0.73 (0.48, 1.11)	0.57 (0.37, 0.90)	0.47 (0.29, 0.77)	0.59 (0.36, 0.99)	0.03

cancer [36], type 2 diabetes [37], and obesity [15]. Results from two recent meta-analyses of cohort studies showed that increasing intake of fruit and vegetable intake was inversely associated with occurrence of stroke and CHD events [2, 5].

Heart Disease and Stroke

The development of heart disease and stroke begins in childhood which is a consequence of modifiable CVD risk factors dietary intake, physical activity, and smoking habits and the non-modifiable risk factors of age, gender, and genetics. The Boyd Orr survey is a longitudinal study of diet and health in 4334 British and Scottish children which began in 1937–1939 with recent follow-up on cardiovascular disease, stroke, and all-cause mortality [38]. After an average 37 years of follow-up, there were 1010 deaths from all-causes with 298 and 83 attributed to CHD and stroke, respectively. Dietary intake was obtained by a 7-day household, weighed inventory at baseline. Consumption of vegetables was significantly and inversely associated with mortality from stroke ($p_{trend} = 0.01$), but not with consumption with fruit. No relation was observed between fruit and vegetable intakes for all-cause or CHD mortality.

Two meta-analyses were performed for the relation of fruit and vegetable intake with incident CHD and stroke using data from 12 to 8 cohort studies, respectively [2, 5]. Cohort studies included in at least one of the meta-analyses were the Adventist Health Study ($n = 26,473$), ARIC (Atherosclerosis Risk from Communities; $n = 11,940$), Baltimore Longitudinal Study ($n = 501$), Danish Diet, Cancer And Health Study ($n = 54,506$), Framingham Study ($n = 832$), Health Professional's Follow-Up Study ($n = 38,683$), Life Span Study from Japan ($n = 37,437$), Mobile Clinic Health Cohort (Finland; $n = 5133$), NHANES I Follow-up Study ($n = 9608$), Nurses' Health Study ($n = 75,596$), Physician's Health Study ($n = 15,220$), PRIME Study (France and Northern Ireland; $n = 7,981$), Women's Health Study ($n = 39,127$), Zutphen Study ($n = 552$), or data from Finland ($n = 25,372$) and UK ($n = 9980$) studies.

Data from these studies were pooled and hazard ratios estimated. Among 247,391 study participants, there were 2195 ischemic stroke events and among 66,666 participants, there were 358 hemorrhagic stroke events. The risk of stroke for those consuming 3–5 and more than 5 servings of fruit and vegetables per day compared to less than 3 servings daily were 0.88 (0.79, 0.98) and 0.72 (0.66, 0.79), respectively, for ischemic stroke and 0.92 (0.81, 1.05) and 0.73 (0.61, 0.87), respectively, for hemorrhagic stroke [5].

Among the 278,459 study participants, there were 9143 incident CHD events. Compared to study participants consuming less than 3 servings of fruit and vegetables per day, the risk of incident CHD was 0.93 (0.86, 1.00) for those consuming 3–5 daily servings and 0.83 (0.77, 0.89) for those consuming more than 5 servings of fruit and vegetables per day [2].

The findings provide strong support for the *Dietary Guidelines for Americans* that consuming more than 5 servings of fruit and vegetables each day is beneficial for cardiovascular health.

Peripheral Artery Disease

Even though fruit and vegetable intake is inversely associated with CHD and stroke in most studies, peripheral artery disease (PAD) was not related to fruit and vegetable intake among over 44,000 male health professionals [39]. Only one study has been published for PAD, therefore, further investigation in this area is warranted.

Type 2 Diabetes

Few studies have examined the relation between fruit and vegetable intake and diabetes. In one national survey of almost 10,000 adults, consumption of 5 or more daily servings of fruit and vegetable intake was associated with a lower risk of developing type 2 diabetes over 20 years of follow-up among women, but not men [6]. In contrast, findings from the Women's Health Study failed to confer a significant relation of fruit and vegetable intake with risk of developing type 2 diabetes in over 38,000 middle-aged women after 8.8 years of follow-up [13].

CVD Risk Factors

Reduction of CVD risk factors lowers the incidence and mortality of CHD. High blood pressure (systolic BP of 140 mm Hg or higher, diastolic BP of 90 mm Hg or higher or taking antihypertensive medicine) is a major risk factor for CHD. About 33% of US adults are hypertensive [40]. Interestingly, about 50% of US adults reported not consuming any fruit or fruit juice and 25% reported not consuming any vegetables every day [18]. Among CARDIA study participants, plant food intake, especially fruit, was inversely related to elevated blood pressure (systolic BP of 130 mm Hg or higher, diastolic BP of 85 mm Hg or higher or taking antihypertensive medicine) over 15 years of follow-up [7]. These study findings are consistent with those of other studies which have examined the relation of fruit, vegetable, fiber, and plant protein with hypertension [8, 41, 42]. In a randomized clinical trial, systolic and diastolic blood pressure were significantly reduced in adults randomized to the intervention group (5 servings of fruit and vegetables daily) compared to those in the control group over 6 months of study [43]. Finally, the dietary approaches to stop hypertension (DASH) feeding study found that a combination diet rich in fruit, vegetables, and low-fat dairy products substantially lowered blood pressure in 459 moderately hypertensive African American and Caucasian men and women [44].

Numerous studies have shown that vegetarians have a lower blood pressure than do nonvegetarians [45] and that the addition of meat to a vegetarian diet increases blood pressure [46].

Elevated LDL-cholesterol (low-density lipoprotein) is a risk factor for CHD and dietary modification may control concentration levels. A plant-based diet lowered plasma lipids in hypercholesterolemic adults [47]. Patients were randomized to one of two diet groups: a low-fat diet (LF) consistent with the former American Heart Association (AHA) Step 1 guidelines and the other a low-fat plus (LFP), including fruit, vegetables, legumes, and whole grains, consistent with the 2000 AHA guidelines. The macronutrient composition for the two diet groups was similar: about 30% of calories from total fat, 10% of calories from saturated fat, 55% of calories from carbohydrate, and 15% of calories from protein. The LF group consumed 2.6 and 2.5 servings per day of fruit and vegetables, respectively; while the LFP group consumed 3.4 and 10.1 servings per day, respectively. A significantly greater reduction in total- and LDL-cholesterol was demonstrated in the LFP diet group compared to the LF group. The difference between groups for change in total cholesterol was -0.22 mg/dl ($p = 0.01$) and -0.18 mg/dl ($p = 0.01$) for LDL-cholesterol. No difference between groups was observed for change in HDL-cholesterol or triglyceride levels. The study was not designed to determine which of the food components promoted the observed cholesterol-lowering effect; however, the difference in number of vegetable servings consumed was substantial. The group with the greatest reduction in cholesterol consumed more vegetables.

Elevated urinary excretion of 8-isoprostane F_{2a} (a metabolite of arachidonic acid) is one measure of lipid peroxidation or oxidative stress that is present in chronic disease, including CHD and type 2 diabetes [48]. Smokers and diabetics have greater levels of isoprostanes than non-smokers and non-diabetics, respectively. In a randomized clinical trial, 8-isoprostane F_{2a} were significantly reduced among women who consumed 9.2 servings of fruit and vegetables daily compared to those consuming 3.6 servings/day [49]. Further, the greatest reductions were seen in women with the highest level of 8-isoprostane F_{2a} at baseline. Dietary intake, including increased fruit and vegetable consumption, may prevent oxidation of LDL thus reducing oxidation stress and also the risk of developing atherosclerosis.

Cancer

Higher intakes of fruits and vegetables and cruciferous vegetables have been associated with lower risk of mortality from cancer, cardiovascular disease, and all-causes [50]. Further, results from the majority of case-control studies showed significant and inverse relations between fruit and vegetable intake and cancers of the esophagus, lung, stomach, and colorectum [10, 51]. Vegetable intake was protective for breast cancer, but not with fruit intake. In contrast to results from studies with case-control study designs and from studies of heart disease and stroke, the findings from prospective studies for most cancer sites are suggestive of protection from fruit and vegetable intake, but are not statistically significant; however the reduction in risk is significant for bladder cancer and lung cancer and only for fruit [10]. According to Potter [11], the relation between dietary intake and cancer risk has yet to be clarified due to differences in study design, heterogeneity of specific cancer outcomes, inadequate sample size of cancer trials, genetic variability, measurement error of both the exposure and outcome, and short follow-up periods. Given the inconsistent evidence based on study design and other limitations, further study of the relations of cancer with fruit and vegetable intake, other modifiable risk factors, and genetic factors is needed.

Bone Health

Osteoporosis is a major public health problem which will affect one in three women, and one in 12 men, at some stage in their lives. Bone health starts in childhood and is influenced by genetic, endocrine, mechanical and nutritional factors. Previous studies focused on calcium and bone health, however, many lifestyle factors affect bone metabolism, including smoking, physical activity, and intakes of caffeine, protein, total energy intake and fruit and vegetables. Markers of bone metabolism, bone mass density, and dietary intake were measured in 62 healthy women aged 44–55 years. Although, the study of New *et al.* did not report the influence of fruit and vegetable intake on bone parameters, bone density was positively associated with intakes of nutrients found in abundance in fruit and vegetables, including magnesium and potassium, as well as a positive association with history of consuming high amounts of fruit and vegetables in childhood [9].

Obesity

The prevalence of overweight and obesity has been increasing over the past 20 years with over 60% of US adults who are overweight or obese [52]; clearly it is unknown which diet pattern best facilitates weight management. Epidemiologic evidence is inconsistent that fruit and vegetable intake is associated with weight gain or maintenance [12, 14, 53]. In over 12 years of follow-up, middle-aged nurses who increased their intake of fruit and vegetables had a 24% lower risk of obesity; and those with the largest increase in fruit and vegetable intake lowered their risk of weight gain by 28% [12]. However, in a study of children and adolescents, fruit and vegetable intake was not related to change in BMI [14]. It seems feasible that greater consumption of fruit and vegetables would facilitate weight management given that lower-energy, nutrient-dense foods might replace more calorie-dense refined grain snack foods or high fat fast foods. In a randomized clinical trial testing the effectiveness of weight loss of two diets: a low-fat/fruit and vegetable (LFFV) and a low-fat (LF) diet in otherwise healthy, overweight women. The women were instructed to eat *ad libitum* amounts of food while following the principles of their respective diet. The LFFV group reduced fat intake and increased fruit and vegetable intake, while the LF group reduced fat intake only. Women randomized to the LFFV weight loss group lost 7.9 kg compared to a loss of 6.4 kg in the LF group after 1 year. The difference in weight loss after 1 year between the groups was 1.5 kg; $p = 0.002$ [53]. The LFFV eating plan is adaptable to individual food preferences and potentially sustainable for lifelong weight management.

HEALTH PROMOTION AND BEHAVIOR CHANGE

Despite the favorable effects of fruit and vegetables on health, the majority of populations, nationally or internationally, are not meeting their country dietary guidelines for fruit and vegetable intake. Even though US adults were aware of the "5 a day for better health" nutrition campaign created in 1991, only 23–26% of adults consume at least 5 servings of fruit and vegetables each day by 2002 [18, 19]. There are still many people missing the message. Several barriers to increasing consumption of fruit and vegetables have been identified, including availability, accessibility, cost, nutrition knowledge, and marketing strategies [54, 55].

Interventions to Promote Fruit and Vegetable Consumption

Both the European Union (EU) and the US have drafted plans, the White Paper in the EU [56] and a similar plan in the US [57], on how to promote healthy diets and physical activity in response to the growing incidence of obesity in youth in the world. The escalating number of obese youth in both US and EU teenagers may translate into tomorrow's heart attack patients [58]. In both regions of the world, awareness has been raised and key stakeholders, including government, industry, communities, and schools, have been asked to commit to coordinate and prioritize limited resources, evaluate policies and programs, monitor progress, and disseminate successful practices to reduce obesity [56, 57].

Many school programs have already successfully designed and implemented programs targeting school children and their parents and school staff to consume less fat and more fruit and vegetables, and to increase physical activity [59, 60]. Learning activities have been developed for the parents, classroom, school cafeteria, and after-school care programs. Other settings in which interventions to increase fruit and vegetable intake were successfully implemented include: churches [61], worksites [62], health care organizations [63], supermarkets [64], community programs [19], and several other adult programs [65]. However, research gaps that need to be filled are (1) to better understand the different intervention components that were effective and how these effects vary in different populations and (2) to better understand the factors influencing fruit and vegetable intake, such as economic, social and environmental factors that influence food availability, individual food choices, and barriers to change (or facilitators to change) eating habits [65].

CONCLUSION

Fruit and vegetables are colorful packages rich in a myriad of nutrients and food compounds beneficial to health. The evidence is consistent for prevention of heart disease and stroke – fruit and vegetable consumption is beneficial. However, the lack of consistency between study findings for other chronic diseases, particularly cancer, may be due to differences in study design, population studied, dietary and outcome assessment methods, environmental and genetic (potentially confounding) factors measured and unmeasured, and follow-up period. No single nutrient or food is responsible for overall health, but a food pattern including five or more fruits and vegetables each day is beneficial and an important strategy for improving the public's health.

So, eat your fruit and vegetables every day!

REFERENCES

1. Lock, K., Pomerleau, J., Causer, L., Altmann, D. R. & McKee, M. (2005). The global burden of disease attributable to low consumption of fruit and vegetables: Implications for the global strategy on diet. *Bulletin of the World Health Organization* **83**, 100–108.
2. He, F. J., Nowson, C. A. & MacGregor, G. A. (2007). Increased consumption of fruit and vegetables is related to a reduce risk of coronary heart disease: Meta-analysis of cohort studies. *J Human Hypertension* **21**, 717–728.
3. Ness, A. R. & Powles, J. W. (1997). Fruit and vegetables, and cardiovascular disease: A review. *Int J Epidemiol* **26**, 1–13.
4. Ness, A. R., Maynard, M., Frankel, S., Smith, G. D., Frobisher, C., Leary, S. D., Emmett, P. M. & Gunnell, D. (2005). Diet in childhood and adult cardiovascular and all cause mortality: The Boyd Orr cohort. *Heart* **91**, 894–898.
5. He, F. J., Nowson, C. A. & MacGregor, G. A. (2006). Fruit and vegetable consumption and stroke: A meta-analysis of cohort studies. *Lancet* **367**, 320–326.
6. Ford, E. S. & Mokdad, A. H. (2001). Fruit and vegetable consumption and diabetes mellitus incidence among US adults. *Prev Med* **32**, 33–39.
7. Steffen, L. M., Kroenke, C. H., Yu, X., Pereira, M. A., Slattery, M. L., Van Horn, L., Gross, M. D. & Jacobs, D. R. (2005). Associations of plant foods, dairy products, and meat consumption with fifteen-year incidence of elevated blood pressure in young black and white adults: The CARDIA Study. *Am J Clin Nutr* **82**, 1169–1177.
8. Miura, K., Greenland, P., Stamler, J., Liu, K., Daviglus, M. L. & Nakagawa, H. (2004). Relation of vegetable, fruit, and meat intake to 7-year blood pressure change in middle-aged men: The Chicago Western Electric Study. *Am J Epidemiol* **159**, 572–580.
9. New, S. A., Robins, S. P., Campbell, M. K., Martin, J. C., Garton, M. J., Bolton-Smith, C., Grubb, D. A., Lee, S. J. & Reid, D. M. (2000). Dietary influences on bone mass and bone metabolism: Further evidence of a positive link between fruit and vegetable consumption and bone health. *Am J Clin Nutr* **71**, 142–151.
10. Riboli, E. & Norat, T. (2003). Epidemiologic evidence of the protective effect of fruit and vegetables on cancer risk. *Am J Clin Nutr* **78**, 559S–569S.
11. Potter, J. D. (2005). Vegetables, fruit, and cancer. *Lancet* **366**, 527–530.
12. He, K., Hu, F. B., Colditz, G. A., Manson, J. E., Willett, W. C. & Liu, S. (2004). Changes in intake of fruits and vegetables in relation to risk of obesity and weight gain among middle-aged women. *Int J Obes Relat Metab Disord* **28**, 1569–1574.
13. Liu, S., Serdula, M., Janket, S. J., Cook, N. R., Sesso, H. D., Willett, W. C., Manson, J. E. & Buring, J. E. (2004). A prospective study of fruit and vegetable intake and the risk of type 2 diabetes in women. *Diabetes Care* **27**, 2993–2996.
14. Field, A. E., Gillman, M. W., Rosner, B., Rockett, H. R. & Colditz, G. A. (2003). Association between fruit and vegetable intake and change in body mass index

among a large sample of children and adolescents in the United States. *Int J Obes Relat Metab Disord* **27**, 821–826.

15. US Department of Health and Human Services and U.S. Department of Agriculture (2005). *Dietary Guidelines for Americans*, 6th ed., US Government Printing Office, Washington, DC.

16. Haven, J., Burns, A., Herring, D. & Britten, P. (2006). MyPryamid gov provides consumers with practical nutrition information at their fingertips. *J Nutr Educ Behav* **38**, S153–S154.

17. Li, R., Serdula, M., Bland, S., Mokdad, A., Bowman, B. & Nelson, D. (2000). Trends in fruit and vegetable consumption among adults in 16 US states: Behavioral risk factor surveillance system, 1990–1996. *Am J Public Health* **90**, 777–781.

18. Casagrand, S. S., Wang, Y., Anderson, C. & Gary, T. L. (2007). Have Americans increased their fruit and vegetable intake? *Am J Prev Med* **32**, 257–263.

19. Forester, S. B., Kizer, K. W., Disogra, L. K., Bal, D. G., Krieg, B. F. & Bunch, K. L. (1995). California's "5-a-day for better health!" campaign: An innovative population-based effort to effect large scale dietary change. *Am J Prev Med* **11**, 124–131.

20. Yngve, A., Wolf, A., Poortvliet, E., Elmadfa, I., Brug, J., Ehrenblad, B., Franchini, B., Haraldsdottir, J., Krolner, R., Maes, L., Perez-Rodrigo, C., Sjostrom, M., Thorsdottir, I. & Klepp, K. I. (2005). Fruit and vegetable intake in a sample of 11-year-old children in 9 European countries: The Pro Children Cross-Sectional Survey. *Ann Nutr Metab* **49**, 236–245.

21. Wolf, A., Yngve, A., Elmadfa, I., Poortvliet, E., Ehrenblad, B., Perez-Rodrigo, C., Thorsdottir, I., Haraldsdottir, J., Brug, J., Maes, L., Vaz de Almeida, M. D., Krolner, R. & Klepp, K. I. (2005). Fruit and vegetable intake of mothers of 11-year-old children in 9 European countries: The Pro Children Cross-Sectional Survey. *Ann Nutr Metab* **49**, 246–254.

22. National Health and Medical Research Council, Commonwealth of Australia. Dietary Guidelines for Australian Adults. Accessed 11/15/07 (http://www.nhmrc.gov.au/publications/synopses/_files/n33.pdf).

23. Jacobs, D. R. & Steffen, L. M. (2003). Nutrients, foods, and dietary patterns as exposures in research: A framework for food synergy. *Am J Clin Nutr* **78**, 508S–513S.

24. Kris-Etherton, P. M., Hecker, K. D., Bonanome, A., Coval, S. M., Binkoski, A. E., Hilpert, K. F., Griel, A. E. & Etherton, T. D. (2002). Bioactive compounds in foods: Their role in the prevention of cardiovascular disease and cancer. *Am J Med* **113**, 71S–88S.

25. Dell'Agli, M., Busciala, A. & Bosisio, E. (2004). Vascular effects of wine polyphenols. *Cardio Res* **63**, 593–602.

26. Zern, T. L. & Fernandez, M. L. (2005). Cardioprotective effects of dietary polyphenols. *J Nutr* **135**, 2291–2294.

27. Gorelik, S., Ligumsky, M., Kohen, R. & Kanner, J. (2008). A novel function of red wine polyphenols in humans: Prevention of absorption of cytotoxic lipid peroxidation products. *FASEB J* **22**, 41–46.

28. Mink, P. J., Scrafford, C. G., Barraj, L. M., Harnack, L., Hong, C. P., Nettleton, J. A. & Jacobs, D. R. (2007). Flavonoid intake and cardiovascular disease mortality: A prospective study in postmenopausal women. *Am J Clin Nutr* **85**, 895–909.

29. Joseph, J. A., Shukitt-Hale, B. & Lau, F. C. (2007). Fruit polyphenols and their effects on neuronal signaling and behavior in senescence. *Ann NY Acad Sci* **1100**, 470–485.

30. Joseph, J. A., Arendash, G., Gordon, M., Diamond, D., Shukitt-Hale, B. & Morgan, D. (2003). Blueberry supplementation enhances signaling and prevents behavioral deficits in an Alzheimer disease model. *Nutr Neurosci* **6**, 153–163.

31. Casadesus, G., Shukitt-Hale, B., Stellwagen, H. M., Zhu, X., Lee, H. G., Smith, M. A. & Joseph, J. A. (2004). Modulation of hippocampal plasticity and cognitive behavior by short-term blueberry supplementation in aged rats. *Nutr Neurosci* **7**, 309–316.

32. Pellegrini, N., Serafini, M., Colombim, B., Del Rio, D., Salvatore, S., Bianchi, M. & Brighenti, F. (2003). Total antioxidant capacity of plant foods, beverages and oils consumed in Italy assessed by three different *in vitro* assays. *J Nutr* **133**, 2812–2819.

33. Brighenti, F., Valtuena, S., Pellegrini, N., Ardigo, D., Del Rio, D., Salvatore, S., Piatti, P. M., Serafini, M. & Zavaroni, I. (2005). Total antioxidant capacity of the diet is inversely and independently related to plasma concentration of high-sensitivity C-reactive protein in adult Italian subjects. *Brit J Nutr* **93**, 619–625.

34. Steffen, L. M., Folsom, A. R., Cushman, M., Jacobs, D. R. & Rosamond, W. D. (2007). Greater fish, fruit, and vegetable intakes are related to lower incidence of venous thromboembolism. The longitudinal investigation of thromboembolism etiology. *Circulation* **115**, 188–195.

35. Lichtenstein, A. H., Appel, L. J., Brands, M., Carnethon, M., Daniels, S., Franch, H. A., Franklin, B., Kris-Etherton, P., Harris, W. S., Howard, B., Karanja, N., Lefevre, M., Rudel, L., Sacks, F., Van Horn, L., Winston, M. & Wylie-Rosett, J. (2006). Diet and lifestyle recommendations revision 2006: A scientific statement from the American Heart Association Nutrition Committee. *Circulation* **114**, 82–96.

36. National Cancer Institute, NCI Dietary Guidelines (http://rex.nci.nih.gov/NCI_Pub_Interface/ActionGd_Web/guidelns.html).

37. Franz, M. J., Bantle, J. P., Beebe, C. A., Brunzell, J. D., Chiasson, J. L., Garg, A., Holzmeister, L. A., Hoogwerf, B., Mayer-Davis, E., Mooradian, A. D., Purnell, J. S. & Wheeler, M. (2002). Evidence-based nutrition principles and recommendations for the treatment and prevention of diabetes and related complications. *Diabetes Care* **25**, 148–198.

38. Ness, A. R., Maynard, M., Frankel, S., Smith, G. D., Frobisher, C., Leary, S. D., Emmett, P. M. & Gunnell, D. (2005). Diet in childhood and adult cardiovascular and all-cause mortality: The Boyd Orr cohort. *Heart* **91**, 894–898.

39. Hung, H. C., Merchant, A., Willett, W., Ascherio, A., Rosner, B. A., Rimm, E. & Joshipura, K. J. (2003). The association between fruit and vegetable consumption and peripheral arterial disease. *Epidemiology* **14**, 659–665.

40. Fields, L. E., Burt, V. L., Cutler, J. A., Hughes, J., Roccella, E. J. & Sorlie, P. (2004). The burden of adult hypertension in the United States, 1999–2000: A rising tide. *Hypertension* **44**, 398–404.

41. Ascherio, A., Rimm, E. B., Giovannucci, E. L., Colditz, G. A., Rosner, B., Willett, W. C., Sacks, F. & Stampfer, M. J. (1992). A prospective study of nutritional factors and hypertension among US men. *Circulation* **86**, 1475–1484.

42. Bietz, R., Mensink, G. B. & Fischer, B. (2000). Blood pressure and vitamin C and fruit and vegetable intake. *Ann Nutr Metab* **47**, 214–220.

43. John, J. H., Ziebland, S., Yudkin, P., Roe, L. S. & Neil, H. A. (2002). Oxford Fruit and Vegetable Study Group. Effects of fruit and vegetable consumption on plasma antioxidant concentrations and blood pressure: A randomised controlled trial. *Lancet* **359**, 1969–1974.

44. Appel, L. J., Moore, T. J., Obarzanek, E., Vollmer, W. M., Svetkey, L. P., Sacks, F. M., Bray, G. A., Vogt, T. M., Cutler, J. A., Windhauser, M. M., Lin, P. H. & Karanja, N. of the DASH Collaborative Research Group (1997). A clinical trial of the effects of dietary patterns on blood pressure. *N Engl J Med* **336**, 1117–1124.

45. Fraser, G. E. (2003). Vegetarianism and obesity, hypertension, diabetes, and arthritis. *In* Diet, Life Expectancy, and Chronic Disease: Studies of Seventh-day Adventists and other Vegetarians (G. E. Fraser, Ed.), Oxford University Press, Inc, New York, NY.

46. Sacks, F. M., Donner, A., Castelli, W. P., Gronemeyer, J., Pletka, P., Margolius, H. S., Landsberg, L. & Kass, E. H. (1981). Effect of ingestion of meat on plasma cholesterol in vegetarians. *JAMA* **246**, 640–644.

47. Gardner, C. D., Coulston, A., Chatterjee, L., Rigby, A., Spiller, G. & Farquhar, J. W. (2005). The effect of a plant based diet on plasma lipids in hypercholesterolemic adults. *Ann Intern Med* **142**, 725–733.

48. Fam, S. S. & Morrow, J. D. (2003). The isoprosotanes: Unique products of arachidonic acid oxidation – a review. *Curr Med Chem* **10**, 1723–1740.

49. Thompson, H. J., Heimendinger, J., Sedlacek, S., Haegele, A., Diker, A., O'Neill, C., Meinecke, B., Wolfe, P., Zhu, Z. & Jiang, W. (2005). 8-isoprostane F_{2a} excretion is reduced in women by increased vegetable and fruit intake. *Am J Clin Nutr* **82**, 768–776.

50. Genkinger, J. M., Platz, E. A., Hoffman, S. C., Comstock, G. W. & Helzlsouer, K. J. (2004). Fruit, vegetable, and antioxidant intake and all-cause, cancer, and cardiovascular disease mortality in a community-dwelling population in Washington County, Maryland. *Am J Epidemiol* **160**, 1223–1233.

51. World Cancer Research Fund Panel (1997). *Food, Nutrition and the Prevention of Cancer: A Global Perspective*, American Institute for Cancer Research, Washington, DC.

52. Flegal, K. M., Carroll, M. D., Ogden, C. L. & Johnson, C. L. (2002). Prevalence and trends in obesity among US adults, 1999–2000. *JAMA* **288**, 1723–1727.

53. Ello-Martin, J. A., Roe, L. S., Ledikwe, J. H., Beach, A. M. & Rolls, B. J. (2007). Dietary energy density in the treatment of obesity: A year-long trial comparing 2 weight-loss diets. *Am J Clin Nutr* **85**, 1465–1477.

54. Glanz, K. & Yaroch, A. L. (2004). Strategies for increasing fruit and vegetable intake in grocery stores and communities: Policy, pricing, and environmental change. *Prev Med* **39**, S75–S80.

55. Drewnowski, A., Darmon, N. & Briend, A. (2004). Replacing fats and sweets with vegetables and fruits – a question of cost. *Am J Public Health* **94**, 1555–1559.

56. Commission to the European Parliament, the Council, the European Economic and Social Committee and the Committee of the Regions (2007). White Paper: A Strategy for Europe on Nutrition, Overweight and Obesity Related Health Issues (accessed November, 15 2007). http://ec.europa. eu/health/ph_determinants/life_style/nutrition/documents/nutrition_wp_cs.pdf).

57. Institute of Medicine, National Academy of Sciences, Food and Nutrition Board (2006). Progress in Preventing Childhood Obesity: How Do We Measure Up? (accessed November, 1 2007). (http://www.iom.edu/?id=37008).

58. Must, A. & Strauss, R. S. (1999). Risks and consequences of childhood and adolescent obesity. *Int J Obes Relat Metab Disord* **23**(Suppl), S2–S11.

59. Trevino, R. P., Pugh, J. A., Hernandez, A. E., Menchaca, V. D., Ramirez, R. R. & Mendoza, M. (1998). Bienestar: A diabetes risk-factor prevention program. *J Sch Health* **68**, 62–67.

60. Teufel, N. I. & Ritenbaugh, C. K. (1998). Development of a primary prevention program: Insight gained in the Zuni Diabetes Prevention Program. *Clin Pediatr* **37**, 131–141.

61. Resnicow, K., Jackson, A., Wang, T., De, A. K., McCarty, F., Dudley, W. N. & Baranowski, T. (2001). A motivational interviewing intervention to increase fruit and vegetable intake through Black churches: Results of the eat for life trial. *Am J Public Health* **91**, 1686–1693.

62. Tilley, B. C., Glanz, K., Kristal, A. R., Hirst, K., Li, S., Vernon, S. W. & Myers, R. (1999). Nutrition intervention for high-risk auto workers: Results of the next step trial. *Prev Med* **28**, 284–292.

63. Jones, H., Edwards, L., Vallis, T. M., Ruggiero, L., Rossi, S. T., Rossi, J. S., Greene, G., Prochaska, J. O. & Zinman, B. (2003). Changes in diabetes self-care behaviors make a difference in glycemic control: The diabetes stages of change (DiSC) study. *Diabetes Care* **26**, 732–737.

64. Kristal, A. R., Goldenhar, L., Muldoon, J. & Morton, R. F. (1997). Evaluation of a supermarket intervention to increase consumption of fruits and vegetables. *Am J Health Promot* **11**, 422–425.

65. Pomerleau, J., Lock, K., Knai, C. & McKee, M. (2005). Interventions designed to increase adult fruit and vegetable intake can be effective: A systematic review of the literature. *J Nutr* **135**, 2486–2495.

Chapter 22

Medicinal Uses of Vinegar[1]

Carol S. Johnston

Department of Nutrition, Arizona State University, Mesa, AZ, USA

Abstract

The use of vinegar to fight infections and other acute conditions dates back to Hippocrates, but recent research suggests that vinegar ingestion favorably influences biomarkers for heart disease, cancer, and diabetes. The acetic acid in vinegar elicits these beneficial effects by altering metabolic processes in the gastrointestinal tract and in the liver. However, there are indications that the direct ingestion of vinegar, as compared to its ingestion as a condiment in foods, may slightly increase body acidity and raise liver enzymes. As a medicinal food, vinegar is affordable and appealing, but future research must better define vinegar's therapeutic value and role in health promotion.

Keywords: *Vinegar, acetic acid, diabetes, chronic disease*

OVERVIEW

For over 2000 years, vinegar has been used not only to flavor and preserve foods, but to heal wounds and fight infections. The Online Archive of American Folk Medicine has over 2000 entries for vinegar cures [1]. Although scientific investigations do not support the use of vinegar as an anti-infective agent [2], recent reports suggest that vinegar may have some medicinal value particularly for the diabetic condition.

Vinegar, from the French "vin aigre" or "sour wine," can be made from any fermentable carbohydrate source including wine, molasses, dates, fruit, coconut, honey, beer, maple syrup, potatoes, beets, grains, and whey. Yeasts ferment the natural food sugars to alcohol, and acetic acid bacteria (*Acetobacter*) convert the alcohol to acetic acid, the organic compound that identifies the product as vinegar. Commercial vinegar is produced by either fast or slow fermentation processes. For the quick methods, the liquid is oxygenated by agitation and the bacteria culture is submerged permitting rapid fermentation.

---

[1]This paper is an update of a previous review "Vinegar: medicinal uses and antiglycemic effect" published online at *Med Gen Med* 2006 May 30, **8**(2), 61.

The slow methods are used for the production of the traditional wine vinegars; the acetic acid bacteria grows on the surface of the liquid and fermentation proceeds slowly over the course of weeks or months. A nontoxic slime, known as *mother*, composed of yeast, acetic acid bacteria, and vinegar eels (*Turbatrix aceti*) accumulate in this naturally fermented vinegar. Most manufacturers filter and pasteurize their product before bottling to prevent these organisms from forming. After opening, *mother* may develop in stored vinegar; it is considered harmless and can be removed by filtering. Many people advocate retaining the *mother* for numerous, but unsubstantiated, health effects.

The sensory qualities of different vinegars are a function of the food source and the fermentation method. Acetic acid is responsible for the tart flavor and pungent, biting odor of vinegars. In the United States, vinegar products generally contain 4–7% acetic acid; Japanese rice vinegars are mild at 2–4% acetic acid, and pickling vinegars are acerbic at 18% acetic acid [3]. Other minor constituents of vinegar include vitamins, mineral salts, amino acids, compounds with antioxidant properties (e.g., catechin and caffeic acid), and other organic acids (e.g., citric, malic, and lactic acids) [4, 5].

Acetic acid, CH_3COOH, is considered a weak acid, and the pH of commercial vinegars (5% acetic acid) is 2.4. Acetic acid is produced naturally in over-ripe fruits and vegetables, presumably to serve as a natural insecticide [6], and it is present in human vaginal fluids perhaps as an antibacterial agent [7]. The antimicrobial properties of vinegar are well documented and relate directly to the pH-lowering effect of acetic acid; yet it is possible that some inhibitory compounds other than acetic acid may be present in vinegar [8]. Vinegar and acetic acid solutions are effective preservatives against food-borne pathogenic bacteria [9, 10]. In freshly ground beef, the effectiveness of a 2% acetic acid treatment at reducing *Escherichia coli* and *Salmonella typhimurium* was sustained over time in refrigerated and frozen storage, and this treatment did not cause adverse sensory changes as detected by a consumer panel [11]. In iceberg lettuce, a 35% vinegar solution (1.9% acetic acid) was effective at reducing bacteria levels including *E. coli*, and although the lettuce was noticeably sour and slightly wilted in appearance, consumer acceptability was maintained [12].

MEDICINAL USES OF VINEGAR

The use of vinegar to fight infections and other acute conditions dates back to Hippocrates (460–377 BC) who recommended a vinegar preparation for cleaning ulcerations and for the treatment of sores. Oxymel, a popular ancient medicine composed of honey and vinegar, was prescribed for persistent coughs by Hippocrates and his contemporaries, and by physicians up to modern day. The formulation of oxymel was detailed in the *British Pharmacopoeia* (1898) and the *German Pharmacopoeia* (1872) and was prepared by mixing virgin honey, four parts, with white wine vinegar, one part, concentrating, and clarifying with paper pulp.

Antimicrobial Properties

Recent scientific investigations clearly demonstrate the antimicrobial properties of vinegar, but mainly in the context of food preparation as discussed above. Experts advise against using vinegar preparations as household disinfectants since they are less effective at inhibiting bacterial growth when compared to commercial disinfectants such as Lysol, Mr. Clean, and Clorox [13]. However, undiluted vinegar may be used effectively for cleaning dentures, and, unlike bleach solutions, vinegar residues left on dentures were not associated with mucosal damage [14]. In the popular media, vinegar is commonly recommended for treating nail fungus, head lice, and warts, yet scientific support for these treatment strategies is lacking. Although investigations have demonstrated the effectiveness of diluted vinegar (2% acetic acid solution at pH 2) for the treatment of ear infections (otitis externa, otitis media, and granular myringitis), the low pH of these solutions may irritate inflamed skin and damage cochlear outer hair cells [15].

Cardiovascular Disease

In spontaneously hypertensive (SHR) rats fed a standard laboratory diet mixed with an acetic acid solution or deionized water, a significant reduction in systolic blood pressure ($\sim$20 mmHg) was noted for the SHR rats fed the acetic acid [16]. The acetic acid-induced decrease in systolic blood pressure was associated with reductions in both plasma renin activity and plasma aldosterone, factors associated with blood vessel constriction. Vinegar ingestion (0.57 mmol acetic acid) also inhibited the renin-angiotensin system in non-hypertensive, Sprague-Dawley rats [17]. Vinegar has been demonstrated to modestly inhibit the angiotensin-converting enzyme (ACE) in rats. Since ACE inhibitors are commonly prescribed to treat hypertension in adults, human trials should be conducted to determine if regular vinegar ingestion alters ACE concentrations and improves blood pressure in adults.

Dietary acetic acid, 0.3% (w/w), reduced serum cholesterol and triglycerides in rats fed a cholesterol-rich diet [18]. Acetic acid treatment reduced liver ATP citrate lyase activity, liver 3-hydroxy-3-methylglutaryl-CoA content, liver mRNA levels of sterol regulatory element binding protein-1, and fatty acid synthase; moreover, fecal bile acid content was significantly higher in the acetic acid-fed rats than controls. These data suggest that acetic acid treatment reduced serum total cholesterol and triacylglycerol via the inhibition of hepatic lipogenesis and the promotion of fecal bile acid excretion. Acetic acid is converted to acetate *in vivo*, and acetate metabolism by tissues activates AMPK which plays a key role in lipid homeostatsis which may explain the lipid-lowering effects of ingested acetic acid in animals [19].

Human trials investigating the effects of vinegar ingestion on blood pressure or blood cholesterol concentrations have not been reported in the literature. Intriguingly, Hu *et al.* reported a significantly lower risk of fatal ischemic heart disease (IHD) among participants in the Nurses' Health Study who consumed oil and vinegar salad dressings frequently (≥5–6 times/week) compared with those who rarely consumed them (multivariate RR: 0.46; CI: 0.27–0.76, *P* for trend = 0.001) [20]. Frequent consumption of mayonnaise or other creamy salad dressings was not significantly associated with risk for IHD in this population (multivariate RR: 0.84; CI: 0.50–1.44, *P* for trend = 0.44).

Cancer

Antitumor properties have been demonstrated for vinegar in cultured cells and in animals. Sugarcane vinegar induced apoptosis in human leukemia cells [21]. A traditional Japanese rice vinegar inhibited the proliferation of human cancer cells in a dose-dependent manner [22] and stimulated the activity natural killer cells that target tumors [23]. Rice vinegar added to drinking water (0.05−0.1% w/v) significantly inhibited the incidence (−60%) and multiplicity (−50%) of azoxymethane-induced colon cancer in rats when compared to the same markers in control animals [24]. Mice fed rice vinegar-fortified feed (0.3−1.5% w/w) had significantly smaller tumor volumes when compared to controls at 40 days after inoculation with sarcoma tumor cells [23].

The antitumor factors in vinegar have not been identified. In the human colonic adenocarcinoma cell line Caco-2, acetate treatment significantly prolonged cell doubling time, promoted cell differentiation, and inhibited cell motility [25], effects that would inhibit tumor growth and metastasis. Vinegars are also a dietary source of polyphenols, compounds synthesized by plants to defend against oxidative stress. Ingestion of polyphenols by man enhances *in vivo* antioxidant protection and reduces cancer risk [26]. The Japanese rice vinegar Kurosu is particularly rich in phenolic compounds; the *in vitro* antioxidant activity of an ethyl acetate extract of Kurosu vinegar was similar to the antioxidant activity of α-tocopherol (vitamin E) and significantly greater than the antioxidant activities of other vinegar extracts, including wine and apple vinegars [27].

Epidemiologic data, however, is scarce and unequivocal. A case-control study conducted in Linzhou, China demonstrated that vinegar ingestion was associated with a decreased risk for esophageal cancer (OR: 0.37) [28]. However, vinegar ingestion was associated with a 4.4-fold greater risk of bladder cancer in a case-control investigation in Serbia [29].

Diabetes

Vinegar has been utilized as diabetic treatment for nearly a century. In the 1920s an Indiana doctor, Charles Kaadt, offered a "wonderful new treatment" for diabetes, an "absolute cure." The formula, Kaadt told his patients, was secret, "disclosed" to him "by an old European woman." The yellow-brown medicine, essentially saltpeter [potassium nitrate] dissolved in vinegar, was proclaimed to "stimulate" digestion. Kaadt maintained that diabetics lacked hydrochloric acid in their stomachs, and that the acetic acid would stimulate "those alkaline glands that empty into the duodenum." Kaadt's assertions that his medicine could replace insulin, however, lead patients to their demise, and he was eventually charged with malpractice, fined, and jailed [30].

Diabetes is characterized by elevated blood glucose, or hyperglycemia, in both the fasted state and following meal consumption. In type 1 diabetes (T1D), the pancreatic cells that produce insulin are destroyed, and the lack of insulin causes hyperglycemia. Individuals with type 2 diabetes (T2D) produce insulin; however, their tissues are resistant to the insulin which leads to elevations in blood glucose. Scientific evidence supporting an antiglycemic effect of vinegar at meal-time was first reported in 1988. In rats, the blood glucose response to a starch load was significantly reduced when co-administered with a 2% acetic acid solution [31]. Several years later, a trial in healthy subjects demonstrated that white vinegar (20 g or ~2 tablespoons) as a salad dressing ingredient reduced the glycemic response to a mixed meal by over 30% [32]. Several placebo-controlled trials have corroborated this meal-time, antiglycemic effect of vinegar in healthy adults [33, 34]. Pickled foods are also a source of acetic acid, ~2.5 acetic acid by weight, and researchers have demonstrated that the substitution of a pickled cucumber (1.6 g acetic acid) for a fresh cucumber (0 g acetic acid) in a test meal (bread, butter, and yogurt) reduced post-meal glycemia by over 30% in healthy subjects [35].

To date, only one trial has examined the antiglycemic effect of vinegar at meal-time in individuals with T2D [36]. This trial also included individuals with "pre-diabetes," a condition characterized by a mild postprandial hyperglycemia. The pre-meal ingestion of apple cider vinegar reduced postprandial glycemia in all subjects, but the effect was most marked in the individuals with prediabetes. Moreover, the vinegar treatment improved insulin sensitivity 19% and 34% in individuals with T2D and prediabetes respectively [36]. These are potentially important findings since reductions in postprandial hyperglycemia may reduce pancreatic stress and slow the progression of diabetes [37]. Also, chronic postprandial hyperglycemia damages blood vessels and is a strong predictor of cardiovascular disease risk in both T2D and prediabetes [38]. Thus, diabetics may be able to moderate meal-time glycemia by including vinegar as a dressing ingredient or condiment, or as a pickled food, in meal plans.

As the diabetic condition worsens, fasting glucose concentrations (e.g., glucose concentrations upon waking) deteriorate reflecting altered hepatic glucose processing [39]. With this in mind, a recent trial examined whether vinegar ingestion at bedtime altered waking glucose concentrations in individuals with T2D [40]. During the two 3-day trial periods, participants consumed a standardized diet and recorded their fasting glucose concentrations in the early mornings. Using a randomized, cross-over study design, 2 tablespoons of apple cider vinegar or 2 tablespoons of water was consumed with 1 oz of cheese at bedtime. Fasting glucose was significantly reduced after 2 days of vinegar treatment, as compared to the water treatment, suggesting that vinegar may exert antiglycemic effects apart from meal time.

It is not known how vinegar alters blood glucose concentrations, but several mechanisms have been proposed. Acetic acid may interfere with the digestion of starch molecules thereby reducing the amount of glucose absorbed into the bloodstream after a meal [41]. This research was conducted in cell culture, and since other dietary acids, such as citric acid or lactic acid, were ineffective, acidity does not seem to be a factor in this inhibition. Others suggest that vinegar slows the rate of gastric emptying which would slow the rate of glucose absorption into the bloodstream [33], or that acetic acid enhances the uptake of glucose from the bloodstream into tissues thereby keeping blood glucose concentrations low [42].

To date, the medicinal use of vinegar by individuals with T1D has not been investigated.

Obesity

Several investigators have reported that vinegar ingestion is associated with satiety and decreased energy intake at subsequent meals; hence, regular vinegar ingestion may reduce the amount of food ingested at meals contributing to weight loss success. In one trial, subjects consumed white bread (50 g carbohydrate) alone or with 3 portions of white vinegar containing 1.1, 1.4, or 1.7 g acetic acid and were asked to rate feelings of hunger/satiety on a scale ranging from extreme hunger (-10) to extreme satiety ($+10$) prior to meal consumption and at 15-minute intervals post-meal [43]. Bread consumption alone scored the lowest rating of satiety (calculated as area under the curve from time 0–120 minutes). Feelings of satiety increased when vinegar was ingested with the bread, and a linear relationship was observed between satiety and the acetic acid content of the test meals ($r = 0.41, p = 0.004$).

In a separate trial, healthy subjects consumed a test meal (bagel and juice) under three treatment conditions: control, vinegar (1 g acetic acid), or peanut ($\sim$1 oz) [44]. One week separated each treatment condition. On treatment days, subjects were instructed to record food and beverage consumption until bedtime. On average, both vinegar and peanut ingestion reduced later energy consumption by 200–275 calories. Statistical analyses indicated that meal-time glyemia explained 15% of the variance in later energy consumption. In other words, if the amount of glucose that enters the blood after a meal can be minimized, the desire to eat at later meals is lessened. Theoretically, a daily 200 calorie deficit would equate to a monthly weight loss of 1-1½ pounds. Only one report has examined the effect of daily vinegar ingestion on body weight. In this small pilot study, healthy adults ingested 2 tablespoons of apple cider vinegar ($\sim$1 g acetic acid) or 2 tablespoons of cranberry juice (control treatment) twice daily for 4 weeks [45]. At the end of the trial, subjects ingesting vinegar lost an average of 1.6 pounds whereas the control subjects gained

0.6 pounds. These data need to be replicated in trials with larger samples and longer durations.

SAFETY AND TOLERANCE OF MEDICINALLY INGESTED VINEGAR

Vinegar's use as a condiment and food ingredient spans thousands of years and is safe; however, when ingested for medicinal purposes (e.g., apart from food and in large quantities), high amounts of acetic acid may have undesired consequences. Acetic acid, at concentrations greater than 20%, is considered a poison and can cause severe injury to the esophagus [46]. Most vinegars purchased for consumption in the US are at 4–7% acidity; however, there are rare reports in the literature regarding adverse reactions to vinegar ingestion. Inflammation of the oropharynx and second-degree caustic injury of the esophagus and cardia were observed in a 39-year-old woman who drank 1 tablespoon of rice vinegar [47], and the unintentional aspiration of vinegar has been associated with laryngospasm and subsequent vasovagal syncope that resolved spontaneously [48]. Hypokalemia was observed in a 28-year-old woman who had reportedly consumed ~250 ml apple cider vinegar daily for 6 years [49].

Recently, the efficacy and safety of medicinally ingested vinegar was examined in type 2 diabetics [50]. Participants ($n = 27$) were stratified by gender, age, and body mass and randomized into three groups: commercial vinegar pills (0.03 g acetic acid daily), pickles (~1.4 g acetic acid daily), or vinegar (2.8 g acetic acid daily). The pill group represented the control group since the pills contained trace amounts of acetic acid, specifically <2% the amount of acetic acid in the pickles or vinegar treatments. Subjects continued their normal eating habits and oral hypoglycemic medication use during the 12-week trial. At baseline and at weeks 6 and 12, fasting blood and urine samples were collected and emergent adverse events were recorded. Hemoglobin A1c concentrations (a marker of recent blood glucose concentrations) fell 2.4% in subjects consuming the vinegar but rose 1.1% and 3.7% in the control group and pickle groups respectively. Reports of adverse events (e.g., burping, flatulence, acid reflux) did not vary significantly by group during the trial; however, 50–56% of subjects consuming either pickles or vinegar reported at least one treatment-emergent adverse event at week 6 as compared to 11% of REF participants. Urine acidity rose significantly in subjects consuming vinegar at week 12 as compared to the other groups (+9% vs. −3% and −2% for the pickle and control groups respectively). At week 6 there was a tendency for liver enzyme concentrations to increase in the subjects consuming the vinegar as compared to the other groups (+17% vs. +8% and −8% for vinegar, pickles, and control groups respectively). These data indicate that chronic vinegar ingestion may favorably influence glucose homeostasis in individuals with type 2 diabetes but may also impact liver function and metabolic pathways aside from glucose metabolism. Since elevations in urine acidity and liver enzymes can signal undesirable changes in metabolism, more trials are needed to better characterize these vinegar-induced alterations in metabolism.

CONCLUSIONS

Much evidence suggests that vinegar has therapeutic value, particularly in the management of blood glucose in diabetic or pre-diabetic populations. As a medicinal food, vinegar is affordable and appealing, but future research must better define vinegar's role in health promotion. Preliminary data suggest that drinking vinegar, as compared to its ingestion as a condiment or ingredient, may be associated with undesirable side effects. Perhaps the health benefits of vinegar are best realized when it is consumed, as it has been through the ages, as a food component, such as a vinaigrette dressing on a leafy green salad or as a pickled vegetable.

REFERENCES

1. Online Archive of American Folk Medicine. http://www.folkmed.ucla.edu/index.html (accessed June, 4, 2007).
2. Johnston, C. S. & Gaas, C. A. (2006). Vinegar: Medicinal uses and antiglyemic effect. *Med Gen Med* **8**, 61.
3. US Food and Drug Administration. Code of Federal Regulations. Available at: http://www.fda.gov/ora/compliance_ref/cpg/cpgfod/cpg525-825.html (accessed March 9, 2006).
4. Natera, R., Castro, R., Garcia-Moreno, M., Hernandez, M. & Garcia-Barroso, C. (2003). Chemometric studies of vinegars from different raw materials and processes of production. *J Agric Food Chem* **51**, 3345–3351.
5. Navarro-Alarcon, M., Velasco, C., Jodral, A., Terres, C., Olalla, M., Lopez, H. & Lopez, M. C. (2007). Copper, zinc, calcium and magnesium content of alcoholic beverages and by-products from Spain: Nutritional supply. *Food Addit Contam* **24**, 685–694.
6. Montooth, K. L., Siebenthall, K. T. & Clark, A. G. (2006). Membrane lipid physiology and toxin catabolism underlie ethanol and acetic acid tolerance in *Drosophila melanogaster*. *J Exp Biol* **209**, 3837–3850.
7. Huggins, G. R. & Preti, G. (1976). Volatile constituents of human vaginal secretions. *Am J Obstet Gynecol* **126**, 129–136.
8. Rhee, M. S., Lee, S. Y., Dougherty, R. H. & Kang, D. H. (2003). Antimicrobial effects of mustard flour and acetic acid against *Escherichia coli* O157:H7, *Listeria monocytogenes*, and *Salmonella enterica serovar Typhimurium*. *Appl Environ Microbiol* **69**, 2959–2963.
9. Entani, E., Asai, M., Taujihata, S., Tsukamoto, Y. & Ohta, M. (1998). Antibacterial action of vinegar against food-borne pathogenic bacteria including *Escherichia coli* O157:H7. *J Food Prot* **61**, 953–959.
10. Medina, E., Romero, C., Brenes, M. & De Castro, A. (2007). Antimicrobial activity of olive oil, vinegar, and various beverages against foodborne pathogens. *J Food Prot* **70**, 1194–1199.

11. Harris, K., Miller, M. F., Loneragan, G. H. & Brashears, M. M. (2006). Validation of the use of organic acids and acidified sodium chlorite to reduce *Escherichia coli* O157 and *Salmonella typhimurium* in beef trim and ground beef in a simulated processing environment. *J Food Prot* **69**, 1802–1807.

12. Vijayakumar, C. & Wolf-Hall, C. E. (2002). Evaluation of household sanitizers for reducing levels of *Escherichia Coli* on iceberg lettuce. *J Food Prot* **65**, 1646–1650.

13. Rutala, W. A., Barbee, S. L., Agular, N. C., Sobsey, M. D. & Weber, D. J. (2000). Antimicrobial activity of home disinfectants and natural products against potential human pathogens. *Infect Control Hosp Epidemiol* **21**, 33–38.

14. Shay, K. (2000). Denture hygiene: A review and update. *J Contemp Dent Pract* **15**, 28–41.

15. Dohar, J. E. (2003). Evolution of management approaches for otitis externa. *Pediatr Infect Dis J* **22**, 299–308.

16. Kondo, S., Tayama, K., Tsukamoto, Y., Ikeda, K. & Yamori, Y. (2001). Antihypertensive effects of acetic acid and vinegar on spontaneously hypertensive rats. *Biosci Biotechnol Biochem* **65**, 2690–2694.

17. Honsho, S., Sugiyama, A., Takahara, A., Satoh, Y., Nakamura, Y. & Hashimoto, K. (2005). A red wine vinegar beverage can inhibit the rennin-angiotensin system: Experimental evidence *in vivo*. *Biol Pharm Bull* **28**, 1208–1210.

18. Fushimi, T., Suruga, K., Oshima, Y., Fukiharu, M., Tsukamoto, Y. & Goda, T. (2006). Dietary acetic acid reduces serum cholesterol and triacylglycerols in rats fed a cholesterol-rich diet. *Br J Nutr* **95**, 916–924.

19. Yamashita, H., Fujisawa, K., Ito, E., Idei, S., Kawaguchi, N., Kimoto, M., Hiemori, M. & Tsuji, H. (2007). Improvement of obesity and glucose tolerance by acetate in Type 2 diabetic Otsuka Long-Evans Tokushima Fatty (OLETF) rats. *Biosci Biotechnol Biochem* **71**, 1236–1243.

20. Hu, F. B., Stampfer, M. J., Manson, J. E., Rimm, E. B., Wolk, A., Colditz, G. A., Hennekens, C. H. & Willett, W. C. (1999). Dietary intake of alpha-linolenic acid and risk of fatal ischemic heart disease among women. *Am J Clin Nutr* **69**, 890–897.

21. Mimura, A., Suzuki, Y., Toshima, Y., Yazaki, S., Ohtsuki, T., Ui, S. & Hyodoh, F. (2004). Induction of apoptosis in human leukemia cells by naturally fermented sugar canevinegar (kibizu) of Amami Ohshima Island. *Biofactors* **22**, 93–97.

22. Nanda, K., Miyoshi, N., Nakamura, Y., Shimoji, Y., Tamura, Y., Nishikawa, Y., Uenakai, K., Kohno, H. & Tanaka, T. (2004). Extract of vinegar "Kurosu" from unpolished rice inhibits the proliferation of human cancer cells. *J Exp Clin Cancer Res* **23**, 69–75.

23. Seki, T., Morimura, S., Shigematsu, T., Maeda, H. & Kida, K. (2004). Antitumor activity of rice-shochu post-distillation slurry and vinegar produced from the post-distillation slurry via oral administration in a mouse model. *Biofactors* **22**, 103–105.

24. Shimoji, Y., Kohno, H., Nanda, K., Nishikawa, Y., Ohigashi, H., Uenakai, K. & Tanaka, T. (2004). Extract of Kurosu, a vinegar from unpolished rice, inhibits azoxymethane-induced colon carcinogenesis in male F344 rats. *Nutr Cancer* **49**, 170–173.

25. Hong, F. U., Ying Qiang, S. H. I. & Shan Jin, M. O. (2004). Effect of short-chain fatty acids on the proliferation and differentiation of the human colonic adenocarcinoma cell line Caco-2. *Chin J Dig Dis* **5**, 115–117.

26. Nishino, H., Murakoshi, M., Mou, X. Y., Wada, S., Masuda, M., Ohsaka, Y., Satomi, Y. & Jinno, K. (2005). Cancer prevention by phytochemicals. *Oncology* **69(Suppl 1)**, 38–40.

27. Nishidai, S., Nakamura, Y., Torikai, K., Yamamoto, M., Ishihara, N., Mori, H. & Ohigashi, H. (2000). Kurosu, a traditional vinegar produced from unpolished rice, suppresses lipid peroxidation *in vitro* and in mouse skin. *Biosci Biotechnol Biochem* **64**, 1909–1914.

28. Xibib, S., Meilan, H., Moller, H., Evans, H. S., Dixin, D., Wenjie, D. & Jianbang, L. (2003). Risk factors for oesophageal cancer in Linzhou, China: A case-control study. *Asian Pac J Cancer Prev* **4**, 119–124.

29. Radosavljevic, V., Jankovic, S., Marinkovic, J. & Dokic, M. (2004). Non-occupational risk factors for bladder cancer: A case-control study. *Tumori* **90**, 175–180.

30. Quackwatch.org [homepage on the Internet]. [cited May 12, 2007] Available from: http://www.quackwatch.org/13Hx/MM/10.html.

31. Ebihara, K. & Nakajima, A. (1988). Effect of acetic acid and vinegar on blood glucose and insulin responses to orally administered sucrose and starch. *Agric Biol Chem* **52**, 1311–1312.

32. Brighenti, F., Castellani, G., Benini, L., Casiraghi, M. C., Leopardi, E., Crovetti, R. & Testolin, G. (1995). Effect of neutralized and native vinegar on blood glucose and acetate responses to a mixed meal in healthy subjects. *Eur J Clin Nutr* **49**, 242–247.

33. Liljeberg, H. & Bjorck, I. (1998). Delayed gastric emptying rate may explain improved glycemia in healthy subjects to a starchy meal with added vinegar. *Eur J Clin Nutr* **64**, 886–893.

34. Leeman, M., Ostman, E. & Bjorck, I. (2005). Vinegar dressing and cold storage of potatoes lowers postprandial glycaemic and insulinaemic responses in healthy subjects. *Eur J Clin Nutr* **59**, 1266–1271.

35. Ostman, E. M., Liljeberg, H., Elmstahl, H. G. & Bjorck, I. M. (2001). Inconsistency between glycemic and insulinemic responses to regular and fermented milk products. *Am J Clin Nutr* **74**, 96–100.

36. Johnston, C. S., Kim, C. M. & Buller, A. J. (2004). Vinegar improves insulin sensitivity to a high-carbohydrate meal in subjects with insulin resistance or type 2 diabetes. *Diabetes Care* **27**, 281–282.

37. Chiasson, J. L., Josse, R. G., Gomis, R., Hanefeld, M., Darasik, A. & Laakso, M. (2002). Acarbose for prevention of type 2 diabetes mellitus: The STOP-NIDDM randomised trial. *Lancet* **359**, 2072–2077.

38. Bonora, E. & Muggeo, M. (2001). Postprandial blood glucose as a risk factor for cardiovascular disease in type II diabetes: The epidemiological evidence. *Diabetiologia* **44**, 2107–2114.

39. Monnier, L., Colette, C., Dunseath, G. J. & Owens, D. R. (2007). The loss of postprandial glycemic control precedes stepwise deterioration of asting with worsening diabetes. *Diabetes Care* **30**, 263–269.

40. White, A. M. & Johnston, C. S. (2007). Vinegar ingestion at bedtime moderates waking glucose concentrations in adults with well-controlled type 2 diabetes. *Diabetes Care* **30**, 2814–2815.

41. Ogawa, N., Satsu, H., Watanabe, H., Fukaya, M., Tsukamoto, Y., Miyamoto, Y. & Shimizu, M. (2000). Acetic acid suppresses the increase in disaccharidase activity that occurs during culture of caco-2 cells. *J Nutr* **130**, 507–513.

42. Fushimi, T., Tayama, K., Fukaya, M., Kitakoshi, K., Nakai, N., Tsukamoto, Y. & Sato, Y. (2001). Acetic acid feeding enhances glycogen repletion in liver and skeletal muscle of rats. *J Nutr* **131**, 1973–1977.

43. Ostman, E., Granfeldt, Y., Persson, L. & Bjorck, I. (2005). Vinegar supplementation lowers glucose and insulin responses and increases satiety after a bread meal in healthy subjects. *Eur J Clin Nutr* **59**, 983–988.

44. Johnston, C. S., Buller, A. J. (2005). Vinegar and peanut products as complementary foods to reduce postprandial glycemia. **105**, 1939–1942.

45. Johnston, C. S. (2006). Strategies for healthy weight loss: From vitamin C to the glycemic response. *J Am Coll Nutr* **25**, 158–165.

46. US Consumer Product Safety Commission: Regulated Products. http://www.cpsc. gov/BUSINFO/reg1.html (accessed Aug 2007).

47. Chung, C. H. (2002). Corrosive oesophageal injury following vinegar ingestion. *Hong Kong Med J* **8**, 365–366.

48. Wrenn, K. (2006). The perils of vinegar and the Heimlich maneuver. *Ann Emerg Med* **47**, 207–208.

49. Lhotta, K., Hofle, G., Gasser, R. & Finkenstedt, G. (1998). Hypokalemia, hyperreninemia and osteoporosis in a patient ingesting large amounts of cider vinegar. *Nephron* **80**, 242–243.

50. Johnston, C. S., White, A. M., Kent, S. M. A (2008) preliminary evaluation of the safety and tolerance of medicinally ingested vinegar in individuals with type 2 diabetes. *J Med Foods* **11**, 179–183.

Chapter 23

Health-Promoting Effects of Grape Bioactive Phytochemicals

Marcello Iriti and Franco Faoro

Istituto di Patologia Vegetale, Università di Milano and Istituto di Virologia Vegetale, Dipartimento Agroalimentare, CNR, Milano, Italy

Everyone serves the good wine first, and then the inferior wine after the guests have become drunk. But you have kept the good wine until now

(John, 2,10–11)

Abstract

The health-promoting effects of dietary styles rich in plant functional foods and beverages have been recently pointed out, emphasizing on the reduced incidence of chronic illnesses, such as cancer, cardiovascular diseases, ischemic stroke and neurodegenerative disorders, relative to the Mediterranean dietary tradition. The observed health benefits can be ascribed to the bioactive phytochemicals occurring in functional foods, also known as "nutraceuticals." Grapevine products (grape and wine), are important components of the Mediterranean diet, whose moderate daily intake can help to prevent the aging-related diseases. Grape chemistry is rather complex, including phenylpropanoids, isoprenoids and alkaloids. The structure–activity relationship of some major phenylpropanoids, such as resveratrol and flavonoids, has been more deeply studied in cancer chemoprevention, cardioprotection and for their free radical-scavenging mechanisms. Nonetheless, the pharmacokinetic of phytochemicals in humans represents a significant topic, whose knowledge is still fragmentary. Only a little amount of these compounds reaches the plasma, in the main as mammalian conjugates after the fermentation by the colonic microflora, a very small fraction being detectable unchanged in the body fluids.

Keywords: *Grape, wine, functional food, functional beverage, nutritional therapy, nutraceutical, phytonutrient, chemoprevention, chronic disease, aging*

INTRODUCTION

Compelling evidences indicate a relationship between human dietary patterns and the etiology of some chronic diseases. Therefore, if on the one hand it has been reported that from 10% up to 70% of human cancer mortality is attributable to dietary constituents, on the other hand healthful changes of dietary patterns, due to a consistently higher intake of plant foodstuffs, represent a first line of defence in the prevention of cancer and other chronic illnesses of aging, such as cardiovascular diseases, ischemic stroke and neurodegenerative disorders [1–3]. Furthermore, according to the modern dietary guidelines, low-saturated fat, high-fiber diets have a lower calorie content and increased nutrient density, on the whole important preventive factors limiting the incidence of type 2 diabetes and obesity. These dietary patterns, including 400–600 g (5–9 servings) of fruits and vegetables/day, legumes, whole cereals, nuts, olive oil and a moderate amounts of wine (two glasses/day) represent the main components of the Mediterranean dietary traditions, hence associated with an array of health benefits [4–6].

The above reported health-promoting effects of plant foods and beverages are ascribed to their particular constituents, that is the chemicals present in some plant tissues and, consequently, occurring in foods. In other words, many plant foods can be considered as functional foods rich in dietary therapeutics or nutraceuticals. A functional food or beverage is a product consumed as part of a normal diet that may provide health benefits beyond basic nutritional functions, by virtue of its nutraceutical content, a restricted group of bioactive phytochemicals [7]. The latter comprise all the secondary metabolites produced by plants in order to defend themselves from biotic and abiotic stresses and, more in general, to interact with the ecosystem [8, 9]. Generally speaking, phytochemicals and nutraceuticals, as well as pharmaconutrients and phytonutrients can be considered as synonyms. They are not classified as nutrients and they do not have to be confused with micronutrients, that is vitamins and minerals. Finally, nutritional therapy is a healing system using functional foods and nutraceuticals as therapeutics. This complementary therapy is based on the fact that food is not only a source of nutrients and energy, but can also provide health benefits [10]. Interestingly, about 2500 years ago, Hippocrates stated: "Let your food be your medicine and your medicine be your foods" [10b].

Grapevine (*Vitis vinifera*) products, important dietary constituents in the Mediterranean area including grape and wine, represent a valuable source of nutraceuticals, as recently emphasized by a growing body of knowledge [11]. The domestication of grapevine, by the early third millennium BC (Early Bronze Age), resulted in the large-scale production of wine for distribution in the Aegean (southern Greece) [12]. Later, in Roman Age, viticulture was an economic matter. The fermented grape was the commonest source of alcohol, in the ancient world, and this created, for wine, a distinctive pattern of demand and consumption associated with a variety of cultural behavior [13]. According to Cato, the annual consumption of wine was very high, about 10 *amphorae* (1 *amphora* ca. 25 liters), although the alcoholic degree of Roman wine remain unknown [13].

This chapter deals with grapevine products, that is grape and wine, as functional foods and sources of nutraceuticals. In particular, the complex grape chemistry will be examined, with emphasis on the health benefits arising from the grape product consumption.

GRAPE CHEMISTRY

The paradigm of the relationship between the chemical diversity of a particular food and the array of its biological activities may be symbolized by grape. Pharmaconutrients of grape, mostly detected in berry skins and seeds, arise from the three metabolic pathways which, on the whole, group nearly all the natural compounds spread in the Plant Kingdom: the phenylpropanoid, the isoprenoid and the alkaloid biosynthetic routes (Fig. 23.1).

Despite the great variety of chemicals in grape and wine, the beneficial effects of these commodities are mostly associated to their content in phenylpropanoids, phenylalanine derivatives commonly named as phenolic compounds or polyphenols, though improperly. Phenylpropanoid biosynthesis leads to simple phenols, or phenolic acids, and polyphenols, including flavonoids, stilbenes and proanthocyanidins (Fig. 23.1). Simple phenols occurring in grape include hydroxybenzoic and hydroxycinnamic acids. Flavonoids are mainly separated into flavonols, flavanols and anthocyanins. Flavanols provide catechin and epicatechin, the monomeric units of proanthocyanidins, whereas anthocyanins are pigments responsible for wine color. Resveratrol is the major stilbene, in addition to the less common piceids, pterostilbenes and viniferins, respectively resveratrol glucosides, dimethylated resveratrol derivatives and resveratrol oligomers. Finally, proanthocyanidins, also known as condensed tannins, are characterized by a polymerization degree (PD) ranging mainly between 3 and 11, up to 17 and more [9, 11].

Wine aroma is largely due to the presence of isoprenoid monoterpens in grape, above all acyclic linalool, geraniol, nerol, citronellol, homotrienol and monocyclic α-terpineol, mostly occurring as glycosides (Fig. 23.1) [14]. Monoterpenes, major components of essential oils, are C_{10} representatives of isoprenoids, arising from geranyl pyrophosphate (GPP) following the head-to-tail condensation of two isoprene residues. Isoprenoids, or terpenoids, are a huge and diversified group of plant chemicals derived from one simple C_5 isoprenoid building unit, isopentenyl pyrophosphate (IPP) (Fig. 23.1). *Sensu lato*, isoprenoids are lipids, coming from acetyl CoA metabolism via hydroxymethylglutaryl coenzyme A (HMG-CoA) synthase and reductase [reviewed in 15].

Carotenoids are isoprenoid tetraterpens (C_{40}) accumulated in ripening grape berries (Fig. 23.1). These compounds originate from the geranylgeranyl pyrophosphate (C_{20}, GGPP), following different reactions of C_5 unit head-to-tail and head-to-head condensation. Oxidation of carotenoids produces volatile fragments, the C_{13}-norisoprenoids (Fig. 23.1). These are strongly odoriferous compounds, such as β-ionone (aroma of viola), damascenone (aroma of exotic fruits) β-damascone (aroma of rose), and β-ionol (aroma of flowers and fruits) [16].

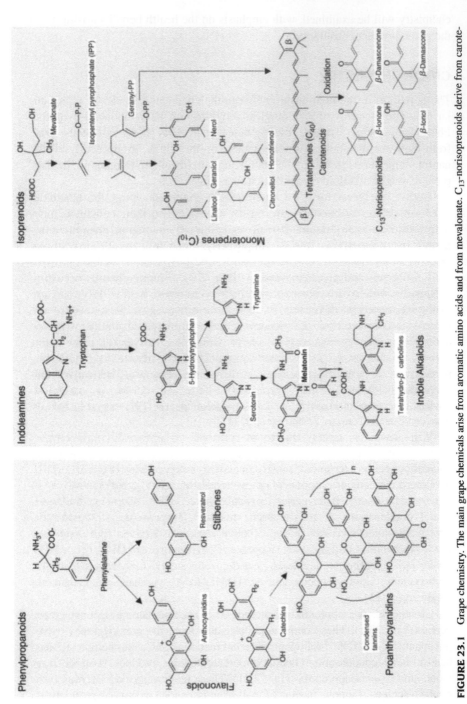

FIGURE 23.1 Grape chemistry. The main grape chemicals arise from aromatic amino acids and from mevalonate. C_{13}-norisoprenoids derive from carotenoid oxidation, while the reaction between indoleamines and aldehydes, in wine, leads to tetrahydro-β-carbolines.

Tetrahydro-β-carbolines are indole alkaloids occurring to a low amount in grape and contributing to its antioxidant power (Fig. 23.1) [17]. Actually, these compounds have been firstly detected in fermented foods, such as cheese, yoghurt, beer and wine, arising from indoleamine (tryptophan derivatives) cyclization with carbonyl substrates, aldheydes typically [18]. Additionally, tetrahydro-β-carbolines are synthesized in mammalian tissues via endogenous condensation [19].

Melatonin (*N*-acetyl-5-methoxytryptamine) has been recently discovered in grape [20]. It was long thought to be a neurohormone found exclusively in vertebrates, up to its recent detection in bacteria, protozoans, algae, plants, fungi and invertebrates [21]. Ever since, melatonin has been detected in edible plants, medicinal herbs and seeds. The essential amino acid tryptophan is the precursor of all the pineal 5-methoxyindoles, or indoleamines/tryptamines, including melatonin, through the intermediate serotonin (5-hydroxytryptamine) and the activity of hydroxyindole-*O*-methyltransferase (Fig. 23.1) [22]. Nevertheless, animals lack the ability to synthesize trypthophan, thus they must obtain it from plant and microbial sources [23].

As for other phytochemicals, particularly polyphenols, melatonin content differs, to a certain extent, among different grapevine cultivars. Nebbiolo and Croatina cultivars contain the highest melatonin concentration, 0.9 and 0.8 ng/g respectively, whereas the lowest level has been detected in Cabernet Franc (0.005 ng/g). Anyway, despite the observed intraspecific variability, melatonin content in grape is slightly higher than that reported for fruits and vegetable (lesser than 0.6 ng/g), with some exceptions such as Brassicaceae and tart cherry, but slightly lower than that found in grains (ranging from 0.9 to 1.9 ng/g) [20].

OXIDATIVE STRESS AND MUTAGENESIS

In metabolism of aerobic organisms, oxygen is essential for providing them with energy through the combustion of nutritive substrates. Because oxygen is the combustive agent, this controlled combustion is an oxidation, that is an aerobic respiration. However, this catabolic route unavoidably and continuously leads to the production of partially reduced oxygen intermediates, more reactive than molecular oxygen in its ground state, including both radical and nonradical forms, collectively termed as reactive oxygen species (ROS) [24]. In mitochondria, leakage of electrons, from their transport chain, leads to the single-electron reduction of oxygen, with the consequent formation of superoxide anion ($^\bullet O_2^-$): approximately 1–5% of oxygen produced by the mitochondria is reduced to this ROS [25]. Other ROS include either non radical, such as hydrogen peroxide (H_2O_2), and radical species, or simply free radicals, such as hydroxyl radical ($^\bullet OH$).

In eukaryotic organisms, damaging prooxidant shift may be the consequence of either an antioxidant-deficient diet or an enhanced prooxidant environment, due to a plethora of external adverse stimuli. Both these conditions may imbalance the prooxidant vs. antioxidant ratio, thus rising the intracellular levels of ROS. External factors that exacerbate the oxidative stress include diseases, pollution, cigarette smoking, radiations and inappropriate activation of phagocytes, such as in chronic inflammatory disease [26]. Pathological conditions mechanistically linked to oxidative stress include inflammation, atherogenesis, carcinogenesis, and foods rich in antioxidant have been shown to play an essential role in the prevention of cancer, cardiovascular diseases, degenerative neurological disorders, such as in Parkinson's and Alzheimer's diseases and aging (Fig. 23.2).

Because of their high reactivity, uncontrolled ROS production may cause injury to the nearest biomacromolecules, if the homeostasis of the oxidation/reduction (redox) state is not preserved (Fig. 23.2). In other words, a disturbance in the prooxidant–antioxidant balance, in favor of the former, may lead to an oxidative stress [27]. Particularly, lipid peroxidation is a free radical-mediated reaction damaging polyunsaturated fatty acid (PUFA), in membranes and plasma lipoprotein particles, such as low-density lipoproteins (LDL) (see the section on atherosclerosis). In order to overcome this side-effect of aerobic life, organisms evolved sophisticated strategies, collectively termed antioxidant defences, to counteract the imbalance of the cellular redox state and keep the ROS concentration under the cytotoxic threshold [28, 29]. Any compound capable of quenching ROS, without itself undergoing conversion to a destructive radical species, can be considered as an antioxidant, such as flavonoids and melatonin.

The basic flavonoid chemical structure is the flavan nucleus, consisting of 15 carbon atoms arranged in three rings (C_6-C_3-C_6): two benzene rings (A and B) combined by an oxygen-containing pyran ring (C) (Fig. 23.3). The various classes of flavonoids differ in the level of oxidation and substitution of the C ring, while individual compounds within a class differ in the pattern of

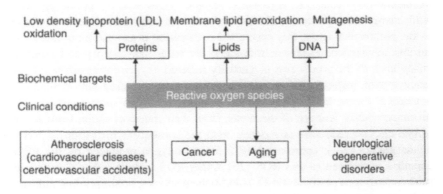

FIGURE 23.2 Oxidative stress. Uncontrolled production of reactive oxygen species (ROS) may cause damage to biomacromolecules, thus resulting involved in the pathogenesis of important aging-related disorders.

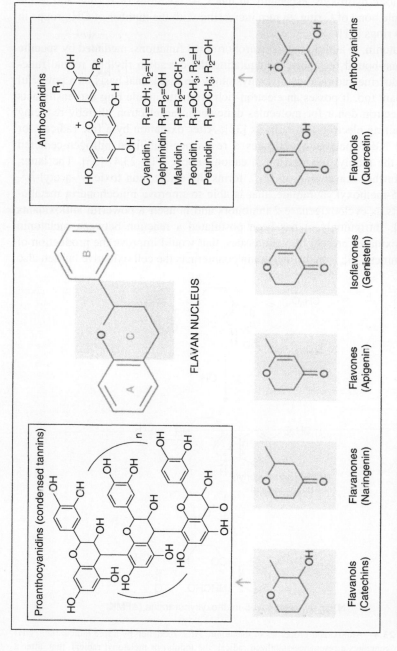

FIGURE 23.3 Flavonoid basic chemical structure. The various classes of flavonoids differ in the level of oxidation and substitution of the C ring, while individual compounds within a class differ in the substitution pattern of A and B rings, as in case of anthocyanidins. Polymerization of flavonoid units, particularly flavanols, leads to proanthocyanidins.

substitution of the A and B ring (Fig. 23.3) [30]. Flavonoids act as antioxidant by donating electrons and stopping radical chains. This activity is attributed to the phenolic hydroxyls, especially in the 3′,4′ positions of B ring, and to the 2,3-double bond of C ring, in turn increasing with the number of OH groups in A and B rings [31].

Melatonin, in addition to its neurohormonal functions, mediated by specific membrane-bound receptors, in regulating the circadian rhythm, retinal function, endocrine and reproductive physiology on a seasonal basis, is a powerful antioxidant too. It posses an electron-rich aromatic indole ring and easily acts as an electron donor for molecules deficient in an electron, thereby reducing and repairing electrophilic radicals [32]. After oxidation by a free radical, for instance ˙OH, melatonin generates a resonance-stabilized nitrogen-centered radical, the indolyl (or melatonyl) cation radical (Fig. 23.4) [33]. The latter, after a further scavenging of $˙O_2^-$, forms the stable, non toxic N^1-acetyl-N^2-formyl-5-methoxykynuramine, that is able to improve mitochondria metabolism, acts as cyclooxigenase-2 inhibitors and is itself a powerful antioxidants [34, 35]. Intriguingly, it has been postulated a reaction between melatonin and peroxidases present in plant tissues, that would improve the production of kynuramines [36]. Finally, melatonin counteracts the cell oxidative burden also

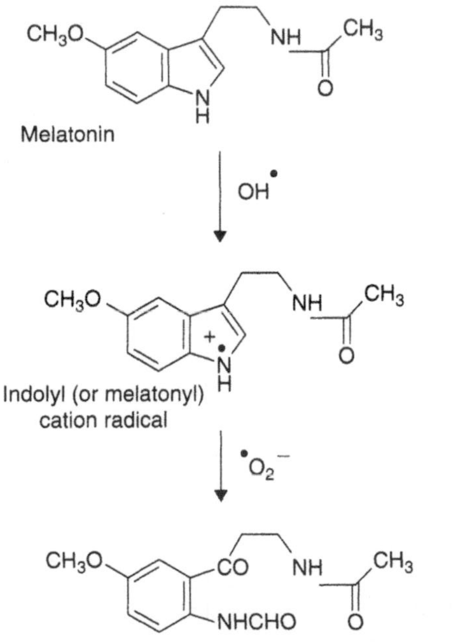

FIGURE 23.4 Antioxidant properties of melatonin. After oxidation by a free radical (i.e., ˙OH) melatonin generates a resonance-stabilized radical, the indolyl or melatonyl radical, that, after a further scavenging of $˙O_2^-$, forms a kynuramine, itself a powerful antioxidant.

indirectly, by enhancing the production of cellular detoxifying enzymes, specifically glutathione peroxidase (GPX), glutathione reductase (GR) and superoxide dismutase (SOD) [37].

Oxidative DNA damage due to modifications of DNA bases is related to mutagenesis, carcinogenesis and aging. The reported data on the antimutagenic activity of grape phytochemicals are still incomplete. In purified calf thymus DNA treated with oxidants, resveratrol exhibited a bimodal response on the formation of 8-hydroxy-2-deoxyguanosine (8-OH-dG), a biomarker of oxidative DNA damage, with a slight prooxidant effect, at lower concentration, while, at higher concentration, resveratrol reduced the 8-OH-dG accumulation in a dose-dependent manner. This biomarker causes $G \rightarrow T$ and $A \rightarrow C$ transversions during DNA replication, thus resulting relevant to carcinogenesis [38]. Intriguingly, melatonin, another grape constituent, besides being more effective than resveratrol, reversed the prooxidant DNA damage induced by low concentration of resveratrol, when added in combination, thus showing a synergistic action [39].

Furthermore, pretreatment with resveratrol prevented the accumulation of DNA strand breaks induced by tobacco smoke condensate in cell lines of different histogenetic origin, as assessed by the comet test [40]. In agreement, in animal cell cultures, resveratrol failed to induce DNA damage, though it slightly increased chromosomal aberrations at the highest assayed doses [41].

However, some prooxidant effects induced by polyphenols have been reported. In particular, resveratrol has been shown to increase oxidative DNA strand breaks, through the generation of copper–peroxide complexes, mainly in the presence of H_2O_2 [42, 43].

CANCER CHEMOPREVENTION

Cancer is a multistage and multifactorial disease. Cancer morbidity and mortality have been steadily rising throughout the last century, with risk increasing with age. Environmental factors, particularly the diet, play a main role in cancer etiology. In westernized countries, cancers of breast, prostate and colon-rectum predominate, because of a diet rich of animal foods and refined carbohydrates and deficient of plant foods. Conversely, in developing countries, where diet is largely based on cereal/starchy foods, esophageal, stomach and liver cancer are more incident [44].

Chemoprevention of cancers is the strategy of preventing, arresting or reversing carcinogenesis with chemopreventive agents, pharmacologically safer than chemotherapeutic agents used in cancer patients. Moreover, the latter may induce time-dependent tumor resistance (chemoresistance) and nonspecific toxicity towards non-target cells [45]. Chemoprevention can interfere with each step of neoplastic progression, which consists of three mechanistically distinct, temporally ordered and closely linked stages: malignancy initiation, promotion and progression (Fig. 23.5) [46–48]. Tumor initiation is a

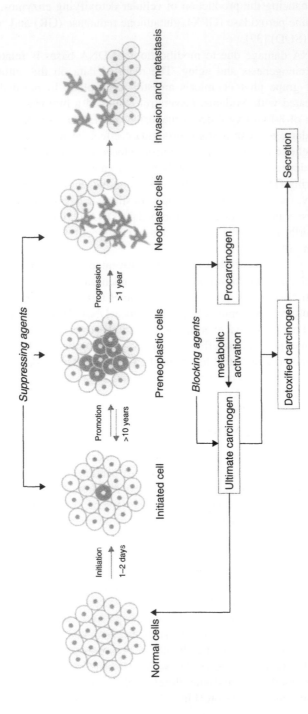

FIGURE 23.5 Carcinogenesis and cancer chemoprevention. Neoplastic progression consists of three distinct, temporally ordered and linked stages: initiation, promotion and progression. Chemopreventive agents are of two types: suppressing agents, that inhibit the malignant transformation of initiated/preneoplastic cells, and blocking agents, that prevent the metabolic activation of procarcinogens.

rapid, mutagenic and irreversible process transforming a normal cell into an initiated cell with a benign tumor phenotype. It includes the exposure to a procarcinogen, its transport and distribution to organs and tissues where metabolic activation and detoxification can occur, and the genotoxic damage due to the covalent interaction of its ultimate electrophilic species with target-cell DNA. The second stage, promotion, is a slow and reversible clonal expansion (proliferation) of preneoplastic cells producing a benign tumor. In the final step, progression, a neoplastic transformation occurs irreversibly, that is the conversion of the benign tumor to a malignant phenotype, with invasive and metastatic potential [46, 48, 49].

Chemopreventive agents can be divided into two categories (Fig. 23.5). Blocking agents arrest the tumor initiation stage, inhibiting the metabolic activation of procarcinogens and preventing their ultimate reactive species to reach the cellular target sites. Blocking agents can also promote the detoxification of procarcinogens, thus stimulating their excretion from the body. Differently, suppressing agents act on the tumor promotion and progression, inhibiting the malignant transformation of initiated cells [48, 50].

Chemopreventive properties of grape products are more likely attributable to the combined effect of their chemicals, rather than to specific molecules [11], although resveratrol represents the most studied example of active phytochemical. Resveratrol is a stilbenic phytoalexin that occurs in grapevine tissues, particularly of leaves, berry skins and petals, as well as in typical grapevine products, wines and grape juice. In plant, phytoalexins, including resveratrol, are synthesized in response to pathogen infections and abiotic stresses, and accumulate in different amounts within tissues [51].

Diverse pathways have been proposed as putative mechanisms for the reported anticarcinogenic activity of grape chemicals, above all the interaction with transcription factors. NF-κB (nuclear factor κB) is a pleiotropic transcription factor involved in different signaling pathways, ranging from inflammation, oncogenesis and apoptosis. Normally, it resides in the cytosol, forming a complex with the inhibitory subunit IκB, whose phosphorylation, ubiquitylation and subsequent degradation, by 26S proteasome, allows NF-κB to move into the nucleus, where it activates gene transcription by binding to specific gene promoter regions. Therefore, aberrant activation of NF-κB, associated with proliferation of malignant cells and inhibition of apoptosis, is causally linked to the neoplastic transformation [52]. The mechanism of resveratrol-induced inhibition of the NF-κB activity includes the suppression of the pathway regulated by the inflammatory mediator TNFα (tumor necrosis factor α) [47, 53, 54]. Additionally, resveratrol inhibits the IKK (IκB kinase) activity and the subsequent IκB phosphorylation, thus blocking its degradation, NF-κB translocation and DNA binding [54b]. Activator protein 1 (AP-1) is another transcription factor that regulates the expression of genes involved in cell adaptation, differentiation and proliferation, whose activation is inhibited by resveratrol and anthocyanidins [53–55].

Androgen receptor (AR) represents an essential mediator of the androgen activity. This transcription factor, belonging to the nuclear steroid hormone receptor family, controls the transcription of androgen-inducible genes, such as PSA (prostate specific antigen), and is implicated in the development of prostate cancer. A decrease in cell proliferation has been reported in androgen-responsive prostate cancer cell lines treated with resveratrol and the flavonoid quercetin, due to the inhibition of the expression and function of AR [56, 57]. Furthermore, the growth of androgen-unresponsive prostate cancer cells was inhibited too, although to a lesser extent than that of the androgen-responsive cell lines [58].

Estrogens play a pivotal role in breast cancer, via their estrogen receptor (ER), another member of the nuclear receptor superfamily. Estrogens regulate gene expression by binding to different intracellular estrogen receptors (ERα and ERβ) with tissue and ligand specificity, influencing the growth, differentiation and function of target tissues. Hence, in non initiated tissues, ligand (estrogen)/receptor (ER) binding leads to the transcription of estrogen responsive target genes, involved in the regulation of different molecular pathways. The phytoestrogen resveratrol has been shown to possess either estrogen agonist and antagonist activity, and these opposing activities have risen some controversy, regarding its therapeutical application against the estrogen-responsive breast cancers [59, 60]. Phytoestrogens are naturally occurring plant metabolites that exert estrogen agonist/antagonist activity. They are diphenolic compounds with structural similarities to natural and synthetic estrogenic steroids and are either hormone-like, with inherent estrogenic activity, or can be converted by the intestinal flora to weakly estrogenic compounds. Other phytoestrogens include lignans and isoflavones, present in whole cereals and legumes respectively, classified as selective estrogen receptor modulators (SERMs) [61].

Inhibition of aromatase activity by red wine components represents another mechanism of breast cancer suppression [62]. Aromatase (estrogen synthetase) is a cytochrome P450 enzyme which converts C19 androgens to aromatic C18 estrogens. Therefore, its overexpression in breast cancer cells may influence the cancer progression itself, because of the major role of estrogens on the breast cancer development [63].

Aryl hydrocarbon receptor (AHR) is a cytosolic protein that translocates to the nucleus upon ligand binding. Metabolic activation of aryl hydrocarbons (AH) results from their binding to AHR, that leads to the transcription of the *CYP1A1* gene, encoding for the cytochrome P450 (CYP450) isozyme CYP1A1. CYP450 isozymes are involved in the metabolism of a wide variety of xenobiotics, including carcinogens such as AH, and are overexpressed in a variety of tumors. The metabolized active forms of carcinogens can subsequently interact with DNA causing mutations. Resveratrol exerts a strong inhibitory effect on the AH-induced *CYP1A1* expression, both at the mRNA and protein level, as well as on other CYP450 isozymes, such as CYP1A2 and CYP3A4 [64–67].

Besides the signaling networks regulated by polyphenols, their anti-proliferative effects can be due to the inhibition of the ribonucleotide reductase, the enzyme that catalyzes the reduction of ribonucleotides into deoxyribo-nucleotides, as well as of the DNA polymerase and ornithine decarboxylase (ODC), the latter a key enzyme of the polyamine synthesis deeply involved in cancer growth [68–70]. Moreover, a number of studies have established that resveratrol blocks cell proliferation by inducing cell cycle arrest at the G1/S and G2/S phase [71–74]. The pro-apoptotic activity and the above described antioxidant power of polyphenols can be other mechanisms involved in the aberrant growth inhibition, as a prooxidant intracellular milieu represents a strong stimulus for cell proliferation [54]. In a variety of tumor cell lines, it has been reported that resveratrol activates the mitochondrial-dependent apop-totic pathway, by the up-regulation of pro-apoptotic p53 and Bax proteins and the down-regulation of the death inhibitory protein Bcl-2 [75–78]. However, in different cell lines, the anticarcinogenic properties of wine polyphenols seem to be mediated by mechanisms other than p53 gene modulation [79].

Apart from the effect on prostate and breast cancers, as above discussed, other tumor types may benefit from regular, moderate wine consumption. Carcinomas of the digestive tract are common and the risk increases with age. Grape polyphenols, mainly quercetin, have been shown to suppress the for-mation of aberrant crypt foci, in animal models of carcinogenesis, by modu-lating both cell proliferation and apoptosis. The crypt is the fundamental unit of epithelial proliferation in the colonic mucosa, where apoptosis removes the genetically damaged stem cells from the epithelium before they undergo clonal expansion. Hence, increased apoptosis in the proliferating zone of the colonic crypt provides a protective mechanism against the crypt cell hyperproliferation and neoplasia [80, 81]. Recently, the growth of human colorectal carcinoma cell has been inhibited by a grape seed extract rich in proanthocyanidins [82].

Photochemoprevention by plant compounds may prevent skin cancer at various stage of carcinogenesis, as shown in animal models. Accordingly, topi-cal application of resveratrol and apigenin, the latter a flavonoid, prior to UV (ultraviolet) exposure, has been shown to be effective in preventing the UV-induced carcinogenesis. Some mechanisms involved in photochemoprevention include the inhibition of the UV-induced ODC activity and NF-κB [83–85].

Among the tumors of the head and neck, the carcinomas of the oral cav-ity, mainly of the squamous cell type, comprise an important group of neoplasia, whose incidence is increasing all over the world. Oral can-cer, including either oral cavity and pharynx cancers, ranks as the sev-enth most common cause of cancer worldwide and represents the 2–4% of all diagnosed cancers, associated with a poor prognosis and survival rate if not early diagnosed [86–88]. Alcohol consumption and tobacco smok-ing account for most of oral cancers, being possible to prevent approxi-mately the 75% of cases avoiding these harmful habits. In particular, alcohol may act as a solvent for the carcinogens thus enhancing the permeability of the oral mucosa to carcinogens, such as those from tobacco. Besides, the ethanol metabolite acetaldehyde has been identified as a tumor promoter [89, 90]. However, the carcinogenic effect of alcohol may depend on drinking habits, though the effect of beverage types on the risk of developing oral cancer remains controversial (see up ahead the section relative to the effects of alcohol on cardiovascular diseases). On the whole, it seems that heavy alcohol consumption is associated to a major incidence of oral cancer, being higher among spirits consumers than wine drinkers [91–93]. Therefore, it seems that red wine, by virtue of its polyphenol content, may have a beneficial effect on the risk of cancers of the upper aerodigestive tracts, specially in a context of Mediterranean diet [94, 95]. In opposition, Maserejian and colleagues observed similar increases in the development of oral premalignant lesions with consumption of spirits, wine and beer, although the association with wine was not statistically significant [96]. Recently, administration of proanthocyanidins, main components of grape seeds, has been shown to suppress the proliferation of human oral squamous cell carcinoma in a dose-dependent manner. More interestingly, proanthocyanidins inhibited the proliferation of cell carcinoma also after transfection with human papillomavirus (HPV), another important risk factor for oral cancer [97].

ALCOHOL

Wine is an alcoholic beverage. The harmful effects of alcohol (ethanol) on the cardiovascular system are not linear, as for cigarette smoking and other risk factors. Several large epidemiological evidences have highlighted a typical correlation between alcohol intake, from whatever source, and all-cause mortality, whereby a regular light to moderate consumption is beneficial and abstinence or a heavy intake are equally detrimental. The biphasic pattern of alcohol–health relationship may be explained, at least in part, by the association of excessive alcohol consumption with systemic hypertension, whereas an established beneficial mechanism, in not heavy drinkers, is the increase in plasma high-density lipoprotein (HDL)-cholesterol levels, due to an enhanced hepatic synthesis [98]. Other effects of ethanol on lipoprotein metabolism include a reduction in HDL-cholesterol degradation and a higher hepatic metabolism of low-density lipoprotein (LDL)-cholesterol. Furthermore, alcohol has a beneficial effect on lipid profile, hemostatic factors and insulin sensitivity [99].

Apart from the hypertension, the ascendant leg of the J-shaped alcohol-linked mortality curve has been explained by the increased risk of cirrhosis, cardiovascular diseases and both hemorrhagic and ischemic stroke, together with higher incidence of certain cancers, mainly those of the oropharynx and oesophagus, as previously described. Conversely, the protection conferred by alcohol consumption strictly depends on the drinking pattern, as well as on the type of beverage [99]. Correlation studies suggest that different types of alcoholic beverages may have dissimilar effects on human health. Mortality from all causes is lower in countries where wine is the predominant type of alcohol than in countries where beer and spirits are mainly drunk [100]. Probably, this is due to the different effects of the diverse types of beverages on the abdominal obesity, that is beer drinkers are at higher risk of developing abdominal obesity than wine consumers [101]. Nevertheless, with regard to the incidence of obesity and type 2 diabetes, it seems that the type of alcoholic beverage is of little importance. The most favorable habit has been shown to be a regular (daily), light to moderate alcohol intake [102].

In view of the above considerations, red wine may be more protective than beer or spirits because of its qualities beyond the alcoholic fraction, whereas white wine seems to be less protective, though there is too little evidence to support this conclusion [103, 104]. The array of the biological activities of the grape phytochemicals, as to a large extent previously described, is thought to be responsible for the protective effect of red wine on the endothelial function and hemostatic factors, inflammation and atherosclerosis, and, finally, on cardiovascular diseases and cerebrovascular accidents [105].

ATHEROSCLEROSIS, CARDIOVASCULAR DISEASES AND CEREBROVASCULAR ACCIDENTS

Atherosclerosis is a chronic, inflammatory, fibro-proliferative process of large and medium-sized arteries that results in the progressive formation of fibrous plaques, which, in turn, impair the blood flow of the vessel. Atherosclerotic lesions, resulting from an eccentric thickening of the intima, can either promote an occlusive thrombosis, in the affected artery, or produce a gradual stenosis of the arterial lumen. In the first case, thrombus formation, due to the disruption of the lesion surface, can lead to an infarction of the organ supplied by the afflicted vessel, such as in a heart attack, when a coronary vessel is suddenly blocked, or in a thrombotic stroke, when a cerebral artery is damaged. In the second case, the stenosis of the vessel limits the blood supply to local tissues, leading to a progressive and gradual injury of the affected organ [106].

Endothelial dysfunction and oxidative modification of LDL are key factors in atherogenesis. Endothelial cells exert multiple physiological functions, maintaining the integrity of the vascular wall and representing a permeable barrier through which diffusion and active transport of several substances occur. Furthermore, endothelial cells constitute a non-thrombotic and non-adherent surface for platelets and leukocytes, they regulate the vascular tone by producing nitric oxide (NO), prostaglandins and endothelins, and, finally, they secrete growth factors and cytokines. Atheroma development begins with the expression of specific glycoproteins by endothelial cells that mediate the adhesion of circulating monocytes and T-lymphocytes (Fig. 23.6). The recruitment of these immune cells and their migration into the subendothelium are triggered by adhesion molecules, such as VCAM (vascular cell adhesion molecules) and ICAM (intracellular adhesion molecules), synthesized in both endothelial and circulating cells, whose secretion is in turn regulated by cytokines released by both endothelium and leukocytes, such as IL-1 (interleukin-1), IL-2, IL6, TNFα and INF γ (interferon γ). After the entry of monocytes through the arterial wall promoted by the monocyte chemotactic protein-1 (MCP-1), atheroma formation continues with the differentiation of monocytes into macrophages, mediated by the macrophage colony-stimulating factor (MCSF), which, in turn, internalize large amounts of oxidized LDL (ox-LDL) particles, thus generating foam cells (Fig. 23.6). Ox-LDL arises from circulating native LDL which undergoes progressive oxidation in the subendothelial space; afterwards, ox-LDL is specifically recognized by the scavenger receptors on the macrophage surface. Additionally, ox-LDL exerts several role other than foam cell formation, by activating the expression of genes for migration and adhesion molecules, such as MCP-1 and MCSF (Fig. 23.6) [107].

At the beginning of the 1990s, the "French paradox" symbolized paradigmatically the health benefits due to a regular and moderate consumption of red wine. This term refers to the low incidence of atherosclerotic cardiovascular disease in the French population, in spite of a diet rich in total and saturated fat, because of moderate daily red wine drinking. Promptly, it was hypothesized, and then extensively demonstrated, that the observed epidemiological

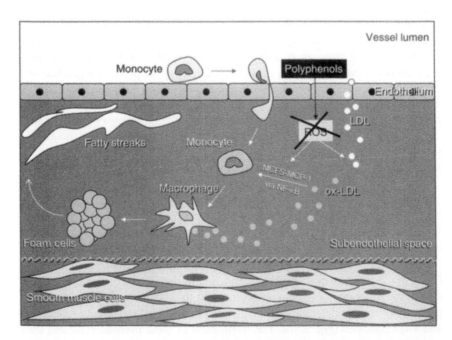

FIGURE 23.6 Atherogenesis. After the entry of monocytes through the arterial wall, promoted by the monocyte chemotactic protein-1 (MCP-1), they differentiate into macrophages, by the macrophage colony-stimulating factor (MCSF), which, in turn, internalize large amounts of oxidized low-density lipoprotein (oxLDL) particles and generate foam cells and fatty streaks. Polyphenols may block either the LDL oxidation and the monocytes activation, by scavenging ROS.

relationship between wine intake and health benefits was attributable to the red wine polyphenolic fraction [108]. Molecular mechanisms by which polyphenols may play a role in the etiology and pathophysiology of atherosclerosis include mainly: (i) the decrease of ET-1 (endothelin-1) production, (ii) the increase of NO synthesis and (iii) the block of NF-κB expression (Fig. 23.7).

Procyanidins, red wine polyphenols, block the production of ET-1 by suppressing the transcription of the gene ET-1, in cultured bovine aortic endothelial cells. ET-1 is a highly potent vasoconstrictor, which also promote leukocyte adhesion, monocyte chemotaxis and smooth muscle cell proliferation, in addition to facilitating the LDL uptake by the endothelial cells [109, 110]. Polyphenols, mainly anthocyanins, trigger an endothelium-dependent, NO-mediated vasorelaxation, besides inhibiting platelet aggregation, modulating primary hemostasis and preventing thrombosis. In addition, red wine increases the expression of human endothelial nitric oxide synthase (eNOS), a mechanism that may further contribute to its beneficial cardiovascular effects [111, 112]. Moreover, delphinidin, an antocyanin, has been shown to inhibit the endothelial cell apoptosis [113]. The NF-κB signaling pathway is subject to a redox regulation. Therefore, it can be evoked by an oxidative stress and inhibited by the antioxidant resveratrol, as already explained [114]. A spectrum of different genes expressed in atherosclerosis has been shown to be upregulated by NF-κB, including those encoding for TNFα, IL-1, MCSF, MCP1, VCAM and ICAM [115]. Finally, increased resistance to LDL oxidation has been documented both experimentally and clinically [116].

The relationship between drinking and stroke is difficult to analyze, because of the available studies are far from being complete, and there is no clear evidence regarding the effect of light to moderate wine drinking on stroke occurrence as a whole. Nonetheless, it is possible that the incidence of ischemic (occlusive) stroke is reduced, while that of hemorrhagic stroke is not, probably because of the different mechanisms involved in these cerebrovascular accidents.

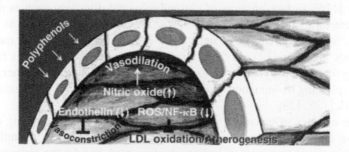

FIGURE 23.7 Endothelial dysfunction. Molecular mechanisms by which polyphenols may play a role in the pathophysiology of endothelial dysfunction include the decrease of endothelin production, the increase of nitric oxide synthesis and the block of either activation of NF-κB (nuclear factor κB) signal transduction pathway and LDL oxidation by scavenging ROS.

Ischemic stroke is due to the atherosclerosis in the carotid or cerebral arteries, resulting from plaque formation and thrombi, whereas hypertension is the main cause of the hemorrhagic stroke. Consequently, in chronic heavy spirits drinkers, hypertension exacerbate the risk for cerebral hemorrhage [117–119].

AGING

Aging is a complex physiological process that involves both morphological and biochemical changes occurring, with the passage of time, in single cells and in the whole organism. Aging is characterized by a diminished ability of responding to stress, because of the decline in the immune function, known as immunosenescence, predisposing to infectious diseases and cancer [120, 121]. Among the many theories proposed to explain the mechanisms of aging at molecular level, the oxidative stress, or free radical, hypothesis has received wide support [122]. Therefore, ROS production and oxidative DNA damage can represent a suitable environment for the development of age-related diseases. For instance, the cumulative risk of cancer increases from the seventh decade of age, and approximately 30% of humans get cancer by age 85. Consequently, in many cases, cancer can be considered a degenerative disease of old age, related to the effects of the continuous exposure to ROS over a lifespan [123].

Recently, it has been reported a significant positive correlation between age and 8-oxo-7,8-dihydroguanosine (8-oxodG) level in leukocyte DNA, with increased levels of this oxidative stress and mutagenesis biomarker in leukocyte DNA of the elderly and middle age group (mean age 67 and 50 years, respectively), in comparison with adults (mean age 31 years) [124]. With this regard, grape phytochemicals resveratrol and melatonin can be considered as promising anti-aging agents, because of their antimutagenic and antioxidant activity [125].

Melatonin, particularly, can counteract the aging process because of its immunomodulatory activity. Melatonin concentration in plasma decreases as aging progresses, and the decline of melatonin with age is coincident with the age-related impairment of the immune system, first appearing around 60 years of age [126]. In fact, an array of chronobiological disorders, such as the general deterioration of cognitive, psychological and social functions, as well as sleep disturbances, can be related to the loss of the amplitude of melatonin rhythmic secretion [127]. A further support to this hypothesis arises from the finding that lymphocytes synthesize melatonin too, in addition to other tissues, thus explaining its immunostimulating affects mediated by the immune-opioid network [128, 129].

The efficacy of melatonin as a potential and promising anti-aging agent is due not only to its immunotherapeutic properties, but also to its antioxidant and antitumoral properties, as previously discussed, besides the antiamyloidogenic activity described in the next section [32, 130].

Old findings suggest that caloric restriction increases the life expectancy [131], but only recent discoveries link this phenomenon with the activation of sirtuins, NAD (nicotinamide adenine dinucleotide)-dependent enzymes that remove acetyl groups from specific lysine residues on various proteins [132]. In *Saccharomyces cerevisiae*, the functional *SIR2* (silent information regulator 2) gene, coding for the Sir2 protein, a NAD-dependent histone deacetylase, is required for caloric restriction to promote an increase in yeast lifespan, by suppressing the genome instability, decreasing the metabolic rate and lowering the production of ROS [133]. Afterwards, in yeasts, other three sirtuins have been discovered (Sir1–4), whereas, in mammals, seven homologs have been identified, SIRT1–7, which deacetylate both histones and nonhistone proteins, implicated in a variety of cellular functions, ranging from the epigenetic regulation of genomic architecture and gene expression, the control of cell cycle and apoptosis, and the regulation of metabolic activity. Mammalian sirtuins are localized in nucleus, cytoplasm and mitochondria, and are ubiquitously expressed in human tissues, with higher levels in the brain and testis. Sirtuin deacetylases are evolutionary conserved and, currently, numerous Sir2 homologs have been identified in archeans, bacteria, plants, protozoans and metazoans [134].

A set of 18 small polyphenolic compounds, including resveratrol and quercetin, has been found to increase the affinity of SIRT1 enzyme for certain protein targets, possibly via an allosteric mechanism. These molecules, referred as sirtuin-activating compounds (STACs), extended the lifespan of *Caenorhabditis elegans*, *Drosophila melanogaster* and *S. cerevisiae*, through the same or a similar pathway as caloric restriction [135, 136]. Accordingly, STACs may increase longevity in mammals too, besides being of therapeutic significance in the treatment of the old age disorders, such as cancer, neurodegeneration and heart failure, as well as diabetes and muscle diseases [137, 138].

NEUROPROTECTION

Several epidemiological studies indicate that a moderate consumption of red wine is associated with a lower incidence of Alzheimer's disease.

In Alzheimer's disease, inhibition of β-fibrillogenesis by melatonin has been reported, that is the ability of the neurotoxic and protease-resistant amyloid β (Aβ) protein to form β-sheet structures or β-amyloid fibrils, deposited within senile plaque in cerebral and meningeal blood vessels. Moreover, it has been suggested that the antiamyloidogenic and neuroprotective effects of melatonin are mostly due to the structural interactions between the hormone and Aβ peptides, rather than to its antioxidant properties exclusively [139,140].

Similarly, in different cell lines, resveratrol has been shown to promote the intracellular degradation of Aβ peptides, via a mechanism that involves the proteasome, without inhibiting directly the enzymes β- and γ-secretases implicated in the Aβ synthesis [141].

More recently, in a mouse model of Alzheimer's disease, the moderate consumption of Cabernet Sauvignon promoted the non-amyloidogenic processing of amyloid precursor proteins mediated by α-secretase, thereby preventing or delaying the generation of Aβ peptides [142]. This different mechanism of neuroprotection is not in disagreement with the results of Marambaud and colleagues [141]. In fact, the resveratrol content in Cabernet Sauvignon used by Wang and colleagues was much lower than the resveratrol concentration employed *in vitro* and, thereby, the observed effect can be presumably ascribed to the pool of phenylpropanoids, including phenolic acids, flavonoids, anthocyanins and stilbenes present in red wine [142].

Protective effect of melatonin in experimental models of Parkinson's disease has been reported too. This disease is a chronic neurodegenerative disorder characterized by the apoptosis of dopaminergic neurons, mainly in the substantia nigra. As oxidative stress seems to be the likely candidate in mediating this process, melatonin, by virtue of its strong antioxidant power, would protect neuronal cells, preventing nigral dopaminergic cell damage, either *in vivo* and *in vitro* [143–145].

Finally, melatonin constitutes a potential and promising new therapeutic agent in degenerative neurological diseases, because of its solubility in both lipids and water, allowing it to easily permeate into any cell compartments and to cross the blood-brain barrier reaching either glial and neuronal cells. Additionally, melatonin has a lower toxicological profile than other antiamyloidogenic drugs [140, 145].

CONCLUSIONS

Plant food pharmaconutritional properties are ascribed to their phytochemical composition. Thus, grape could represent the paradigm of the great variety of compounds synthesized and contained in plant tissues. These natural products, namely phenylpropanoids, isoprenoids and alkaloids, combined together, contribute to the beneficial effects derived from the large fruit and vegetable consumption, especially in a Mediterranean dietary style.

A good understanding of the absorption and bioavailability of phytochemicals is critical before evaluating their bioactivity (Fig. 23.8). However, despite the extensive amount of indications on the bioactivity of phytochemicals, there is, up to now, only sparse information on their bioavailability. Particularly, biokinetic data on their absorption, distribution, metabolism and excretion in humans are still fragmentary and sometimes controversial [146, 147]. For instance, flavonoids occur in plants both as glycosides and aglycones. Glycosylation, mainly with glucose, galactose, rhamnose, xylose and arabinose residues, increases their water solubility, allowing flavonoids storage in the plant cell vacuole. After ingestion, both glycosides and aglycones can be absorbed [148, 149]. Glycosylated flavonoids are deglycosylated by lactase phlorizin hydrolase [150], a membrane-bound enzyme located in the luminal side of the brush border in the small intestine, whereas free aglycones in the lumen can diffuse into the epithelial cells, either passively or by facilitated

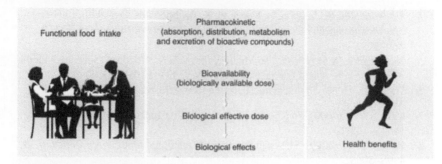

FIGURE 23.8 Bioavailability. Health benefits arising from a correct dietary style depend on the biologically available dose of bioactive components present in functional foods. Health-promoting effects due to functional food intake are difficult to be evaluated properly, because of the scarce information on their pharmacokinetic.

diffusion [151]. An alternative mechanism involves glycoside transport into the cell by sodium-dependent glucose transporter (SGLT1) and, then, deglycosylation by cytosolic β-glucosidase [152]. Moreover, aglycones may be released by the colon microflora into the large intestine [153], though, in any case, the flavonoid bioavailability is only partial, with the absorbed proportion of the ingested amount that is absorbed varying from 0.2% to 20% [149, 154, 155]. Another promising and interesting aspect is the development of reliable and sensitive intake biomarkers, in order to assess the response to functional foods and their active components at organism level [7].

In conclusion, the amount of evidence presented here clearly points out the potential of grape products as remedies in the field of the complementary and alternative medicine, by virtue of the biological activities of the grape constituents as a whole. Additionally, the recent discovery of melatonin in grape opens a new field of knowledge that, in the future, will certainly contribute to explain the plethora of the health benefits arising from the regularly moderate wine consumption [20].

ACKNOWLEDGMENTS

The authors apologize to the colleagues whose excellent works, in the field of grape sciences, could not have been cited for brevity in this chapter.

REFERENCES

1. Doll, R. & Peto, R. (1981). The causes of cancer: Quantitative estimates of avoidable risks of cancer in the United States today. *J Natl Cancer Inst* **66**, 1191–1308.
2. Visioli, F., Grande, S., Bogani, P. & Galli, C. (2004). The role of antioxidants in the Mediterranean diets: Focus on cancer. *Eur J Cancer Prev* **13**, 337–343.
3. Olatunde Farombi, E. (2004). Diet-related cancer and prevention using anticarcinogens. *Afr J Biotech* **3**, 651–661.

4. Trichopoulou, A., Lagiou, P., Kuper, H. & Trichopoulos, D. (2000). Cancer and Mediterranean dietary traditions. *Cancer Epidemiol Biomarkers Prev* **9**, 869–873.

5. Simopoulos, A. P. (2001). The Mediterranean diets: What is so special about the diet of Greece? The scientific evidence. *J Nutr* **131**, S3065–S3073.

6. Heber, D. (2004). Phytochemicals beyond antioxidation. *J. Nutr* **134**, 3175S–3176S.

7. Milner, J. A. (2000). Functional foods: The US perspective. *Am J Clin Nutr* **71**, 1654S–1659S.

8. Hasler, C. M. (2000). The changing face of functional foods. *J Am Coll Nutr* **19**, 499S–506S.

9. Iriti, M. & Faoro, F. (2004). Plant defense and human nutrition: The phenylpropanoids on the menù. *Curr Top Nutr Res* **2**, 47–65.

10. Zhao, J. (2007). Nutraceuticals, nutritional therapy, phytonutrients and hytotherapy for improvement of human health: A perspective on plant biotechnology application. *Rec Pat Biotech* **1**, 75–97.

10b. Nicolao Leoniceno Vincentino (1549). Aphorismi Hippocratis. graecae et latinae, unaa cum Galeni commentariis. Ed. Lvgdvni, apud Gulielmum Rouillium, 521 pp.

11. Iriti, M. & Faoro, F. (2006). Grape phytochemicals: A bouquet of old and new nutraceuticals for human health. *Med Hypot* **67**, 833–838.

12. Hansen, J. M. (1988). Agriculture in the prehistoric Aegean: Data versus speculation. *Am J Archaeol* **92**, 39–52.

13. Purcell, N. (1985). Wine and wealth in ancient Italy. *J Roman Stud* **75**, 1–19.

14. Pisarnitskii, A. F. (2001). Formation of wine aroma: Tones and imperfections caused by minor components. *Appl Biochem Microbiol* **37**, 552–560.

15. Iriti, M. & Faoro, F. (2006). Lipids biosynthesis in spermatophyta. *In* Floriculture, Ornamental and Plant Biotechnology: Advances and Topical Issues (J. A. Teixeira da Silva, Ed.), Vol. I, pp. 359–372, Global Science Books, London, UK.

16. Baumes, R., Wirth, J., Bureau, S., Gunata, Y. & Razungles, A. (2002). Biogeneration of C13-norisoprenoid compounds: Experiment supportive for an apo-carotenoid pathway in grapevines. *Anal Chim Acta* **458**, 3–14.

17. Herraiz, T. & Galisteo, J. (2003). Tetrahydro-β-carboline alkaloids occur in fruits and fruit juice. Activity as antioxidant and radical scavengers. *J Agric Food Chem* **51**, 7156–7161.

18. Herraiz, T. (1996). Occurrence of tetrahydro-β-carboline-3-carboxylic acids in commercial foodstuffs. *J Agric Food Chem* **44**, 3057–3065.

19. Brossi, A., Focella, A. & Teitel, S. (1973). Alkaloids in mammalian tissues. 3. Condensation of L-tryptophan and L-5-hydroxytryptophan with formaldehyde and acetaldehyde. *J Med Chem* **16**, 418–420.

20. Iriti, M., Rossoni, M. & Faoro, F. (2006). Melatonin content in grape: Myth or panacea? *J Sci Food Agric* **86**, 1432–1438.

21. Hardeland, R. & Poeggeler, B. (2003). Non-vertebrate melatonin. *J Pineal Res* **34**, 233–241.

22. Axelrod, J. & Weissbach, H. (1961). Purification and properties of hydroxyindole-O-methyltransferase. *J Biol Chem* **236**, 211–213.

23. Crawford, I. P. (1989). Evolution of a biosynthetic pathway: The tryptophan paradigm. *Ann Rev Microbiol* **43**, 567–600.

24. Lee, J., Koo, N. & Min, D. B. (2004). Reactive oxygen species, aging, and antioxidant nutraceuticals. *Compr Rev Food Sci Food Saf* **3**, 21–33.
25. Ames, B. N., Shigenaga, M. K. & Hagen, T. M. (1993). Oxidants, antioxidants, and the degenerative diseases of aging. *Proc Natl Acad Sci USA* **90**, 7915–7922.
26. Halliwell, B. (1997). Antioxidants and human disease: A general introduction. *Nutr Rev* **55**, S44–S49.
27. Wiseman, H. (1996). Dietary influences on membrane function: Importance in protection against oxidative damage and disease. *J Nutr Biochem* **7**, 2–15.
28. Yu, B. P. (1994). Cellular defenses against damage from reactive oxygen species. *Physiological Rev* **74**, 139–162.
29. Tadolini, C., Juliano, L., Piu, F., Franconi, F. & Cabrini, L. (2000). Resveratrol inhibition of lipid peroxidation. *Free Radic Res* **33**, 105–114.
30. Pietta, P.-G. (2000). Flavonoids as antioxidants. *J Nat Prod* **63**, 1035–1042.
31. Frankel, E. N. (1999). Food antioxidants and phytochemicals: Present and future perspectives. *Fett/Lipid* **101**, 450–455.
32. Reiter, R. (1998). Cytoprotective properties of melatonin: Presumed association with oxidative damage and aging. *Nutrition* **14**, 691–696.
33. Reiter, R. J., Tan, D.-X., Pilar Terron, M., Flores, L. J. & Czarnocki, Z. (2007). Melatonin and its metabolites: New findings regarding their production and their radical scavenging action. *Acta Biochim Pol* **54**, 1–9.
34. Burkhardt, S., Reiter, R. J., Tan, D.-X., Hardeland, R., Cabrera, J. & Karbownik, M. (2001). DNA oxidatively damaged by chromium(III) and H_2O_2 is protected by melatonin, N^1-acetyl-N^2-formyl-5-methoxykynuramine, resveratrol and uric acid. *Int J Biochem Cell Biol* **33**, 775–783.
35. Mayo, J. C., Sainz, R. M., Tan, D.-X., Hardeland, R., Leon, J., Rodriguez, C. & Reiter, R. J. (2005). Anti-inflammatory actions of melatonin and its metabolites, N^1-acetyl-N^2-formyl-5-methoxykynuramine (AFMK) and N^1-acetyl-5-methoxykynuramine (AMK), in macrophages. *J Neuroimmunol* **165**, 139–149.
36. Ximenes, V. F., Fernandes, J. R., Bueno, V. B., Catalani, L. H., Oliveira, G. H. & Machado, R. G. P. (2007). The effect of pH on horseradish peroxidase-catalyzed oxidation of melatonin: Production of N^1-acetyl-N^2-formyl-5-methoxykynuramine versus radical-mediated degradation. *J Pineal Res* **42**, 291–296.
37. Antolín, I., Rodríguez, C., Sáinz, R. M., Mayo, J. C., Uría, H., Kotler, M. L., Rodríguez-Colunga, M. J., Tolivia, D. & Menéndez-Peláez, A. (1996). Neurohormone melatonin prevents cell damage: Effect on gene expression for antioxidant enzymes. *FASEB J* **10**, 882–890.
38. Cheng, K. C., Cahill, D. S., Kasai, H., Nishimura, S. & Loeb, L. A. (1992). 8-Hydroxyguanine, an abundant form of oxidative DNA damage, causes G----T and A----C substitutions. *J Biol Chem* **267**, 166–172.
39. López-Burillo, S., Tan, D.-X., Mayo, J. C., Sainz, R. M., Manchester, L. C. & Reiter, R. J. (2003). Melatonin, xanthurenic acid, resveratrol, EGCG Vitamin C and alpha-lipoic acid differentially reduce oxidative DNA damage induced by fenton reagents: A study of their individual and synergistic actions. *J Pineal Res* **34**, 269–277.
40. Sgambato, A., Ardito, R., Faraglia, B., Boninsegna, A., Wolf, F. I. & Cittadini, A. (2001). Resveratrol, a natural phenolic compound, inhibits cell proliferation and prevents oxidative DNA damage. *Mutat Res* **496**, 171–180.

41. De Salvia, R., Festa, F., Ricordy, R., Particone, P. & Cozzi, R. (2002). Resveratrol affects in a different way primary versus fixed DNA damage induced by $H_{(2)}O_{(2)}$ in mammalian cells *in vitro*. *Toxicol Lett* **135**, 1–9.

42. Fukuhara, K. & Miyata, N. (1998). Resveratrol as a new type of DNA-cleaving agent. *Bioorg Med Chem Lett* **8**, 3187–3193.

43. Win, W., Cao, Z., Peng, X., Trush, M. A. & Li, Y. (2002). Different effects of genistein and resveratrol on oxidative DNA damage *in vitro*. *Mutat Res* **513**, 113–120.

44. Young, G. & Le Leu, R. (2002). Preventing cancer: Dietary lifestyle or clinical intervention? *Asian Pac J Clin Nutr* **11**, S618–S631.

45. Garg, A. K., Buchholz, T. A. & Aggarwal, B. B. (2005). Chemosensitization and radiosensitization of tumors by plant polyphenols. *Antiox Redox Signal* **7**, 1630–1647.

46. Greewald, P. (2002). Cancer chemoprevention. *Br Med J* **324**, 714–718.

47. Suhr, Y.-J. (2003). Cancer chemoprevention with dietary phytochemicals. *Nat Rev Cancer* **3**, 768–780.

48. Fresco, P., Borges, F., Diniz, C. & Marques, M. P. M. (2006). New insights on the anticancer properties of dietary polyphenols. *Med Res Rev* **26**, 747–766.

49. Manson, M. M. (2003). Cancer prevention: The potential for diet to modulate molecular signalling. *Trends Mol Med* **9**, 11–18.

50. Wattenberg, L. W. (1985). Chemoprevention of cancer. *Cancer Res* **45**, 1–8.

51. Jeandet, P., Douillet-Breuil, A. C., Bessis, R., Debord, S., Sbaghi, M. & Adrian, M. (2002). Phytoalexins from the Vitaceae: Biosynthesis, phytoalexin gene expression in transgenic plants, antifungal activity and metabolism. *J Agric Food Chem* **50**, 2731–2741.

52. Bharti, A. C. & Aggarwal, B. B. (2002). Nuclear factor-κB and cancer: Its role in prevention and therapy. *Biochem Pharmacol* **64**, 883–888.

53. Manna, S. K., Mukhopadhyay, A. & Aggarwal, B. B. (2000). Resveratrol suppresses TNF-induced activation of nuclear transcription factors NF-κB, activator protein-1, and apoptosis: Potential role of reactive oxygen intermediates and lipid peroxidation. *J Immunol* **164**, 6509–6519.

54. Pervaiz, S. (2003). Resveratrol: From grapevines to mammalian biology. *FASEB J* **17**, 1975–1985.

54b. Holmes-McNary, M. & Baldwin Jr, A. S. (2000). Chemopreventive properties of trans-resveratrol are associated with inhibition or activation of the IkappaB kinase. *Cancer Res* **60**, 3477–3483.

55. Hou, D.-X., Kai, K., Li, J. J., Lin, S., Terahara, N., Wakamatsu, M., Fujii, M., Young, M. R. & Colburn, N. (2004). Anthocyanidins inhibit activator protein 1 activity and cell transformation: Structure-activity relationship and molecular mechanisms. *Carcinogenesis* **25**, 29–36.

56. Mitchell, S. H., Zhu, W. & Young, C. Y. (1999). Resveratrol inhibits the expression and function of the androgen receptor in LNCaP prostate cancer cells. *Cancer Res* **59**, 5892–5895.

57. Xing, N., Chen, Y., Mitchell, S. H. & Young, C. Y. (2001). Quercetin inhibits the expression and function of the androgen receptor in LNCaP prostate cancer cells. *Carcinogenesis* **22**, 409–414.

58. Hsieh, T. C. & Wu, J. M. (1999). Differential effects on growth, cell cycle arrest, and induction of apoptosis by resveratrol in human prostate cancer cell lines. *Exp Cell Res* **249**, 109–115.

59. Lu, R. & Serrero, G. (1999). Resveratrol, a natural product derived from grape, exhibits antiestrogenic activity and inhibits the growth of human breast cancer cells. *J Cell Physiol* **179**, 297–304.

60. Basly, P., Marre-Fournier, F., Le Bail, J. C., Habrioux, G. & Chulia, A. J. (2000). Estrogenic/antiestrogenic and scavenging properties of (E)- and (Z)-resveratrol. *Life Sci* **66**, 769–777.

61. Ososki, A. L. & Kennelly, E. J. (2003). Phytoestrogens: A review of the present state of reaserch. *Phytother Res* **17**, 845–869.

62. Eng, E. T., Williams, D., Mandava, U., Kirma, N., Tekmal, R. R. & Chen, S. (2001). Suppression of aromatase (estrogen synthetase) by red wine phytochemicals. *Breast Cancer Res Treat* **67**, 133–146.

63. Sun, X. Z., Zhou, D. & Chen, S. (1997). Autocrine and paracrine actions of breast tumor aromatase. A three-dimensional cell culture study involving aromatase transfected MCF-7 and T-47D cells. *J Steroid Biochem Mol Biol* **63**, 29–36.

64. Ciolino, H. P., Daschner, P. J. & Yeh, G. C. (1998). Resveratrol inhibits transcription of CYP1A1 *in vitro* by preventing activation of the aryl hydrocarbon receptor. *Cancer Res* **58**, 5707–5712.

65. Ciolino, H. P. & Yeh, G. C. (1999). Inhibition of aryl hydrocarbon-induced cytochrome P-450 1A1 enzyme activity and CYP1A1 expression by resveratrol. *Mol Pharmacol* **56**, 760–767.

66. Chan, W. K. & Delucchi, A. B. (2000). Resveratrol, a red wine constituent, is a mechanism-based inactivator of cytochrome P450 3A4. *Life Sci* **67**, 3103–3112.

67. Chang, T. K., Chen, J. & Lee, W. B. (2001). Differential inhibition and inactivation of human CYP1 enzymes by trans-resveratrol: Evidence for mechanism-based inactivation of CYP1A2. *J Pharmacol Exp Ther* **299**, 874–882.

68. Fontecave, M., Lepoivre, M., Elleingand, E., Gerez, C. & Guittet, O. (1998). Resveratrol, a remarkable inhibitor of ribonucleotide reductase. *FEBS Lett* **421**, 277–279.

69. Schneider, Y., Vincent, F., Duranton, B., Badolo, L., Gosse, F., Bergmann, C., Seiler, N. & Raul, F. (2000). Anti-proliferative effect of resveratrol, a natural component of grapes and wine, on human colonic cancer cells. *Cancer Lett* **158**, 85–91.

70. Tsan, M. F., White, J. E., Maheshwari, J. G. & Chikkappa, G. (2002). Anti-leukemia effect of resveratrol. *Leuk Lymphoma* **43**, 983–987.

71. Ragione, F. D., Cucciolla, V., Borriello, A., Pietra, V. D., Racioppi, L., Soldati, G., Manna, C., Galletti, P. & Zappia, V. (1998). Resveratrol arrests the cell division cycle at S/G2 phase transition. *Biochem Biophys Res Commun* **250**, 53–58.

72. Hsieh, T. C., Burfeind, P., Laud, K., Backer, J. M., Traganos, F., Darzynkiewicz, Z. & Wu, J. M. (1999). Cell cycle effects and control of gene expression by resveratrol in human breast carcinoma cell lines with different metastatic potentials. *Int J Oncol* **15**, 245–252.

73. Bernhard, D., Tinhofer, I., Tonko, M., Hubl, H., Ausserlechner, M. J., Greil, R., Kofler, R. & Csordas, A. (2000). Resveratrol causes arrest in the S-phase prior to Fas-independent apoptosis in CEM-C7H2 acute leukemia cells. *Cell Death Differ* **7**, 834–842.

74. Joe, A. K., Liu, H., Suzui, M., Vural, M. E., Xiao, D. & Weinstein, I. B. (2002). Resveratrol induces growth inhibition, S-phase arrest, apoptosis, and changes in biomarker expression in several human cancer cell lines. *Clin Cancer Res* **8**, 893–903.

75. Clement, M. V., Ponton, A. & Pervaiz, S. (1998). Apoptosis induced by hydrogen peroxide is mediated by decreased superoxide anion concentration and reduction of intracellular milieu. *FEBS Lett* **440**, 13–18.

76. Dorrie, J., Gerauer, H., Wachter, Y. & Zunino, S. J. (2001). Resveratrol induces extensive apoptosis by depolarizing mitochondrial membranes and activating caspase-9 in acute lymphoblastic leukemia cells. *Cancer Res* **61**, 4731–4739.

77. Tinhofer, I., Bernhard, D., Senfter, M., Anether, G., Loeffler, M., Kroemer, G., Kofler, R., Csordas, A. & Greil, R. (2001). Resveratrol, a tumor-suppressive compound from grapes, induces apoptosis via a novel mitochondrial pathway controlled by Bcl-2. *FASEB J* **15**, 1613–1615.

78. Roman, V., Billard, C., Kern, C., Ferry-Dumazet, H., Izard, J. C., Mohammad, R., Mossalayi, D. M. & Kolb, J. P. (2002). Analysis of resveratrol-induced apoptosis in human B-cell chronic leukaemia. *Br J Haematol* **117**, 842–851.

79. Soleas, G. J., Goldberg, D. M., Grass, L., Levesque, M. & Diamandis, E. P. (2001). Do wine polyphenols modulate p53 gene expression in human cancer cell lines? *Clin Biochem* **34**, 415–420.

80. Johnson, I. T. (2002). Anticarcinogenic effects of diet-related apoptosis in the colorectal mucosa. *Food Chem Tox* **40**, 1171–1178.

81. Dolora, P., Luceri, C., De Filippo, C., Pietro Femia, A., Giovannelli, L., Caderni, G., Cecchini, C., Silvi, S., Orpianesi, C. & Cresci, A. (2005). Red wine polyphenols influence carcinogenesis, oxidation damage, intestinal microflora and colonic gene expression profiles in F344 rats. *Mutat Res* **591**, 237–246.

82. Kaur, M., Singh, R. P., Gu, M., Agarwal, R. & Agarwal, C. (2006). Grape seed extract inhibits *in vitro* and *in vivo* growth of human colorectal carcinoma cells. *Clin Cancer Res* **12**, 6194–6202.

83. Birt, D. F., Mitchell, D., Gold, B., Pour, P. & Pinch, H. C. (1997). Inhibition of ultraviolet light induced skin carcinogenesis in SKH-1 mice by apigenin, a plant flavonoid. *Anticancer Res* **17**, 85–91.

84. Afaq, F., Adhami, V. M., Ahmad, N. & Mukhtar, H. (2003). Green tea constituent (–)– epigallocatechin-3-gallate inhibits ultraviolet B-mediated activation of nuclear factor kappa B signaling pathway in normal human epidermal keratinocytes. *Oncogene* **22**, 1035–1044.

85. Adhami, V. M., Afaq, F. & Ahmad, N. (2003). Prevention of skin neoplasia by resveratrol: Involvement of nuclear transcription factor NF-κB. *Neoplasia* **5**, 74–82.

86. Jane-Salas, E., Chimenos-Kustner, E., Lopez-Lopez, J. & Rosello-Llabres, X. (2003). Importance of diet in the prevention of oral cancer. *Med Oral* **8**, 260–268.

87. Davies, L. & Welch, H. G. (2006). Epidemiology of head and neck cancer in the United States. *Otolaryngol Head Neck Surg* **135**, 451–457.

88. Pavia, M., Pileggi, C., Nobile, C. G. & Angelillo, I. F. (2006). Association between fruit and vegetable consumption and oral cancer: A meta-analysis of observational studies. *Am J Clin Nutr* **83**, 1126–1134.

89. Pöschl, G. & Seitz, H. K. (2004). Alcohol and cancer. *Alcohol* **39**, 155–165.

90. Mehrotra, R. & Yadav, S. (2006). Oral squamous cell carcinoma: Etiology, pathogenesis and prognostic value of genomic alterations. *Ind J Cancer* **43**, 60–66.

91. Castellsagué, X., Quintana, M. J., Martínez, M. C., Nieto, A., Sánchez, M. J., Juan, A., Monner, A., Carrera, M., Agudo, A., Quer, M., Muñoz, N., Herrero, R., Franceschi, S. & Bosch, F. X. (2004). The role of type of tobacco and type of alcoholic beverage in oral carcinogenesis. *Int J Cancer* **108**, 741–749.

92. Petti, S. & Scully, C. (2005). Oral cancer: The association between nation-based alcohol-drinking profiles and oral cancer mortality. *Oral Oncol* **41**, 828–834.

93. Güneri, P., Çankaya, H., Yavuzer, A., Güneri, E. A., Erişen, L., Özkul, D., Nehir El, S., Karakaya, S., Arican, A. & Boyacioğlu, H. (2005). Primary oral cancer in a Turkish population sample: Association with sociodemographic features, smoking, alcohol, diet and dentition. *Oral Oncol* **41**, 1005–1012.

94. Bosetti, C., Gallus, S., Trichopoulou, A., Talamini, R., Franceschi, S., Negri, E. & La Vecchia, C. (2003). Influence of the Mediterranean diet on the risk of cancers of the upper aerodigestive tract. *Cancer Epidemiol Biomarkers Prev* **12**, 1091–1094.

95. Rossi, M., Garavello, W., Salamini, R., Negri, E., Borsetti, C., Dal Maso, L., Lagiou, P., Tafani, A., Polesel, J., Barman, L., Ramazzotti, V., Franceschi, S. & La Vecchia, C. (2007). Flavonoids and the risk of oral and pharyngeal cancer: A case-control study from Italy. *Cancer Epidemiol Biomarkers Prev* **16**, 1621–1625.

96. Maserejian, N. N., Joshipura, K. J., Rosner, B. A., Giovannucci, E. & Zavras, A. I. (2006). Prospective study of alcohol consumption and risk of oral premalignant lesions in men. *Cancer Epidemiol Biomarkers Prev* **15**, 774–781.

97. King, M., Chatelain, K., Farris, D., Jensen, D., Pickup, J., Swapp, A., O'Malley, S. & Kingsley, K. (2007). Oral squamous cell carcinoma proliferative phenotype is modulated by proanthocyanidins: A potential prevention and treatment alternative for oral cancer. *BMC Complem Altern Med* **7**, 22.

98. Beilin, L. J. & Puddey, I. B. (2006). Alcohol and hypertension: An update. *Hypertension* **47**, 1035–1038.

99. Grønbaek, M. (2006). Alcohol/disease risk and beneficial effects. *In* Encyclopaedia of Human Nutrition (B. Caballero, Ed.), pp. 57–62, Elsevier, St. Louis, MO, USA.

100. Grønbaek, M., Becker, U., Johansen, D., Gottschau, A., Schnohr, P., Hein, H. O., Jensen, G. & Sørensen, T. I. A. (2000). Type of alcohol consumed and mortality from all causes, coronary heart disease, and cancer. *Ann Intern Med* **133**, 411–419.

101. Vadstrup, E. S., Petersen, L., Sørensen, T. I. A. & Grønbæk, M. (2003). Waist circumference in relation to history of amount and type of alcohol. *Int J Obesity* **27**, 238–246.

102. Klatsky, A. L. (2007). Alcohol, cardiovascular diseases and diabetes mellitus. *Pharmacol Res* **55**, 237–247.

103. Vogel, R. A. (2003). Vintners and vasodilators: Are French red wines more cardioprotective? *J Am Coll Cardiol* **41**, 479–481.

104. Zilkens, R. R., Burke, V., Hodgson, J. M., Barden, A., Beilin, L. J. & Puddey, I. B. (2005). Red wine and beer elevate blood pressure in normotensive men. *Hypertension* **45**, 874–879.

105. Opie, L. H. & Lecour, S. (2007). The red wine hypothesis: From concepts to protective signalling molecules. *Eur Heart J* **28**, 1683–1693.

106. Berliner, J. A., Navab, M., Fogelman, A. M., Frank, J. S., Demer, L. L., Edward, P. A., Watson, A. D. & Lusis, A. J. (1995). Atherosclerosis: Basic mechanisms. Oxidation, inflammation, and genetics. *Circulation* **91**, 2488–2496.

107. da Luz, P. L. & Coimbra, S. R. (2004). Wine, alcohol and atherosclerosis: Clinical evidences and mechanisms. *Braz J Med Biol Res* **37**, 1275–1295.

108. Renaud, S. & de Lorgeril, M. (1992). Wine, alcohol, platelets, and the French paradox for coronary heart disease. *Lancet* **339**, 1523–1526.

109. Corder, R., Douthwaite, J. A., Lees, D. M., Khan, N. Q., Viseu Dos Santos, A. C., Wood, E. G. & Carrier, M. J. (2001). Endothelin-1 synthesis reduced by red wine. *Nature* **414**, 863–864.

110. Corder, R., Mullen, W., Khan, N. Q., Marks, S. C., Wood, E. G., Carrier, M. J. & Crozier, A. (2006). Oenology: Red wine procyanidins and vascular health. *Nature* **444**, 566.

111. Wallerath, T., Poleo, D., Li, H. & Förstermann, U. (2003). Red wine increases the expression of human endothelial nitric oxide synthase, a mechanism that may contribute to its beneficial cardiovascular effects. *J Am Coll Cardiol* **41**, 471–478.

112. Fumagalli, F., Rossoni, M., Iriti, M., Di Gennaro, A., Faoro, F., Borroni, E., Borgo, M., Scienza, A., Sala, A. & Folco, G. (2006). From field to health: A simple way to increase the nutraceutical content of grape as shown by NO-dependent vascular relaxation. *J Agric Food Chem* **54**, 5344–5349.

113. Martin, S., Giannone, G., Andriantsitohaina, R. & Martinez, M. C. (2003). Delphinidin, an active compound of red wine, inhibits endothelial cell apoptosis via nitric oxide pathway and regulation of calcium homeostasis. *Br J Pharmacol* **139**, 1095–1102.

114. Csiszar, A., Smith, K., Labinskyy, N., Orosz, Z., Rivera, A. & Ungvari, Z. (2006). Resveratrol attenuates TNF-alpha-induced activation of coronary arterial endothelial cells: Role of NF-kappaB inhibition. *Am J Physiol Heart Circ Physiol* **291**, H1694–H1699.

115. Brand, K., Page, S., Walli, A. K., Neumeier, D. & Bauerle, P. A. (1997). Role of nuclear factor NF-kB in atherogenesis. *Exp Physiol* **82**, 297–304.

116. Stein, J. H., Keevil, J. G., Wiebe, D. A., Aeschlimann, S. & Foltz, J. D. (1999). Purple grape juice improves endothelial function and reduces the susceptibility of LDL cholesterol to oxidation in patients with coronary artery disease. *Circulation* **100**, 1050–1055.

117. Truelsen, T., Grønbaek, M., Schnohr, P. & Boysen, G. (1998). Intake of beer, wine and spirits and risk of stroke: The Copenhagen City Heart Study. *Stroke* **29**, 2467–2472.

118. Romelsjo, A. & Eifman, A. (1999). Association between alcohol consumption and mortality, myocardial infarction, and stroke in 25 year follow up of 49,618 young Swedish men. *Br Med J* **319**, 821–822.

119. Hart, C. L., Smith, G. D., Hole, D. J. & Hawthorme, V. M. (1999). Alcohol consumption and mortality from all causes, coronary heart disease, and stroke: Results from a prospective cohort study of Scottish men with 21 years of follow up. *Br Med J* **318**, 1725–1729.

120. Weinert, B. T. & Timiras, P. S. (2003). Theories of aging. *J Appl Physiol* **95**, 1706–1716.

121. Hakim, F. T., Flomerfelt, F. A., Boyiadzis, M. & Gress, R. E. (2004). Aging, immunity and cancer. *Curr Opin Immunol* **16**, 151–156.

122. Olinski, R., Siomek, A., Rozalski, R., Gackowski, D., Foksinski, M., Guz, J., Dziaman, T., Szpila, A. & Tudek, B. (2007). Oxidative damage to DNA and antioxidant status in aging and age-related diseases. *Acta Biochim Pol* **54**, 11–26.

123. Ames, B. N. (1989). Endogenous oxidative DNA damage, aging, and cancer. *Free Radic Res Commun* **7**, 121–128.

124. Siomek, A., Gackowski, D., Rozalski, R., Dziaman, T., Szpila, A., Guz, J. & Olinski, R. (2007). Higher leukocyte 8-oxo-7,8-dihydro-2′-deoxyguanosine and lower plasma ascorbate in aging humans? *Antioxid Redox Signal* **9**, 143–150.

125. Micallef, M., Lexis, L. & Lewandowski, P. (2007). Red wine consumption increases antioxidant status and decreases oxidative stress in the circulation of both young and old humans. *Nutr J* **6**, 27.

126. Srinivasan, V., Maestroni, G. J. M., Cardinali, D. P., Esquifino, A. I., Pandi-Perumal, S. R. & Miller, S. C. (2005). Melatonin, immune function and aging. *Immunity & Ageing* **2**, 17.

127. Pandi-Perumal, S. R., Seils, L. K., Kayumov, L., Ralph, M. R., Lowe, A., Moller, H. & Swaab, D. F. (2002). Senescence, sleep, and circadian rhythms. *Ageing Res Rev* **1**, 559–604.

128. Maestroni, G. J. & Conti, A. (1991). Anti-stress role of the melatonin-immuno-opioid network: Evidence for a physiological mechanism involving T cell-derived, immunoreactive beta-endorphin and MET-enkephalin binding to thymic opioid receptors. *Int J Neurosci* **61**, 289–298.

129. Carrillo-Vico, A., Calvo, J. R., Abreu, P., Lardone, P. J., Garcia-Maurino, S., Reiter, R. J. & Guerrero, J. M. (2004). Evidence of melatonin synthesis by human lymphocytes and its physiological significance: Possible role as intracrine, autocrine, and/or paracrine substance. *FASEB J* **18**, 537–539.

130. Maestroni, G. J. (2001). The immunotherapeutic potential of melatonin. *Expert Opin Investig. Drugs* **10**, 467–476.

131. McCay, C. M., Crowell, M. F. & Maynard, L. A. (1935). The effect of restricted growth upon the length of life and upon the ultimate body size. *J Nutr* **10**, 63–79.

132. Lin, S.-J., Defossez, P. A. & Guarente, L. (2000). Requirment of NAD and *Sir2* for life-span extension by caloric restriction in *Saccharomyces cerevisiae*. *Science* **289**, 2126–2128.

133. Masoro, E. J. (2004). Role of sirtuin proteins in life extension by caloric restriction. *Mech Ageing Dev* **125**, 591–594.

134. Yamamoto, H., Schoonjans, K. & Auwerx, J. (2007). Sirtuin functions in health and disease. *Mol Endocrinol* **21**, 1745–1755.

135. Howitz, K. T., Bitterman, K. J., Cohen, H. Y., Lamming, D. W., Lavu, S., Wood, J. G., Zipkin, R. E., Chung, P., Kisielewski, A., Zhang, L.-L., Scherer, B. & Sinclair, D. A. (2003). Small molecule activators of sirtuins extend Saccharomyces cerevisiae lifespan. *Nature* **425**, 191–196.

136. Wood, J. G., Rogina, B., Lavu, S., Howitz, K., Helfand, S. L., Tartar, M. & Sinclair, D. A. (2004). Sirtuin activators mimic caloric restriction and delay ageing in metazoans. *Nature* **430**, 686–689.

137. Sinclair, D. A. (2005). Sirtuins for healthy neurons. *Nat Gen* **37**, 339–340.

138. Porcu, M. & Chiarugi, A. (2005). The emerging therapeutic potential of sirtuin-interacting drugs: From cell death to lifespan extension. *Trends Pharmacol Sci* **26**, 94–103.

139. Pappolla, M., Bozner, P., Soto, C., Shao, H., Robakis, N. K., Zagorski, M., Frangione, B. & Ghiso, J. (1998). Inhibition of Alzheimer beta-fibrillogenesis by melatonin. *J Biol Chem* **273**, 7185–7188.

140. Pappolla, M. A., Chyan, Y., Poeggeler, B., Frangione, B., Wilson, G., Ghiso, J. & Reiter, R. J. (2000). An assessment of the antioxidant and the antiamyloidogenic

properties of melatonin: Implications for Alzheimer's disease. *J Neural Transm* **107**, 203–231.

141. Marambaud, P., Zhao, H. & Davies, P. (2005). Resveratrol promotes clearance of Alzheimer's disease amyloid-β peptides. *J Biol Chem* **280**, 37377–37382.

142. Wang, J., Ho, L., Zhao, Z., Seror, I., Humala, N., Dickstein, D. L., Thiyagarajan, M., Percival, S. S., Talcott, S. T. & Pasinetti, G. M. (2006). Moderate consumption of Cabernet Sauvignon attenuates Abeta neuropathology in a mouse model of Alzheimer's disease. *FASEB J* **20**, 2313–2320.

143. Acuña-Castroviejo, D., Coto-Montes, A., Gaia Monti, M., Ortiz, G. G. & Reiter, R. J. (1997). Melatonin is protective against MPTP-induced striatal and hippocampal lesions. *Life Sci* **60**, PL23–PL29.

144. Ortiz, G. G., Crespo-López, M. E., Moran-Moguel, C., Garcia, J. J., Reiter, R. J. & Acuña-Castroviejo, D. (2001). Protective role of melatonin against MPTP-induced mouse brain cell DNA fragmentation and apoptosis *in vivo*. *Neuroendocrinol Lett* **22**, 101–108.

145. Antolin, I., Mayo, J. C., Sainz, R. M., del Brio, M. L., Herrera, F., Martin, V. & Rodriquez, C. (2002). Protective effect of melatonin in a chronic experimental model of Parkinson's disease. *Brain Res* **943**, 163–173.

146. Clifford, M. N. (2004). Diet-derived phenols in plasma and tissues and their implications for health. *Planta Med* **70**, 1103–1114.

147. Karakaya, S. (2004). Bioavailability of phenolic compounds. *Crit Rev Food Sci Nutr* **44**, 453–464.

148. Paganga, G. & Rice-Evans, C. A. (1997). The identification of flavonoids as glycosides in human plasma. *FEBS Lett* **401**, 78–82.

149. Hollman, P. C., Bijsman, M. N., van Gameren, Y., Cnossen, E. P., de Vries, J. H. & Katan, M. B. (1999). The sugar moiety is a major determinant of the absorption of dietary flavonoid glycosides in man. *Free Rad Res* **31**, 569–573.

150. Day, A. J., Canada, F. J., Diaz, J. C., Kroon, P. A., McLauchlan, W. R., Faulds, C. B., Plumb, G. W., Morgan, M. R. A. & Williamson, G. (2000). Dietary flavonoid and isoflavone glycosides are hydrolysed by the lactase phlorizin hydrolase. *FEBS Lett* **468**, 166–170.

151. Gee, J. M., DuPont, M. S., Day, A. J., Plumb, J. W., Williamson, G. & Johnson, I. T. (2000). Intestinal transport of quercetin glycosides in rats involves both deglycosylation and interaction with hexose transport pathway. *J Nutr* **130**, 2765–2771.

152. Day, A. J., Du Pont, M. S., Ridley, S., Rhodes, M. J. C., Morgan, M. R. A. & Williamson, G. (1998). Deglycosylation of flavonoid and isoflavonoid glycosides by human small intestine and liver β-glucosidase activity. *FEBS Lett* **436**, 71–75.

153. Aura, A. M., O'Leary, K. A., Williamson, G., Ojala, M., Bailey, M., Puupponnen-Pimiaa, R., Nuutila, A. M., Oksman-Caldentey, K.-M. & Poutanen, K. (2002). Quercetin derivatives are deconjugated and converted to hydroxyphenylacetic acids but not methylated by human fecal flora *in vitro*. *J Agric Food Chem* **50**, 1725–1730.

154. Scalbert, A. & Williamson, G. (2000). Dietary intake and bioavailability of polyphenols. *J Nutr* **130**, 2073S–2080S.

155. Scalbert, A., Morand, C., Manach, C. & Rémésy, C. (2002). Absorption and metabolism of polyphenols in the gut and impact on health. *Biomed Pharmacother* **56**, 276–282.

Chapter 24

Isoflavones Made Simple – Agonist Activity for the Beta-Type Estrogen Receptor May Mediate Their Health Benefits

Mark F. McCarty

NutriGuard Research Encinitas, CA, USA

Abstract

Soy isoflavones, the focus of much research and controversy, are often referred to as "weak estrogens." In fact, genistein is a relatively potent agonist for the recently characterized beta isoform of the estrogen receptor (ERbeta). The low nanomolar serum concentrations of unconjugated free genistein achieved with high-nutritional intakes of soy isoflavones are near the binding affinity of genistein for this receptor, but are about an order of magnitude lower than genistein's affinity for the "classical" alpha isoform of the estrogen receptor (ERalpha). Moreover, these concentrations are far too low to inhibit tyrosine kinases or topoisomerase II, *in vitro* activities of genistein often cited as potential mediators of its physiological effects. S-Equol, derived from bacterial metabolism of daidzein in some individuals, is also a relatively selective agonist for ERbeta. The thesis that the physiological effects of high-dietary levels of soy isoflavones are in fact mediated by ERbeta activation provides a satisfying rationale for the clinical activities of these agents. Hepatocytes do not express ERbeta; this explains why soy isoflavones, unlike oral estrogen, neither modify serum lipids nor provoke the prothrombotic effects associated with increased risk for thromboembolic disorders. The lack of uterotrophic activity of soy isoflavones reflects the fact that ERalpha is the exclusive mediator of estrogen's impact in this regard. Vascular endothelium expresses both ERalpha and ERbeta, each of which has the potential to induce and activate nitric oxide synthase; this may account for the favorable influence of soy isoflavones on endothelial function in postmenopausal women and ovariectomized rats. The ERbeta expressed in osteoblasts may mediate the reported beneficial impact of soy isoflavones on bone metabolism. Suggestive evidence that soy-rich diets decrease prostate cancer risk, and possibly colorectal cancer risk as well, accords well with the observations that ERbeta appears to play an antiproliferative role in healthy prostate, and likely mediates the reduction in colorectal cancer risk associated with hormone replacement therapy.

In the breast, ERalpha promotes epithelial proliferation, whereas ERbeta has a restraining influence in this regard – consistent with the emerging view that soy isoflavones do not increase breast cancer risk, and possibly may diminish it. Premenopausal women enjoy a relative protection from kidney failure; since ERbeta is an antagonist of TGF-β signaling in mesangial cells, soy isoflavones may have nephroprotective potential. Estrogen also appears to protect women from left ventricular hypertrophy and hepatic fibrosis, and recent evidence suggests that these effect are mediated by ERbeta. In conjunction with reports that isoflavones may have a modestly beneficial impact on menopausal symptoms – perhaps reflecting the presence of ERbeta in the hypothalamus – these considerations suggest that soy isoflavone regimens of sufficient potency may represent a safe and moderately effective alternative to HRT in postmenopausal women. Further clinical research is required to characterize the impact of optimal genistein intakes on endothelial and bone function in men. Studies with ERbeta-knockout mice could be helpful for clarifying the role of this receptor in mediating the effects of soy-rich diets.

Keywords: *Soy, isoflavones, genistein, ERalpha, ERbeta*

PHYSIOLOGICAL CONCENTRATIONS OF FREE GENISTEIN ACTIVATE ESTROGEN RECEPTOR-BETA

The key to understanding the health-protective potential of soy isoflavones may have been provided by Kuiper and colleagues, who first established the existence of a "novel" estrogen receptor, now known as estrogen receptor beta (ERbeta) to distinguish it from the "classical" estrogen receptor alpha (ERalpha) [1, 2] These workers assessed the affinity of these receptors for a range of xenobiotic and phytochemical estrogenic compounds, including the soy isoflavones [3, 4]. They established that genistein has agonist activity for both ERalpha and ERbeta, but that genistein's affinity for ERbeta is considerably greater; genistein's affinities for ERbeta and ERalpha were determined to be 8.4 nM and 145 nM, respectively. For daidzein, the corresponding values were 100 nM and 420 nM, indicative of its much lower affinity for these receptors. At saturating concentrations, both genistein and daidzein could interact with either of these receptors to activate transcription from estrogen response elements, at least as effectively as the physiological ligand 17β-estradiol.

A number of subsequent studies have examined genistein's comparative abilities to bind to and promote transcription from the two estrogen receptor isoforms [5–12]. Although the absolute values obtained in these studies differ, genistein's binding affinity for ERbeta consistently emerges as 7–30-fold greater than its affinity for ERalpha; this is paralleled by genistein's ability to activate transcription with ERbeta at a lower concentration than with ERalpha. As a rule, ERbeta-mediated transcription is approximately half-maximal at a genistein concentration of 10 nM, whereas ERalpha-mediated transcription is minimal at this concentration, only becoming substantial as genistein rises above 100 nM.

One recent study has examined the impact of isoflavones on the rate at which the ER isoforms bind to the estrogen response element in DNA; they determined the isoflavone concentration which would increase this binding rate by 50% [13]. For genistein, this value was determined to be 30 nM for ERbeta and 15 μM for ERalpha – once again indicative of marked selectivity for ERbeta. The corresponding values for daidzein were 350 nM for ERbeta and >300 μM for ERalpha.

Some of the key effects of estrogen result not from transcriptional activation at estrogen response elements, but from transcriptional repression of certain promoters that bind NF-kappaB, such as the IL-6 promoter [14]. This latter effect reflects interaction of the activated estrogen receptor with NF-kappaB in a manner that does not entail binding of the estrogen receptor to DNA. Genistein has been shown to activate ERbeta such that it is capable of inhibiting the TNF response element; this effect was half-maximal at a genistein concentration of only 8.5 nM [7]. In contrast, in cells overexpressing ERalpha, only a moderate transrepression was seen with a genistein concentration of 1 μM.

Estrogen receptors can also influence the transcriptional activity of AP-1, Sp1, and certain c-AMP response elements, through interactions that do not entail direct binding to DNA [15–17]. In particular, agonist-activated ERalpha often increases the transcriptional activation mediated by AP-1, possibly by binding to coactivators that interact with fos/jun [15, 18]. In contrast, activated ERbeta has the opposite effect, suppressing AP-1-mediated transcription [15, 19–22]. Since AP-1 exerts various pro-proliferative effects, these findings may help to rationalize the opposing effects of ERalpha and ERbeta on cell proliferation in certain tissues, as cited below. In particular, ERalpha activates the cyclin D1 promoter through its AP-1 and c-AMP response elements, whereas ERbeta has a suppressive effect in this regard [21]. These considerations suggest that low nanomolar concentrations of genistein may have the potential to exert certain effects opposite to those of the classical estrogen receptor – including anti-proliferative effects.

The relevance of these findings becomes evident when one considers the plasma genistein concentration in subjects who habitually consume a soy-rich diet. Adlercreutz et al. reported that the mean concentration of total genistein (free plus conjugated) was 276 nM in Japanese men; however, only about 4% of this was in free or sulfated form, the balance consisting of the glucuronate conjugate which presumably has limited intracellular access [23, 24]. More recent studies have specifically measured unconjugated plasma isoflavones; one of these found that unconjugated genistein constituted only about 1.1–1.5% of the total plasma pool of genistein – the higher percentage being observed transiently in the first 2 hours after soy ingestion [25]. The low content of unconjugated isoflavones is presumed to reflect rapid glucuronidation (and to a lesser extent, sulfation) of these compounds in the liver and intestinal mucosa [26]. Since total serum genistein concentrations of around 1.5 μM are noted during prolonged supplementation with high-physiological doses of genistein [27], this would correspond to an unconjugated genistein concentration of about 20 nM if 1.3% of total genistein were in free form. After several subjects ingested a meal providing 125 g (dry weight) of whole soybeans, free serum genistein rose to about 20–40 nM within about 2 hours, persisting at this level at 8 hours, but returning to baseline after 24 hours [28]. About half of the unconjugated genistein in serum is bound to serum proteins, so the effective concentration available to cells may be about 50% of the measured total concentration [29]; in other words, the physiological impact of 20 nM serum genistein may be comparable to that observed with 10 nM genistein *in vitro*.

These findings encourage the speculation that high-physiological serum levels of free genistein – i.e. those achievable by ingesting a soy-rich diet – will achieve ample activation of ERbeta, but only minimal or modest activation of ERalpha. As we shall see, this thesis appears capable of rationalizing both the safety and the physiological benefits of dietary soy isoflavones.

S-EQUOL ALSO ACTS AS ERBETA AGONIST

Although daidzein *per se* would not be expected to exert estrogenic activity in plasma concentrations achievable by ingestion of high-nutritional doses of soy isoflavones, about a third of humans possess a colonic bacterial flora capable of converting daidzein to *S*-equol [30–32]. This latter compound is readily absorbed and, like genistein, is rapidly and almost quantitatively converted to glucuronide and sulfate conjugates [30]. Also like genistein, *S*-equol is a relatively selective agonist for ERbeta; Katzenbogen and colleagues measured a K_i of 16 nM for *S*-equol's interaction with ERbeta (as contrasted to 6.7 nM for genistein) [33]. *S*-Equol's K_i for ERalpha was reported to be 200 nM; thus, *S*-equol's isoform selectivity appears to be comparable to that of genistein. Nonetheless, these authors found that the transcriptional bioactivity of *S*-equol – measured in an endometrial carcinoma cell line transfected with ER expression vectors – was less potent and less selective than that of genistein. In any case, since total plasma *S*-equol concentrations (free + conjugated) in excess of 1 μM can be achieved in equol producers consuming diets rich in soy isoflavones [34], it is reasonable to suspect that equol could contribute to the physiological estrogen activity observed after soy isoflavone ingestion in equol producers. Indeed, several studies have concluded that soy isoflavones tend to exert greater physiological effects in equol producers than in non-producers [30, 31, 35, 36]. A relatively high proportion (about 60%) of people habitually consuming low-fat vegetarian diets are equol producers [37]; however, whether long-term adoption of such a diet could turn equol non-producers into producers remains to be seen.

IRRELEVANCE OF OTHER SUSPECTED EFFECTS

Much of the speculation regarding the physiological effects of isoflavones makes reference to *in vitro* studies in which genistein has been shown to inhibit tyrosine kinases or topoisomerase II, or to modulate activation of mitogenic signaling pathways in cultured cells. The effects of genistein on tyrosine kinase or topoisomerase activity require concentrations well into the micromolar range [38, 39]. Similarly, the great majority of studies showing that genistein is a signal modulator in cells have used micromolar concentrations of this agent. These effects thus have no conceivable relevance to the physiological impact of genistein. To the best of my knowledge, activation of estrogen receptors is the only effect of genistein that has been documented in the low nanomolar range.

There is a recent report that genistein, as well as daidzein and biochanin A, have agonist activity for the so-called estrogen-related receptors (ERRs) [40]. These receptors are structural relatives of genuine estrogen receptors, and can activate transcription from estrogen response elements, but do not bind estrogen, and possess constitutive activity. Although isoflavones can bind to ERR and modestly enhance their transactivational activity, this effect is minimal and statistically insignificant at a genistein concentration of $1\,\mu M$ – nor are daidzein or biochanin A much more active in this regard. Thus, interaction of soy isoflavones with ERRs is unlikely to be of physiological significance.

SOY ISOFLAVONES HAVE NO DIRECT HEPATIC EFFECTS

Studies in rats, primates, and humans demonstrate that hepatocytes express ERalpha, but not ERbeta [41–45]. Many of the notable physiological effects of oral estrogen are mediated in the liver. Thus, oral estrogen lowers LDL cholesterol, raises serum triglycerides, boosts synthesis of angiotensinogen and sex hormone-binding globulin, and decreases hepatic production of IGF-I – effects which are thought to reflect direct estrogenic activity in hepatocytes [46–53]. Moreover, oral estrogen up-regulates thrombotic mechanisms by modulating hepatic production of a range of plasma proteins which regulate thrombosis. Thus, oral estrogen increases plasma concentrations of clotting factors VII and IX, activated protein C, and C-reactive protein, while decreasing those of antithrombin, proteins C and S, and tissue factor pathway inhibitor [54–58]. These effects are much less substantial when estrogens are administered transdermally; this is thought to explain the observation that risk for venous thromboembolism is increased far more by oral estrogen than by transdermal estrogen [56, 59]. Since physiological concentrations of genistein can be expected to have only a modest impact on ERalpha activity, it is not surprising that none of these effects are observed when soy isoflavones are ingested [60–65].

Gallstone risk is higher for women than men, and this has been traced to the fact that activated ERalpha boosts cholesterol output to the bile. In mice, ERalpha-selective agonists, but not ERbeta-selective agonists, have this effect [66]. It can be deduced that soy isoflavones will not increase risk for gallstones.

The modest impact of soy protein-rich diets on elevated LDL cholesterol in some studies presumably reflects replacement of "high-quality" animal protein (such as casein) with "lower-quality" plant protein [67]. Indeed, Sirtori, who first established the utility of soy protein-based diets for cholesterol reduction, pointed out that the soy protein isolate he used to first demonstrate this effect was devoid of isoflavones! [68] He maintained that the utility of his regimen was contingent on replacing animal protein with plant protein [69]. The studies which document reduction of elevated LDL cholesterol with supplemental soy protein have typically used comparable intakes of milk protein for the placebo group [70]; there is little evidence that simply adding soy protein to a diet that remains high in animal protein will lower elevated LDL.

While it may be disappointing to concede that soy isoflavones cannot lower LDL cholesterol, or diminish cancer risk by suppressing plasma IGF-I, it is nonetheless comforting to realize that isoflavones will not increase thrombotic risk in the way that oral estrogens do. Conceivably, the prothrombotic hepatic effects of oral estrogen are largely if not wholly responsible for the unanticipated increase in risk for myocardial infarction observed during recent prospective trials of oral hormone replacement therapy – despite the favorable influence of estrogen activity on vascular endothelium and LDL cholesterol [71].

NO UTEROTROPHIC ACTIVITY

Physiological concentrations of soy isoflavones can also be expected to be safe for the uterine endometrium, as the uterotrophic effect of estrogens appears to be mediated solely by ERalpha. This has been demonstrated elegantly in ERalpha-knockout mice, in which estrogens fail to exert a uterotrophic effect [72]. As would be expected, soy isoflavones have shown no impact on endometrial proliferation in clinical studies [73–77]. Although endometrium expresses both alpha and beta receptors, synthetic agonists specific for ERbeta do not decrease uterine weight in rats or prevent the proliferative response to a concurrently administered ERalpha-specific agonist [45]. In women, soy isoflavones do not suppress the endometrial proliferative response to estrogen [78]. Based on these observations, ingestion of genistein within the nutritional range would not be expected to either increase or decrease endometrial cancer risk.

Nonetheless, when rats are fed doses of genistein that could be considered pharmacological – for example, 750 mg/kg diet, resulting in a free serum genistein level of 400 nM – uterotrophic activity is indeed seen [79]. This finding is consistent with the responsiveness of ERalpha to high nanomolar concentrations of genistein. The implication is that genistein doses which greatly exceed the nutritional range should not be presumed to be safe from the standpoint of endometrial cancer risk.

GENISTEIN UP-REGULATES ENOS ACTIVITY IN VASCULAR ENDOTHELIUM

One of the chief reasons for suspecting that hormone replacement therapy would decrease cardiovascular risk is that estrogens have a favorable impact on endothelial function, promoting the activity of the endothelial isoform of nitric oxide synthase (eNOS); this results both from increased transcription, and also from extranuclear effects of activated extrogen receptors (both ERalpha and ERbeta) exerted at the plasma membrane [80–85]. Estrogen can also enhance the bioactivity of nitric oxide by down-regulating NADPH oxidase expression – more specifically, that of its gp91phox subunit – in human endothelial cells [86]. Vascular endothelium expresses both ERalpha and ERbeta, and their effects on human umbilical vein endothelial cells appear to be quite comparable [87]. Studies point to a role for ERalpha in the induction of eNOS and/or NO production in the endothelial cells of diverse species [88–93]; the impact of ERbeta in this regard is less clear. Whereas estrogen increased the expression of eNOS in the coronary arteries of ovariectomized ERalpha-knockout mice [94], consistent with a role for ERbeta in eNOS induction, no such effect was seen in their cerebrovascular arteries [90]. Induction of eNOS by ERbeta in rat cardiac myocytes and in human myometrium has been reported [95, 96]. In the vascular smooth muscle cells of rodents, ERbeta exerts both antihyperplastic and antihypertensive effects [97, 98].

Clinical observations appear consistent with the possibility that ERbeta supports endothelial eNOS activity in at least some vascular beds. Adequate oral intakes of genistein have been reported to improve endothelium-dependent vasodilation – as well as other markers for endothelial NO production – in postmenopausal women [99–102]. The most striking findings in this regard have been reported by Squadrito and colleagues, who administered either 54 mg free genistein daily, a typical oral hormone replacement regimen, or a placebo, to 90 postmenopausal women for 1 year [100]. Genistein treatment increased brachial endothelium-dependent vasodilation and post-occlusive blood flow relative to placebo; the effects of the hormone replacement regimen were quite similar. Moreover, plasma levels of nitric oxide metabolites were doubled, and plasma levels of endothelin-1 virtually halved, in both the genistein and hormone replacement groups. (This suppression of endothelin-1 may reflect the ability of NO to inhibit endothelial secretion of endothelin.) [103] Other studies have likewise reported favorable effects of soy isoflavone supplementation (or administration of isoflavone-rich soy protein) on vascular endothelial function in women – albeit a few studies have failed to observe such an effect [104, 105]. One study reported an improvement in arterial compliance, but not in acetylcholine-mediated vasodilation [106]. In ovariectomized rats, dietary genistein has been shown to improve endothelium-dependent, but not endothelium-independent, vasodilation [107–109].

Squadrito suggests that lower intakes of genistein, or shorter duration of supplementation, might account for the two negative reports. Indeed, each of these studies administered 80 mg of mixed conjugated soy isoflavones daily [104, 105]; it would take about 150 mg of such a preparation to provide the 54 mg of pure genistein used in the Squadrito study. The fact that Squadrito administered free genistein, rather than the genistein glycoside (genistin) that occurs natively in unfermented soy foods, might also have some bearing in this regard. There are conflicting reports regarding the relative bioavailabilities of free iso-flavones and conjugated isoflavones; one Japanese study concluded that, during long-term administration, administration of free isoflavones yielded plasma concentrations of total isoflavones that were roughly twice as high as those achieved during administration of conjugated isoflavones [110]. On the other hand, three recent American and Swiss studies conclude that, after single oral doses, the availabilities of the two forms of isoflavones are roughly comparable [111–113]. Although isoflavone glycosides are not taken up by intestinal cells [114], these compounds are readily converted to free glycosides by membrane-bound or bacterial β-glucosidases in the intestinal tract [115]; the resulting free isoflavones are absorbable [116]. The propensity of gut bacteria to degrade isoflavones varies from person to person and influences their bioavailability – slow metabolizers achieve higher plasma levels of genistein and daidzein [117]. Since free isoflavones should be absorbed more rapidly, one would suspect that they would be more effective than conjugates in rapid metabolizers – but this has not been documented. Evidently, more research is needed to evaluate the relative impact of free vs. conjugated isoflavones on plasma isoflavone levels during long-term administration.

The favorable effects of genistein on endothelial function might be operative in men as well, in light of a report that intrabrachial administration of genistein led to a nitric oxide-mediated increase in forearm blood flow in male volunteers; infusion of 17 β-estradiol – but not daidzein – had a comparable effect [118]. On the other hand, one study reported a modest reduction in endothelium-dependent vasodilation after men had ingested isoflavone-rich soy protein (40 g daily, providing 118 mg isoflavones) for 3 months [119]. The impact of dietary genistein on endothelial function in males should be studied further. Estrogen can boost endothelium-dependent vasodilation in males [120–122], and studies in aromatase-knockout male mice indicate that endogenous estrogen improves endothelial function in the males of this species [123].

In light of the versatile role which endothelial nitric oxide production plays in preservation of vascular health, it seems likely that genistein's ability to up-regulate eNOS function could be exploited to decrease vascular risk. Epidemiological evidence suggests that estrogen may be largely responsible for the relative protection from cardiovascular disease enjoyed by premenopausal women [124–126]. It would be a fortunate development indeed if men could use genistein to achieve at least a portion of this benefit without incurring typical estrogenic side effects.

Sadly, induction of eNOS is not always an unalloyed benefit; in endotheliopathies associated with increased superoxide production, tetrahydrobiopterin deficiency leads to an "uncoupling" of eNOS that impairs its activity while turning it into a superoxide generator [127–129]. Fortunately, there is recent evidence that high-dose folic acid can restore the proper protective function of eNOS when tetrahydrobiopterin is deficient [130–134]. Thus, it is reasonable to suggest that concurrent administration of high-dose folate could be a prudent adjuvant to genistein supplementation in patients at risk for endothelial dysfunction. Supplemental arginine, as well as various measures which lessen superoxide production by NADPH oxidase, may also help to optimize the bio-efficacy of the eNOS expressed by dysfunctional endothelium [134–136].

IMPROVED INSULIN SENSITIVITY

More recently, Squadrito and colleagues have reported the results of a 2-year study in which osteopenic postmenopausal women were randomized to receive 54 mg genistein daily or placebo [137]. A range of cardiovascular risk factors was evaluated. The most striking finding was a significant improvement in insulin sensitivity (HOMA-IR), coupled with reductions in fasting levels of both insulin and glucose, in the genistein-treated group. These findings are consistent with those of a previous controlled study in which isoflavone-rich soy protein had been administered to postmenopausal type 2 diabetics [138]. Although the mechanistic basis of this benefit is not clear, one likely possibility is that it reflects an improved capacity of insulin to dilate resistance arteries feeding skeletal muscle. The vasodilatory impact of post-prandial insulin – which aids storage of meal-derived glucose – is mediated by nitric oxide [139, 140]; it is reasonable to expect that genistein's up-regulatory impact on endothelial expression of eNOS could potentiate this effect.

Intriguingly, Squadrito also noted significant reductions in plasma levels of fibrinogen, F2-isoprostanes, and endothelial adhesion proteins in the genistein-treated group; blood lipid levels were not influenced [137].

FAVORABLE EFFECTS ON BONE METABOLISM

Both ERalpha and ERbeta are expressed in the main cell types present in human bone: osteoblasts, osteoclasts, and osteocytes [141–143]. Studies with osteoblast-derived cell lines indicate that these two receptors modulate the transcription of distinctly different sets of genes, with only a modest amount of overlap [144]. The effects of ERalpha on gene expression tend to be amplified in ERbeta-knockout mice, suggesting that ERbeta down-regulates some responses to ERalpha [145]. Cortical bone density is greater, and age-related loss of trabecular density is lower, in ERbeta-knockout mice as compared to wild type [146]. Yet in ovariectomized ERalpha-knockout mice, estrogen promotes increased bone density – albeit not as effectively as it does in ERbeta knockouts; evidently, both types of estrogen receptor can act to preserve bone integrity [147]. Indeed, trabecular bone density tends to be increased in ERalpha-knockout female mice [148]. These effects may be sex-specific, as estrogen did not improve bone density in orchidectomized ERalpha-knockout mice [147]. In a human osteoblast-derived cell line (MG63) in which ERalpha had been silenced with antisense plasmids, estrogen increased collagen and alkaline phosphatase secretion, demonstrating an anabolic effect of ERbeta in these cells [149].

The increase in bone osteoclastic activity and bone resorption ushered in by menopause is thought to stem primarily from an alteration of osteoblast function; soluble mediators produced by osteoblasts have a major impact on the functional status of nearby osteoclasts. Estrogen inhibits osteoblast production of IL-6, an important trophic factor for osteoclasts; it also boosts production of osteoprotegerin, a soluble "false receptor" which inhibits activity of RANKL, another important trophic factor for osteoclasts [14, 150, 151]. It is thus of particular interest that, in physiological concentrations, genistein has been shown to suppress IL-6 production, and boost osteoprotegerin production, in human osteoblast-derived cell lines [152, 153]. These effects are inhibited by concurrent incubation with an estrogen receptor antagonist. These findings strongly suggest that genistein can interact with ERbeta to achieve transrepression of the IL-6 promoter – as it does with the TNF promoter [7].

Genistein also has the potential to improve bone metabolism through its impact on vascular eNOS, in light of recent evidence that this enzyme is a mediator of the osteogenic impact of estrogen on osteoblasts [154–156].

In light of these considerations, it is not surprising that, in non-uterotrophic doses, genistein has repeatedly been shown to promote maintenance of bone density in ovariectomized rats and mice [157–162]. Whether this effect would be lost in ERbeta-knockout mice – thus confirming that ERbeta mediates the effect – has not been determined. Surprisingly, two drugs said to be potent and selective ERbeta agonists did not inhibit bone loss in ovariectomized rats [45, 163]. However, the fact that these agents have agonist activity for transcriptional promotion in some contexts, does not necessarily imply that they will have such activity in other contexts – nor that they will interact with ERbeta in a manner that achieves transrepression of the IL-6 promoter.

Clinical studies of supplementation with soy isoflavones or isoflavone-rich soy protein in postmenopausal women have reached divergent conclusions: some find that such supplementation has a favorable effect on markers of bone metabolism and on preservation of bone density [27, 164–169], whereas others do not [170–172]. These disparities prompted a recent meta-analysis, which included nine randomized controlled studies involving a total of 432 subjects; isoflavones were administered either as tablets or as isoflavone-rich soy protein [173]. This analysis concluded that isoflavone supplementation does indeed suppress bone resorption – as assessed by urinary levels of deoxypyridinoline – while also stimulating bone formation – as assessed by serum levels of bone-specific alkaline phosphatase.

Perhaps the most impressive study in this regard was that of Squadrito and colleagues [27]. These researchers recruited 90 postmenopausal women, 47–57 years of age, who were randomized to receive either genistein (54 mg daily), a standard HRT combination (17β-estradiol/norethisterone acetate), or a matching placebo; response was evaluated at 6 and 12 months. Genistein treatment was found to decrease excretion of pyridinium cross-links (a marker for collagen catabolism in bone) at both 6 and 12 months; this response was quite comparable to that achieved with HRT. In contrast to HRT, however, genistein increased serum levels of bone alkaline phosphatase and osteocalcin, markers for osteoblastic activity. At 12 months, the serum RANKL/osteoprotegerin ratio was notably reduced in the genistein group, to a greater extent than in the HRT group [169]. Finally, after 12 months, bone mineral density in the femoral neck and lumbar spine had increased by 3–4% in both the genistein and HRT group, as contrasted to modest losses of density noted in the placebo group. This study is notable for its comparatively long duration – sufficient to evaluate changes in bone density – and for its use of a fairly ample dose of free genistein. The total serum genistein (conjugated plus free) in the genistein-supplemented group, measured during a morning fast, was $1.5\,\mu M$ at 6 months and $1.7\,\mu M$ at 12 months; assuming that about 1.3% of the genistein pool was unconjugated, this would be expected to correspond to a free genistein concentration of about $20\,nM$, presumably sufficient to activate ERbeta.

Isoflavone supplementation has also been assessed in premenopausal women and in men; no impact on bone metabolism or bone density was noted in these studies [174, 175]. However, soy isoflavones were found to decrease loss of bone mass in orchidectomized male rats [176]. The possibility that isoflavones might influence bone metabolism in elderly men merits further examination.

Since East Asian women often consume ample amounts of soy isoflavones in their habitual diets, several studies have attempted to correlate habitual isoflavone intake or serum isoflavone level with postmenopausal bone density and/or bone metabolism in such women. Two studies – one each from Japan and China – have reported that women in the highest quartile of soy intake, as contrasted to the lowest quartile, had higher bone density [177, 178]. Several other studies, including those in the United States or Europe, where soy intake is comparatively low, did not observe such a correlation [179–181], albeit a Southern California study had a positive outcome [182].

REDUCING PROSTATE AND COLORECTAL CANCER RISKS

Human prostatic epithelium expresses ERbeta, but not ERalpha – whereas prostate stroma expresses ERalpha [183, 184]. There is reason to believe that ERbeta activity has an antiproliferative impact both in healthy prostate and in prostate cancers [185, 186]. Prostatic hypertrophy is common in aging ERbeta-knockout mice, whereas knockout of ERalpha has no such effect [187, 188]. Furthermore, transfection of ERbeta into human prostate cancer cell lines induces apoptosis [189]. As prostate cancers progress, ERbeta expression tends to decrease – consistent with the possibility that this receptor exerts a restraining effect on proliferation [184, 190, 191]. In prostate cancer cell lines which express ERbeta, a variety of estrogens and anti-estrogens – including genistein and the drug raloxifene – have an antiproliferative, pro-apoptotic effect [192–195].

Genistein has been shown to decrease expression of the androgen receptor in the human prostate cancer-derived LNCaP cell line, an effect mediated by activation of ERbeta [196]. Moreover, soy phytochemical concentrates slow the growth of LNCaP in nude mice [195, 197, 198]. Genistein feeding likewise down-regulates androgen receptor expression in rat prostate [199], and reduces the yield of prostate cancer in carcinogen-treated rats as well as in transgenic "TRAMP" mice that have a high spontaneous incidence of this cancer [200, 201]. Pilot clinical studies evaluating the impact of oral genistein on early stage prostate cancer have achieved a moderate reduction of PSA in a minority of patients, and an apparent reduction in cancer growth rate in others [202, 203]. Case-control studies from the Orient are reasonably consistent with the thesis that diets high in soy products are associated with lower risk for prostate cancer [204–206] – albeit high soy intake may be a marker for diets and lifestyles that are more traditional.

Although the increased risk of breast cancer among women who use postmenopausal hormone replacement therapy (HRT) has occasioned considerable comment, less attention has been paid to evidence that current or recent use of HRT markedly decreases risk for colon cancer; a meta-analysis concludes that such therapy reduces colorectal cancer risk by about 30% [207, 208]. In light of the fact that colonic epithelium expresses ERbeta (but little ERalpha), it is reasonable to suspect that this protective effect is mediated by a direct estrogenic effect on this epithelium [209]. The possibility that an adequate dietary intake of soy isoflavones could provide comparable protection evidently merits consideration. Although epidemiological studies evaluating the association of soy consumption with colorectal cancer risk have yielded inconsistent results, some of these studies support a protective role for soy in this regard [210–214]. Moreover, dietary soy isoflavones have reduced colon cancer yields in some though not all rodent models of colon carcinogenesis [214–217].

Of related interest are recent studies correlating good vitamin D status with a decidedly lower risk for colorectal cancer [218, 219]. This phenomenon appears to reflect the fact that healthy colon epithelium expresses CYP27B1, the hydroxylase which converts 25-hydroxycholecalciferol to the active hormone calcitriol [220]; since circulating levels of 25-hydroxycholesterol are reflective of vitamin D status (unlike circulating calcitriol levels), it follows that that good vitamin D status should be associated with increased calcitriol production in colonic epithelium [221]. However, increased vitamin D activity provokes a compensatory up-regulation of CYP24, which eliminates calcitriol's hormonal activity by catalyzing its 24-hydroxylation. There is now evidence that estrogenic (ERbeta) activity in colonic epithelial cells or colorectal cancers promotes increased vitamin D activity in these cells by boosting the expression of CYP27B1, while decreasing the expression of CYP24; this phenomenon has demonstrated in the colonic epithelium of mice fed genistein or isoflavone-rich soy protein [222]. These considerations suggest that dietary soy isoflavones might potentiate the protective impact of good vitamin D status on colorectal cancer risk. A similar phenomenon may obtain in breast and prostate tissue, as genistein can modulate CYP27B1 and CYP24 expression in an analogous way in human mammary and prostate cells [222].

ISOFLAVONES AND THE BREAST – SAFE AND POSSIBLY PROTECTIVE

How dietary soy isoflavones influence breast cancer risk is also a matter of considerable interest. In the normal human breast, both types of estrogen receptor are expressed in epithelial cells [223]; ERbeta predominates in adult human mammary fibroblasts [224]. In ERalpha-knockout mice, the breast is atrophic; conversely, in ERbeta-knockout mice, epithelium is hyperproliferative and the mice are prone to severe cystic breast disease as they age [225, 226]. Transfection of ERbeta into an ERalpha-expressing human breast cancer cell line (MCF-7) results in a suppression of proliferation associated with up-regulation of cdk inhibitors p21 and p27, and down-regulation of c-myc and cyclins D1 and A; however, these effects are only partially ligand dependent [227]. ERbeta transfection also slows the estrogen-stimulated growth of the estrogen-sensitive T47D mammary cancer cell line [228], but has a pro-proliferative impact on the MDA-MB-435 tumor [229]. In the main, these findings suggest that ERalpha and ERbeta may have a "yin-yang" role in breast development, with ERbeta opposing the proliferative impact of ERalpha; however, they do not necessarily imply that ERbeta-specific ligands will have an antiproliferative effect.

ERbeta is expressed by the majority of human breast cancers – even those considered "estrogen negative" [230, 231]; the standard assays for breast cancer "estrogen receptors" are ERalpha-specific. The prognostic significance of ERbeta expression in breast cancer has been the subject of conflicting reports [227].

A number of studies have examined the impact of soy isoflavones on breast cancer risk or growth in rodents, but some of these are of limited interest owing to their use of high-parenteral doses that would likely have ERalpha-agonist activity. High-dose genistein, administered pre-pubertally, induces a premature differentiation of breast tissue that diminishes susceptibility of adult rats to carcinogen-induced breast cancer [232–234]; this effect is also seen with estrogen administration, and there is no evidence that physiological levels of genistein could achieve a comparable effect. There are however several studies which conclude that more modest intakes of genistein can favorably influence breast cancer induction. When administered at 250 mg/kg diet, either genistein or daidzein was found to slow the onset of breast cancer in cancer-prone MMTV-neu mice; however, they did not influence the growth of established tumors [235]. A functional food rich in unconjugated genistein slowed the growth of the MDA-MB-231 human breast cancer in nude mice; this was associated with increased apoptosis in the tumor [236]. In the mouse mammary tumor virus-induced spontaneous breast cancer model, oral administration of biochanin A – but not daidzein – reduced tumor incidence at 15 months; this effect was not seen in germ-free animals, and thus presumably was contingent on conversion of biochanin A to genistein by intestinal bacteria [237].

On the other hand, a number of studies show that dietary genistein can increase the growth of estrogen-dependent MCF-7 tumors in ovariectomized nude mice; this effect appears to hinge on activation of ERalpha [238–241]. This cell line seems to be exquisitely sensitive to ERalpha activation, inasmuch as genistein concentrations as low as 10 nM can modestly increase its rate of proliferation *in vitro* [238, 242]. Nonetheless, a much more substantial response is seen with genistein concentrations in the high nanomolar range, consistent with the known affinity of genistein for ERalpha; responsiveness at 10 nM presumably reflects that fact that activation of only a small minority of ERalpha receptors can have a discernible impact on proliferation in this cell line. Administered at 750 mg/kg of diet to rats pretreated with the carcinogen MNU, genistein increases the size of MNU-induced mammary tumors in ovariectomized rats [243]; this dose of genistein also increases uterus size, pointing to an ERalpha-mediated effect on estrogen-sensitive tumors. In DMBA-treated mice, 1 g/kg dietary genistein increases the yield of malignant adenocarcinomas – whereas no cancers develop with ERalpha-knockout mice [244]. Overall, these findings suggest that moderate intakes of genistein may slow the onset or progression of certain mammary tumors, but that very high intakes can be expected to boost the growth of estrogen-dependent tumors, and even moderate intakes may have the potential to at least modestly influence the growth of certain tumors that are highly sensitive to ERalpha activation.

The impact of soyfood ingestion on breast cancer incidence has been examined in a number of case-control as well as prospective epidemiological studies. Although many of these studies find no link between breast cancer and soy consumption [245–249], four case-control studies found an inverse association between soy intake and risk for premenopausal breast cancer in Asian populations, and two such studies found a similar association with postmenopausal breast cancer [250–254]. One recent prospective Japanese study found that high intakes of miso or of isoflavones – but not of soyfoods *per se* – were associated with decreased risk for pre- or postmenopausal breast cancer [255]. Other prospective studies have had a negative outcome. One case-control study in Asian-Americans focused on soy consumption during adolescence, and found that high soy intake during this time predicted a lower risk for postmenopausal breast cancer; such risk was lowest for those who maintained high soy consumption in adult life [254]. Given the fact that most Asian diets provide suboptimal isoflavone intakes from the standpoint of ERbeta activation, these findings are reasonably consistent with the possibility that somewhat higher supplemental intakes of genistein might be protective in regard to breast cancer risk; however, they certainly don't prove this proposition. A conservative but optimistic perspective is that, as contrasted with HRT, there is little reason to suspect that genistein intakes in the high *nutritional* range would *increase* breast cancer risk – and some reason to suspect that such a measure might decrease this risk.

On the other hand, in women who have been diagnosed with estrogen-sensitive breast cancers, the possibility cannot be excluded that nutritional intakes of genistein will modestly boost cancer growth by promoting low-level activation of ERalpha. Theoretically, selective activation of ERbeta with moderate-dose genistein might slow the growth of certain estrogen-sensitive mammary cancers which express this receptor – but this is speculative. Until further evidence is forthcoming, it might be prudent for women with estrogen-sensitive breast cancer to refrain from frequent soy ingestion or isoflavone supplementation.

MODESTLY EFFECTIVE FOR HOT FLASHES

A number of clinical studies have assessed the impact of supplemental soy isoflavones – with or without soy protein – on postmenopausal hot flashes. A recent overview notes that four of these studies had a positive outcome, five were negative, and one showed a positive trend that missed statistical significance [256]. This overview could not include a more recent study by Squadrito and colleagues [257]. These researchers nested a hot flash study into their bone metabolism study by enrolling only women who were troubled by this complication; since this study achieved free genistein concentrations sufficient to benefit bone metabolism, and since it included an HRT arm, its findings may be particularly illuminating. At baseline, the daily hot flash score was very similar in the three groups, averaging 4.5–4.7/day. After 3 months, as contrasted with the placebo group, this score was 22% lower in the genistein group and 53% lower in the HRT group; these differences were statistically significant. The findings at 12 months were similar – relative to placebo response, the score was 24% lower with genistein and 54% lower with HRT. Response to HRT was significantly greater than that to genistein.

The available findings appear consistent with the proposition that soy isoflavone regimens which achieve an adequate plasma level of free genistein are mildly beneficial with respect to hot flashes – though less effective in this regard than HRT. The inconsistency of the results of clinical studies examining this issue, may reflect the fact that the benefit to be expected is modest, as well as the likelihood that some of the isoflavone regimens tested failed to achieve adequate free genistein concentrations in some subjects. It seems highly unlikely that about half of the clinical studies to date examining this issue would find statistically significant benefit, if in fact isoflavones had no genuine potential for controlling hot flashes. Soy isoflavones have access to the brain, and certain regions of the hypothalamus express ERbeta [258–260]; conceivably, some of these receptors mediate the impact of genistein on hot flashes.

POTENTIAL FOR PREVENTION OF GLOMERULOSCLEROSIS

Chronic renal disease, of either diabetic or non-diabetic origin, tends to progress less rapidly in women than in men [261–263]. The relative protection enjoyed by women appears to be confined to the premenopausal period, and thus is likely to be mediated by estrogen [263, 264]. Indeed, estrogen ameliorates, whereas ovariectomy exacerbates, the progression of glomerulosclerosis in various rodent models of this disorder [265–271]. Contrary findings have been reported in certain hyperlipidemic strains of rodents, presumably because estrogen treatment exacerbates nephrotoxic hyperlipidemia in these animals [272–275]; an estrogen-evoked increase in growth hormone secretion can also exert a countervailing negative effect in this regard [276–278]. However, these latter findings do not appear to be germane to the impact of endogenously produced estrogen in women.

The various agents and circumstances which provoke glomerulosclerosis – such as hyperglycemia, glomerular hypertension, angiotensin II, advanced glycation endproducts, thromboxane, and oxidized LDL – appear to do so by boosting glomerular production of transforming growth factor-beta (TGF-β); activation of AP-1 response elements in the TGF-β promoter, often in response to PKC/MAP kinase activation, plays a role in these inductions [279–292]. This increased autocrine/paracrine production of TGF-β, in turn, activates mesangial receptors for this hormone, leading to increased production of various ground substance proteins – including collagen types I and IV, laminin, and fibronectin – decreased production of the collagenases MMP-2 and MMP-9, and increased production of protease inhibitors such as TIMP-1 [293–303]; the net effect is an accumulation of mesangial ground substance and a thickening of glomerular basement membranes. TGF-β is also a mediator of the proteinuria characteristically seen in glomerular disorders [304–308]. Injection of anti-TGF-β antibodies into diabetic rodents can prevent and in some measure reverse glomerulosclerosis – demonstrating the central role of TGF-β in this syndrome [308–311].

Mesangial cells express both ERalpha and ERbeta [263, 312]; it is noteworthy that expression of both types of ER is diminished in this mesangial cells of a strain of mouse prone to glomerulosclerosis [263]. Physiological concentrations of estrogen have been shown to suppress the response of mesangial cells to TGF-β [313, 314]. This effect appears to reflect the ability of activated estrogen receptors of both types to bind to, and suppress the transactivating activity of, the transcription factor SMAD3 [315], whose phosphorylation and activation by TGF-β receptors mediates most effects of TGF-β [316] (not surprisingly, SMAD3-knockout mice are virtually immune to diabetic glomerulopathy) [307]. Moreover, estrogen can also suppress glomerular production of TGF-β, by boosting the NO production of glomerular endothelial cells [317]. NO's suppressive impact on TGF-β production is poorly understood; the fact that eNOS inhibitors up-regulate glomerular TGF-β synthesis suggests that this mechanism is of physiological significance. It does not appear to be known whether glomerular endothelial cells express ERbeta, or whether this receptor can enhance eNOS activity in these cells. A further theoretical possibility is that activated ERbeta could inhibit transcription of TGF-β by interfering with

AP-1 activity in its promoter; on the other hand, ERalpha would be expected to enhance AP-1 activity [15, 20]. In any case, there is reason to suspect that high-physiological concentrations of genistein, via activation of ERbeta, could inhibit the effects of TGF-β on mesangial cells, thereby helping to prevent glomerulosclerosis. Whether activation of ERbeta could also increase glomerular NO production and/or interfere with AP-1 activity – resulting in suppression of glomerular TGF-β production – is more speculative.

In fact, many rodent studies conclude that soy-based diets – in comparison to casein-based diets – are associated with slower progression of glomerulosclerosis [318–326]. Two recent clinical studies in type 2 diabetics likewise report that proteinuria is lower during soy protein supplementation than during casein supplementation [327, 328]. At least a portion of this effect reflects the fact that soy is of "poorer quality" than casein. It is well established that diets rich in "high quality" protein promote glomerulosclerosis by increasing glomerular pressure and thereby increasing glomerular filtration rate; this presumably represents a homeostatic response which helps the body to cope with increased nitrogenous waste [322, 329, 330]. Soy and other plant proteins have a less substantial effect in this regard [331–333]. Thus, diets low but adequate in protein content have been used clinically to slow the progression of glomerular disease [334, 335]; in particular, quasi-vegan diets, some featuring soy protein, have been used for this purpose [332, 336–339].

The possibility that phytochemical components of soy – such as isoflavones – contribute to the nephroprotection afforded by soy-based diets has been suggested by Valasquez and Bhathena [322, 340]. Indeed, a subsequent study with hypercholesterolemic rats prone to glomerulosclerosis demonstrated that addition of an isoflavone-rich soy ethanol extract to their casein-based diets ameliorated subsequent renal damage; the interpretation of this study is complicated by the fact that serum lipids declined in the isoflavone-supplemented rats [341]. Also of particular interest in this regard is a study by Neugarten and colleagues [342]. These researchers demonstrated that, in concentrations as low as 1–10 nM, genistein markedly inhibits synthesis of both type I and type IV collagen by murine mesangial cells; the authors propose that ERbeta mediates this effect. Conceivably, this finding simply reflects the fact that genistein-activated ERbeta can block the impact of autocrine TGF-β on mesangial cells [315]. Whether physiological concentrations of genistein can also influence glomerular production of TGF-β remains to be seen. Of related interest is a report that a diet supplemented with red clover isoflavones decreases production of TGF-β by prostatic epithelium in mice [343].

If subsequent animal and clinical studies prove that soy isoflavones can indeed reduce risk for, or slow progression of, glomerulosclerosis, it won't necessarily follow that a diet high in soy protein should be recommended. Most likely, the most nephroprotective diet will be a vegan diet relatively low in protein content, supplemented with soy isoflavones. In this regard, adding soy protein to a diet already rich in casein did not protect hypercholesterolemic rats from glomerular injury – albeit addition of a comparable surplus of casein exacerbated this injury [324].

POTENTIAL FOR PREVENTION OF LEFT VENTRICULAR HYPERTROPHY AND HEPATIC FIBROSIS

The intracellular signaling mechanisms which mediate left ventricular hypertrophy (LVH) appear to be very similar to those that evoke glomerulosclerosis [344, 345]; moreover, NO has an antagonistic impact on development of LVH analogous to its impact on glomerulosclerosis [346]. Premenopausal women are relatively protected from LVH, and estrogen replacement has been shown to limit expansion of ventricular mass in postmenopausal women and ovariectomized rodents at risk for this disorder [347–354]. Cardiac myocytes and fibroblasts express both isoforms of the estrogen receptor, but, in neonatal rat cardiac myocytes, only ERbeta has an inductive effect on eNOS [355, 356]. A very recent study examining ERalpha- and ERbeta-knockout mice demonstrates that ERbeta mediates the protective effect of estrogen on cardiac hypertrophy [357]. Thus, it is reasonable to suspect that genistein has the potential to protect postmenopausal women, and possibly men, from LVH.

There is growing epidemiological evidence that premenopausal women afflicted with fibrogenic liver diseases such as hepatitis C are at lower risk for fibrosis and cirrhosis than are postmenopausal women or men with this disorder; furthermore, in postmenopausal women with hepatitis C, concurrent hormone replacement therapy is associated with slower progression of fibrosis [358–360]. This conclusion accords well with studies demonstrating that administration of estrogen or of estrogenic drugs attenuates hepatic fibrosis in rodents treated with hepatotoxic agents – whereas ovariectomy has the opposite effect [360–364]. A likely site of estrogen's action in this regard is the hepatic stellate cell, which, in response to numerous hepatotoxic agents, converts to a myofibroblast phenotype and proliferates, depositing the excessive collagen and other ground substance proteins observed in hepatic fibrosis [365]. *In vitro*, estrogen suppresses the proliferation and activation of stellate cells induced by various agents [360, 366, 367]. In aggregate, these findings have prompted suggestions that postmenopausal women with hepatitis C or other fibrogenic liver disorders should be treated with hormone replacement therapy (HRT) [358, 359].

Studies with cultured rat hepatic stellate cells have concluded that these cells do in fact express estrogen receptors – but these receptors are of the beta isoform; these cells do not express ERalpha [368]. Thus, the antifibrogenic hepatic effects of estrogen are likely to be mediated by ERbeta receptors. It is therefore reasonable to suspect that soy isoflavones could have potential for prevention of hepatic fibrosis. Indeed, Chinese researchers have demonstrated that concentrations of genistein as low as 10 nM reduce the basal and PDGF-induced proliferation of stellate cells in culture, while also inhibiting their transformation to a myofibroblast phenotype – that is blocking α-smooth muscle actin expression

[369]. (While these investigators interpreted this effect as reflecting genistein's tyrosine kinase inhibitory activity, such activity in fact require micromolar concentrations of genistein that are of no physiological relevance [370].) To date, there do not appear to be any published studies evaluating the impact of soy phytoestrogens or soy-rich diets on hepatic fibrosis in rodents. Nor have epidemiological studies examined the impact of soy-rich diets on susceptibility to hepatic fibrosis in humans.

DIRECTIONS FOR FUTURE RESEARCH

The thesis that ERbeta mediates the favorable physiological effects of moderate-dose isoflavones on bone metabolism and endothelial function can best be tested in ovariectomized ERbeta knockout rodents, using dietary concentrations of isoflavones that will achieve a free genistein plasma concentration not in excess of 50 nM. If these effects largely persist in the ERbeta knockouts, the thesis of this chapter will be falsified, and it will be necessary to identify further molecular targets that respond to free isoflavones in the low nanomolar range. In light of current evidence, however, the contention that ERbeta is the key target of dietary isoflavones is credible and brings a satisfying unity to the diverse research literature on these compounds.

The fact that clinical studies with soy isoflavone supplementation have yielded inconsistent results may reflect, at least in part, variations in the plasma levels of free genistein (and possibly equol) achieved by the diverse supplementation regimens that have been assessed. Is genistin truly as effective as equimolar intakes of genistein during long-term administration in most subjects? Or do variations in GI metabolism of genistin render supplementation with genistein a more fail-safe proposition? Too few studies have assessed the long-term impact of various isoflavone regimens on equilibrium concentrations of free genistein; we should bear in mind that acute pharmacokinetic studies do not take into account possible adaptive changes in enzyme expression that could influence achieved plasma levels. In light of the markedly beneficial effects on endothelial function and bone metabolism achieved by Squadrito *et al.* with 54 mg genistein daily, efforts to confirm these results in larger and more diverse populations are clearly warranted.

As a safer substitute for HRT in postmenopausal women, supplemental genistein would appear to have great promise; in Squadrito's studies, the impact of supplemental genistein on endothelium and bone was fully comparable to that of HRT, and the relief from hot flashes noted was worthwhile though less substantial. Whether premenopausal women would benefit is less clear, since the impact of genistein on endothelium or bone may be modest compared to that of ambient estrogen levels. However, the epidemiological and rodent literature provides just a hint that, by shifting the balance toward ERbeta activity in mammary tissue, premenopausal soy isoflavone ingestion may in fact be protective in regard to breast cancer risk. In this regard, more rodent chemoprevention studies, using moderate genistein doses that will selectively activate ERbeta, would be desirable; in regard to epidemiology, more attention should be focused on the possible impact of adolescent isoflavone intake on subsequent breast cancer risk.

Could supplemental genistein improve endothelial function and bone metabolism in men? Too few studies have examined this issue to allow any conclusions to be drawn. However, even if genistein cannot protect men in these respects, its likely favorable impact on risk for prostate cancer (and possibly colorectal cancer as well) may make genistein supplementation a very worthwhile option for men. Ongoing clinical studies with genistein in early prostate cancer may shed further light on this issue. The fact that ERbeta expression tends to be lost as prostate cancer progresses probably means that, as a therapy for pre-existing prostate cancer, genistein will have at best transient efficacy; thus, its greater potential may be for chemoprevention.

With respect to expectations that isoflavone-rich diets may decrease risk for certain common cancers, a proviso is in order. Commentators frequently note that risks for certain "Western" cancers are comparatively low in East Asian cultures which make frequent use of soy products. However, these rates are equally low in many other Third World rural societies in Africa and South America where soy consumption is minimal [371–373]. The traditional diets of these societies tend to be low in fat and animal products, and moderate in total protein; lifelong consumption of such diets is likely to be associated with reduced serum levels of insulin and of free IGF-I – now known to have important cancer promotional activity [374–376]. High intakes of soy protein can actually boost serum IGF-I [377–379]; thus, heavy use of soy protein *per se* may be inadvisable from the standpoint of cancer risk. These considerations suggest that ample intakes of soy isoflavones may best be achieved through supplementation rather than through heavy consumption of protein-rich soy products. Furthermore, we should take care not to encourage the delusion that simply adding soy products – or soy isoflavones – to a meat-rich omnivore diet will reproduce the full measure of cancer protection associated with quasi-vegan Third World diets. The popular focus on soy protein runs the risk of obscuring the broader and deeper truth that diets featuring "low quality" plant protein can have an important anti-promotional impact on many types of cancer [376, 380, 381].

ACKNOWLEDGMENT

This chapter is an update and expansion of a review originally published in the journal *Medical Hypotheses* [382].

REFERENCES

1. Kuiper, G. G., Enmark, E., Pelto-Huikko, M., Nilsson, S. & Gustafsson, J. A. (1996 June 11). Cloning of a novel receptor expressed in rat prostate and ovary. *Proc Natl Acad Sci USA.* **93**(12), 5925–5930.

2. Kuiper, G. G. & Gustafsson, J. A. (1997 June 23). The novel estrogen receptor-beta subtype: Potential role in the cell- and promoter-specific actions of estrogens and anti-estrogens. *FEBS Lett* **410**(1), 87–90.

3. Kuiper, G. G., Carlsson, B., Grandien, K., Enmark, E., Haggblad, J., Nilsson, S. & Gustafsson, J. A. (1997). Comparison of the ligand binding specificity and transcript tissue distribution of estrogen receptors alpha and beta. *Endocrinology* **138**(3), 863–870.

4. Kuiper, G. G., Lemmen, J. G., Carlsson, B., Corton, J. C., Safe, S. H., van der Saag, P. T., van Der, B. B. & Gustafsson, J. A. (1998). Interaction of estrogenic chemicals and phytoestrogens with estrogen receptor beta. *Endocrinology* **139**(10), 4252–4263.

5. Barkhem, T., Carlsson, B., Nilsson, Y., Enmark, E., Gustafsson, J. & Nilsson, S. (1998). Differential response of estrogen receptor alpha and estrogen receptor beta to partial estrogen agonists/antagonists. *Mol Pharmacol* **54**(1), 105–112.

6. Routledge, E. J., White, R., Parker, M. G. & Sumpter, J. P. (2000 Nov 17). Differential effects of xenoestrogens on coactivator recruitment by estrogen receptor (ER) alpha and ERbeta. *J Biol Chem* **275**(46), 35986–35993.

7. An, J., Tzagarakis-Foster, C., Scharschmidt, T. C., Lomri, N. & Leitman, D. C. (2001 May 25). Estrogen receptor beta-selective transcriptional activity and recruitment of coregulators by phytoestrogens. *J Biol Chem* **276**(21), 17808–17814.

8. Morito, K., Hirose, T., Kinjo, J., Hirakawa, T., Okawa, M., Nohara, T., Ogawa, S., Inoue, S., Muramatsu, M. & Masamune, Y. (2001). Interaction of phytoestrogens with estrogen receptors alpha and beta. *Biol Pharm Bull* **24**(4), 351–356.

9. Liu, J., Knappenberger, K. S., Kack, H., Andersson, G., Nilsson, E., Dartsch, C. & Scott, C. W. (2003). A homogeneous *in vitro* functional assay for estrogen receptors: Coactivator recruitment. *Mol Endocrinol* **17**(3), 346–355.

10. Muthyala, R. S., Ju, Y. H., Sheng, S., Williams, L. D., Doerge, D. R., Katzenellenbogen, B. S., Helferich, W. G. & Katzenellenbogen, J. A. (2004 Mar 15). Equol, a natural estrogenic metabolite from soy isoflavones: Convenient preparation and resolution of R- and S-equols and their differing binding and biological activity through estrogen receptors alpha and beta. *Bioorg Med Chem* **12**(6), 1559–1567.

11. Bovee, T. F., Helsdingen, R. J., Rietjens, I. M., Keijer, J. & Hoogenboom, R. L. (2004). Rapid yeast estrogen bioassays stably expressing human estrogen receptors alpha and beta, and green fluorescent protein: A comparison of different compounds with both receptor types. *J Steroid Biochem Mol Biol* **91**(3), 99–109.

12. Mueller, S. O., Simon, S., Chae, K., Metzler, M. & Korach, K. S. (2004). Phytoestrogens and their human metabolites show distinct agonistic and antagonistic properties on estrogen receptor alpha (ERalpha) and ERbeta in human cells. *Toxicol Sci* **80**(1), 14–25.

13. Kostelac, D., Rechkemmer, G. & Briviba, K. (2003 Dec 17). Phytoestrogens modulate binding response of estrogen receptors alpha and beta to the estrogen response element. *J Agric Food Chem* **51**(26), 7632–7635.

14. Kurebayashi, S., Miyashita, Y., Hirose, T., Kasayama, S., Akira, S. & Kishimoto, T. (1997). Characterization of mechanisms of interleukin-6 gene repression by estrogen receptor. *J Steroid Biochem Mol Biol* **60**(1–2), 11–17.

15. Paech, K., Webb, P., Kuiper, G. G., Nilsson, S., Gustafsson, J., Kushner, P. J. & Scanlan, T. S. (1997 Sept 5). Differential ligand activation of estrogen receptors ERalpha and ERbeta at AP1 sites. *Science* **277**(5331), 1508–1510.

16. Saville, B., Wormke, M., Wang, F., Nguyen, T., Enmark, E., Kuiper, G., Gustafsson, J. A. & Safe, S. (2000 Feb 25). Ligand-, cell-, and estrogen receptor subtype (alpha/beta)-dependent activation at GC-rich (Sp1) promoter elements. *J Biol Chem* **275**(8), 5379–5387.

17. Sabbah, M., Courilleau, D., Mester, J. & Redeuilh, G. (1999 Sept 28). Estrogen induction of the cyclin D1 promoter: Involvement of a cAMP response-like element. *Proc Natl Acad Sci U S A* **96**(20), 11217–11222.

18. Kushner, P. J., Agard, D. A., Greene, G. L., Scanlan, T. S., Shiau, A. K., Uht, R. M. & Webb, P. (2000 Nov 30). Estrogen receptor pathways to AP-1. *J Steroid Biochem Mol Biol* **74**(5), 311–317.

19. Wu, J. J., Geimonen, E. & Andersen, J. (2000). Increased expression of estrogen receptor beta in human uterine smooth muscle at term. *Eur J Endocrinol* **142**(1), 92–99.

20. Maruyama, S., Fujimoto, N., Asano, K. & Ito, A. (2001). Suppression by estrogen receptor beta of AP-1 mediated transactivation through estrogen receptor alpha. *J Steroid Biochem Mol Biol* **78**(2), 177–184.

21. Liu, M. M., Albanese, C., Anderson, C. M., Hilty, K., Webb, P., Uht, R. M., Price, R. H., Jr., Pestell, R. G. & Kushner, P. J. (2002 Jul 5). Opposing action of estrogen receptors alpha and beta on cyclin D1 gene expression. *J Biol Chem* **277**(27), 24353–24360.

22. Kanda, N. & Watanabe, S. (2003). 17Beta-estradiol inhibits MCP-1 production in human keratinocytes. *J Invest Dermatol* **120**(6), 1058–1066.

23. Adlercreutz, H., Markkanen, H. & Watanabe, S. (1993 Nov 13). Plasma concentrations of phyto-oestrogens in Japanese men. *Lancet* **342**(8881), 1209–1210.

24. Adlercreutz, H., Fotsis, T., Lampe, J., Wahala, K., Makela, T., Brunow, G. & Hase, T. (1993). Quantitative determination of lignans and isoflavonoids in plasma of omnivorous and vegetarian women by isotope dilution gas chromatography-mass spectrometry. *Scand J Clin Lab Invest Suppl* **215**, 5–18.

25. Setchell, K. D., Brown, N. M., Desai, P., Zimmer-Nechemias, L., Wolfe, B. E., Brashear, W. T., Kirschner, A. S., Cassidy, A. & Heubi, J. E. (2001). Bioavailability of pure isoflavones in healthy humans and analysis of commercial soy isoflavone supplements. *J Nutr* **131**(4 Suppl), 1362S–1375S.

26. Doerge, D. R., Chang, H. C., Churchwell, M. I. & Holder, C. L. (2000). Analysis of soy isoflavone conjugation *in vitro* and in human blood using liquid chromatography-mass spectrometry. *Drug Metab Dispos* **28**(3), 298–307.

27. Morabito, N., Crisafulli, A., Vergara, C., Gaudio, A., Lasco, A., Frisina, N., D'Anna, R., Corrado, F., Pizzoleo, M. A., Cincotta, M., Altavilla, D., Ientile, R. & Squadrito, F. (2002). Effects of genistein and hormone-replacement therapy on bone loss in early postmenopausal women: A randomized double-blind placebo-controlled study. *J Bone Miner Res* **17**(10), 1904–1912.

28. Lapcik, O., Hampl, R., Hill, M., Wahala, K., Maharik, N. A. & Adlercreutz, H. (1998). Radioimmunoassay of free genistein in human serum. *J Steroid Biochem Mol Biol* **64**(5–6), 261–268.

29. Nagel, S. C., vom Saal, F. S. & Welshons, W. V. (1998). The effective free fraction of estradiol and xenoestrogens in human serum measured by whole cell uptake assays: Physiology of delivery modifies estrogenic activity. *Proc Soc Exp Biol Med* **217**(3), 300–309.

30. Setchell, K. D., Brown, N. M. & Lydeking-Olsen, E. (2002). The clinical importance of the metabolite equol-a clue to the effectiveness of soy and its isoflavones. *J Nutr* **132**(12), 3577–3584.

31. Yuan, J. P., Wang, J. H. & Liu, X. (2007). Metabolism of dietary soy isoflavones to equol by human intestinal microflora – implications for health. *Mol Nutr Food Res* **51**(7), 765–781.

32. Setchell, K. D., Clerici, C., Lephart, E. D., Cole, S. J., Heenan, C., Castellani, D., Wolfe, B. E., Nechemias-Zimmer, L., Brown, N. M., Lund, T. D., Handa, R. J. & Heubi, J. E. (2005). *S*-Equol, a potent ligand for estrogen receptor beta, is the exclusive enantiomeric form of the soy isoflavone metabolite produced by human intestinal bacterial flora. *Am J Clin Nutr* **81**(5), 1072–1079.

33. Muthyala, R. S., Ju, Y. H., Sheng, S., Williams, L. D., Doerge, D. R., Katzenellenbogen, B. S., Helferich, W. G. & Katzenellenbogen, J. A. (2004 Mar 15). Equol, a natural estrogenic metabolite from soy isoflavones: Convenient preparation and resolution of R- and S-equols and their differing binding and biological activity through estrogen receptors alpha and beta. *Bioorg Med Chem* **12**(6), 1559–1567.

34. Vedrine, N., Mathey, J., Morand, C., Brandolini, M., Davicco, M. J., Guy, L., Remesy, C., Coxam, V. & Manach, C. (2006). One-month exposure to soy isoflavones did not induce the ability to produce equol in postmenopausal women. *Eur J Clin Nutr* **60**(9), 1039–1045.

35. Wu, J., Oka, J., Ezaki, J., Ohtomo, T., Ueno, T., Uchiyama, S., Toda, T., Uehara, M. & Ishimi, Y. (2007). Possible role of equol status in the effects of isoflavone on bone and fat mass in postmenopausal Japanese women: A double-blind, randomized, controlled trial. *Menopause* **14**(5), 866–874.

36. Vatanparast, H. & Chilibeck, P. D. (2007). Does the effect of soy phytoestrogens on bone in postmenopausal women depend on the equol-producing phenotype? *Nutr Rev* **65**(6 Pt 1), 294–299.

37. Setchell, K. D. & Cole, S. J. (2006). Method of defining equol-producer status and its frequency among vegetarians. *J Nutr* **136**(8), 2188–2193.

38. Akiyama, T., Ishida, J., Nakagawa, S., Ogawara, H., Watanabe, S., Itoh, N., Shibuya, M. & Fukami, Y. (1987 Apr 25). Genistein, a specific inhibitor of tyrosine-specific protein kinases. *J Biol Chem* **262**(12), 5592–5595.

39. Markovits, J., Linassier, C., Fosse, P., Couprie, J., Pierre, J., Jacquemin-Sablon, A., Saucier, J. M., Le Pecq, J. B. & Larsen, A. K. (1989 Sept 15). Inhibitory effects of the tyrosine kinase inhibitor genistein on mammalian DNA topoisomerase II. *Cancer Res* **49**(18), 5111–5117.

40. Suetsugi, M., Su, L., Karlsberg, K., Yuan, Y. C. & Chen, S. (2003). Flavone and isoflavone phytoestrogens are agonists of estrogen-related receptors. *Mol Cancer Res* **1**(13), 981–991.

41. Pau, C. Y., Pau, K. Y. & Spies, H. G. (1998 Nov 25). Putative estrogen receptor beta and alpha mRNA expression in male and female rhesus macaques. *Mol Cell Endocrinol* **146**(1–2), 59–68.

42. Alvaro, D., Alpini, G., Onori, P., Perego, L., Svegliata, B. G., Franchitto, A., Baiocchi, L., Glaser, S. S., Le Sage, G., Folli, F. & Gaudio, E. (2000). Estrogens

stimulate proliferation of intrahepatic biliary epithelium in rats. *Gastroenterology* **119**(6), 1681–1691.

43. Taylor, A. H. & Al Azzawi, F. (2000). Immunolocalisation of oestrogen receptor beta in human tissues. *J Mol Endocrinol* **24**(1), 145–155.

44. Pelletier, G. (2000). Localization of androgen and estrogen receptors in rat and primate tissues. *Histol Histopathol* **15**(4), 1261–1270.

45. Hillisch, A., Peters, O., Kosemund, D., Muller, G., Walter, A., Schneider, B., Reddersen, G., Elger, W. & Fritzemeier, K. H. (2004). Dissecting physiological roles of estrogen receptor alpha and beta with potent selective ligands from structure-based design. *Mol Endocrinol* **18**(7), 1599–1609.

46. Vehkavaara, S., Silveira, A., Hakala-Ala-Pietila, T., Virkamaki, A., Hovatta, O., Hamsten, A., Taskinen, M. R. & Yki-Jarvinen, H. (2001). Effects of oral and transdermal estrogen replacement therapy on markers of coagulation, fibrinolysis, inflammation and serum lipids and lipoproteins in postmenopausal women. *Thromb Haemost* **85**(4), 619–625.

47. Hemelaar, M., van der Mooren, M. J., Mijatovic, V., Bouman, A. A., Schijf, C. P., Kroeks, M. V., Franke, H. R. & Kenemans, P. (2003). Oral, more than transdermal, estrogen therapy improves lipids and lipoprotein(a) in postmenopausal women: A randomized, placebo-controlled study. *Menopause* **10**(6), 550–558.

48. Nanda, S., Gupta, N., Mehta, H. C. & Sangwan, K. (2003). Effect of oestrogen replacement therapy on serum lipid profile. *Aust N Z J Obstet Gynaecol* **43**(3), 213–216.

49. Schunkert, H., Danser, A. H., Hense, H. W., Derkx, F. H., Kurzinger, S. & Riegger, G. A. (1997 Jan 7). Effects of estrogen replacement therapy on the renin-angiotensin system in postmenopausal women. *Circulation* **95**(1), 39–45.

50. Helle, S. I., Omsjo, I. H., Hughes, S. C., Botta, L., Huls, G., Holly, J. M. & Lonning, P. E. (1996). Effects of oral and transdermal oestrogen replacement therapy on plasma levels of insulin-like growth factors and IGF binding proteins 1 and 3: A cross-over study. *Clin Endocrinol (Oxf)* **45**(6), 727–732.

51. Paassilta, M., Karjalainen, A., Kervinen, K., Savolainen, M. J., Heikkinen, J., Backstrom, A. C. & Kesaniemi, Y. A. (2000). Insulin-like growth factor binding protein-1 (IGFBP-1) and IGF-I during oral and transdermal estrogen replacement therapy: Relation to lipoprotein(a) levels. *Atherosclerosis* **149**(1), 157–162.

52. Cardim, H. J., Lopes, C. M., Giannella-Neto, D., da Fonseca, A. M. & Pinotti, J. A. (2001). The insulin-like growth factor-I system and hormone replacement therapy. *Fertil Steril* **75**(2), 282–287.

53. Biglia, N., Ambroggio, S., Ponzone, R., Sgro, L., Ujcic, E., Dato, F. A. & Sismondi, P. (2003 Aug 20). Modification of serum IGF-I, IGFBPs and SHBG levels by different HRT regimens. *Maturitas* **45**(4), 283–291.

54. Scarabin, P. Y., Alhenc-Gelas, M., Plu-Bureau, Taisne, P., Agher, R. & Aiach, M. (1997). Effects of oral and transdermal estrogen/progesterone regimens on blood coagulation and fibrinolysis in postmenopausal women. A randomized controlled trial. *Arterioscler Thromb Vasc Biol* **17**(11), 3071–3078.

55. Lowe, G. D., Upton, M. N., Rumley, A., McConnachie, A., O'Reilly, D. S. & Watt, G. C. (2001). Different effects of oral and transdermal hormone replacement therapies on factor IX, APC resistance, t-PA, PAI and C-reactive protein: A cross-sectional population survey. *Thromb Haemost* **86**(2), 550–556.

56. Lowe, G. D. (2002). Hormone replacement therapy: Prothrombotic vs. protective effects. *Pathophysiol Haemost Thromb* **32**(5–6), 329–332.

57. Post, M. S., Christella, M., Thomassen, L. G., van der Mooren, M. J., van Baal, W. M., Rosing, J., Kenemans, P. & Stehouwer, C. D. (2003 June 1). Effect of oral and transdermal estrogen replacement therapy on hemostatic variables associated with venous thrombosis: A randomized, placebo-controlled study in postmenopausal women. *Arterioscler Thromb Vasc Biol* **23**(6), 1116–1121.

58. Oger, E., Alhenc-Gelas, M., Lacut, K., Blouch, M. T., Roudaut, N., Kerlan, V., Collet, M., Abgrall, J. F., Aiach, M., Scarabin, P. Y. & Mottier, D. (2003 Sept 1). Differential effects of oral and transdermal estrogen/progesterone regimens on sensitivity to activated protein C among postmenopausal women: A randomized trial. *Arterioscler Thromb Vasc Biol* **23**(9), 1671–1676.

59. Scarabin, P. Y., Oger, E. & Plu-Bureau, (2003 Aug 9). Differential association of oral and transdermal oestrogen-replacement therapy with venous thromboembolism risk. *Lancet* **362**(9382), 428–432.

60. Greaves, K. A., Parks, J. S., Williams, J. K. & Wagner, J. D. (1999). Intact dietary soy protein, but not adding an isoflavone-rich soy extract to casein, improves plasma lipids in ovariectomized cynomolgus monkeys. *J Nutr* **129**(8), 1585–1592.

61. Lichtenstein, A. H., Jalbert, S. M., Adlercreutz, H., Goldin, B. R., Rasmussen, H., Schaefer, E. J. & Ausman, L. M. (2002 Nov 1). Lipoprotein response to diets high in soy or animal protein with and without isoflavones in moderately hypercholesterolemic subjects. *Arterioscler Thromb Vasc Biol* **22**(11), 1852–1858.

62. Weggemans, R. M. & Trautwein, E. A. (2003). Relation between soy-associated isoflavones and LDL and HDL cholesterol concentrations in humans: A meta-analysis. *Eur J Clin Nutr* **57**(8), 940–946.

63. Demonty, I., Lamarche, B. & Jones, P. J. (2003). Role of isoflavones in the hypocholesterolemic effect of soy. *Nutr Rev* **61**(6 Pt 1), 189–203.

64. Adams, K. F., Newton, K. M., Chen, C., Emerson, S. S., Potter, J. D., White, E. & Lampe, J. W. (2003). Soy isoflavones do not modulate circulating insulin-like growth factor concentrations in an older population in an intervention trial. *J Nutr* **133**(5), 1316–1319.

65. Teede, H. J., Dalais, F. S. & McGrath, B. P. (2004). Dietary soy containing phytoestrogens does not have detectable estrogenic effects on hepatic protein synthesis in postmenopausal women. *Am J Clin Nutr* **79**(3), 396–401.

66. Wang, H. H., Afdhal, N. H. & Wang, D. Q. (2004). Estrogen receptor alpha, but not beta, plays a major role in 17beta-estradiol-induced murine cholesterol gallstones. *Gastroenterology* **127**(1), 239–249.

67. Carroll, K. K. (1982). Hypercholesterolemia and atherosclerosis: Effects of dietary protein. *Fed Proc* **41**(11), 2792–2796.

68. Sirtori, C. R., Gianazza, E., Manzoni, C., Lovati, M. R. & Murphy, P. A. (1997). Role of isoflavones in the cholesterol reduction by soy proteins in the clinic. *Am J Clin Nutr* **65**(1), 166–167.

69. Sirtori, C. R., Agradi, E., Conti, F., Mantero, O. & Gatti, E. (1977 Feb 5). Soybean-protein diet in the treatment of type-II hyperlipoproteinaemia. *Lancet* **1**(8006), 275–277.

70. Anderson, J. W., Johnstone, B. M. & Cook-Newell, M. E. (1995 Aug 3). Meta-analysis of the effects of soy protein intake on serum lipids [see comments]. *N Engl J Med* **333**(5), 276–282.

71. Shah, S. H. & Alexander, K. P. (2003). Hormone replacement therapy for primary and secondary prevention of heart disease. *Curr Treat Options Cardiovasc Med* **5**(1), 25–33.

72. Couse, J. F. & Korach, K. S. (2001). Contrasting phenotypes in reproductive tissues of female estrogen receptor null mice. *Ann N Y Acad Sci* **948**, 1–8.

73. Duncan, A. M., Underhill, K. E., Xu, X., Lavalleur, J., Phipps, W. R. & Kurzer, M. S. (1999). Modest hormonal effects of soy isoflavones in postmenopausal women. *J Clin Endocrinol Metab* **84**(10), 3479–3484.

74. Kurzer, M. S. (2002). Hormonal effects of soy in premenopausal women and men. *J Nutr* **132**(3), 570S–573S.

75. Balk, J. L., Whiteside, D. A., Naus, G., DeFerrari, E. & Roberts, J. M. (2002). A pilot study of the effects of phytoestrogen supplementation on postmenopausal endometrium. *J Soc Gynecol Investig* **9**(4), 238–242.

76. Penotti, M., Fabio, E., Modena, A. B., Rinaldi, M., Omodei, U. & Vigano, P. (2003). Effect of soy-derived isoflavones on hot flushes, endometrial thickness, and the pulsatility index of the uterine and cerebral arteries. *Fertil Steril* **79**(5), 1112–1117.

77. Sammartino, A., Di Carlo, C., Mandato, V. D., Bifulco, G., Di Stefano, M. & Nappi, C. (2003). Effects of genistein on the endometrium: Ultrasonographic evaluation. *Gynecol Endocrinol* **17**(1), 45–49.

78. Murray, M. J., Meyer, W. R., Lessey, B. A., Oi, R. H., DeWire, R. E. & Fritz, M. A. (2003). Soy protein isolate with isoflavones does not prevent estradiol-induced endometrial hyperplasia in postmenopausal women: A pilot trial. *Menopause* **10**(5), 456–464.

79. Santell, R. C., Chang, Y. C., Nair, M. G. & Helferich, W. G. (1997). Dietary genistein exerts estrogenic effects upon the uterus, mammary gland and the hypothalamic/pituitary axis in rats. *J Nutr* **127**(2), 263–269.

80. Chambliss, K. L. & Shaul, P. W. (2002). Estrogen modulation of endothelial nitric oxide synthase. *Endocr Rev* **23**(5), 665–686.

81. McNeill, A. M., Kim, N., Duckles, S. P., Krause, D. N. & Kontos, H. A. (1999). Chronic estrogen treatment increases levels of endothelial nitric oxide synthase protein in rat cerebral microvessels. *Stroke* **30**(10), 2186–2190.

82. Yang, S., Bae, L. & Zhang, L. (2000). Estrogen increases eNOS and NOx release in human coronary artery endothelium. *J Cardiovasc Pharmacol* **36**(2), 242–247.

83. Stirone, C., Chu, Y., Sunday, L., Duckles, S. P. & Krause, D. N. (2003 Sept 30). 17 Beta-estradiol increases endothelial nitric oxide synthase mRNA copy number in cerebral blood vessels: Quantification by real-time polymerase chain reaction. *Eur J Pharmacol* **478**(1), 35–38.

84. Haynes, M. P., Li, L., Sinha, D., Russell, K. S., Hisamoto, K., Baron, R., Collinge, M., Sessa, W. C. & Bender, J. R. (2003 Jan 24). Src kinase mediates phosphatidylinositol 3-kinase/Akt-dependent rapid endothelial nitric-oxide synthase activation by estrogen. *J Biol Chem* **278**(4), 2118–2123.

85. Chambliss, K. L., Yuhanna, I. S., Anderson, R. G., Mendelsohn, M. E. & Shaul, P. W. (2002). ERbeta has nongenomic action in caveolae. *Mol Endocrinol* **16**(5), 938–946.

86. Wagner, A. H., Schroeter, M. R. & Hecker, M. (2001). 17beta-estradiol inhibition of NADPH oxidase expression in human endothelial cells. *FASEB J* **15**(12), 2121–2130.

87. Evans, M. J., Harris, H. A., Miller, C. P., Karathanasis, S. K. & Adelman, S. J. (2002). Estrogen receptors alpha and beta have similar activities in multiple endothelial cell pathways. *Endocrinology* **143**(10), 3785–3795.

88. Rubanyi, G. M., Freay, A. D., Kauser, K., Sukovich, D., Burton, G., Lubahn, D. B., Couse, J. F., Curtis, S. W. & Korach, K. S. (1997 May 15). Vascular estrogen receptors and endothelium-derived nitric oxide production in the mouse aorta, Gender difference and effect of estrogen receptor gene disruption. *J Clin Invest* **99**(10), 2429–2437.

89. Tan, E., Gurjar, M. V., Sharma, R. V. & Bhalla, R. C. (1999 Aug 15). Estrogen receptor-alpha gene transfer into bovine aortic endothelial cells induces eNOS gene expression and inhibits cell migration. *Cardiovasc Res* **43**(3), 788–797.

90. Geary, G. G., McNeill, A. M., Ospina, J. A., Krause, D. N., Korach, K. S. & Duckles, S. P. (2001). Selected contribution: Cerebrovascular nos and cyclooxygenase are unaffected by estrogen in mice lacking estrogen receptor-alpha. *J Appl Physiol* **91**(5), 2391–2399.

91. Rubanyi, G. M., Kauser, K. & Johns, A. (2002). Role of estrogen receptors in the vascular system. *Vascul Pharmacol* **38**(2), 81–88.

92. Darblade, B., Pendaries, C., Krust, A., Dupont, S., Fouque, M. J., Rami, J., Chambon, P., Bayard, F. & Arnal, J. F. (2002 Mar 8). Estradiol alters nitric oxide production in the mouse aorta through the alpha-, but not beta-, estrogen receptor. *Circ Res* **90**(4), 413–419.

93. Widder, J., Pelzer, T., Poser-Klein, C., Hu, K., Jazbutyte, V., Fritzemeier, K. H., Hegele-Hartung, C., Neyses, L. & Bauersachs, J. (2003). Improvement of endothelial dysfunction by selective estrogen receptor-alpha stimulation in ovariectomized SHR. *Hypertension* **42**(5), 991–996.

94. Muller-Delp, J. M., Lubahn, D. B., Nichol, K. E., Philips, B. J., Price, E. M., Curran, E. M. & Laughlin, M. H. (2003). Regulation of nitric oxide-dependent vasodilation in coronary arteries of estrogen receptor-alpha-deficient mice. *Am J Physiol Heart Circ Physiol* **285**(5), H2150–H2157.

95. Nuedling, S., Karas, R. H., Mendelsohn, M. E., Katzenellenbogen, J. A., Katzenellenbogen, B. S., Meyer, R., Vetter, H. & Grohe, C. (2001 Aug 3). Activation of estrogen receptor beta is a prerequisite for estrogen-dependent upregulation of nitric oxide synthases in neonatal rat cardiac myocytes. *FEBS Lett* **502**(3), 103–108.

96. Kakui, K., Itoh, H., Sagawa, N., Yura, S., Korita, D., Takemura, M., Miyamoto, Y., Saito, Y., Nakao, K. & Fujii, S. (2004). Augmented endothelial nitric oxide synthase (eNOS) protein expression in human pregnant myometrium: Possible involvement of eNOS promoter activation by estrogen via both estrogen receptor (ER)alpha and ERbeta. *Mol Hum Reprod* **10**(2), 115–122.

97. Zhu, Y., Bian, Z., Lu, P., Karas, R. H., Bao, L., Cox, D., Hodgin, J., Shaul, P. W., Thoren, P., Smithies, O., Gustafsson, J. A. & Mendelsohn, M. E. (2002 Jan 18). Abnormal vascular function and hypertension in mice deficient in estrogen receptor beta. *Science* **295**(5554), 505–508.

98. Makela, S., Savolainen, H., Aavik, E., Myllarniemi, M., Strauss, L., Taskinen, E., Gustafsson, J. A. & Hayry, P. (1999 June 8). Differentiation between vasculoprotective and uterotrophic effects of ligands with different binding affinities to estrogen receptors alpha and beta. *Proc Natl Acad Sci U S A* **96**(12), 7077–7082.

99. Squadrito, F., Altavilla, D., Morabito, N., Crisafulli, A., D'Anna, R., Corrado, F., Ruggeri, P., Campo, G. M., Calapai, G., Caputi, A. P. & Squadrito, G. (2002). The effect of the phytoestrogen genistein on plasma nitric oxide concentrations, endothelin-1 levels and endothelium dependent vasodilation in postmenopausal women. *Atherosclerosis* **163**(2), 339–347.

100. Squadrito, F., Altavilla, D., Crisafulli, A., Saitta, A., Cucinotta, D., Morabito, N., D'Anna, R., Corrado, F., Ruggeri, P., Frisina, N. & Squadrito, G. (2003 Apr 15). Effect of genistein on endothelial function in postmenopausal women: A randomized, double-blind, controlled study. *Am J Med* **114**(6), 470–476.

101. Steinberg, F. M., Guthrie, N. L., Villablanca, A. C., Kumar, K. & Murray, M. J. (2003). Soy protein with isoflavones has favorable effects on endothelial function that are independent of lipid and antioxidant effects in healthy postmenopausal women. *Am J Clin Nutr* **78**(1), 123–130.

102. Lissin, L. W., Oka, R., Lakshmi, S. & Cooke, J. P. (2004). Isoflavones improve vascular reactivity in post-menopausal women with hypercholesterolemia. *Vasc Med* **9**(1), 26–30.

103. Vanhoutte, P. M. (2000 July 3). Say NO to ET. *J Auton Nerv Syst* **81**(1–3), 271–277.

104. Simons, L. A., Von Konigsmark, M., Simons, J. & Celermajer, D. S. (2000 June 1). Phytoestrogens do not influence lipoprotein levels or endothelial function in healthy, postmenopausal women. *Am J Cardiol* **85**(11), 1297–1301.

105. Hale, G., Paul-Labrador, M., Dwyer, J. H. & Merz, C. N. (2002). Isoflavone supplementation and endothelial function in menopausal women. *Clin Endocrinol (Oxf)* **56**(6), 693–701.

106. Nestel, P. J., Yamashita, T., Sasahara, T., Pomeroy, S., Dart, A., Komesaroff, P., Owen, A. & Abbey, M. (1997). Soy isoflavones improve systemic arterial compliance but not plasma lipids in menopausal and perimenopausal women. *Arterioscler Thromb Vasc Biol* **17**(12), 3392–3398.

107. Squadrito, F., Altavilla, D., Squadrito, G., Saitta, A., Cucinotta, D., Minutoli, L., Deodato, B., Ferlito, M., Campo, G. M., Bova, A. & Caputi, A. P. (2000 Jan 14). Genistein supplementation and estrogen replacement therapy improve endothelial dysfunction induced by ovariectomy in rats. *Cardiovasc Res* **45**(2), 454–462.

108. Catania, M. A., Crupi, A., Firenzuoli, F., Parisi, A., Sturiale, A., Squadrito, F., Caputi, A. P. & Calapai, G. (2002). Oral administration of a soy extract improves endothelial dysfunction in ovariectomized rats. *Planta Med* **68**(12), 1142–1144.

109. Khemapech, S., Monsiri, K., Patumraj, S. & Siriviriyakul, P. (2003). Genistein replacement therapy for vasodilation disorder in bilateral ovariectomized rats. *Clin Hemorheol Microcirc* **29**(3–4), 271–277.

110. Izumi, T., Piskula, M. K., Osawa, S., Obata, A., Tobe, K., Saito, M., Kataoka, S., Kubota, Y. & Kikuchi, M. (2000). Soy isoflavone aglycones are absorbed faster and in higher amounts than their glucosides in humans. *J Nutr* **130**(7), 1695–1699.

111. Setchell, K. D., Brown, N. M., Desai, P., Zimmer-Nechemias, L., Wolfe, B. E., Brashear, W. T., Kirschner, A. S., Cassidy, A. & Heubi, J. E. (2001). Bioavailability of pure isoflavones in healthy humans and analysis of commercial soy isoflavone supplements. *J Nutr* **131**(4 Suppl), 1362S–1375S.

112. Richelle, M., Pridmore-Merten, S., Bodenstab, S., Enslen, M. & Offord, E. A. (2002). Hydrolysis of isoflavone glycosides to aglycones by beta-glycosidase does not alter plasma and urine isoflavone pharmacokinetics in postmenopausal women. *J Nutr* **132**(9), 2587–2592.

113. Zubik, L. & Meydani, M. (2003). Bioavailability of soybean isoflavones from aglycone and glucoside forms in American women. *Am J Clin Nutr* **77**(6), 1459–1465.

114. Setchell, K. D., Brown, N. M., Zimmer-Nechemias, L., Brashear, W. T., Wolfe, B. E., Kirschner, A. S. & Heubi, J. E. (2002). Evidence for lack of absorption of soy isoflavone glycosides in humans, supporting the crucial role of intestinal metabolism for bioavailability. *Am J Clin Nutr* **76**(2), 447–453.

115. Day, A. J., DuPont, M. S., Ridley, S., Rhodes, M., Rhodes, M. J., Morgan, M. R. & Williamson, G. (1998 Sept 25). Deglycosylation of flavonoid and isoflavonoid glycosides by human small intestine and liver beta-glucosidase activity. *FEBS Lett* **436**(1), 71–75.

116. Murota, K., Shimizu, S., Miyamoto, S., Izumi, T., Obata, A., Kikuchi, M. & Terao, J. (2002). Unique uptake and transport of isoflavone aglycones by human intestinal caco-2 cells: Comparison of isoflavonoids and flavonoids. *J Nutr* **132**(7), 1956–1961.

117. Xu, X., Harris, K. S., Wang, H. J., Murphy, P. A. & Hendrich, S. (1995). Bioavailability of soybean isoflavones depends upon gut microflora in women. *J Nutr* **125**(9), 2307–2315.

118. Walker, H. A., Dean, T. S., Sanders, T. A., Jackson, G., Ritter, J. M. & Chowienczyk, P. J. (2001 Jan 16). The phytoestrogen genistein produces acute nitric oxide-dependent dilation of human forearm vasculature with similar potency to 17beta-estradiol. *Circulation* **103**(2), 258–262.

119. Teede, H. J., Dalais, F. S., Kotsopoulos, D., Liang, Y. L., Davis, S. & McGrath, B. P. (2001). Dietary soy has both beneficial and potentially adverse cardiovascular effects: A placebo-controlled study in men and postmenopausal women. *J Clin Endocrinol Metab* **86**(7), 3053–3060.

120. McCrohon, J. A., Walters, W. A., Robinson, J. T., McCredie, R. J., Turner, L., Adams, M. R., Handelsman, D. J. & Celermajer, D. S. (1997). Arterial reactivity is enhanced in genetic males taking high dose estrogens. *J Am Coll Cardiol* **29**(7), 1432–1436.

121. New, G., Duffy, S. J., Harper, R. W. & Meredith, I. T. (2000). Long-term oestrogen therapy is associated with improved endothelium-dependent vasodilation in the forearm resistance circulation of biological males. *Clin Exp Pharmacol Physiol* **27**(1–2), 25–33.

122. Sader, M. A., McCredie, R. J., Griffiths, K. A., Wishart, S. M., Handelsman, D. J. & Celermajer, D. S. (2001). Oestradiol improves arterial endothelial function in healthy men receiving testosterone. *Clin Endocrinol (Oxf)* **54**(2), 175–181.

123. Kimura, M., Sudhir, K., Jones, M., Simpson, E., Jefferis, A. M. & Chin-Dusting, J. P. (2003 Dec 12). Impaired acetylcholine-induced release of nitric oxide in the aorta of male aromatase-knockout mice: Regulation of nitric

oxide production by endogenous sex hormones in males. *Circ Res* **93**(12), 1267–1271.

124. Hanke, H., Hanke, S., Ickrath, O., Lange, K., Bruck, B., Muck, A. O., Seeger, H., Zwirner, M., Voisard, R., Haasis, R. & Hombach, V. (1997). Estradiol concentrations in premenopausal women with coronary heart disease. *Coron Artery Dis* **8**(8–9), 511–515.

125. Christian, R. C., Harrington, S., Edwards, W. D., Oberg, A. L. & Fitzpatrick, L. A. (2002). Estrogen status correlates with the calcium content of coronary atherosclerotic plaques in women. *J Clin Endocrinol Metab* **87**(3), 1062–1067.

126. Bairey Merz, C. N., Johnson, B. D., Sharaf, B. L., Bittner, V., Berga, S. L., Braunstein, G. D., Hodgson, T. K., Matthews, K. A., Pepine, C. J., Reis, S. E., Reichek, N., Rogers, W. J., Pohost, G. M., Kelsey, S. F. & Sopko, G. (2003 Feb 5). Hypoestrogenemia of hypothalamic origin and coronary artery disease in premenopausal women: A report from the NHLBI-sponsored WISE study. *J Am Coll Cardiol* **41**(3), 413–419.

127. Vasquez-Vivar, J., Kalyanaraman, B., Martasek, P., Hogg, N., Masters, B. S., Karoui, H., Tordo, P. & Pritchard, K. A., Jr. (1998 Aug 4). Superoxide generation by endothelial nitric oxide synthase: The influence of cofactors. *Proc Natl Acad Sci U S A* **95**(16), 9220–9225.

128. Milstien, S. & Katusic, Z. (1999 Oct 5). Oxidation of tetrahydrobiopterin by peroxynitrite: Implications for vascular endothelial function. *Biochem Biophys Res Commun* **263**(3), 681–684.

129. Vasquez-Vivar, J., Kalyanaraman, B. & Martasek, P. (2003). The role of tetrahydrobiopterin in superoxide generation from eNOS: Enzymology and physiological implications. *Free Radic Res* **37**(2), 121–127.

130. Stroes, E. S., van Faassen, E. E., Yo, M., Martasek, P., Boer, P., Govers, R. & Rabelink, T. J. (2000 June 9). Folic acid reverts dysfunction of endothelial nitric oxide synthase. *Circ Res* **86**(11), 1129–1134.

131. Verhaar, M. C., Stroes, E. & Rabelink, T. J. (2002). Folates and cardiovascular disease. *Arterioscler Thromb Vasc Biol* **22**(1), 6–13.

132. Hyndman, M. E., Verma, S., Rosenfeld, R. J., Anderson, T. J. & Parsons, H. G. (2002). Interaction of 5-methyltetrahydrofolate and tetrahydrobiopterin on endothelial function. *Am J Physiol Heart Circ Physiol* **282**(6), H2167–H2172.

133. Doshi, S. N., McDowell, I. F., Moat, S. J., Payne, N., Durrant, H. J., Lewis, M. J. & Goodfellow, J. (2002 Jan 1). Folic acid improves endothelial function in coronary artery disease via mechanisms largely independent of homocysteine lowering. *Circulation JID – 0147763* **105**(1), 22–26.

134. McCarty, M. F. (2004). Coping with endothelial superoxide: Potential complementarity of arginine and high-dose folate. *Med Hypotheses* **63**(4), 709–718.

135. Cooke, J. P. & Oka, R. K. (2002). Atherogenesis and the arginine hypothesis. *Curr Atheroscler Rep JID – 100897685* **3**(3), 252–259.

136. Boger, R. H. (2003 Oct 1). The emerging role of asymmetric dimethylarginine as a novel cardiovascular risk factor. *Cardiovasc Res* **59**(4), 824–833.

137. Atteritano, M., Marini, H., Minutoli, L., Polito, F., Bitto, A., Altavilla, D., Mazzaferro, S., D'Anna, R., Cannata, M. L., Gaudio, A., Frisina, A., Frisina, N., Corrado, F., Cancellieri, F., Lubrano, C., Bonaiuto, M., Adamo, E. B. & Squadrito, F. (2007). Effects of the phytoestrogen genistein on some predictors of cardiovascular risk in osteopenic, postmenopausal women: A two-year

randomized, double-blind, placebo-controlled study. *J Clin Endocrinol Metab* **92**(8), 3068–3075.

138. Jayagopal, V., Albertazzi, P., Kilpatrick, E. S., Howarth, E. M., Jennings, P. E., Hepburn, D. A. & Atkin, S. L. (2002). Beneficial effects of soy phytoestrogen intake in postmenopausal women with type 2 diabetes. *Diabetes Care* **25**(10), 1709–1714.

139. Steinberg, H. O., Brechtel, G., Johnson, A., Fineberg, N. & Baron, A. D. (1994). Insulin-mediated skeletal muscle vasodilation is nitric oxide dependent. A novel action of insulin to increase nitric oxide release. *J Clin Invest* **94**(3), 1172–1179.

140. Muniyappa, R. & Quon, M. J. (2007). Insulin action and insulin resistance in vascular endothelium. *Curr Opin Clin Nutr Metab Care* **10**(4), 523–530.

141. Vidal, O., Kindblom, L. G. & Ohlsson, C. (1999). Expression and localization of estrogen receptor-beta in murine and human bone. *J Bone Miner Res* **14**(6), 923–929.

142. Bord, S., Horner, A., Beavan, S. & Compston, J. (2001). Estrogen receptors alpha and beta are differentially expressed in developing human bone. *J Clin Endocrinol Metab* **86**(5), 2309–2314.

143. Batra, G. S., Hainey, L., Freemont, A. J., Andrew, G., Saunders, P. T., Hoyland, J. A. & Braidman, I. P. (2003). Evidence for cell-specific changes with age in expression of oestrogen receptor (ER) alpha and beta in bone fractures from men and women. *J Pathol* **200**(1), 65–73.

144. Monroe, D. G., Getz, B. J., Johnsen, S. A., Riggs, B. L., Khosla, S. & Spelsberg, T. C. (2003 Oct 1). Estrogen receptor isoform-specific regulation of endogenous gene expression in human osteoblastic cell lines expressing either ERalpha or ERbeta. *J Cell Biochem* **90**(2), 315–326.

145. Lindberg, M. K., Moverare, S., Skrtic, S., Gao, H., Dahlman-Wright, K., Gustafsson, J. A. & Ohlsson, C. (2003). Estrogen receptor (ER)-beta reduces ERalpha-regulated gene transcription, supporting a "ying yang" relationship between ERalpha and ERbeta in mice. *Mol Endocrinol* **17**(2), 203–208.

146. Windahl, S. H., Hollberg, K., Vidal, O., Gustafsson, J. A., Ohlsson, C. & Andersson, G. (2001). Female estrogen receptor beta-/- mice are partially protected against age-related trabecular bone loss. *J Bone Miner Res* **16**(8), 1388–1398.

147. Sims, N. A., Clement-Lacroix, P., Minet, D., Fraslon-Vanhulle, C., Gaillard-Kelly, M., Resche-Rigon, M. & Baron, R. (2003). A functional androgen receptor is not sufficient to allow estradiol to protect bone after gonadectomy in estradiol receptor-deficient mice. *J Clin Invest* **111**(9), 1319–1327.

148. Sims, N. A., Dupont, S., Krust, A., Clement-Lacroix, P., Minet, D., Resche-Rigon, M., Gaillard-Kelly, M. & Baron, R. (2002). Deletion of estrogen receptors reveals a regulatory role for estrogen receptors-beta in bone remodeling in females but not in males. *Bone* **30**(1), 18–25.

149. Cao, L., Bu, R., Oakley, J. I., Kalla, S. E. & Blair, H. C. (2003 May 1). Estrogen receptor-beta modulates synthesis of bone matrix proteins in human osteoblast-like MG63 cells. *J Cell Biochem* **89**(1), 152–164.

150. Koka, S., Petro, T. M. & Reinhardt, R. A. (1998). Estrogen inhibits interleukin-1beta-induced interleukin-6 production by human osteoblast-like cells. *J Interferon Cytokine Res* **18**(7), 479–483.

151. Bord, S., Ireland, D. C., Beavan, S. R. & Compston, J. E. (2003). The effects of estrogen on osteoprotegerin, RANKL, and estrogen receptor expression in human osteoblasts. *Bone* **32**(2), 136–141.

152. Chen, X., Garner, S. C., Quarles, L. D. & Anderson, J. J. (2003). Effects of genistein on expression of bone markers during MC3T3-E1 osteoblastic cell differentiation. *J Nutr Biochem* **14**(6), 342–349.

153. Viereck, V., Grundker, C., Blaschke, S., Siggelkow, H., Emons, G. & Hofbauer, L. C. (2002). Phytoestrogen genistein stimulates the production of osteoprotegerin by human trabecular osteoblasts. *J Cell Biochem* **84**(4), 725–735.

154. Aguirre, J., Buttery, L., O'Shaughnessy, M., Afzal, F., Fernandez, dM. I., Hukkanen, M., Huang, P., MacIntyre, I. & Polak, J. (2001). Endothelial nitric oxide synthase gene-deficient mice demonstrate marked retardation in postnatal bone formation, reduced bone volume, and defects in osteoblast maturation and activity. *Am J Pathol* **158**(1), 247–257.

155. Samuels, A., Perry, M. J., Gibson, R. L., Colley, S. & Tobias, J. H. (2001). Role of endothelial nitric oxide synthase in estrogen-induced osteogenesis. *Bone* **29**(1), 24–29.

156. McFarlane, S. I., Muniyappa, R., Shin, J. J., Bahtiyar, G. & Sowers, J. R. (2004). Osteoporosis and cardiovascular disease: Brittle bones and boned arteries, is there a link? *Endocrine* **23**(1), 1–10.

157. Anderson, J. J., Ambrose, W. W. & Garner, S. C. (1998). Biphasic effects of genistein on bone tissue in the ovariectomized, lactating rat model. *Proc Soc Exp Biol Med* **217**(3), 345–350.

158. Fanti, P., Monier-Faugere, M. C., Geng, Z., Schmidt, J., Morris, P. E., Cohen, D. & Malluche, H. H. (1998). The phytoestrogen genistein reduces bone loss in short-term ovariectomized rats. *Osteoporos Int* **8**(3), 274–281.

159. Ishimi, Y., Miyaura, C., Ohmura, M., Onoe, Y., Sato, T., Uchiyama, Y., Ito, M., Wang, X., Suda, T. & Ikegami, S. (1999). Selective effects of genistein, a soybean isoflavone, on B-lymphopoiesis and bone loss caused by estrogen deficiency. *Endocrinology* **140**(4), 1893–1900.

160. Wu, J., Wang, X. X., Takasaki, M., Ohta, A., Higuchi, M. & Ishimi, Y. (2001). Cooperative effects of exercise training and genistein administration on bone mass in ovariectomized mice. *J Bone Miner Res* **16**(10), 1829–1836.

161. Nakajima, D., Kim, C. S., Oh, T. W., Yang, C. Y., Naka, T., Igawa, S. & Ohta, F. (2001). Suppressive effects of genistein dosage and resistance exercise on bone loss in ovariectomized rats. *J Physiol Anthropol Appl Human Sci* **20**(5), 285–291.

162. Li, B. & Yu, S. (2003). Genistein prevents bone resorption diseases by inhibiting bone resorption and stimulating bone formation. *Biol Pharm Bull* **26**(6), 780–786.

163. Harris, H. A., Albert, L. M., Leathurby, Y., Malamas, M. S., Mewshaw, R. E., Miller, C. P., Kharode, Y. P., Marzolf, J., Komm, B. S., Winneker, R. C., Frail, D. E., Henderson, R. A., Zhu, Y. & Keith, J. C., Jr. (2003). Evaluation of an estrogen receptor-beta agonist in animal models of human disease. *Endocrinology* **144**(10), 4241–4249.

164. Potter, S. M., Baum, J. A., Teng, H., Stillman, R. J., Shay, N. F. & Erdman, J. W., Jr. (1998). Soy protein and isoflavones: Their effects on blood lipids and bone density in postmenopausal women. *Am J Clin Nutr* **68**(6 Suppl), 1375S–1379S.

165. Uesugi, T., Fukui, Y. & Yamori, Y. (2002). Beneficial effects of soybean isoflavone supplementation on bone metabolism and serum lipids in postmenopausal japanese women: A four-week study. *J Am Coll Nutr* **21**(2), 97–102.

166. Yamori, Y., Moriguchi, E. H., Teramoto, T., Miura, A., Fukui, Y., Honda, K. I., Fukui, M., Nara, Y., Taira, K. & Moriguchi, Y. (2002). Soybean isoflavones reduce postmenopausal bone resorption in female Japanese immigrants in Brazil: A ten-week study. *J Am Coll Nutr* **21**(6), 560–563.

167. Chen, Y. M., Ho, S. C., Lam, S. S., Ho, S. S. & Woo, J. L. (2003). Soy isoflavones have a favorable effect on bone loss in Chinese postmenopausal women with lower bone mass: A double-blind, randomized, controlled trial. *J Clin Endocrinol Metab* **88**(10), 4740–4747.

168. Chen, Y. M., Ho, S. C., Lam, S. S., Ho, S. S. & Woo, J. L. (2004). Beneficial effect of soy isoflavones on bone mineral content was modified by years since menopause, body weight, and calcium intake: A double-blind, randomized, controlled trial. *Menopause* **11**(3), 246–254.

169. Crisafulli, A., Altavilla, D., Squadrito, G., Romeo, A., Adamo, E. B., Marini, R., Inferrera, M. A., Marini, H., Bitto, A., D'Anna, R., Corrado, F., Bartolone, S., Frisina, N. & Squadrito, F. (2004). Effects of the phytoestrogen genistein on the circulating soluble receptor activator of nuclear factor kappaB ligand-osteoprotegerin system in early postmenopausal women. *J Clin Endocrinol Metab* **89**(1), 188–192.

170. Hsu, C. S., Shen, W. W., Hsueh, Y. M. & Yeh, S. L. (2001). Soy isoflavone supplementation in postmenopausal women. Effects on plasma lipids, antioxidant enzyme activities and bone density. *J Reprod Med* **46**(3), 221–226.

171. Gallagher, J. C., Satpathy, R., Rafferty, K. & Haynatzka, V. (2004). The effect of soy protein isolate on bone metabolism. *Menopause* **11**(3), 290–298.

172. Kreijkamp-Kaspers, S., Kok, L., Grobbee, D. E., de Haan, E. H., Aleman, A., Lampe, J. W. & van der Schouw, Y. T. (2004 July 7). Effect of soy protein containing isoflavones on cognitive function, bone mineral density, and plasma lipids in postmenopausal women: A randomized controlled trial. *JAMA* **292**(1), 65–74.

173. Ma, D. F., Qin, L. Q., Wang, P. Y. & Katoh, R. (2007 Mar 28). Soy isoflavone intake inhibits bone resorption and stimulates bone formation in menopausal women: meta-analysis of randomized controlled trials. *Eur J Clin Nutr*.

174. Anderson, J. J., Chen, X., Boass, A., Symons, M., Kohlmeier, M., Renner, J. B. & Garner, S. C. (2002). Soy isoflavones: No effects on bone mineral content and bone mineral density in healthy, menstruating young adult women after one year. *J Am Coll Nutr* **21**(5), 388–393.

175. Khalil, D. A., Lucas, E. A., Juma, S., Smith, B. J., Payton, M. E. & Arjmandi, B. H. (2002). Soy protein supplementation increases serum insulin-like growth factor-I in young and old men but does not affect markers of bone metabolism. *J Nutr* **132**(9), 2605–2608.

176. Khalil, D. A., Lucas, E. A., Smith, B. J., Soung, D. Y., Devareddy, L., Juma, S., Akhter, M. P., Recker, R. & Arjmandi, B. H. (2005). Soy isoflavones may protect against orchidectomy-induced bone loss in aged male rats. *Calcif Tissue Int* **76**(1), 56–62.

177. Somekawa, Y., Chiguchi, M., Ishibashi, T. & Aso, T. (2001). Soy intake related to menopausal symptoms, serum lipids, and bone mineral density in postmenopausal Japanese women. *Obstet Gynecol* **97**(1), 109–115.

178. Ho, S. C., Woo, J., Lam, S., Chen, Y., Sham, A. & Lau, J. (2003). Soy protein consumption and bone mass in early postmenopausal Chinese women. *Osteoporos Int* **14**(10), 835–842.

179. Kardinaal, A. F., Morton, M. S., Bruggemann-Rotgans, I. E. & van Beresteijn, E. C. (1998). Phyto-oestrogen excretion and rate of bone loss in postmenopausal women. *Eur J Clin Nutr* **52**(11), 850–855.

180. Kim, M. K., Chung, B. C., Yu, V. Y., Nam, J. H., Lee, H. C., Huh, K. B. & Lim, S. K. (2002). Relationships of urinary phyto-oestrogen excretion to BMD in postmenopausal women. *Clin Endocrinol (Oxf)* **56**(3), 321–328.

181. Nagata, C., Shimizu, H., Takami, R., Hayashi, M., Takeda, N. & Yasuda, K. (2002). Soy product intake and serum isoflavonoid and estradiol concentrations in relation to bone mineral density in postmenopausal Japanese women. *Osteoporos Int* **13**(3), 200–204.

182. Kritz-Silverstein, D. & Goodman-Gruen, D. L. (2002). Usual dietary isoflavone intake, bone mineral density, and bone metabolism in postmenopausal women. *J Womens Health Gend Based Med* **11**(1), 69–78.

183. Royuela, M., de Miguel, M. P., Bethencourt, F. R., Sanchez-Chapado, M., Fraile, B., Arenas, M. I. & Paniagua, R. (2001). Estrogen receptors alpha and beta in the normal, hyperplastic and carcinomatous human prostate. *J Endocrinol* **168**(3), 447–454.

184. Fixemer, T., Remberger, K. & Bonkhoff, H. (2003). Differential expression of the estrogen receptor beta (ERbeta) in human prostate tissue, premalignant changes, and in primary, metastatic, and recurrent prostatic adenocarcinoma. *Prostate* **54**(2), 79–87.

185. Signoretti, S. & Loda, M. (2001). Estrogen receptor beta in prostate cancer: Brake pedal or accelerator? *Am J Pathol* **159**(1), 13–16.

186. Ho, S. M. (2004 Feb 15). Estrogens and anti-estrogens: Key mediators of prostate carcinogenesis and new therapeutic candidates. *J Cell Biochem* **91**(3), 491–503.

187. Krege, J. H., Hodgin, J. B., Couse, J. F., Enmark, E., Warner, M., Mahler, J. F., Sar, M., Korach, K. S., Gustafsson, J. A. & Smithies, O. (1998 Dec 22). Generation and reproductive phenotypes of mice lacking estrogen receptor beta. *Proc Natl Acad Sci U S A* **95**(26), 15677–15682.

188. Weihua, Z., Makela, S., Andersson, L. C., Salmi, S., Saji, S., Webster, J. I., Jensen, E. V., Nilsson, S., Warner, M. & Gustafsson, J. A. (2001 May 22). A role for estrogen receptor beta in the regulation of growth of the ventral prostate. *Proc Natl Acad Sci U S A* **98**(11), 6330–6335.

189. Cheng, J., Lee, E. J., Madison, L. D. & Lazennec, G. (2004 May 21). Expression of estrogen receptor beta in prostate carcinoma cells inhibits invasion and proliferation and triggers apoptosis. *FEBS Lett* **566**(1–3), 169–172.

190. Zhu, X., Leav, I., Leung, Y. K., Wu, M., Liu, Q., Gao, Y., McNeal, J. E. & Ho, S. M. (2004). Dynamic regulation of estrogen receptor-beta expression by DNA methylation during prostate cancer development and metastasis. *Am J Pathol* **164**(6), 2003–2012.

191. Linja, M. J., Savinainen, K. J., Tammela, T. L., Isola, J. J. & Visakorpi, T. (2003 May 15). Expression of ERalpha and ERbeta in prostate cancer. *Prostate* **55**(3), 180–186.

192. Lau, K. M., LaSpina, M., Long, J. & Ho, S. M. (2000 June 15). Expression of estrogen receptor (ER)-alpha and ER-beta in normal and malignant prostatic epithelial cells: Regulation by methylation and involvement in growth regulation. *Cancer Res* **60**(12), 3175–3182.

193. Kim, I. Y., Seong, D. H., Kim, B. C., Lee, D. K., Remaley, A. T., Leach, F., Morton, R. A. & Kim, S. J. (2002 July 1). Raloxifene, a selective estrogen receptor modulator, induces apoptosis in androgen-responsive human prostate cancer cell line LNCaP through an androgen-independent pathway. *Cancer Res* **62**(13), 3649–3653.

194. Kim, I. Y., Kim, B. C., Seong, D. H., Lee, D. K., Seo, J. M., Hong, Y. J., Kim, H. T., Morton, R. A. & Kim, S. J. (2002 Sept 15). Raloxifene, a mixed estrogen agonist/antagonist, induces apoptosis in androgen-independent human prostate cancer cell lines. *Cancer Res* **62**(18), 5365–5369.

195. Bemis, D. L., Capodice, J. L., Desai, M., Buttyan, R. & Katz, A. E. (2004 Aug 1). A concentrated aglycone isoflavone preparation (GCP) that demonstrates potent anti-prostate cancer activity *in vitro* and *in vivo*. *Clin Cancer Res* **10**(15), 5282–5292.

196. Bektic, J., Berger, A. P., Pfeil, K., Dobler, G., Bartsch, G. & Klocker, H. (2004). Androgen receptor regulation by physiological concentrations of the isoflavonoid genistein in androgen-dependent LNCaP cells is mediated by estrogen receptor beta. *Eur Urol* **45**(2), 245–251.

197. Zhou, J. R., Gugger, E. T., Tanaka, T., Guo, Y., Blackburn, G. L. & Clinton, S. K. (1999). Soybean phytochemicals inhibit the growth of transplantable human prostate carcinoma and tumor angiogenesis in mice. *J Nutr* **129**(9), 1628–1635.

198. Aronson, W. J., Tymchuk, C. N., Elashoff, R. M., McBride, W. H., McLean, C., Wang, H. & Heber, D. (1999). Decreased growth of human prostate LNCaP tumors in SCID mice fed a low-fat, soy protein diet with isoflavones. *Nutr Cancer* **35**(2), 130–136.

199. Fritz, W. A., Wang, J., Eltoum, I. E. & Lamartiniere, C. A. (2002 Jan 15). Dietary genistein down-regulates androgen and estrogen receptor expression in the rat prostate. *Mol Cell Endocrinol* **186**(1), 89–99.

200. Wang, J., Eltoum, I. E. & Lamartiniere, C. A. (2002 Dec 1). Dietary genistein suppresses chemically induced prostate cancer in Lobund-Wistar rats. *Cancer Lett* **186**(1), 11–18.

201. Mentor-Marcel, R., Lamartiniere, C. A., Eltoum, I. E., Greenberg, N. M. & Elgavish, A. (2001 Sept 15). Genistein in the diet reduces the incidence of poorly differentiated prostatic adenocarcinoma in transgenic mice (TRAMP). *Cancer Res* **61**(18), 6777–6782.

202. Hussain, M., Banerjee, M., Sarkar, F. H., Djuric, Z., Pollak, M. N., Doerge, D., Fontana, J., Chinni, S., Davis, J., Forman, J., Wood, D. P. & Kucuk, O. (2003). Soy isoflavones in the treatment of prostate cancer. *Nutr Cancer* **47**(2), 111–117.

203. deVere White, R. W., Hackman, R. M., Soares, S. E., Beckett, L. A., Li, Y. & Sun, B. (2004). Effects of a genistein-rich extract on PSA levels in men with a history of prostate cancer. *Urology* **63**(2), 259–263.

204. Messina, M. J. (2003). Emerging evidence on the role of soy in reducing prostate cancer risk. *Nutr Rev* **61**(4), 117–131.

205. Lee, M. M., Gomez, S. L., Chang, J. S., Wey, M., Wang, R. T. & Hsing, A. W. (2003). Soy and isoflavone consumption in relation to prostate cancer risk in China. *Cancer Epidemiol Biomarkers Prev* **12**(7), 665–668.

206. Ozasa, K., Nakao, M., Watanabe, Y., Hayashi, K., Miki, T., Mikami, K., Mori, M., Sakauchi, F., Washio, M., Ito, Y., Suzuki, K., Wakai, K. & Tamakoshi, A. (2004). Serum phytoestrogens and prostate cancer risk in a nested case-control study among Japanese men. *Cancer Sci* **95**(1), 65–71.

207. Nanda, K., Bastian, L. A., Hasselblad, V. & Simel, D. L. (1999). Hormone replacement therapy and the risk of colorectal cancer: A meta-analysis. *Obstet Gynecol* **93**(5 Pt 2), 880–888.

208. La, V. C., Gallus, S. & Fernandez, E. (2005). Hormone replacement therapy and colorectal cancer: An update. *J Br Menopause Soc* **11**(4), 166–172.

209. Wada-Hiraike, O., Warner, M. & Gustafsson, J. A. (2006). New developments in oestrogen signalling in colonic epithelium. *Biochem Soc Trans* **34**(Pt 6), 1114–1116.

210. Messina, M. & Bennink, M. (1998). Soyfoods, isoflavones and risk of colonic cancer: A review of the *in vitro* and *in vivo* data. *Baillieres Clin Endocrinol Metab* **12**(4), 707–728.

211. Lechner, D., Kallay, E. & Cross, H. S. (2005). Phytoestrogens and colorectal cancer prevention. *Vitam Horm* **70**, 169–198.

212. Cotterchio, M., Boucher, B. A., Manno, M., Gallinger, S., Okey, A. & Harper, P. (2006). Dietary phytoestrogen intake is associated with reduced colorectal cancer risk. *J Nutr* **136**(12), 3046–3053.

213. Oba, S., Nagata, C., Shimizu, N., Shimizu, H., Kametani, M., Takeyama, N., Ohnuma, T. & Matsushita, S. (2007). Soy product consumption and the risk of colon cancer: A prospective study in Takayama, Japan. *Nutr Cancer* **57**(2), 151–157.

214. Badger, T. M., Ronis, M. J., Simmen, R. C. & Simmen, F. A. (2005). Soy protein isolate and protection against cancer. *J Am Coll Nutr* **24**(2), 146S–149S.

215. Hakkak, R., Korourian, S., Ronis, M. J., Johnston, J. M. & Badger, T. M. (2001 May 10). Soy protein isolate consumption protects against azoxymethane-induced colon tumors in male rats. *Cancer Lett* **166**(1), 27–32.

216. Bennink, M. R. (2001). Dietary soy reduces colon carcinogenesis in human and rats. Soy and colon cancer. *Adv Exp Med Biol* **492**, 11–17.

217. Guo, J. Y., Li, X., Browning, J. D., Jr., Rottinghaus, G. E., Lubahn, D. B., Constantinou, A., Bennink, M. & MacDonald, R. S. (2004). Dietary soy isoflavones and estrone protect ovariectomized ERalphaKO and wild-type mice from carcinogen-induced colon cancer. *J Nutr* **134**(1), 179–182.

218. Gorham, E. D., Garland, C. F., Garland, F. C., Grant, W. B., Mohr, S. B., Lipkin, M., Newmark, H. L., Giovannucci, E., Wei, M. & Holick, M. F. (2007). Optimal vitamin D status for colorectal cancer prevention: A quantitative meta analysis. *Am J Prev Med* **32**(3), 210–216.

219. Grant, W. B., Garland, C. F. & Gorham, E. D. (2007). An estimate of cancer mortality rate reductions in Europe and the US with 1,000 IU of oral vitamin D per day. *Recent Results Cancer Res* **174**, 225–234.

220. Cross, H. S., Peterlik, M., Reddy, G. S. & Schuster, I. (1997). Vitamin D metabolism in human colon adenocarcinoma-derived Caco-2 cells: Expression

of 25-hydroxyvitamin D3-1alpha-hydroxylase activity and regulation of side-chain metabolism. *J Steroid Biochem Mol Biol* **62**(1), 21–28.

221. Cross, H. S., Kallay, E., Khorchide, M. & Lechner, D. (2003). Regulation of extrarenal synthesis of 1,25-dihydroxyvitamin D3 – relevance for colonic cancer prevention and therapy. *Mol Aspects Med* **24**(6), 459–465.

222. Cross, H. S., Kallay, E., Lechner, D., Gerdenitsch, W., Adlercreutz, H. & Armbrecht, H. J. (2004). Phytoestrogens and vitamin D metabolism: A new concept for the prevention and therapy of colorectal, prostate, and mammary carcinomas. *J Nutr* **134**(5), 1207S–1212S.

223. Pelletier, G. & El Alfy, M. (2000). Immunocytochemical localization of estrogen receptors alpha and beta in the human reproductive organs. *J Clin Endocrinol Metab* **85**(12), 4835–4840.

224. Palmieri, C., Saji, S., Sakaguchi, H., Cheng, G., Sunters, A., O'Hare, M. J., Warner, M., Gustafsson, J. A., Coombes, R. C. & Lam, E. W. (2004). The expression of oestrogen receptor (ER)-beta and its variants, but not ERalpha, in adult human mammary fibroblasts. *J Mol Endocrinol* **33**(1), 35–50.

225. Couse, J. F. & Korach, K. S. (1999). Estrogen receptor null mice: What have we learned and where will they lead us? *Endocr Rev* **20**(3), 358–417.

226. Gustafsson, J. A. & Warner, M. (2000 Nov 30). Estrogen receptor beta in the breast: Role in estrogen responsiveness and development of breast cancer. *J Steroid Biochem Mol Biol* **74**(5), 245–248.

227. Paruthiyil, S., Parmar, H., Kerekatte, V., Cunha, G. R., Firestone, G. L. & Leitman, D. C. (2004 Jan 1). Estrogen receptor beta inhibits human breast cancer cell proliferation and tumor formation by causing a G2 cell cycle arrest. *Cancer Res* **64**(1), 423–428.

228. Strom, A., Hartman, J., Foster, J. S., Kietz, S., Wimalasena, J. & Gustafsson, J. A. (2004 Feb 10). Estrogen receptor beta inhibits 17beta-estradiol-stimulated proliferation of the breast cancer cell line T47D. *Proc Natl Acad Sci U S A* **101**(6), 1566–1571.

229. Hou, Y. F., Yuan, S. T., Li, H. C., Wu, J., Lu, J. S., Liu, G., Lu, L. J., Shen, Z. Z., Ding, J. & Shao, Z. M. (2004 July 29). ERbeta exerts multiple stimulative effects on human breast carcinoma cells. *Oncogene* **23**(34), 5799–5806.

230. Dotzlaw, H., Leygue, E., Watson, P. H. & Murphy, L. C. (1997). Expression of estrogen receptor-beta in human breast tumors. *J Clin Endocrinol Metab* **82**(7), 2371–2374.

231. Fuqua, S. A., Schiff, R., Parra, I., Moore, J. T., Mohsin, S. K., Osborne, C. K., Clark, G. M. & Allred, D. C. (2003 May 15). Estrogen receptor beta protein in human breast cancer: Correlation with clinical tumor parameters. *Cancer Res* **63**(10), 2434–2439.

232. Murrill, W. B., Brown, N. M., Zhang, J. X., Manzolillo, P. A., Barnes, S. & Lamartiniere, C. A. (1996). Prepubertal genistein exposure suppresses mammary cancer and enhances gland differentiation in rats. *Carcinogenesis* **17**(7), 1451–1457.

233. Lamartiniere, C. A., Murrill, W. B., Manzolillo, P. A., Zhang, J. X., Barnes, S., Zhang, X., Wei, H. & Brown, N. M. (1998). Genistein alters the ontogeny of mammary gland development and protects against chemically-induced mammary cancer in rats. *Proc Soc Exp Biol Med* **217**(3), 358–364.

234. Cabanes, A., Wang, M., Olivo, S., DeAssis, S., Gustafsson, J. A., Khan, G. & Hilakivi-Clarke, L. (2004). Prepubertal estradiol and genistein exposures

up-regulate BRCA1 mRNA and reduce mammary tumorigenesis. *Carcinogenesis* **25**(5), 741–748.

235. Jin, Z. & MacDonald, R. S. (2002). Soy isoflavones increase latency of spontaneous mammary tumors in mice. *J Nutr* **132**(10), 3186–3190.

236. Yuan, L., Wagatsuma, C., Yoshida, M., Miura, T., Mukoda, T., Fujii, H., Sun, B., Kim, J. H. & Surh, Y. J. (2003). Inhibition of human breast cancer growth by GCP (genistein combined polysaccharide) in xenogeneic athymic mice: involvement of genistein biotransformation by beta-glucuronidase from tumor tissues. *Mutat Res* **523–524**, 55–62.

237. Mizunuma, H., Kanazawa, K., Ogura, S., Otsuka, S. & Nagai, H. (2002). Anticarcinogenic effects of isoflavones may be mediated by genistein in mouse mammary tumor virus-induced breast cancer. *Oncology* **62**(1), 78–84.

238. Hsieh, C. Y., Santell, R. C., Haslam, S. Z. & Helferich, W. G. (1998 Sept 1). Estrogenic effects of genistein on the growth of estrogen receptor-positive human breast cancer (MCF-7) cells *in vitro* and *in vivo*. *Cancer Res* **58**(17), 3833–3838.

239. Allred, C. D., Allred, K. F., Ju, Y. H., Virant, S. M. & Helferich, W. G. (2001 July 1). Soy diets containing varying amounts of genistein stimulate growth of estrogen-dependent (MCF-7) tumors in a dose-dependent manner. *Cancer Res* **61**(13), 5045–5050.

240. Ju, Y. H., Allred, C. D., Allred, K. F., Karko, K. L., Doerge, D. R. & Helferich, W. G. (2001). Physiological concentrations of dietary genistein dose-dependently stimulate growth of estrogen-dependent human breast cancer (MCF-7) tumors implanted in athymic nude mice. *J Nutr* **131**(11), 2957–2962.

241. Ju, Y. H., Doerge, D. R., Allred, K. F., Allred, C. D. & Helferich, W. G. (2002 May 1). Dietary genistein negates the inhibitory effect of tamoxifen on growth of estrogen-dependent human breast cancer (MCF-7) cells implanted in athymic mice. *Cancer Res* **62**(9), 2474–2477.

242. Maggiolini, M., Bonofiglio, D., Marsico, S., Panno, M. L., Cenni, B., Picard, D. & Ando, S. (2001). Estrogen receptor alpha mediates the proliferative but not the cytotoxic dose-dependent effects of two major phytoestrogens on human breast cancer cells. *Mol Pharmacol* **60**(3), 595–602.

243. Allred, C. D., Allred, K. F., Ju, Y. H., Clausen, L. M., Doerge, D. R., Schantz, S. L., Korol, D. L., Wallig, M. A. & Helferich, W. G. (2004). Dietary genistein results in larger MNU-induced, estrogen-dependent mammary tumors following ovariectomy of Sprague-Dawley rats. *Carcinogenesis* **25**(2), 211–218.

244. Day, J. K., Besch-Williford, C., McMann, T. R., Hufford, M. G., Lubahn, D. B. & MacDonald, R. S. (2001). Dietary genistein increased DMBA-induced mammary adenocarcinoma in wild-type, but not ER alpha KO, mice. *Nutr Cancer* **39**(2), 226–232.

245. Hirohata, T., Shigematsu, T., Nomura, A. M., Nomura, Y., Horie, A. & Hirohata, I. (1985). Occurrence of breast cancer in relation to diet and reproductive history: A case-control study in Fukuoka, Japan. *Natl Cancer Inst Monogr* **69**, 187–190.

246. Yuan, J. M., Wang, Q. S., Ross, R. K., Henderson, B. E. & Yu, M. C. (1995). Diet and breast cancer in Shanghai and Tianjin, China. *Br J Cancer* **71**(6), 1353–1358.

247. Key, T. J., Sharp, G. B., Appleby, P. N., Beral, V., Goodman, M. T., Soda, M. & Mabuchi, K. (1999). Soya foods and breast cancer risk: A prospective study in Hiroshima and Nagasaki, Japan. *Br J Cancer* **81**(7), 1248–1256.

248. Horn-Ross, P. L., John, E. M., Lee, M., Stewart, S. L., Koo, J., Sakoda, L. C., Shiau, A. C., Goldstein, J., Davis, P. & Perez-Stable, E. J. (2001 Sept 1). Phytoestrogen consumption and breast cancer risk in a multiethnic population: the Bay Area Breast Cancer Study. *Am J Epidemiol* **154**(5), 434–441.

249. Horn-Ross, P. L., Hoggatt, K. J., West, D. W., Krone, M. R., Stewart, S. L., Anton, H., Bernstei, C. L., Deapen, D., Peel, D., Pinder, R., Reynolds, P., Ross, R. K., Wright, W. & Ziogas, A. (2002). Recent diet and breast cancer risk: The California Teachers Study (USA). *Cancer Causes Control* **13**(5), 407–415.

250. Lee, H. P., Gourley, L., Duffy, S. W., Esteve, J., Lee, J. & Day, N. E. (1992). Risk factors for breast cancer by age and menopausal status: A case-control study in Singapore. *Cancer Causes Control* **3**(4), 313–322.

251. Hirose, K., Tajima, K., Hamajima, N., Inoue, M., Takezaki, T., Kuroishi, T., Yoshida, M. & Tokudome, S. (1995). A large-scale, hospital-based case-control study of risk factors of breast cancer according to menopausal status. *Jpn J Cancer Res* **86**(2), 146–154.

252. Wu, A. H., Ziegler, R. G., Horn-Ross, P. L., Nomura, A. M., West, D. W., Kolonel, L. N., Rosenthal, J. F., Hoover, R. N. & Pike, M. C. (1996). Tofu and risk of breast cancer in Asian-Americans. *Cancer Epidemiol Biomarkers Prev* **5**(11), 901–906.

253. Dai, Q., Shu, X. O., Jin, F., Potter, J. D., Kushi, L. H., Teas, J., Gao, Y. T. & Zheng, W. (2001 Aug 3). Population-based case-control study of soyfood intake and breast cancer risk in Shanghai. *Br J Cancer* **85**(3), 372–378.

254. Wu, A. H., Wan, P., Hankin, J., Tseng, C. C., Yu, M. C. & Pike, M. C. (2002). Adolescent and adult soy intake and risk of breast cancer in Asian-Americans. *Carcinogenesis* **23**(9), 1491–1496.

255. Yamamoto, S., Sobue, T., Kobayashi, M., Sasaki, S. & Tsugane, S. (2003 June 18). Soy, isoflavones, and breast cancer risk in Japan. *J Natl Cancer Inst* **95**(12), 906–913.

256. Huntley, A. L. & Ernst, E. (2004 Jan 20). Soy for the treatment of perimenopausal symptoms – a systematic review. *Maturitas* **47**(1), 1–9.

257. Crisafulli, A., Marini, H., Bitto, A., Altavilla, D., Squadrito, G., Romeo, A., Adamo, E. B., Marini, R., D'Anna, R., Corrado, F., Bartolone, S., Frisina, N. & Squadrito, F. (2004). Effects of genistein on hot flushes in early postmenopausal women: A randomized, double-blind EPT- and placebo-controlled study. *Menopause* **11**(4), 400–404.

258. Shughrue, P. J., Komm, B. & Merchenthaler, I. (1996). The distribution of estrogen receptor-beta mRNA in the rat hypothalamus. *Steroids* **61**(12), 678–681.

259. Kruijver, F. P., Balesar, R., Espila, A. M., Unmehopa, U. A. & Swaab, D. F. (2003 Nov 10). Estrogen-receptor-beta distribution in the human hypothalamus: Similarities and differences with ER alpha distribution. *J Comp Neurol* **466**(2), 251–277.

260. Forsling, M. L., Kallo, I., Hartley, D. E., Heinze, L., Ladek, R., Coen, C. W. & File, S. E. (2003). Oestrogen receptor-beta and neurohypophysial hormones: Functional interaction and neuroanatomical localisation. *Pharmacol Biochem Behav* **76**(3–4), 535–542.

261. Silbiger, S. R. & Neugarten, J. (1995). The impact of gender on the progression of chronic renal disease. *Am J Kidney Dis* **25**(4), 515–533.

262. Neugarten, J., Acharya, A. & Silbiger, S. R. (2000). Effect of gender on the progression of nondiabetic renal disease: a meta-analysis. *J Am Soc Nephrol* **11**(2), 319–329.

263. Potier, M., Karl, M., Zheng, F., Elliot, S. J., Striker, G. E. & Striker, L. J. (2002). Estrogen-related abnormalities in glomerulosclerosis-prone mice: reduced mesangial cell estrogen receptor expression and prosclerotic response to estrogens. *Am J Pathol* **160**(5), 1877–1885.

264. Neugarten, J., Gallo, G., Silbiger, S. & Kasiske, B. (1999). Glomerulosclerosis in aging humans is not influenced by gender. *Am J Kidney Dis* **34**(5), 884–888.

265. Sakemi, T., Toyoshima, H., Shouno, Y. & Morito, F. (1995). Estrogen attenuates progressive glomerular injury in hypercholesterolemic male Imai rats. *Nephron* **69**(2), 159–165.

266. Sakemi, T., Ohtsuka, N., Tomiyoshi, Y. & Morito, F. (1997). Testosterone does not eliminate the attenuating effect of estrogen on progressive glomerular injury in estrogen-treated hypercholesterolemic male Imai rats. *Kidney Blood Press Res* **20**(1), 51–56.

267. Xiao, S., Gillespie, D. G., Baylis, C., Jackson, E. K. & Dubey, R. K. (2001). Effects of estradiol and its metabolites on glomerular endothelial nitric oxide synthesis and mesangial cell growth. *Hypertension* **37**(2 Part 2), 645–650.

268. Elliot, S. J., Karl, M., Berho, M., Potier, M., Zheng, F., Leclercq, B., Striker, G. E. & Striker, L. J. (2003). Estrogen deficiency accelerates progression of glomerulosclerosis in susceptible mice. *Am J Pathol* **162**(5), 1441–1448.

269. Antus, B., Hamar, P., Kokeny, G., Szollosi, Z., Mucsi, I., Nemes, Z. & Rosivall, L. (2003). Estradiol is nephroprotective in the rat remnant kidney. *Nephrol Dial Transplant* **18**(1), 54–61.

270. Gross, M. L., Adamczak, M., Rabe, T., Harbi, N. A., Krtil, J., Koch, A., Hamar, P., Amann, K. & Ritz, E. (2004). Beneficial effects of estrogens on indices of renal damage in uninephrectomized SHRsp rats. *J Am Soc Nephrol* **15**(2), 348–358.

271. Maric, C., Sandberg, K. & Hinojosa-Laborde, C. (2004). Glomerulosclerosis and tubulointerstitial fibrosis are attenuated with 17beta-estradiol in the aging Dahl salt sensitive rat. *J Am Soc Nephrol* **15**(6), 1546–1556.

272. Sakemi, T., Ohtsuka, N., Shouno, Y. & Morito, F. (1996). Effect of ovariectomy on glomerular injury in hypercholesterolemic female Imai rats. *Nephron* **72**(1), 72–78.

273. Joles, J. A., van Goor, H. & Koomans, H. A. (1998). Estrogen induces glomerulosclerosis in analbuminemic rats. *Kidney Int* **53**(4), 862–868.

274. Stevenson, F. T., Wheeldon, C. M., Gades, M. D., Kaysen, G. A., Stern, J. S. & van Goor, H. (2000). Estrogen worsens incipient hypertriglyceridemic glomerular injury in the obese Zucker rat. *Kidney Int* **57**(5), 1927–1935.

275. Tomiyoshi, Y., Sakemi, T., Aoki, S. & Miyazono, M. (2002). Different effects of castration and estrogen administration on glomerular injury in spontaneously hyperglycemic Otsuka Long-Evans Tokushima Fatty (OLETF) rats. *Nephron* **92**(4), 860–867.

276. Sakemi, T., Ohtsuka, N., Shouno, Y. & Morito, F. (1996). Ovariectomy attenuates proteinuria and glomerular injury in unilaterally nephrectomized female Sprague-Dawley rats. *Nephron* **73**(2), 251–257.

277. Ohtsuka, N., Sakemi, T., Tomiyoshi, Y. & Morito, F. (1997). Different effect of estrogen administration from castration on glomerular injury in unilaterally nephrectomized male Sprague-Dawley rats. *Nephron* **77**(4), 445–451.

278. Ikeda, Y., Sakemi, T., Tomiyoshi, Y. & Miyazono, M. (2000). Combined therapy with estrogen and testosterone eliminates the aggravating effect of estrogen replacement therapy on glomerular injury in hypercholesterolemic female Imai rats. *Kidney Blood Press Res* **23**(1), 27–34.

279. Studer, R. K., Craven, P. A. & DeRubertis, F. R. (1997). Antioxidant inhibition of protein kinase C-signaled increases in transforming growth factor-beta in mesangial cells. *Metabolism* **46**(8), 918–925.

280. Toyoda, M., Suzuki, D., Honma, M., Uehara, G., Sakai, T., Umezono, T. & Sakai, H. (2004). High expression of PKC-MAPK pathway mRNAs correlates with glomerular lesions in human diabetic nephropathy. *Kidney Int* **66**(3), 1107–1114.

281. Weigert, C., Sauer, U., Brodbeck, K., Pfeiffer, A., Haring, H. U. & Schleicher, E. D. (2000). AP-1 proteins mediate hyperglycemia-induced activation of the human TGF-beta1 promoter in mesangial cells. *J Am Soc Nephrol* **11**(11), 2007–2016.

282. Koya, D., Jirousek, M. R., Lin, Y. W., Ishii, H., Kuboki, K. & King, G. L. (1997 July 1). Characterization of protein kinase C beta isoform activation on the gene expression of transforming growth factor-beta, extracellular matrix components, and prostanoids in the glomeruli of diabetic rats. *J Clin Invest* **100**(1), 115–126.

283. Ishii, H., Tada, H. & Isogai, S. (1998). An aldose reductase inhibitor prevents glucose-induced increase in transforming growth factor-beta and protein kinase C activity in cultured mesangial cells. *Diabetologia* **41**(3), 362–364.

284. Ikehara, K., Tada, H., Kuboki, K. & Inokuchi, T. (2003). Role of protein kinase C-angiotensin II pathway for extracellular matrix production in cultured human mesangial cells exposed to high glucose levels. *Diabetes Res Clin Pract* **59**(1), 25–30.

285. Yasuda, T., Kondo, S., Homma, T. & Harris, R. C. (1996). Regulation of extracellular matrix by mechanical stress in rat glomerular mesangial cells. *J Clin Invest* **98**(9), 1991–2000.

286. Hirakata, M., Kaname, S., Chung, U. G., Joki, N., Hori, Y., Noda, M., Takuwa, Y., Okazaki, T., Fujita, T., Katoh, T. & Kurokawa, K. (1997). Tyrosine kinase dependent expression of TGF-beta induced by stretch in mesangial cells. *Kidney Int* **51**(4), 1028–1036.

287. Weigert, C., Brodbeck, K., Klopfer, K., Haring, H. U. & Schleicher, E. D. (2002). Angiotensin II induces human TGF-beta 1 promoter activation: Similarity to hyperglycaemia. *Diabetologia* **45**(6), 890–898.

288. Chen, S., Cohen, M. P., Lautenslager, G. T., Shearman, C. W. & Ziyadeh, F. N. (2001). Glycated albumin stimulates TGF-beta 1 production and protein kinase C activity in glomerular endothelial cells. *Kidney Int* **59**(2), 673–681.

289. Kim, Y. S., Kim, B. C., Song, C. Y., Hong, H. K., Moon, K. C. & Lee, H. S. (2001). Advanced glycosylation end products stimulate collagen mRNA synthesis in mesangial cells mediated by protein kinase C and transforming growth factor-beta. *J Lab Clin Med* **138**(1), 59–68.

290. Studer, R. K., Negrete, H., Craven, P. A. & DeRubertis, F. R. (1995). Protein kinase C signals thromboxane induced increases in fibronectin synthesis and TGF-beta bioactivity in mesangial cells. *Kidney Int* **48**(2), 422–430.

291. Wu, Z., Zhou, Q., Lan, Y., Wang, Y., Xu, X. & Jin, H. (2004). AP-1 complexes mediate oxidized LDL-induced overproduction of TGF-beta(1) in rat mesangial cells. *Cell Biochem Funct* **22**(4), 237–247.

292. Lee, H. S., Kim, B. C., Hong, H. K. & Kim, Y. S. (1999). LDL stimulates collagen mRNA synthesis in mesangial cells through induction of PKC and TGF-beta expression. *Am J Physiol* **277**(3 Pt 2), F369–F376.

293. Singh, L. P., Green, K., Alexander, M., Bassly, S. & Crook, E. D. (2004). Hexosamines and TGF-beta1 use similar signaling pathways to mediate matrix protein synthesis in mesangial cells. *Am J Physiol Renal Physiol* **286**(2), F409–F416.

294. Weiss, R. H. & Ramirez, A. (1998). TGF-beta- and angiotensin-II-induced mesangial matrix protein secretion is mediated by protein kinase C. *Nephrol Dial Transplant* **13**(11), 2804–2813.

295. Tada, H. & Isogai, S. (1998). The fibronectin production is increased by thrombospondin via activation of TGF-beta in cultured human mesangial cells. *Nephron* **79**(1), 38–43.

296. Runyan, C. E., Schnaper, H. W. & Poncelet, A. C. (2003). Smad3 and PKCdelta mediate TGF-beta1-induced collagen I expression in human mesangial cells. *Am J Physiol Renal Physiol* **285**(3), F413–F422.

297. Zdunek, M., Silbiger, S., Lei, J. & Neugarten, J. (2001). Protein kinase CK2 mediates TGF-beta1-stimulated type IV collagen gene transcription and its reversal by estradiol. *Kidney Int* **60**(6), 2097–2108.

298. Singh, R., Song, R. H., Alavi, N., Pegoraro, A. A., Singh, A. K. & Leehey, D. J. (2001). High glucose decreases matrix metalloproteinase-2 activity in rat mesangial cells via transforming growth factor-beta1. *Exp Nephrol* **9**(4), 249–257.

299. Baricos, W. H., Cortez, S. L., Deboisblanc, M. & Xin, S. (1999). Transforming growth factor-beta is a potent inhibitor of extracellular matrix degradation by cultured human mesangial cells. *J Am Soc Nephrol* **10**(4), 790–795.

300. Poncelet, A. C. & Schnaper, H. W. (1998). Regulation of human mesangial cell collagen expression by transforming growth factor-beta1. *Am J Physiol* **275** (3 Pt 2), F458–F466.

301. Marti, H. P., Lee, L., Kashgarian, M. & Lovett, D. H. (1994). Transforming growth factor-beta 1 stimulates glomerular mesangial cell synthesis of the 72-kd type IV collagenase. *Am J Pathol* **144**(1), 82–94.

302. Xin, C., Ren, S., Kleuser, B., Shabahang, S., Eberhardt, W., Radeke, H., Schafer-Korting, M., Pfeilschifter, J. & Huwiler, A. (2004 Aug 20). Sphingosine 1-phosphate cross-activates the Smad signaling cascade and mimics transforming growth factor-beta-induced cell responses. *J Biol Chem* **279**(34), 35255–35262.

303. Kaizuka, M., Yamabe, H., Osawa, H., Okumura, K. & Fujimoto, N. (1999). Thrombin stimulates synthesis of type IV collagen and tissue inhibitor of metalloproteinases-1 by cultured human mesangial cells. *J Am Soc Nephrol* **10**(7), 1516–1523.

304. Kopp, J. B., Factor, V. M., Mozes, M., Nagy, P., Sanderson, N., Bottinger, E. P., Klotman, P. E. & Thorgeirsson, S. S. (1996). Transgenic mice with increased plasma levels of TGF-beta 1 develop progressive renal disease. *Lab Invest* **74**(6), 991–1003.

305. Ali, S. M., Laping, N. J., Fredrickson, T. A., Contino, L. C., Olson, B., Anderson, K. & Brooks, D. P. (1998). Angiotensin-converting enzyme inhibition attenuates proteinuria and renal TGF-beta 1 mRNA expression in rats with chronic renal disease. *Pharmacology* **57**(1), 20–27.

306. Sharma, R., Khanna, A., Sharma, M. & Savin, V. J. (2000). Transforming growth factor-beta1 increases albumin permeability of isolated rat glomeruli via hydroxyl radicals. *Kidney Int* **58**(1), 131–136.

307. Fujimoto, M., Maezawa, Y., Yokote, K., Joh, K., Kobayashi, K., Kawamura, H., Nishimura, M., Roberts, A. B., Saito, Y. & Mori, S. (2003 June 13). Mice lacking Smad3 are protected against streptozotocin-induced diabetic glomerulopathy. *Biochem Biophys Res Commun* **305**(4), 1002–1007.

308. Benigni, A., Zoja, C., Corna, D., Zatelli, C., Conti, S., Campana, M., Gagliardini, E., Rottoli, D., Zanchi, C., Abbate, M., Ledbetter, S. & Remuzzi, G. (2003). Add-on anti-TGF-beta antibody to ACE inhibitor arrests progressive diabetic nephropathy in the rat. *J Am Soc Nephrol* **14**(7), 1816–1824.

309. Sharma, K., Jin, Y., Guo, J. & Ziyadeh, F. N. (1996). Neutralization of TGF-beta by anti-TGF-beta antibody attenuates kidney hypertrophy and the enhanced extracellular matrix gene expression in STZ-induced diabetic mice. *Diabetes* **45**(4), 522–530.

310. Ziyadeh, F. N., Hoffman, B. B., Han, D. C., Iglesias-de la Cruz, M. C., Hong, S. W., Isono, M., Chen, S., McGowan, T. A. & Sharma, K. (2000 July 5). Long-term prevention of renal insufficiency, excess matrix gene expression, and glomerular mesangial matrix expansion by treatment with monoclonal antitransforming growth factor-beta antibody in db/db diabetic mice. *Proc Natl Acad Sci U S A* **97**(14), 8015–8020.

311. Chen, S., Iglesias-de la Cruz, M. C., Jim, B., Hong, S. W., Isono, M. & Ziyadeh, F. N. (2003 Jan 3). Reversibility of established diabetic glomerulopathy by anti-TGF-beta antibodies in db/db mice. *Biochem Biophys Res Commun* **300**(1), 16–22.

312. Potier, M., Elliot, S. J., Tack, I., Lenz, O., Striker, G. E., Striker, L. J. & Karl, M. (2001). Expression and regulation of estrogen receptors in mesangial cells: Influence on matrix metalloproteinase-9. *J Am Soc Nephrol* **12**(2), 241–251.

313. Lei, J., Silbiger, S., Ziyadeh, F. N. & Neugarten, J. (1998). Serum-stimulated alpha 1 type IV collagen gene transcription is mediated by TGF-beta and inhibited by estradiol. *Am J Physiol* **274**(2 Pt 2), F252–F258.

314. Silbiger, S., Lei, J., Ziyadeh, F. N. & Neugarten, J. (1998). Estradiol reverses TGF-beta1-stimulated type IV collagen gene transcription in murine mesangial cells. *Am J Physiol* **274**(6 Pt 2), F1113–F1118.

315. Matsuda, T., Yamamoto, T., Muraguchi, A. & Saatcioglu, F. (2001 Nov 16). Cross-talk between transforming growth factor-beta and estrogen receptor signaling through Smad3. *J Biol Chem* **276**(46), 42908–42914.

316. Derynck, R., Zhang, Y. & Feng, X. H. (1998 Dec 11). Smads: Transcriptional activators of TGF-beta responses. *Cell* **95**(6), 737–740.

317. Craven, P. A., Studer, R. K., Felder, J., Phillips, S. & DeRubertis, F. R. (1997). Nitric oxide inhibition of transforming growth factor-beta and collagen synthesis in mesangial cells. *Diabetes* **46**(4), 671–681.

318. Williams, A. J., Baker, F. & Walls, J. (1987). Effect of varying quantity and quality of dietary protein intake in experimental renal disease in rats. *Nephron* **46**(1), 83–90.

319. Williams, A. J. & Walls, J. (1987). Metabolic consequences of differing protein diets in experimental renal disease. *Eur J Clin Invest* **17**(2), 117–122.

320. Iwasaki, K., Gleiser, C. A., Masoro, E. J., McMahan, C. A., Seo, E. J. & Yu, B. P. (1988). The influence of dietary protein source on longevity and age-related disease processes of Fischer rats. *J Gerontol* **43**(1), B5–12.

321. Aukema, H. M. & Housini, I. (2001). Dietary soy protein effects on disease and IGF-I in male and female Han:SPRD-cy rats. *Kidney Int* **59**(1), 52–61.

322. Velasquez, M. T. & Bhathena, S. J. (2001). Dietary phytoestrogens: A possible role in renal disease protection. *Am J Kidney Dis* **37**(5), 1056–1068.

323. Maddox, D. A., Alavi, F. K., Silbernick, E. M. & Zawada, E. T. (2002). Protective effects of a soy diet in preventing obesity-linked renal disease. *Kidney Int* **61**(1), 96–104.

324. Sakemi, T., Ikeda, Y. & Shimazu, K. (2002). Effect of soy protein added to casein diet on the development of glomerular injury in spontaneous hypercholesterolemic male Imai rats. *Am J Nephrol* **22**(5–6), 548–554.

325. Fair, D. E., Ogborn, M. R., Weiler, H. A., Bankovic-Calic, N., Nitschmann, E. P., Fitzpatrick-Wong, S. C. & Aukema, H. M. (2004). Dietary soy protein attenuates renal disease progression after 1 and 3 weeks in Han:SPRD-cy weanling rats. *J Nutr* **134**(6), 1504–1507.

326. Trujillo, J., Ramirez, V., Perez, J., Torre-Villalvazo, I., Torres, N., Tovar, A. R., Munoz, R. M., Uribe, N., Gamba, G. & Bobadilla, N. A. (2005). Renal protection by soy diet in obese Zucker rats is associated with restoration of nitric oxide generation. *Am J Physiol Renal Physiol* **288**, F108–F116.

327. Azadbakht, L., Shakerhosseini, R., Atabak, S., Jamshidian, M., Mehrabi, Y. & Esmaill-Zadeh, A. (2003). Beneficiary effect of dietary soy protein on lowering plasma levels of lipid and improving kidney function in type II diabetes with nephropathy. *Eur J Clin Nutr* **57**(10), 1292–1294.

328. Teixeira, S. R., Tappenden, K. A., Carson, L., Jones, R., Prabhudesai, M., Marshall, W. P. & Erdman, J. W., Jr. (2004). Isolated soy protein consumption reduces urinary albumin excretion and improves the serum lipid profile in men with type 2 diabetes mellitus and nephropathy. *J Nutr* **134**(8), 1874–1880.

329. Brenner, B. M., Meyer, T. W. & Hostetter, T. H. (1982 Sept 9). Dietary protein intake and the progressive nature of kidney disease: The role of hemodynamically mediated glomerular injury in the pathogenesis of progressive glomerular sclerosis in aging, renal ablation, and intrinsic renal disease. *N Engl J Med* **307**(11), 652–659.

330. Klahr, S., Buerkert, J. & Purkerson, M. L. (1983). Role of dietary factors in the progression of chronic renal disease. *Kidney Int* **24**(5), 579–587.

331. Nakamura, H., Takasawa, M., Kashara, S., Tsuda, A., Momotsu, T., Ito, S. & Shibata, A. (1989). Effects of acute protein loads of different sources on renal function of patients with diabetic nephropathy. *Tohoku J Exp Med* **159**(2), 153–162.

332. Kontessis, P., Jones, S., Dodds, R., Trevisan, R., Nosadini, R., Fioretto, P., Borsato, M., Sacerdoti, D. & Viberti, G. (1990). Renal, metabolic and hormonal responses to ingestion of animal and vegetable proteins. *Kidney Int* **38**(1), 136–144.

333. Anderson, J. W., Smith, B. M. & Washnock, C. S. (1999). Cardiovascular and renal benefits of dry bean and soybean intake. *Am J Clin Nutr* **70**(3 Suppl), 464S–474S.

334. Fouque, D., Laville, M., Boissel, J. P., Chifflet, R., Labeeuw, M. & Zech, P. Y. (1992 Jan 25). Controlled low protein diets in chronic renal insufficiency: Meta-analysis. *BMJ* **304**(6821), 216–220.

335. Pedrini, M. T., Levey, A. S., Lau, J., Chalmers, T. C. & Wang, P. H. (1996). The effect of dietary protein restriction on the progression of diabetic and nondiabetic renal diseases: A meta-analysis. *Ann Intern Med* **124**(7), 627–632.

336. Jibani, M. M., Bloodworth, L. L., Foden, E., Griffiths, K. D. & Galpin, O. P. (1991). Predominantly vegetarian diet in patients with incipient and early clinical diabetic nephropathy: Effects on albumin excretion rate and nutritional status. *Diabet Med* **8**(10), 949–953.

337. D'Amico, G. & Gentile, M. G. (1993). Influence of diet on lipid abnormalities in human renal disease. *Am J Kidney Dis* **22**(1), 151–157.

338. Barsotti, G., Morelli, E., Cupisti, A., Meola, M., Dani, L. & Giovannetti, S. (1996). A low-nitrogen low-phosphorus Vegan diet for patients with chronic renal failure. *Nephron* **74**(2), 390–394.

339. Soroka, N., Silverberg, D. S., Greemland, M., Birk, Y., Blum, M., Peer, G. & Iaina, A. (1998). Comparison of a vegetable-based (soya) and an animal-based low-protein diet in predialysis chronic renal failure patients. *Nephron* **79**(2), 173–180.

340. Ranich, T., Bhathena, S. J. & Velasquez, M. T. (2001). Protective effects of dietary phytoestrogens in chronic renal disease. *J Ren Nutr* **11**(4), 183–193.

341. Sakemi, T., Ikeda, Y., Shimazu, K. & Uesugi, T. (2001). Attenuating effect of a semipurified alcohol extract of soy protein on glomerular injury in spontaneous hypercholesterolemic male Imai rats. *Am J Kidney Dis* **37**(4), 832–837.

342. Neugarten, J., Acharya, A., Lei, J. & Silbiger, S. (2000). Selective estrogen receptor modulators suppress mesangial cell collagen synthesis. *Am J Physiol Renal Physiol* **279**(2), F309–F318.

343. Slater, M., Brown, D. & Husband, A. (2002). In the prostatic epithelium, dietary isoflavones from red clover significantly increase estrogen receptor beta and E-cadherin expression but decrease transforming growth factor beta1. *Prostate Cancer Prostatic Dis* **5**(1), 16–21.

344. McCarty, M. F. (2004). Adjuvant strategies for prevention of glomerulosclerosis. *Med Hypotheses* **24**, submitted for publication.

345. Higuchi, Y., Otsu, K., Nishida, K., Hirotani, S., Nakayama, H., Yamaguchi, O., Hikoso, S., Kashiwase, K., Takeda, T., Watanabe, T., Mano, T., Matsumura, Y., Ueno, H. & Hori, M. (2003 June 6). The small GTP-binding protein Rac1 induces cardiac myocyte hypertrophy through the activation of apoptosis signal-regulating kinase 1 and nuclear factor-kappa B. *J Biol Chem* **278**(23), 20770–20777.

346. Simko, F. & Simko, J. (2000). The potential role of nitric oxide in the hypertrophic growth of the left ventricle. *Physiol Res* **49**(1), 37–46.

347. Lim, W. K., Wren, B., Jepson, N., Roy, S. & Caplan, G. (1999 Apr 1). Effect of hormone replacement therapy on left ventricular hypertrophy. *Am J Cardiol* **83**(7), 1132–1134, A9.

348. du, C. G., Ribstein, J., Pasquie, J. L. & Mimran, A. (1999). Determinant of left ventricular hypertrophy in the hypertensive woman, Influence of hormone replacement therapy for menopause. *Arch Mal Coeur Vaiss* **92**(8), 975–977.

349. Modena, M. G., Molinari, R., Muia, N., Jr., Castelli, A., Pala, F. & Rossi, R. (1999). Double-blind randomized placebo-controlled study of transdermal

estrogen replacement therapy on hypertensive postmenopausal women. *Am J Hypertens* **12**(1O Pt 1), 1000–1008.

350. Modena, M. G., Muia, N., Jr., Aveta, P., Molinari, R. & Rossi, R. (1999). Effects of transdermal 17beta-estradiol on left ventricular anatomy and performance in hypertensive women. *Hypertension* **34**(5), 1041–1046.

351. Light, K. C., Hinderliter, A. L., West, S. G., Grewen, K. M., Steege, J. F., Sherwood, A. & Girdler, S. S. (2001). Hormone replacement improves hemodynamic profile and left ventricular geometry in hypertensive and normotensive postmenopausal women. *J Hypertens* **19**(2), 269–278.

352. Hayward, C. S., Webb, C. M. & Collins, P. (2001 Apr 28). Effect of sex hormones on cardiac mass. *Lancet* **357**(9265), 1354–1356.

353. Miya, Y., Sumino, H., Ichikawa, S., Nakamura, T., Kanda, T., Kumakura, H., Takayama, Y., Mizunuma, H., Sakamaki, T. & Kurabayashi, M. (2005). Effects of hormone replacement therapy on left ventricular hypertrophy and growth-promoting factors in hypertensive postmenopausal women. *Hypertens Res* **25**(2), 153–159.

354. Agabiti-Rosei, E. & Muiesan, M. L. (2002). Left ventricular hypertrophy and heart failure in women. *J Hypertens* **20**(Suppl 2), S34–S38.

355. Grohe, C., Kahlert, S., Lobbert, K., Stimpel, M., Karas, R. H., Vetter, H. & Neyses, L. (1997 Oct 13). Cardiac myocytes and fibroblasts contain functional estrogen receptors. *FEBS Lett* **416**(1), 107–112.

356. Nuedling, S., Karas, R. H., Mendelsohn, M. E., Katzenellenbogen, J. A., Katzenellenbogen, B. S., Meyer, R., Vetter, H. & Grohe, C. (2001 Aug 3). Activation of estrogen receptor beta is a prerequisite for estrogen-dependent upregulation of nitric oxide synthases in neonatal rat cardiac myocytes. *FEBS Lett* **502**(3), 103–108.

357. Skavdahl, M., Steenbergen, C., Clark, J., Myers, P., Demianenko, T., Mao, L., Rockman, H. A., Korach, K. S. & Murphy, E. (2005). The beta estrogen receptor mediates male-female differences in the development of pressure overload hypertrophy. *Am J Physiol Heart Circ Physiol* **288**, H469–H476

358. Di, M. V., Lebray, P., Myers, R. P., Pannier, E., Paradis, V., Charlotte, F., Moussalli, J., Thabut, D., Buffet, C. & Poynard, T. (2004). Progression of liver fibrosis in women infected with hepatitis C: Long-term benefit of estrogen exposure. *Hepatology* **40**(6), 1426–1433.

359. Codes, L., Asselah, T., Cazals-Hatem, D., Tubach, F., Vidaud, D., Parana, R., Bedossa, P., Valla, D. & Marcellin, P. (2007). Liver fibrosis in women with chronic hepatitis C: Evidence for the negative role of menopause and steatosis and the potential benefit of hormone replacement therapy. *Gut* **56**, 390–395.

360. Shimizu, I. (2003). Impact of oestrogens on the progression of liver disease. *Liver Int* **23**(1), 63–69.

361. Xu, J. W., Gong, J., Chang, X. M., Luo, J. Y., Dong, L., Hao, Z. M., Jia, A. & Xu, G. P. (2002). Estrogen reduces CCL4-induced liver fibrosis in rats. *World J Gastroenterol* **8**(5), 883–887.

362. Liu, Q. H., Li, D. G., Huang, X., Zong, C. H., Xu, Q. F. & Lu, H. M. (2004 May 1). Suppressive effects of 17beta-estradiol on hepatic fibrosis in CCl4-induced rat model. *World J Gastroenterol* **10**(9), 1315–1320.

363. Lu, G., Shimizu, I., Cui, X., Itonaga, M., Tamaki, K., Fukuno, H., Inoue, H., Honda, H. & Ito, S. (2004 Jan 2). Antioxidant and antiapoptotic activities of idoxifene and estradiol in hepatic fibrosis in rats. *Life Sci* **74**(7), 897–907.

364. Zhou, Y. J., Yin, D. M., Chen, H. S., Shi, J. H., Sha, B. X. & Wang, X. (2005). Inhibitory effects of idoxifene on hepatic fibrosis in rats. *Acta Pharmacol Sin* **26**(5), 581–586.

365. Wu, J. & Zern, M. A. (2000). Hepatic stellate cells: A target for the treatment of liver fibrosis. *J Gastroenterol* **35**(9), 665–672.

366. Shimizu, I., Mizobuchi, Y., Yasuda, M., Shiba, M., Ma, Y. R., Horie, T., Liu, F. & Ito, S. (1999). Inhibitory effect of oestradiol on activation of rat hepatic stellate cells *in vivo* and *in vitro*. *Gut* **44**(1), 127–136.

367. Itagaki, T., Shimizu, I., Cheng, X., Yuan, Y., Oshio, A., Tamaki, K., Fukuno, H., Honda, H., Okamura, Y. & Ito, S. (2005). Opposing effects of oestradiol and progesterone on intracellular pathways and activation processes in the oxidative stress induced activation of cultured rat hepatic stellate cells. *Gut* **54**(12), 1782–1789.

368. Zhou, Y., Shimizu, I., Lu, G., Itonaga, M., Okamura, Y., Shono, M., Honda, H., Inoue, S., Muramatsu, M. & Ito, S. (2001 Sept 7). Hepatic stellate cells contain the functional estrogen receptor beta but not the estrogen receptor alpha in male and female rats. *Biochem Biophys Res Commun* **286**(5), 1059–1065.

369. Liu, X. J., Yang, L., Mao, Y. Q., Wang, Q., Huang, M. H., Wang, Y. P. & Wu, H. B. (2002). Effects of the tyrosine protein kinase inhibitor genistein on the proliferation, activation of cultured rat hepatic stellate cells. *World J Gastroenterol* **8**(4), 739–745.

370. McCarty, M. F. (2006). Isoflavones made simple – genistein's agonist activity for the beta-type estrogen receptor mediates their health benefits. *Med Hypotheses* **66**(6), 1093–1114.

371. Armstrong, B. & Doll, R. (1975 Apr 15). Environmental factors and cancer incidence and mortality in different countries, with special reference to dietary practices. *Int J Cancer* **15**(4), 617–631.

372. Hebert, J. R., Hurley, T. G., Olendzki, B. C., Teas, J., Ma, Y. & Hampl, J. S. (1998 Nov 4). Nutritional and socioeconomic factors in relation to prostate cancer mortality: A cross-national study [see comments]. *J Natl Cancer Inst* **90**(21), 1637–1647.

373. Hebert, J. R. & Rosen, A. (1996). Nutritional, socioeconomic, and reproductive factors in relation to female breast cancer mortality: Findings from a cross-national study. *Cancer Detect Prev* **20**(3), 234–244.

374. McCarty, M. F. (2001). Mortality from Western cancers rose dramatically among African-Americans during the 20th century: Are dietary animal products to blame? *Med Hypotheses* **57**(2), 169–174.

375. Giovannucci, E. (2003). Nutrition, insulin, insulin-like growth factors and cancer. *Horm Metab Res* **35**(11–12), 694–704.

376. McCarty, M. F. (2004). Insulin and IGF-I as determinants of low "Western" cancer rates in the rural third world. *Int J Epidemiol* **33**(4), 908–910.

377. Khalil, D. A., Lucas, E. A., Juma, S., Smith, B. J., Payton, M. E. & Arjmandi, B. H. (2002). Soy protein supplementation increases serum insulin-like growth factor-I in young and old men but does not affect markers of bone metabolism. *J Nutr* **132**(9), 2605–2608.

378. Allen, N. E., Appleby, P. N., Davey, G. K., Kaaks, R., Rinaldi, S. & Key, T. J. (2002). The associations of diet with serum insulin-like growth factor I and its main binding proteins in 292 women meat-eaters, vegetarians, and vegans. *Cancer Epidemiol Biomarkers Prev* **11**(11), 1441–1448.

379. Arjmandi, B. H., Khalil, D. A., Smith, B. J., Lucas, E. A., Juma, S., Payton, M. E. & Wild, R. A. (2003). Soy protein has a greater effect on bone in postmenopausal women not on hormone replacement therapy, as evidenced by reducing bone resorption and urinary calcium excretion. *J Clin Endocrinol Metab* **88**(3), 1048–1054.

380. Schulsinger, D. A., Root, M. M. & Campbell, T. C. (1989 Aug 16). Effect of dietary protein quality on development of aflatoxin B1-induced hepatic preneoplastic lesions. *J Natl Cancer Inst* **81**(16), 1241–1245.

381. Campbell, T. C. & Junshi, C. (1994). Diet and chronic degenerative diseases: Perspectives from China. *Am J Clin Nutr* **59**(5 Suppl), 1153S–1161S.

382. McCarty, M. F. (2006). Isoflavones made simple – genistein's agonist activity for the beta-type estrogen receptor mediates their health benefits. *Med Hypotheses* **66**(6), 1093–1114.

Chapter 25

Signal Therapy: Propolis and Pepper Extracts as Cancer Therapeutics

Hiroshi Maruta[1] and Toshiro Ohta[2]

[1]University Hospital at Eppendorf (UKE), Hamburg, Germany; University of Maryland at Baltimore (UMB), Baltimore, USA

[2]School of Food and Nutritional Sciences, University of Shizuoka, Shizuoka, Japan

Abstract

A variety of tumors are caused by either abnormal activation of proto-oncoproteins or dysfunction of tumor suppressors. The majority of these proteins are signal transducers such as G proteins, protein kinases and transcription factors that control the cell growth positively or negatively. Thus, recently several chemical compounds called signal therapeutics (STs) such as Gleevec emerged as a new generation of effective cancer therapeutics that selectively block the oncogenic signal pathways, to which tumors are highly addicted for their growth, but not for the normal cell growth. Unlike the conventional anti-cancer drugs such as DNA/microtubule poisons, these STs show far less side effects. Interestingly, many natural plant products inexpensively available in the market such as fruits, vegetables and healthcare food supplements also contain a series of STs useful for cancer therapy. Here we discuss a few emerging examples of these natural STs such as propolis (bee wax) and pepper extracts that block the major oncogenic signal transducer "PAK1," a unique Ser/Thr kinase, which is responsible for the development of more than 70% of human cancers/tumors.

Keywords: *Signal, therapeutic, cancer, neurofibromatosis, PAK1, kinase, propolis, pepper*

INTRODUCTION

PAK1 and Cancers

Discovery of many different oncogenes and tumor suppressor genes during last three decades has completely changed both our understanding of cancers and approach to cancer therapy. For most of these gene products were found signal transducers that regulate cell proliferation positively or negatively. Many onco-gene products are abnormally activated GTPases (GTP-dependent proteins) such as RAS, or protein kinases such as SRC. Similarly, many tumor suppressor gene products are transcription factors such as p53 and RB, and inhibitors of GTPases or kinases, such as NF1 and NF2/merlin, respectively. Thus, it became possible to generate specific chemical inhibitors of these oncogenic signal transducers or mimetics (agonists) of these anti-oncogenic signals, which would be useful for the systemic treatment of a variety of malignant or benign tumors.

Here we call such a new generation of anti-cancer drugs "signal (blocking) ther-apeutics," to distinguish them from a series of the conventional anti-cancer drugs which target mainly DNA or microtubules (MT), thereby handling mainly the fast-growing cancers. These DNA/MT poisons such as cisplatin, 5-FU, and Taxol have been successful for the treatment of a variety of cancers, but failed to suppress the growth of pancreatic cancers and slowly growing tumors such as NF (neurofibromatosis). Furthermore, the DNA/MT poisons cause inevita-bly a series of side effects such as hair loss and immuno-suppression. These side effects are due to damaging the fast-growing normal cells such as hair and bone marrow cells.

Among the first signal therapeutics, so far Gleevec (STI-571) appears to be most successful. Gleevec is a specific inhibitor of the Tyr-kinases BCL-ABL, PDGF receptor (PDGFR), and Kit [1]. It is an ATP antagonist which binds the ATP-binding pocket of these kinases. Since CML (chronic myeloid leukemia) and GIST (gastrointestinal stromal tumors) are caused by abnormal activation of BCL-ABL and Kit, respectively, Gleevec (400–600 mg daily) has been used for the treatment of these rather rare cancers [1]. However, the remaining vast major-ity of cancers and NF cannot be treated by Gleevec, simply because either BCL-ABL, PDGFR or Kit is not essential for the growth of these cancers/tumors.

Which signal transducer is essential for the majority of those remain-ing cancers/tumors? A systematic study by our group and a few others has recently led us to a conclusion that the Ser/Thr-kinase PAK1 is essential for more than 70% of cancers (including major cancers such as breast and pros-tate cancers, and pancreatic cancer) and even slowly growing tumors such as NF [2–7]. These tumors are highly addicted to this kinase for their anchorage-independent growth, but not for the normal (anchorage-dependent) cell growth. So we call them PAK1-dependent tumors (PDTs). PAK1 is a Rac/CDC42-dependent kinase that phosphorylates several effectors such as the kinase Raf, LIM kinase 1, BAD, and the kinase aurora [8–9]. Thus, PAK1 is involved in several different features of tumorigenesis, including cell division, anti-apoptosis (cell survival), metastasis/invasion, and angiogenesis (Fig. 25.1).

First of all, PAK1 phosphorylates Ser 338 of Raf to activate this kinase [10], and eventually through the down-stream MEK-ERK signal pathway up-regulates cyclin D1 that activates CDKs (cyclin-dependent kinases), which in turn push the cell cycle from G1 to S phase for DNA replication [11]. Secondly, PAK1 phosphorylates Thr 508 of LIM kinase 1 for the activation,

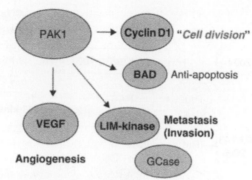

>70% of human cancers are addicted to PAK1!

FIGURE 25.1   Roles of PAK1 in tumorigenesis.

and in return LIM kinase 1 inactivates cofilin by phosphorylating at Ser 3 [12]. Since cofilin is an F-actin severing protein, fragmenting actin filaments, and the phosphorylation blocks its actin-binding, the PAK1-LIM kinase pathway leads to actin polymerization (stabilization of actin filaments) and stimulation of cell migration, and eventually metastasis of malignant tumors.

PAK1 also blocks apoptosis (programmed cell death) by phosphorylating and inactivating a pro-apoptotic protein called BAD [13]. Furthermore, PAK1 activates *VEGF* gene which is essential for the tumor-induced angiogenesis [14]. In other words, anti-PAK1 drugs can block not only cell division, but also metastasis, and angiogenesis, and cause apoptosis of tumors as well. Among anti-PAK1 drugs, so far a ring peptide called FK228 is the most potent anti-cancer drug (IC_{50} around 5 pM). Its direct target is HDAC (histone deacetylase) [15]. However, as shown in Fig. 25.2, FK228 blocks both down-stream and up-stream of PAK1, by up-regulating two tumor suppressors, p21/WAF1 and Rap1A, respectively [16–17]. p21 is an inhibitor of CDKs, thereby antagonizing cyclin D1 that activates CDKs. Rap1A is a GTPase, that antagonizes RAS, thereby blocking the oncogenic RAS-PI-3 kinase pathway essential for PAK1 activation. FK228 is currently in clinical trials for a variety of PAK1-dependent cancers (phase 2), but it would still take several more years for FK228 to enter the market.

So recently we have started exploring anti-PAK1 drugs among natural products available in the market, hopefully being able to give an immediate benefit to those who are currently suffering from these formidable cancers/NF (PDTs). The followings are a few examples of those which block the oncogenic PAK1 signaling.

PROPOLIS

Propolis from bee hives (also called "bee wax") is a 100 million years' wisdom of bee society protecting their larva from a variety of diseases (Fig. 25.3).

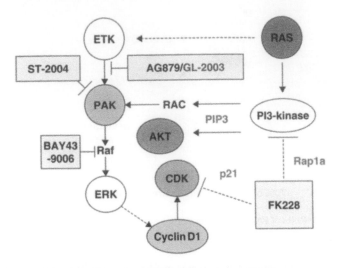

FIGURE 25.2   FK228 blocks both down-stream and up-stream of PAK1.

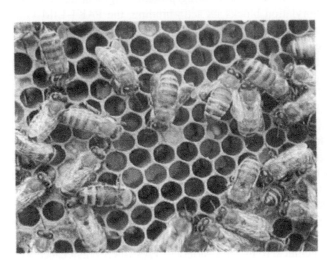

FIGURE 25.3   Propolis is an extract of the honey cum (bee wax) that protects larva.

Propolis has been used since the ancient Egypt as a traditional/folk medicine for the treatment of infection, wound and inflammation as well as preparing mummies. Entering our modern era, propolis was first identified as an anti-cancer remedy in a late 1980s when Dezider Grunberger's group at Columbia University found that CAPE (caffeic acid phenethyl ester) is the major anti-cancer ingredient in a propolis sample from Israel [18]. As shown in Fig. 25.4, CAPE is a derivative of CA (caffeic acid) that down-regulates the GTPase Rac, a direct activator of PAK1 [19]. Thus, it would inactivate PAK1 eventually.

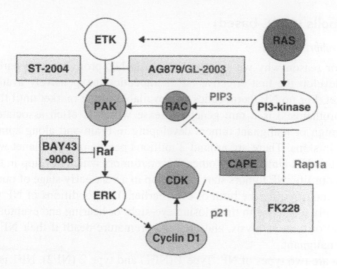

FIGURE 25.4   CAPE inactivates PAK1 by down-regulating RAC.

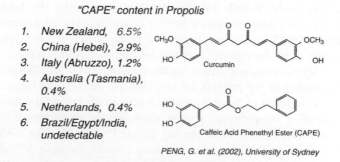

FIGURE 25.5   CAPE content of various propolis samples.

Interestingly, NZ (New Zealand) propolis reportedly showed the highest CAPE content (6–7% of extract) among a variety of propolis samples around the world (Fig. 25.5), whereas Brazilian propolis samples (either green or red) contain no CAPE. Nevertheless the latter are also known to have an anti-cancer property, and the biochemical nature of the major anti-cancer ingredient in green propolis will be discussed in detail later.

The major source of CAPE in propolis is known to be young buds of poplar trees. Thus, most of propolis samples harvested in the Temperate Zone including Europe and East Asia (China, Korea, and Japan) are expected to be relatively rich in CAPE. Like many other anti-PAK1 drugs, CAPE has been shown to block both angiogenesis and metastasis, in addition to anchorage-independent growth of cancer cells [20, 21].

NZ Propolis (CAPE-based)

NF (Neurofibromatosis)

The major reason why we started to work on NZ propolis in an early 2006 was to develop the first effective NF therapeutics inexpensively available in the market. For no NF therapeutics was available in the market until then. NF (neurofibromatosis) is a rare genetic disease which is often associated with either benign or malignant tumors developing in brain and along spinal cord and also in skins. There are around 2 millions people on this planet who suffer from this NF. Unlike many other cancers/tumors which develop in the later stages of our life, NF tumors start to develop in a very early stage of our life, in around 6 months after the birth or even earlier. The conditions of NF patients get gradually worsen with time, losing eye-sight or hearing and eventually facing partial or total paralysis, and even the premature death if their NF tumors become malignant.

There are two types of NF: Type 1 (NF1) and type 2 (NF2). NF1 is caused by dysfunction (loss-of-function mutation) of a tumor suppressor (*NF1* gene product) which is a RAS GAP of 2818 amino acids [22]. NF2 is caused by dysfunction of another tumor suppressor, a *NF2* gene product of 595 amino acids called merlin, which was found recently to inhibit the kinase PAK1 directly [3]. NF1 tumors include benign neurofibromas, plexiform, and the malignant MPNST (malignant peripheral nerve sheath tumor), representing around 90% of NF tumors. NF2 tumors include mainly two tumors, meningiomas and Schwannomas, representing the remaining 10% of NF tumors. Since the total number of NF patients are less than 1% of the total cancer patients, the progress in R&D of NF therapeutics has been far behind the those of cancer therapeutics. Nevertheless, several years ago the development of an NF1 tumor was found to depend on the key kinase PAK1 [23], like RAS-induced cancers such as pancreatic, colon and lung cancers, because *NF1*-deficiency leads to abnormal activation of normal RAS, which in turn activates PAK1 constitutively (Fig. 25.6). More recently, we found that NF2 tumors also require the same kinase for their growth, mainly because *NF2*-deficiency causes the abnormal activation of PAK1 [3]. Subsequently we confirmed that FK228, the most potent anti-PAK1 drugs, is effective for the treatment of a human NF tumor (MPNST) xenograft in mice [4]. Unfortunately, however, it turned out that FK228 would not be available for NF patients until the on-going clinical trials for cancer patients are completed, and this drug would enter the market with the FDA approval. Thus, an alternative NF therapeutics has been explored among the inexpensive and safe healthcare food supplements freely available in the market.

Among such alternatives we found that a water-miscible CAPE-rich extract of New Zealand (NZ) propolis called Bio 30 is the most effective NF therapeutics, using human NF1 and NF2 tumor xenografts in mice [24].

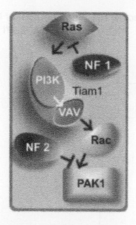

FIGURE 25.6 Oncogenic RAS-PAK1 signaling pathway blocked by NF1 and NF2 gene products.

TABLE 25.1 Content of Major Anti-Cancer Polyphenols in Bio 30

	(mg/g)
Galangin	60
Chrysin	30
CAPE	12
Caffeic acid	12
Apigenin	12

NZ Propolis as NF/Cancer Therapeutics

First of all, Bio 30 (alcohol-free liquid) was found to contain not only CAPE but also several other anti-cancer ingredients such as galangin, chrysin, apigenin and CA (caffeic acid) (see Table 25.1). The IC_{50} of CAPE alone for the growth of *NF1*-deficient MPNST and *NF2*-deficient Schwannoma cells is 25 and 36 μM, respectively. However, the IC_{50} of Bio 30 for Schwannoma cells turned out to be 1.5 μg/ml. Since the CAPE content of Bio 30 is around 12 mg/g, its contribution to 1.5 μg/ml is only 0.018 μg/ml, which is around 0.06 μM, meaning that the anti-mitotic activity of CAPE is potentiated by around 600 times with several other anti-cancer ingredients in this extract [24]. Furthermore, this propolis extract contains a lot of lipids which solubilize the water-insoluble CAPE. Although CAPE has been shown to have an anti-cancer activity, its bioavailability is very poor (mainly due to its poor water-solubility) *in vivo*, and therefore it has never been in clinical trials. Thus, Bio 30 potentiates not only the anti-mitotic ability per se but also the bio-availability of CAPE.

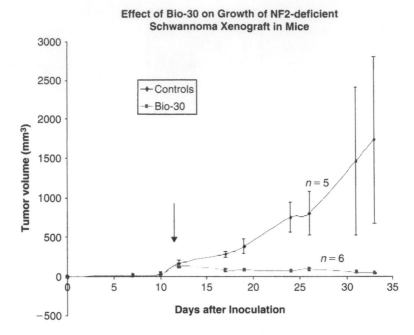

FIGURE 25.7   Bio 30 suppresses the growth of NF tumors (Schwannoma) grafted in mice.

To determine its *in vivo* effect, we have treated nude mice bearing either human MPNST or Schwannoma xenografts with Bio 30 (100 mg/kg, i.p., twice a week). Over 100 days the slow growth of MPNST was suppressed by 90%, while the fast-growing Schwannoma was almost completely regressed over 30 days (Fig. 25.7) [24]. Furthermore, when Bio 30 was supplemented with an extra CAPE (5 mg/kg), in four out of six mice, MPNST was completely regressed, and also its metastasis was significantly delayed and reduced to around 15% of the control.

Thus, Bio 30 has been proved to be the first effective NF therapeutics available in the market. Furthermore, 5 ml of Bio 30 required for daily treatment of each adult NF patient (weighing 50–60 kg) costs only a dollar. Thus, it would be economically quite feasible even for a life-long treatment of both NF1 and NF2 tumors. So far Bio 30 shows no side effect at this dose, except that only 5% of population is known to be allergic to the CAPE-based propolis such as Bio 30.

Using a similar xenograft system, we have confirmed that Bio 30 is effective to suppress the growth of at least human pancreatic and breast cancers as well (Demestre, M. *et al.*, unpublished data).

Brazilian Propolis (ARC-based)

Artepillin C (ARC)

Generally speaking, propolis contains several distinct anti-cancer ingredients: not only CA and CAPE, but also artepillin C, chrysin, and propolins. In the case of Brazilian green propolis, it has no detectable CAPE, but instead a phenolic acid called artepillin C (ARC), whose content is 6–7%, appears to be the primary anti-cancer ingredient in this propolis [25, 26]. ARC was first isolated as an antibiotic from this propolis by Masashi Kurimoto and his colleagues at Hayashibara Biochem Lab in Okayama, Japan [27]. Brazilian green propolis at the oral dose of 160 mg/kg strongly suppresses the growth of colon cancer xenograft in mice, as much as 10 mg/kg of ARC does, according to a recent report from a Japanese group led by Kazuki Kanazawa at Kobe University [28]. In other words, unlike the NZ propolis, there is no synergy between ARC and the remaining ingredients in the green propolis for tumor suppression.

Interestingly, like CAPE and other anti-PAK1 drugs, ARC up-regulates p21, but not p27 [29], suggesting the possibility that ARC also might block the PAK1 signal cascade which is required for down-regulation of p21 (but not p27). The down-regulation of p27 by the oncogenic RAS/PI-3 kinase signaling appears to depend on the kinase AKT, and not PAK1. Several years ago two groups led by Takashi Tsuruo at Tokyo University in Japan, and by Carlos Arteaga at Vanderbilt University Medical School in Nashville, independently showed that AKT phosphorylates p27 at Thr 157 or 198, and this phosphorylation blocks the importin-dependent nuclear localization of p27, causing a rapid degradation of p27 in the cytoplasm [30, 31]. Two years later our group in Melbourne, Australia, found that both up-regulation of cyclin D1 and down-regulation of p21, but not p27, requires PAK1 [11]. In an early 2007 our group in Hamburg, Germany, found that ARC inhibits the growth of NF1-deficient (PAK1-dependent) MPNST cells with the IC_{50} around 25 μM [32], suggesting that like the CAPE-rich NZ propolis, Brazilian green propolis is also useful for the treatment of PAK1-dependent cancers and NF. Furthermore, almost simultaneously, another group of ours in Shizuoka, Japan, found that ARC inhibits angiogenesis both *in vitro* and *in vivo* [33], again supporting the notion that like CAPE, ARC blocks PAK1 activation somehow. Finally, during 2007–2008, we confirmed that ARC indeed blocks the PAK1/Raf/ERK pathway, but not the AKT pathway (see Fig. 25.8), and that both ARC alone and ARC-rich extract of Brazilian green propolis can suppress almost completely the growth of NF2 tumor xenograft in mice [32].

Thus, ARC alone or ARC-rich extract of Brazilian green propolis appears to share a common pharmacological property with Chinese (Sichuan) pepper extract that selectively blocks PAK1 signaling, without affecting AKT signaling, and suppresses the growth of NF1-deficient cancer cells *in vitro* and *in vivo* [34]. Thus, it would be of great interest to determine whether the major anti-PAK1 ingredient in the Chinese pepper extract is ARC or a new compound.

As summarized in Fig. 25.9, the chemical synthesis of ARC was conducted by Hitoshi Hori's group at Tokushima University in 2002 [35]. Thereafter they have synthesized a series of ARC derivatives to study their structure–function relationship, hoping to develop a much more potent and water-soluble anti-PAK1 drug from ARC derivatives useful for PDTs such as pancreatic cancers and NF.

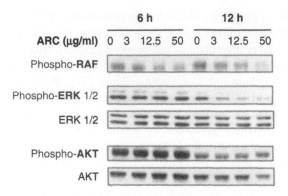

ARC (Artepillin C) blocks PAK1(Raf-ERK), but not AKT, pathways.

FIGURE 25.8 ARC blocks PAK1-Raf-ERK, but not AKT, pathways.

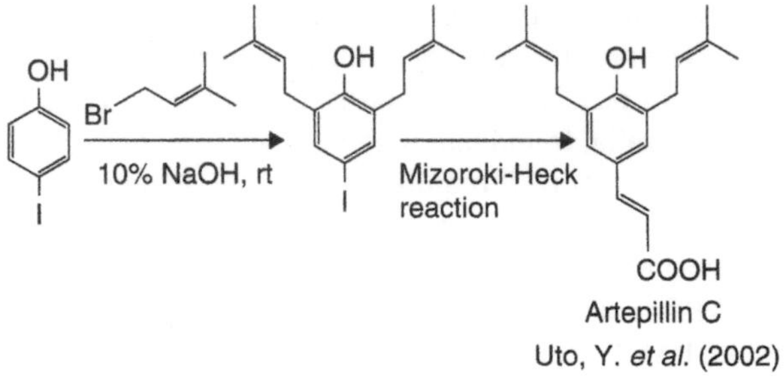

FIGURE 25.9 Chemical synthesis of ARC.

PEPPER EXTRACTS

Chinese (Sichuan) pepper extract

Chinese pepper from Sichuan Province called Hua Jiao (Fig. 25.10) has been used for a few thousands years as one of the two seasonings (spices) for cooking a popular Chinese (Sichuan) dish called Mapo Tofu, a combination of bean curd and minced beef. Hua Jiao belongs to the genus *Zanthoxylum*, a member of Citrus family, and the ripe peppercorn is red-colored. It is closely related to a Japanese pepper called Sansho whose ripe pepper corn is green-colored. The latter also has been used as both a seasoning for a popular Japanese eel dish and a Chinese traditional (herb) medicine for several centuries.

A few years ago we found that 70% ethanol (or warm water) extract of both Hua Jiao and Sansho shows an anti-mitotic activity towards both breast and prostate cancer cells as well as MPNST cells, but not normal cells [34].

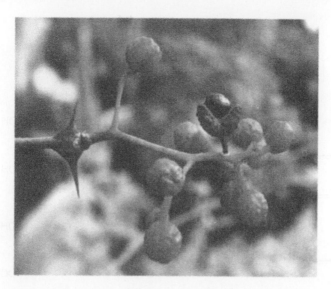

FIGURE 25.10   Chinese peppercorns (Hua Jiao) from Sichuan.

The IC_{50} of Hua Jiao extract is around $10\,\mu g/ml$, whereas that of Sancho extract is around $100\,\mu g/ml$. Interestingly, both pepper extracts selectively blocks PAK1 activation, but not the activation of another kinase called AKT. Both kinases act down stream of PI-3 kinase. Thus, the target of this pepper extract must be somewhere down-stream of PI-3 kinase, but up-stream of PAK1. We found that Hua Jiao extract ($110\,mg/kg$, i.p. twice a week) suppresses the growth of NF1-deficient breast cancer xenograft in mice by 50%. However, it still remains to be clarified which ingredient of this extract is responsible for this anti-PAK1 activity.

Chili Pepper Extract

Another spice used for cooking the Mapo tofu is chili pepper.

It is a red fruit of the plant Capsicum from the nightshade family, Solanaceae. Chili peppers have been a part of the human diet in the Americas since at least 7500 BC and perhaps earlier. There is archaeological evidence at sites located in southwestern Ecuador that chili peppers were already well domesticated more than 6000 years ago, and is one of the first cultivated crops in the Americas (http://en.wikipedia.org/wiki/Chili_pepper).

Capsaicin was first isolated in 1816 by P. A. Buchtholz and again 30 years later by L. T. Tresh in crystalline form, who also gave it the name capsaicin (see the chemical structure in Fig. 25.11). In 1878 Hungarian doctor Endre Hogyes, who called it capsicol, proved that this substance is the cause of the burning feeling when in contact with mucous membrane and it also increases secretion of gastric juice. Capsaicin was first synthesized in 1930 by E. Spath and

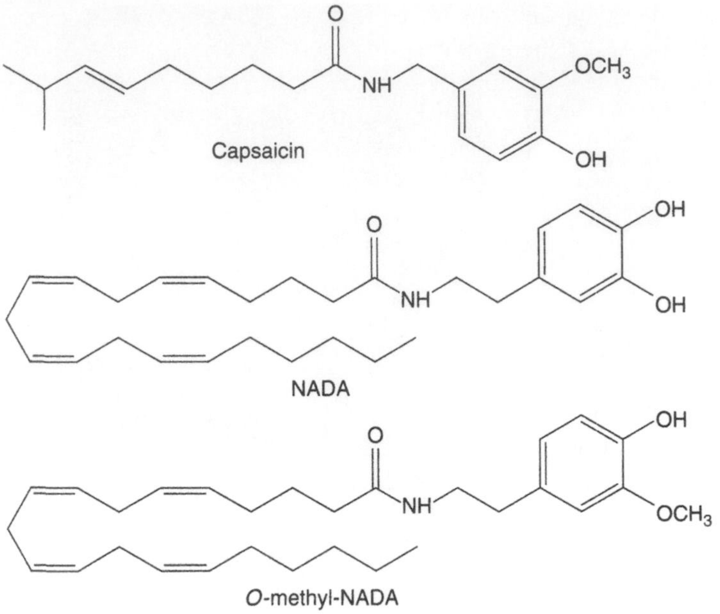

FIGURE 25.11   Chemical structure of Capsaicin and NADA.

F. S. Darling. Later similar substances were isolated from chili pepper by two Japanese chemists S. Kosuge and Y. Inagaki in 1964, who named them capsaicinoids. Capsaicin is a homovanillic acid derivative (8-methyl-N-vanillyl-6-nonenamide), and binds the capsaicin receptor TRPV1 (transient receptor potential vanilloid 1, VR1), a non-selective cation channel, and causes a heat-sensation.

For 400 years, Kimchi has been the keystone spicy food of the Korean diet. It consists mainly of fermented vegetables such as Chinese cabbage in brine with spicy seasonings. The most common seasonings include garlic, scallions, and chili pepper. Thus, Korean people were delighted when a Korean group led by Taik-koo Yun of Korea Cancer Center Hospital in Seoul found that Capsaicin suppresses the growth of MDBA-induced lung cancer in mice [36]. How does capsaicin block the cancer growth? In 2003 Aree Moon's group at Duksung Women's University in Seoul, Korea, found that capsaicin inhibits the growth of RAS-transformants, but not its normal parental cells, and requires the oncogenic RAS-PAK1-p38 signaling pathway for its anti-cancer potential [37]. Why does capsaicin require the RAS pathway?

The answer came independently from two groups in England: Janet Winter's group at Novartis Institute for Medical Research in London, and Peter McNaughton's group at University Cambridge. In 2003, they found that NGF (nerve growth factor) induces the up-regulation of VR1 in dorsal root ganglion (DRG) neurons through the RAS-PI-3 kinase-PAK signaling pathway [38, 39].

This would explain well why more than 70% of cancer cells, where the onco-genic RAS-PAK1 signaling is constitutively activated and VR1 is up-regulated, are much more sensitive to the anti-mitotic action of capsaicin than the normal cells where RAS-PAK1 signaling is transient, and the VR1 level is kept low.

In 2006, Phillip Koeffler's group at UCLA demonstrated that the oral administration of capsaicin (5 mg/kg, 3 times a week) suppresses the growth of human PC-3 prostate cancer xenograft in nude mice by 80% [40]. In this cancer cell line the tumor suppressor PTEN is missing, and therefore PAK1 is abnormally activated. It would be of great interest to see the possible combined effect of Bio 30 and capsaicin (or Sichuan pepper extract) on NF tumors.

Capsiate

Since capsaicin is spicy, it would be better for clinical application if a non-spicy derivative of capsaicin becomes available. In 1989 a Japanese group led by Susumu Yazawa at Kyoto University selected a unique non-pungent cultivar from a pungent pepper called CH-19 from Thailand [41]. This sweet cultivar called "CH-19 Sweet" contains a capsaicin derivative called capsiate [42]. In capsiate, the amide bond of capsaicin is replaced by an ester bond. In other words, the nitrogen (NH) in the latter is substituted with an oxygen (O) in cap-siate. Nevertheless, like capsaicin, capsiate still binds TPVR1. Interestingly, however, in 2003 Giovanni Appendino's group in Spain/Italy found that capsi-ate also suppresses the growth of cancer cells and causes their apoptosis, but in a TPVR1-independent manner [43]. Furthermore, capsiate was recently found to boost the endurance swimming capacity of mice through TPVR1 by stimu-lating their lipid metabolism [44]. Actually in Japan capsiate has been widely used to lose the body weight or an extra fat by stimulating the resting lipid metabolism (oxidation). Thus, capsiate appears to be potentially useful not only for cancer therapy but also for preventing the obesity.

NADA as an Endogenous Capsaicin

Furthermore, in 2003, the collaborative work by Vincenzo Di Marzo's group at National Research Council in Napoli, Italy, and Mike Walker's group at Brown University in Providence, US, discovered an endogenous "capsaicin-like" molecule called NADA (N-arachidonoyl-dopamine) (see the chemical structure in Fig. 25.11) in mammalian brain tissues, in particular the striatum, which stimulates TPVR1 with the EC_{50} around 50 nM [45, 46]. Thus, in a long term, it is worth looking for the optimal "mental" (or physiological) conditions which would induce the biosynthesis of NADA in NF/cancer patients so that each patient can cure the NF/cancer through his or her "meditation," instead of any exogenous medication such as Capsaicin or other anti-PAK1 drugs. This entirely new approach might be called self-cure, natural-healing or even "placebo" therapy.

NADA could be synthesized by the condensation of dopamine (or tyrosine) and arachidonic acid through arachidonoyl-CoA. Since dopamine is the major pleasure hormone in human brains, perhaps the best conditions for self-cure would be those which make NF or cancer patients feel most pleasant, such as listening to his or her favorite classic music, disco dancing, hot bath, swimming or walking/running, and sexual pleasure, like "runner's high" or euphoria. For the moment, it still remains uncertain whether or not these conditions alone are sufficient for curing NF or other tumors, but they would surely improve at least the patients' QOL (quality of life) without any apparent side effect.

OGF (OPIOID GROWTH FACTOR)

Interestingly, more than two decades ago, another pleasure hormone called Met-enkephalin (also called OGF for opioid growth factor) was discovered by a group at University of Houston to inhibit the growth of (Raf-mediated) melanoma xenograft in mice [47]. OGF is a pentapeptide that carries Met at the terminus, and also blocks metastasis of cancers. A decade ago Ian Zagon's group at Pennsylvania State University found that OGF inhibits the growth of pancreatic cancer xenograft in mice [48], and blocks the angiogenesis, strongly suggesting that OGF and its receptor somehow block the oncogenic RAS-PAK1 pathways. In 2006 OGF entered the phase 2 of clinical trials for pancreatic cancers. These findings all together hint the existence of a self-curing system for PAK1-dependent cancers and NF in our own brain.

ACKNOWLEDGMENT

Our work on herbal medicines was supported in part by funds from DGF (to HM) and Japanese ministry of education, culture sports, science and technology (to TO). We are very grateful to Drs. Yuan Luo of UMB, Tatsuo Watanabe and Shigenori Kumazawa of Shizuoka University for their critical reading of this manuscript.

REFERENCES

1. Jones, R. L. & Judson, I. R. (2005). The development and application of imatinib (Gleevec). *Expert Opin. Drug Saf* **4**, 183–191.
2. Sasakawa, Y., Naoe, Y., Inoue, T., Sasakawa, T. *et al.* (2003). Effects of FK228, a novel histone deacetylase inhibitor, on tumor growth and expression of p21 and c-myc genes *in vivo*. *Cancer Lett* **195**, 161–168.
3. Hirokawa, Y., Tikoo, A., Huynh, J., Utermark, T. *et al.* (2004). A clue to the therapy of neurofibromatosis type 2: NF2/merlin is a PAK1 inhibitor. *Cancer J* **10**, 20–26.
4. Hirokawa, Y., Nakajima, H., Hanemann, O., Kurtz, A. *et al.* (2005). Signal therapy of Nf1-deficient tumor xenograft in mice. *Cancer Biol Ther* **4**, 379–381.

5. Hirokawa, Y., Arnold, M., Nakajima, H., Zalcberg, J. & Maruta, H. (2005). Signal therapy of breast cancer xenograft in mice by the HDAC inhibitor FK228 that blocks the activation of PAK1 and abrogates the tamoxifen-resistance. *Cancer Biol Ther* **4**, 956–960.

6. Wang, R. A., Zhang, H., Balasenthil, S., Medina, D. & Kumar, R. (2006). PAK1 hyperactivation is sufficient for mammary gland tumor formation. *Oncogene* **25**, 2931–2936.

7. Hirokawa, Y., Levitzki, A., Lessene, G., Baell, J. & Maruta, H. (2007). Signal therapy of human pancreatic cancer and NF1-deficient breast cancer xenograft in mice by a combination of PP1 and GL-2003, Anti-PAK1 Drugs (Tyr-kinase Inhibitors). *Cancer Lett* **245**, 242–251.

8. Zhao, Z. S. & Manser, E. (2005). PAK and other Rho-associated kinases – effectors with surprisingly diverse mechanisms of regulation. *Biochem J* **386**, 201–214.

9. Zhao, Z. S., Lim, J. P., Ng, Y. W., Lim, L. & Manser, E. (2005). The GIT-associated kinase PAK targets to the centrosome and regulates Aurora-A. *Mol Cell* **20**, 237–249.

10. Chaudhary, A., King, W. G., Mattaliano, M., Frost, J. *et al.* (2000). Phosphatidylinositol 3-kinase regulates Raf1 through Pak phosphorylation of serine 338. *Curr Biol* **10**, 551–554.

11. Nheu, T., He, H., Hirokawa, Y., Walker, F., Wood, J. & Maruta, H. (2004). PAK is essential for RAS-induced up-regulation of cyclin D1 during the G1 to S transition. *Cell Cycle* **3**, 71–74.

12. Edwards, D. C., Sanders, L., Bokoch, G. & Gill, G. (1999). Activation of LIM-kinase by Pak1 couples Rac/Cdc42 GTPase signalling to actin cytoskeletal dynamics. *Nat Cell Biol* **1**, 253–259.

13. Schurmann, A., Mooney, A., Sanders, L., Sells, M., Wang, H. G. *et al.* (2000). p21-activated kinase 1 phosphorylates the death agonist Bad and protects cells from apoptosis. *Mol Cell Biol* **20**, 453–461.

14. Bagheri-Yarmand, R., Vadlamudi, R., Wang, R. A., Mendelsohn, J. & Kumar, R. (2000). Vascular endothelial growth factor up-regulation via p21-activated kinase-1 signaling regulates heregulin-beta1-mediated angiogenesis. *J Biol Chem* **275**, 39451–39457.

15. Nakajima, H., Kim, Y. B., Terano, H., Yoshida, M. & Horinouchi, S. (1998). FR901228, a potent antitumor antibiotic, is a novel histone deacetylase inhibitor. *Exp Cell Res* **241**, 126–133.

16. Rajgolikar, G., Chan, K. K. & Wang, H. C. (1998). Effects of a novel antitumor depsipeptide, FR901228, on human breast cancer cells. *Breast Cancer Res Treat* **51**, 29–38.

17. Kobayashi, Y., Ohtsuki, M., Murakami, T., Kobayashi, T. *et al.* (2006). Histone deacetylase inhibitor FK228 suppresses the Ras-MAP kinase signaling pathway by upregulating Rap1 and induces apoptosis in malignant melanoma. *Oncogene* **25**, 512–524.

18. Grunberger, D., Banerjee, R., Eisinger, K., Oltz, E. *et al.* (1988). Preferential cytotoxicity on tumor cells by caffeic acid phenethyl ester isolated from propolis. *Experientia* **44**, 230–232.

19. Xu, J. W., Ikeda, K., Kobayakawa, A., Ikami, T. *et al.* (2005). Down-regulation of Rac1 activation by caffeic acid in aortic smooth muscle cells. *Life Sci* **76**, 2861–2872.

20. Nagaoka, T., Banskota, A., Tezuka, Y., Harimaya, Y. *et al.* (2003). Inhibitory effects of caffeic acid phenethyl ester analogues on experimental lung metastasis of murine colon 26-L5 carcinoma cells. *Biol Pharm Bull* **26**, 638–641.

21. Liao, H. F., Chen, Y. Y., Liu, J. J. *et al.* (2003). Inhibitory effect of caffeic acid phenethyl ester on angiogenesis, tumor invasion, and metastasis. *J Agric Food Chem* **51**, 7907–7912.

22. Maruta, H. & Burgess, A. W. (1994). Regulation of the Ras signalling network. *Bioessays* **16**, 489–496.

23. Tang, Y., Marwaha, S., Rutkowski, J., Tennekoon, G. *et al.* (1998). A role for Pak protein kinases in Schwann cell transformation. *Proc Natl Acad Sci USA* **95**, 5139–5144.

24. Demestre, M., Messerli, S., Celli, N., Shahhossini, M. *et al.* (2008). CAPE (Caffeic Acid Phenethyl Ester) – based Propolis Extract (Bio 30) Suppresses the Growth of Human Neuro–fibromatosis (NF) Tumor Xenografts in Mice. Phytother. Res., in press.

25. Matsuno, T., Jung, S. K., Matsumoto, Y., Saito, M. *et al.* (1997). Preferential cytotoxicity to tumor cells of Artepillin C isolated from propolis. *Anticancer Res* **17**, 3565–3568.

26. Kimoto, T., Arai, S., Kohguchi, M., Aga, M. *et al.* (1998). Apoptosis and suppression of tumor growth by artepillin C extracted from Brazilian propolis. *Cancer Detect Prev* **22**, 506–515.

27. Aga, M., Shibuya, T., Sugimoto, T., Kurimoto, M. *et al.* (1994). Isolation and identification of anti-microbial compounds in Brazilian propolis. *Biosci Biotechnol Biochem* **58**, 945–946.

28. Shimizu, K., Das, S. K., Baba, M., Matsuura, Y. & Kanazawa, K. (2006). Dietary artepillin C suppresses the formation of aberrant crypt foci induced by azoxymethane in mouse colon. *Cancer Lett* **240**, 135–142.

29. Shimizu, K., Das, S. K., Hashimoto, T., Sowa, Y., Yoshida, T., Sakai, T., Matsuura, Y. & Kanazawa, K. (2005). Artepillin C in Brazilian propolis induces G(0)/G(1) arrest via stimulation of Cip1/p21 expression in human colon cancer cells. *Mol Carcinog* **44**, 293–299.

30. Fujita, N., Sato, S., Katayama, K. & Tsuruo, T. (2002). Akt-dependent phosphorylation of p27Kip1 promotes binding to 14-3-3 and cytoplasmic localization. *J Biol Chem* **277**, 28706–28713.

31. Shin, I., Yakes, F., Rojo, F., Shin, N. Y., Bakin, A., Baselga, J. & Arteaga, C. (2002). PKB/Akt mediates cell-cycle progression by phosphorylation of p27(Kip1) at threonine 157 and modulation of its cellular localization. *Nat Med* **8**, 1145–1152.

32. Messerli, S., Ahn, M. R., Kunimasa, K., Yanagihara, M. *et al.* (2008). Artepillin C (ARC) in Brazilian Green Propolis Selectively Blocks the Oncogenic PAK1 Signaling and Suppresses the Growth of NF Tumors in Mice. Phytother. Res., in press.

33. Ahn, M. R., Kunimasa, K., Ohta, T., Kumazawa, S. *et al.* (2007). Suppression of tumor–induced angiogenesis by Brazilian propolis: Major component artepillin C inhibits in vitro tube formation and endothelial cell proliferation. *Cancer Lett* **252**, 235–243.

34. Hirokawa, Y., Nheu, T., Grimm, K., Mautner, V. *et al.* (2006). Sichuan pepper extracts block the PAK1/Cyclin D1 pathway and the growth of NF1-deficient cancer xenograft in mice. *Cancer Biol Ther* **5**, 305–309.

35. Uto, Y., Hirata, A., Fujita, T., Takubo, S. *et al.* (2002). First total synthesis of artepillin C established by *o,o* -diprenylation of *p*-halophenols in water. *J Org Chem* **67**, 2355–2357.

36. Jang, J. J., Kim, S. H. & Yun, T. K. (1989). Inhibitory effect of capsaicin on mouse lung tumor development. *In Vivo* **3**, 49–53.

37. Kang, H. J., Soh, Y., Kim, M. S., Lee, E. J. *et al.* (2003). Roles of JNK-1 and p38 in selective induction of apoptosis by capsaicin in ras-transformed human breast epithelial cells. *Int J Cancer* **103**, 475–482.

38. Bonnington, J. & McNaughton, P. (2003). Signalling pathways involved in the sensitisation of mouse nociceptive neurones by nerve growth factor. *J Physiol* **551**, 433–446.

39. Bron, R., Klesse, L., Shah, K., Parada, L. & Winter, J. (2003). Activation of Ras is necessary and sufficient for upregulation of vanilloid receptor type 1 in sensory neurons by neurotrophic factors. *Mol Cell Neurosci* **22**, 118–132.

40. Mori, A., Lehmann, S., O'Kelly, J., Kumagai, T. *et al.* (2006). Capsaicin, a component of red peppers, inhibits the growth of androgen-independent, p53 mutant prostate cancer cells. *Cancer Res* **66**, 3222–3229.

41. Yazawa, S., Suetome, N., Okamoto, K. & Namiki, T. (1989). Content of capsaicinoids and capsaicinoid-like substances in fruit of pepper (*Capsicum annuum* L.) hybrids made with CH-19 Sweet as a parent. *Jpn Soc Hortic Sci (in Japanese)* **58**, 601–607.

42. Kobata, K., Todo, T., Yazawa, S., Iwai, K. & Watanabe, T. (1998). Novel capsaicinoid-like substances, capsiate and dihydrocapsiate, from the fruits of a non-pungent cultivar, CH-19 Sweet, of pepper (*Capsicum annuum* L.). *J Agric Food Chem* **46**, 1695–1697.

43. Macho, A., Lucena, C., Sancho, R., Daddario, N. *et al.* (2003). Non-pungent capsaicinoids from sweet pepper synthesis and evaluation of the chemopreventive and anticancer potential. *Eur J Nutr* **42**, 2–9.

44. Haramizu, S., Mizunoya, W., Masuda, Y., Ohnuki, K. *et al.* (2006). Capsiate, a nonpungent capsaicin analog, increases endurance swimming capacity of mice by stimulation of vanilloid receptors. *Biosci Biotechnol Biochem* **70**, 774–781.

45. Huang, S. M., Bisogno, T., Trevisani, M., Al-Hayani, A. *et al.* (2002). An endogenous capsaicin-like substance with high potency at recombinant and native vanilloid VR1 receptors. *Proc Natl Acad Sci USA* **99**, 8400–8405.

46. Chu, C. J., Huang, S. M., De Petrocellis, L., Bisogno, T. *et al.* (2003). *N*-oleoyldopamine, a novel endogenous capsaicin-like lipid that produces hyperalgesia. *J Biol Chem* **278**, 13633–13639.

47. Zagon, I. S. & McLaughlin, P. (1985). Stereospecific modulation of tumorigenicity by opioid antagonists. *Eur J Pharmacol* **113**, 115–120.

48. Zagon, I. S., Hytrek, S. & McLaughlin, P. (1996). Opioid growth factor tonically inhibits human colon cancer cell proliferation in tissue culture. *Am J Physiol* **271**, R511–R518.

Chapter 26

Health Benefits of Traditional Culinary and Medicinal Mediterranean Plants

Stephanie C. Degner, Andreas J. Papoutsis and Donato F. Romagnolo

Department of Nutritional Sciences, The University of Arizona, Tucson, AZ, USA

Abstract

The Mediterranean diet is rich in fruits and vegetables, monounsaturated fatty acids from olive oil, and is complemented with the traditional use of culinary and medicinal herbs and spices. An important feature of this diet is the negative association with the incidence of metabolic syndrome, which is characterized by increased risk of cardiovascular disease. Conformity to the Mediterranean diet has also been linked to a decreased risk of cardiovascular disease and cancer in US populations. Plants that originated in the Mediterranean basin have been used for centuries in botanical therapies. Many of these plants are believed to prevent and/or cure a wide spectrum of ailments based on their content in bioactive components that exert anti-oxidant, anti-inflammatory, anti-carcinogenic, anti-diabetic, and anti-thrombotic functions. This chapter underlines the health benefits that may derive from utilization through dietary assumption or medicinal applications of a selected group of plant products including extracts and specific bioactive components found in rosemary, licorice, chamomile, and olive oil. Each section provides a scientific analysis of the most recent literature and attempts to highlight the mechanisms of action and molecular targets of bioactive components derived from these plants.

Keywords: *Mediterranean plants, health, disease, culinary, medicinal*

INTRODUCTION

In recent history, the Mediterranean diet has been the subject of much interest because of its association in Mediterranean populations with reduced incidence of some chronic diseases including cancer, coronary heart disease (CHD), and cardiovascular disease (CVD), which represent in industrialized countries, ~75% of deaths for individuals of age 65 and older [1]. The beneficial effects of the Mediterranean diet have been ascribed at least in part to high intake of antioxidants from fruits and vegetables, nuts, the prevalent consumption of monounsaturated fatty acids from olive oil, a moderately high intake of fish, and a regular but moderate intake of wine primarily during meals [2,3]. The health benefits of the Mediterranean diet have also been attributed to ingestion of a variety of botanical preparations from herbs and spices, which provide rich sources of flavor-giving and bioactive components including phenolic compounds that possess antioxidant properties [4]. The literature concerning the cultivation and culinary use of vegetables, herbs, and spices in the Mediterranean area date back to the ancient Egyptian, Greek, and Roman civilizations [5]. In modern history, there has been an increasing research focus to define the health benefits of dietary constituents found in traditional Mediterranean foods [6] with the objective of identifying bioactive components and develop strategies for their functional use in preventive medicine and maintenance of health [7, 8]. Traditionally, herbs are referred to as leafy parts of plants, whereas the term spices is generally adopted for preparations from roots, seeds, root bark, berries, flower parts, fruits, or other plant parts. The main objective of this chapter is to discuss the health benefits of a selected group of traditional culinary and medicinal Mediterranean plants for which we deemed sufficient scientific literature information is available to support their potential use in food preparations or for preventative and therapeutic applications (Table 26.1). Purposely, we have not covered vegetables and herbs that have been covered extensively in previous scientific reviews and limited our focus to selected traditional Mediterranean plants. Specific emphasis is given to the profile of bioactive components; the chemistry and mechanisms of action of bioactive compounds; the health benefits associated with intake; potential toxicity; and recommendations for consumption.

ROSEMARY

Rosemary (*Rosmarinus officinalis* Linn. Family Labiatae) is a perennial plant native of the Mediterranean area. Rosemary extracts are used routinely for cooking, preservation of foods, cosmetics, or in herbal medicine for anti-inflammatory and antimicrobial applications [9, 10], and for the prevention and treatment of diabetic and cardiovascular diseases [11]. At least 30 components have been identified in essential oils, which have been shown to possess olfactory properties that influence cognitive performance including memory [12]. Rosemary extracts contain many bioactive components including phenolic mono-terpenes (α-pinene, camphene, limonene) [13], diterpenes (carnosic acid, carnosol), flavones (genkwanin, isoscutellarein 7-O-glucoside), and caffeolyl derivatives (rosmarinic acid). The highest accumulation of these groups of compounds occurs in leaves and it is related to young stages of plant development

TABLE 26.1 Mediterranean Plants and Health Benefits

Plant extracts and bioactive food components	Health benefits	References
Rosemary (R. *officinalis*)	Anti-oxidant	15, 18, 19
Extracts	Reduced hepato-toxicity	20
	Anti-viral (H. *simplex*)	25
	Anti-microbial (H. *pylori*)	26
	Anti-thrombotic	28
	Food packaging	55–57
Rosmarinic acid	Epidermal anti-inflammatory	34
	Anti-allergic	35, 36
	Inhibits angiogenesis	37
Carnosol, Carnosic acid	Anti-oxidant, anti-inflammatory	41, 42
	Anti-diabetic	50
Licorice (G. *glabra*)	Anti-inflammatory, anti-allergenic	67
Extracts	Anti-viral	59
Glycyrrhizic acid	Inhibits cortisol metabolism	63
Isoliquiritigenin	Anti-oxidant	68
Chamomile (M. *recutita* and A. *nobilis*)		
Extracts	Treatment of gastro-intestinal spasm, anti-inflammatory, bacterial skin disease, wound healing	65, 72, 79
Apigenin	Anti-cancer	74
Olive oil (O. *europea*)	Cardio-protective	99
Extracts	Anti-oxidant, anti-inflammatory	97, 100
Oleic acid, phenolic compounds	Reduce hypertension, anti-thrombotic	108–110
	Anticancer (prostate, breast, colon, oral cavity)	114–117
	Anti-diabetic	126

[14]. In general, rosmarinic acid is present at the highest concentration in all rosemary plant organs. Carnosic acid and carnosol are found in stems during young stages, but their concentrations decrease in the vascular system following aging. However, high levels of phenolic diterpenes and rosmarinic acid are found in flowers as a result of *in situ* biosynthesis and transport from other plant organs. Rosemary extracts in both aqueous and lipid medium have been shown to possess antioxidant activity, which is due to the presence of a catechol group in the aromatic ring of the phenolic terpenes, and cathecols conjugated with a carboxylic acid group in rosmarinic acid. Interestingly, rosmarinic acid is more effective as antioxidant in bulk oil whereas carnosol and carnosic acid perform better in oil-in-water emulsions. These differences in antioxidant efficacy have been attributed to interfacial partitioning of these compounds [15].

Many studies have investigated the health benefits of extracts from rosemary plants and documented that extracts exhibited protective effects against oxidative damage to DNA by scavenging hydroxyl and singlet oxygen radicals [16], and prevented the activation of carcinogens by members of P450 family of metabolizing enzymes while increasing detoxification [17, 18]. Aqueous extracts of the young sprouts of rosemary were found to exert anti-lipoperoxidant activity, and protected against radiation-induced hepatotoxicity in Swiss albino mice [19]. Similarly, the oral administration (250 mg/kg body weight) of rosemary extracts to male Sprague-Dawley rats reduced tetrachloride-induced acute hepatotoxicity [20]. Moreover, dietary rosemary extracts at doses ranging from 0.5% to 1.0% were reported to suppress the binding of dimethylbenz[a]anthracene (DMBA) metabolites to DNA in female Sprague-Dawley rats [21, 22], DNA damage by the carcinogen benzo[a]pyrene [23], and at doses of 500 mg/kg body weight DMBA-induced skin tumors in mice [24]. Extracts of rosemary have also been shown to possess antiviral effects against *Herplex simplex* [25] and inhibited the growth of the gram-negative bacterium *Helicobacter pylori*, which is recognized as the primary etiological factor in the development of gastritis and peptic ulcer disease [26]. In association with vitamin D3, rosemary preparations and carnosic acid enhanced differentiation of HL60 cells *in vitro* and exerted antileukemic activity in Balb/c mice [27]. A recent study that screened herb extracts for antithrombotic effects *in vitro* and in a mouse model reported that rosemary along with thyme extracts showed significant antithrombotic activity possibly through an inhibitory effect on platelet reactivity [28]. Interestingly, the same study reported that the anti-platelet activity of rosemary was heat-stable suggesting that the active components may remain preserved after cooking.

Rosmarinic acid, which was first isolated from *Rosmarinus officinalis* by two Italian scientists [29], is an esterification product of caffeic acid which originates from the amino acid phenylalanine, and 3,4-dihydroxyphenyllactic acid which is produced from tyrosine [30]. However, other medicinal herbs have been shown to contain rosmarinic acid including lemon balm (*Melissa officinalis*), sage (Salvia *officinalis, Salvia aegyptiaca* L.), olives (*Olea europea* L), tobacco (*Nicotiana tabacuum*), and peppermint (*Mentha piperita* L.) [31]. In plants, rosmarinic acid may exert a protective role against pathogens and herbivores. In humans, rosmarinic acid is absorbed, conjugated, and methylated in the intestine and liver and it is present in plasma and urine in a conjugated form (glucuronide and/or sulfated). Metabolites of rosmarinic acid have been shown to be excreted within few hours [32, 33].

Studies have investigated in animal models the biological activity of rosmarinic acid and reported that it inhibited epidermal inflammatory responses by reducing neutrophil infiltration, myeloperoxidase activity, cyclooxygenase-2 mRNA expression, and reactive oxygen radical production [34]. In humans, rosmarinic acid reduced the incidence of allergic rhinoconjunctivitis by inhibiting the inflammatory response and scavenging of reactive oxygen species

(ROS) [35, 36]. Recent studies have documented that rosmarinic acid inhibited a number of processes involved in angiogenesis and ROS-associated VEGF expression and Il-8 release [37].

Several studies have investigated the mechanisms of action of rosmarinic acid. In B16 melanoma cells, it induced melanin synthesis (melanogenesis) through activation of CREB via PKA signaling in a cAMP-independent manner [38]. Other effects of rosmarinic acid included protection against adriamycin-induced apoptosis in H9c2 cardiac muscle cells [39] and inhibition of Ca^{2+}-dependent pathways of T-cell antigen receptor-mediated signaling [40].

Carnosol and carnosic acid are diterpenes, which contribute to the antioxidant and anti-inflammatory activity of rosemary extracts [41, 42]. In rosemary plants, carnosic acid protects chloroplasts from oxidative stress by scavenging free radicals [43]. Studies documented that carnosol exerted a variety of preventative effects by reducing DMBA-induced rat mammary tumorigenesis and *in vivo* DMBA–DNA adduct formation [44], skin tumorigenesis [45], the invasion of melanoma cells [46], progression through the cell cycle [47], aflatoxin B1-induced oxidative stress [48], and platelet aggregatation [49]. Both carnosol and carnosic acid have been shown to be activators of the human peroxisome proliferators-activated receptor gamma [50] thus raising the possibility these compounds may exert hypoglycemic and anti-diabetic effects.

Toxicity related to rosemary has been reported for skin applications of rosemary alcohol which induced contact dermatitis in one patient [51]. The dietary administration to Sprague-Dawley rats of rosemary at levels of 500 mg/kg of body weight for 63 days was associated with reduced fertility in females and a decline in spermatogenesis [52]. However, the clinical implications of these results to traditional dietary consumption of rosemary in human populations of the Mediterranean basin remain unknown.

These cumulative data suggest that rosemary extracts contain several bioactive components including phenolic diterpenes, phenolic acids, and flavonoids that may enhance the health benefits of the Mediterranean diet by acting as antioxidants and improving the detoxification systems [20, 53]. Also, rosemary extracts or selected constituents exert anti-inflammatory, anti-thrombotic, and anti-tumor actions [54] which could be exploited for the routine preparation of foods as well as for the development of prophylactic dietary protocols.

Rosemary extracts have been used in a variety of applications. The addition of rosemary to ground chicken had an overall positive effect on raw meat appearance during storage and cooked meat flavor, and improved redness [55]. Similarly, antioxidant films have been developed to incorporate a natural extract of rosemary and are intended for contact with foods [56]. A study that examined the clinical safety and efficacy of NG440, a phytochemical-based anti-inflammatory formula consisting of a combination of rho iso-alpha acids from hops, rosemary, and oleanolic acid, concluded that NG440 reduced pain scores in patients with joint discomfort suggesting that phytochemical preparations containing rosemary may be used as an alternative to specific

COX2 inhibitors [57]. Aromatherapy acupressure in stroke patients with lavender, rosemary, and peppermint exerted a positive effect on hemiplegic shoulder pain compared to acupressure alone [58].

LICORICE (OR LIQUORICE)

The first documented use of licorice (*Glycyrrhiza glabra*) in Europe is provided by the Greek botanist and pharmacologist Theophrastus in the third century BC. who was a disciple of Plato and Aristotle [59]. The genus name of the licorice plant, *Glycyrrhiza*, is derived from the ancient Greek words for "sweet root" (*glykos* = sweet and *rhiza* = root) [60]. The sweetness of licorice is from the glycyrrhizin contained in the root and is 50 times sweeter than sucrose [61]. Native to southeastern Europe, the licorice root was used as something sweet to chew on and the black juice extract was taken as a refreshing drink by both the Greeks and Romans. Today licorice is found in candies, soft drinks, tobacco products, cough syrups, Guinness beer, and sambuca [60]. Medicinal uses of licorice throughout antiquity included treatment for asthma, cough, skin lesions, ulcers (bladder, stomach, and kidney pain), and diseases of the liver and arteries. Licorice also shows anti-inflammatory and mineralocorticoid properties due to the activity of glycyrrhizinic acid and its metabolite glycyrrhetinic acid, which inhibit cortisol metabolism. Recent studies have shown licorice to possess antiatherogenic effects, and that the presence of saponins and flavonoids in the root provide antioxidant activity [59]. Modern research has verified these uses finding licorice to be an effective expectorant and antiviral agent, as well as an aid for healing stomach and duodenal ulcers [61].

The principle chemical component of the licorice root is glycyrrhizin. Glycyrrhizin is a triterpenoid saponin glycoside which occurs as a mixture of calcium and potassium salts of glycyrrhizic acid. Following hydrolysis, glycyrrhizin is converted to two molecules of glucuronic acid and the aglycone glycyrrhetinic acid [59]. Glycyrrhizic acid and glycyrrhetinic acid competitively inhibit the enzyme 11β-hydroxysteroid dehydrogenase [62]. 11β-Hydroxysteroid dehydrogenase normally catalyzes the oxidation of the active cortisol in the kidney, to the inactive cortisone. The inhibition of cortisol metabolism by glycyrrhizic/glycyrrhetinic acid increases cortisol activity in the kidney. Cortisol has the same affinity to the aldosterone receptors as aldosterone and the effects mimic aldosterone excess [63]. The resulting hypermineralocorticoidism is characterized by sodium retention, hypokalemia, and hypertension [64].

Licorice may be used as a demulcent for sore throats and as an expectorant in facilitating the discharge of mucus from the upper respiratory tract [65]. Licorice is useful in treating gastric and duodenal ulcers as it reduces stomach secretions and produces protective mucus for the lining of the digestive tract [66]. The anti-inflammatory and anti-allergenic activity of licorice arises mainly from the presence of the flavones liquiritin and liquiritigenin which can treat rheumatism and arthritis. These properties are further extended to the treatment of atopic dermatitis; reducing erythema, edema, and itching [67]. Licorice possesses anti-viral properties and has long been used in the treatment of chronic viral hepatitis [61]. *In vitro* studies have reported anti-viral effects for the influenza virus, the severe acute respiratory syndrome (SARS) corona virus, the Hepatitis B virus, and the Epstein Barr virus [59]. The antioxidant activity of licorice stems from the presence of saponins and flavonoids which are known for their antioxidant activity. Of the flavonoids present in the root, isoliquiritigenin is among the most potent [68]. Licorice is also useful as a gentle laxative [66].

The most widely reported side effects from licorice are caused by the inhibition of cortisol metabolism by glycyrrhetinic acid causing hypertension and edema. Prolonged use and excessive consumption (more than 20 g/day) not only produce hypertension and edema, but can also induce hypokalemia and reduce plasma aldosterone levels [65]. These symptoms are reversible with withdrawal from the herb. The acceptable daily intake of the active component glycyrrhizin is 0.015–0.229 mg/kg body weight [61].

CHAMOMILE

Chamomile is derived from the Greek words chamos (ground) in reference to its low-growing characteristics and melos (apple), in reference to the apple scent of fresh chamomile blossoms. The two primary types of chamomile are German chamomile (*Maricaria recutita*) and Roman chamomile (*Anthemis nobilis*). References to chamomile are found in medicinal writings of the ancient Egyptian, Greek, and Romans. The writings of Hippocrates, Dioscorides, and Galen contain descriptions of the chamomile plant. The Greeks and Egyptians used crushed chamomile flowers to treat the skin conditions erythema and xerosis caused by dry, harsh weather [69]. Chamomile is one of the most widely used herbs and has been traditionally used for its mild sedative, spasmolytic, anti-inflammatory, and wound healing properties [70]. The German E Commission has approved chamomile for internal use to treat gastrointestinal spasms and inflammatory diseases of the gastrointestinal tract. In addition, the German E Commission has approved external use of chamomile for inflammation of the skin and bacterial skin diseases, and respiratory tract inflammation [65]. In the United States, chamomile is one of the most widely consumed tea ingredients [70].

Over 120 different components have been identified in the chamomile flower [71]. One of the primary bioactive components of chamomile is levomenol (α-bisabolol) and its oxides. Other components of chamomile include apigenin, azulenes, farnesene, spathuleno, and spiroethers [72]. Teas brewed from chamomile contain approximately 10–15% of the essential oils available from the flowers [72]. The coumarins herniarin and umbelliferone make up approximately 0.1% of the total constituents of the flower [73]. Apigenin is found in relatively high amounts in chamomile (840 mg/100 g) and it has been reported to possess a number of anti-cancer properties *in vitro* [74]. Chamomile has also been shown to possess antioxidant properties, although to a lesser degree compared to other medicinal and culinary herbs [75]. Essential oils extracted from chamomile have also been reported to exert antimicrobial properties against certain species of bacteria, fungi, and viruses [72].

Despite its widespread use in traditional medicine, only a few clinical trials have been conducted to evaluate the traditional medicinal claims of chamomile. In young Japanese males, one serving of chamomile tea decreased heart rate and ratings of sadness and depression compared to the placebo group [76]. In heart disease patients hospitalized for cardiac catheterization ($n = 12$), two cups of chamomile significantly decreased the mean brachial arterial pressure [77]. In children with acute, non-complicated diarrhea, a chamomile/apple pectin preparation significantly decreased the duration of the diarrhea compared to the placebo [78].

Several clinical studies have examined the effects of topical preparations of chamomile. A randomized, placebo-controlled trial investigated whether or not chamomile influenced skin reactions induced by radiation treatment. Treatment with chamomile appeared to delay the onset and reduce the frequency of skin reactions, however the results were not statistically significant [79]. Topical preparations of chamomile have been reported to enhance wound healing [80, 81]. In a double-blind study of 14 patients with weeping wounds from dermabrasion following tattoo removal, a compress made of chamomile extract significantly increased would healing and increased the drying of the wound [80]. Another randomized double-blind study investigated whether a chamomile spray relieved post-operative sore throat from intubation. The patients who received the chamomile extract spray (111 mg) did not report any differences from patients receiving a placebo spray [82].

Chamomile is most commonly prepared as a tea using the dried flowers. Tea infusions can be prepared by taking 3 g of the whole flower head into 150 ml of water. For inflammation of the upper respiratory tract, steam vapor from aqueous infusions of chamomile can be inhaled. In other cases, compresses can be made with chamomile.

In rare cases, chamomile may result in an allergic reaction or irritation upon contact [83, 84]. Individuals who are allergic to other members of the aster family (ragweed, asters, chrysanthemums) may also be allergic to chamomile [85]. Chamomile has also been reported to interact with cyclosporine in three renal transplant patients [86]. In addition, coumarin, which is a component of chamomile, may potentiate the effects of warfarin [73, 87].

OLIVE OIL

Olive oil has been used for centuries in Greece and other Mediterranean countries for its beneficial health properties. Ancient Egyptians and Romans used olive oil to soothe wounds. Olive oil is extracted from the fruit (*Olea europea*) by crushing the fruit to create a pomace, which is subsequently homogenized before it is pressed to produce the oil [88]. Unlike other oils that are extracted by solvents, virgin olive oil is obtained solely from mechanical or physical means. The leftover pomace is sometimes processed again to extract a lower quality refined virgin olive oil.

The percentage of dietary vegetable fat obtained from olive oil in Mediterranean countries is 71% in Greece, 42% in Italy, and 37% in Spain [89]. Since non-Mediterranean countries have relatively low consumption of olive oil compared to Mediterranean countries, the majority of studies investigating the beneficial health effects of olive oil arise from countries of the Mediterranean basin. In non-Mediterranean countries, monounsaturated fatty acid intake comes primarily from meat and dairy products along with other plant oils. Therefore, it may not be appropriate to equate the health benefits of olive oil intake with those of monounsaturated fatty acids intake in non-Mediterranean populations [90].

The saponifiable fraction of olive oil consists of 98.5–99.5% of olive oil and the remainder accounts for the unsaponifiable fraction [91]. Olive oil consists primarily of oleic acid (55.0–83.0%) [91]. Additional fatty acids present in olive oil include palmitic acid (7.5–20.0%), stearic (0.5–5.0%), linoleic (3.5–21.0%), linolenic (0.0–0.9%), and palmitoleic acid (0.3–3.5%) [91]. Oleic acid (18:1 $n9$) is a monounsaturated fatty acid containing one double bond, making it less susceptible to oxidation compared to polyunsaturated fatty acids with multiple double bonds. Therefore, olive oil tends to have a longer shelf-life than many other oils containing higher amounts of polyunsaturated fatty acids [92]. In addition, antioxidant phenolic compounds increase the stability of extra-virgin olive oils compared to refined virgin olive oil [93]. Long-term storage and heating can lead to degradation and changes in the composition of olive oil.

Phenolic compounds also contribute to the health benefits of olive oil, of which 30 have been identified. The major phenolic compounds identified in olive oil belong to five different classes: simple phenols (hydroxytyrosol, tyrosol), secoiridoids (oleuropein, ligstroside, and their hydrolysis derivatives), lignans (pinoresinol and acetoxypinoresinol), flavonoids (luteolin and apigenin), and phenolic acids (*p*-coumaric acid, vanillic acid). The reported total amount of phenolic compounds contained in olive oils ranges widely in the literature (between 200 mg/kg and 1500 mg/kg). The phenolic compounds are found in higher amounts in the less processed extra virgin olive oil [91]. In addition, the concentration of phenolic compounds depends on the cultivar, degree of maturation, climate, and extraction procedures [91, 94]. The phenolic compound that has been implicated for the bitter taste of olive oil is oleuropein [95]. In dried, unripe olives oleuropein accounts for approximately 14% of the dried weight. However, as the olive matures oleuropein undergoes hydrolysis to several simple phenols that contribute to the complex taste of olive oil. The phenols in the olive fruit are present in the more polar and hydrophobic glycoside form, whereas the phenols present in olive oil are found in the more lipid-soluble aglyconic form. Mediterranean diets rich in olive oil supply approximately 10–20 mg of phenolic compounds per day [96]. In addition to fatty acids and phenolic compounds, olive oil contains thousands of other components including tocopherols (α-, β-, γ-, and δ-) and β-carotene (which along with chlorophylls is responsible for the color of the oil). Olive oil also contains approximately 0.7% squalene [88].

The antioxidant properties of the phenolic compounds in olive oil have been the subject of numerous investigations and may contribute to the healthy properties through a variety of mechanisms. For example, olive oil has been suggested to reduce oxidative stress that leads to lipid peroxidation and formation of DNA adducts [97]. Other mechanisms of action that may contribute to the health benefits of olive oil include modulation of signal transduction pathways, regulation of gene expression, alteration of the immune system, and modification of cell membrane structure and function [98].

The cardioprotective effects of the Mediterranean diet were brought to light through results from the Seven Countries Study led by Keys [99]. These studies demonstrated that dietary intake of saturated fatty acid was associated with increased serum cholesterol levels and coronary artery diseases. Furthermore, these studies revealed the cardioprotective effect of virgin olive oil. Since then numerous investigations have studied the role of olive oil in cardiovascular diseases. Consumption of olive oil has been associated with several beneficial biological and clinical effects related to lipoprotein metabolism, oxidative damage, endothelial dysfunction, blood pressure, inflammation, thrombosis, and carbohydrate metabolism [100].

In Mediterranean countries, there is a strong correlation between olive oil consumption and reduced hypertension. In the Greek European Prospective Investigation into Cancer and Nutrition (EPIC) study of 20,343 men and women, olive oil consumption and the monounsaturated fatty acid to saturated fatty acid ratio were inversely associated with systolic and dystolic blood pressure [101]. Results from the cross-sectional Italian Nine Communities Study with 4903 men and women, olive oil consumption was also associated with decreased blood pressure [102]. The Suguimiento Universidad de Navarra (SUN) study in Spain with 6863 men and women noted an inverse association of olive oil consumption and blood pressure in men but not women [103]. However, several cohort or cross-sectional studies conducted in the United States to examine the effects of monounsaturated fat consumption and hypertension have produced conflicting results, possibly due to the fact that meat is the primary source of monounsaturated fatty acids in the Western diet [104].

Several clinical trials have been conducted in controlled environments to examine the effects of olive oil on hypertension. A double-blind, randomized crossover study evaluated the effects of monounsaturated (MUFA) (extra-virgin olive oil) and polyunsaturated fatty acids (PUFA) (sunflower oil) on blood pressure in 23 hypertensive patients. Resting blood pressure was significantly lowered in patients after 6 months of receiving the MUFA diet (30–40 g/day) compared to PUFA diet along with reduced use of anti-hypertensive medications [105]. In several cross-over trials where olive oil replaced either polyunsaturated fatty acids or carbohydrate, olive oil significantly reduced systolic and dystolic blood pressure [104]. However, not all studies have reported a beneficial effect of olive oil on blood pressure in short-term clinical trials [104].

Olive oil may also influence hemostasis by altering components of platelet function, thrombogenesis, and fibrinolysis [106]. Plasminogen activator inhibitor-1 (PAI-1) is a procoagulant factor that has been linked to coronary heart disease (CHD). Several short-term clinical trials have investigated the effects of olive oil on PAI-1 and overall olive oil or MUFA diets lowered PAI-levels compared to diets rich in saturated fatty acids [106,107]. Furthermore, human clinical trials have reported that interventions with olive oil reduced production of thromboxane A2 (TXA2), which is produced by platelets to increase aggregation [108–110].

Oxidation of the lipids and lipoprotein in LDL is thought to play a major role in development of cardiovascular disease and atherosclerosis. One mechanism through which olive oil may be cardioprotective is by inhibiting of LDL oxidation [96]. Diets high in MUFA reduced the susceptibility of LDL oxidation in comparison to carbohydrate-rich diets [111]. Diets containing extra virgin olive oil increased the resistance of LDL to oxidation [112]. Numerous randomized, controlled, crossover human studies have examined the effects of phenolic compounds from olive oil on markers of DNA and lipid damage [summarized in 100]. Cumulatively, these studies have produced conflicting results in regards to the antioxidant effects of the phenolic olive oil compounds *in vivo*. However, recent results from the EUROLIVE study provided evidence that phenolic compounds from olive possess *in vivo* antioxidant properties. The EUROLIVE study was a large, crossover trial conducted with 200 individuals from five different European countries [113]. Participants were given 3 similar olive oils (25 ml/day) with different phenolic contents for intervals of 3 weeks followed by 2-week washout periods. The greatest increases in HDL cholesterol levels and greatest decreases in lipid oxidative damage were observed during ingestion of olive oil containing the highest phenolic content [113].

The clinical efficacy of olive oil on the cancer process is highly controversial. Numerous epidemiological studies have reported an inverse correlation between olive oil consumption and the incidence of cancers of the prostate [114], breast [115], colon [116], and oral cavity [117]. In comparison to other types of fatty acids, fewer experimental animal studies have investigated the role olive oil on tumor development and have produced inconsistent results [118]. Several mechanisms of action have been investigated *in vitro* for the anti-cancer properties of olive oil and its constituents including modulation of signal transduction pathways, regulation of gene expression, alteration of the immune system, and modification of cell membrane structure and function [118]. Furthermore, the antioxidant properties of olive oil may reduce the formation of DNA adducts by decreasing oxidative stress from lipid peroxidation [97]. *In vitro* experiments documented that olive oil down-regulated the expression of cyclooxygenase 2 (COX2) and Bcl-2 [119]. Minor polar compounds from olive oil inhibited NF-kappaB translocation in monocytes and monocyte-derived-macrophages isolated from healthy volunteers [120]. Oleuropeuin aglycone isolated from extra virgin olive oil was found to inhibit cleavage of the HER2 extracellular domain (ECD) and subsequent HER2 expression in breast cancer cells resistant to trastuzumab (Herceptin) [121]. In addition, the oleuropeuin aglycone enhanced the trastuzumab-induced down-regulation of HER2 expression [121]. Phenolic extracts from olive oil inhibited the invasion of HT115 human colon carcinoma cells in the Matrigel invasion assay [122]. In HL-60 human promyelocytic leukemia cells, hydroxytyrosol inhibited cell cycle progression and altered expression levels of proteins associated with cell cycle regulation including cyclin-dependent kinase (CDK) 6, cyclin D3, p21, and p27 [123]. In colon cancer cells lines, pinoresinol-rich olive oil induced the ATM-p53 cascade [124].

A meta-analysis that compared low-saturated-fat, high-carbohydrate diets vs. high-monounsaturated-fat diets in type 2 diabetic patients reported that the high-monounsaturated fat diets improved lipoprotein profiles and glycemic control [125]. In a prospective cross-over study, obese and type 2 diabetes patients ($n = 11$) were placed on three different diets including a diet high in saturated fat, a diet rich in monounsaturated fat in the form of extra virgin olive oil, and a diet rich in carbohydrates [126]. The diet rich in olive oil decreased postprandial glucose and insulin concentrations, increased HDL cholesterol, and glucagon-like peptide 1 (GLP-1) concentrations as compared with the carbohydrate rich diet. In another study, the effects of virgin olive oil consumption on changes in membrane fatty acids and signaling proteins were examined in elderly patients with type 2 diabetes ($n = 16$) compared to a control group ($n = 28$). After 4 weeks of olive oil consumption, significant modifications were noted in the fatty acid composition of plasma membrane and there was a reduction in G-protein subunits (Gαs and Gβ) and protein kinase C alpha (PKCα). These results suggest that diets rich in olive oil may influence glycemic homeostasis through alteration of membrane lipids and signaling proteins [127].

In addition to protective cardiovascular and anti-cancer effects, olive oil has also been investigated for its antimicrobial properties [128]. In particular, the phenolic compounds hydroxytyrosol and oleuropein have been noted for their inhibitory properties against selected standard bacterial strains [129]. In addition, virgin olive oil extract was reported to exhibit antibacterial effects against eight strains of *Helicobacter pylori,* which has been linked to peptic ulcers and some types of gastric cancers [130]. These reports also demonstrated that several of the phenolic compounds from the olive oil are stable for hours in an acidic environment similar to that of gastric juices.

Besides dietary consumption, olive oil exerts beneficial effects in topical applications [69]. Skin application of olive oil after UVB exposure reduced 8-hydroxy-2'-deoxyguanosine (8-OHdG), a measure of DNA damage, and decreased the subsequent formation of UVB-induced skin tumors in mice [131]. A topical application of olive oil in combination with honey and beeswax has been shown to be effective in a number of skin and fungal infections including pityriasis versicolor, tinea cruris, tinea corporis, and tinea faciei [132].

In 2004, the United States Food and Drug Administration released a report stating that two teaspoonfuls of olive oil (23 g) per day that replace other saturated fats had the potential to reduce coronary disease [133]. There are no adverse effects associated with consumption of olive oil. However, one concern is the high energy density of olive oil could promote weight gain. Therefore, it is recommended to replace other fatty acids and simple carbohydrates with olive oil, rather than add olive oil in addition to the normal diet [90].

REFERENCES

Rosemary
1. Knoops, K. T., de Groot, L. C., Kromhout, D., Perrin, A. E., Moreiras-Varela, O., Menotti, A. & van Staveren, W. A. (2004). Mediterranean diet, lifestyle factors, and 10-year mortality in elderly European men and women: The HALE project. *JAMA* **292**(12), 1433–1439.
2. Trichopoulou, A., Costacou, T., Bamia, C. & Trichopoulos, D. (2003). Adherence to a Mediterranean diet and survival in a Greek population. *N Engl J Med* **348**(26), 2599–2608.
3. Fitó, M., Guxens, M., Corella, D., Sáez, G., Estruch, R., de la Torre, R., Francés, F., Cabezas, C., López-Sabater Mdel, C., Marrugat, J., García-Arellano, A., Arós, F., Ruiz-Gutierrez, V., Ros, E., Salas-Salvadó, J., Fiol, M., Solá, R. & Covas, M. I.for the PREDIMED Study Investigators (2007). Effect of a traditional Mediterranean diet on lipoprotein oxidation: A randomized controlled trial. *Arch Intern Med* **167**(11), 1195–1203.
4. Ninfali, P., Mea, G., Giorgini, S., Rocchi, M. & Bacchiocca, M. (2005). Antioxidant capacity of vegetables, spices and dressings relevant to nutrition. *Br J Nutr* **93**(2), 257–266.
5. Hemphill, I. & Cobiac, L. (2006). Health benefits of herbs and spices: The past, the present, the future. The historical and cultural use of herbs and spices. *Med J Aust* **185**(4 Suppl), S5.
6. Trichopoulou, A. & Critselis, E. (2004). Mediterranean diet and longevity. *Eur J Cancer Prev,* **13**(5), 453–456.
7. Tapsell, L. C. (2006). Health benefits of herbs and spices: The past, the present, the future. Herbs and spices as functional foods. *Med J Aust* **185**(4 Suppl), S6.
8. Patch, C. S. & Sullivan, D. R. (2006). Health benefits of herbs and spices: Health benefits of herbs and spices: The past, the present, the future. Cardiovascular disease. *Med J Aust* **185**(4 Suppl), S7.

9. Bozin, B., Mimica-Dukic, N., Samojlik, I. & Jovin, E. (2007). Antimicrobial and antioxidant properties of rosemary and sage (*Rosmarinus officinalis* L. and *Salvia officinalis* L., Lamiaceae) essential oils. *J Agric Food Chem* **55**(19), 7879–7885.

10. Cheung, S. & Tai, J. (2007). Anti-proliferative and antioxidant properties of rosemary *Rosmarinus officinalis*. *Oncol Rep* **17**(6), 1525–1531.

11. Hsieh, C. L., Peng, C. H., Chyau, C. C., Lin, Y. C., Wang, H. E. & Peng, R. Y. Low-density lipoprotein, collagen, and thrombin models reveal that Rosemarinus officinalis L. exhibits potent antiglycative effects. J Agric Food Chem. 2007;55(8), 2884–2891 (Epub 2007 Mar 27. Erratum in: J Agric Food Chem. 2007;55(11), 4624).

12. Moss, M., Cook, J., Wesnes, K. & Duckett, P. (2003). Aromas of rosemary and lavender essential oils differentially affect cognition and mood in healthy adults. *Int J Neurosci* **113**(1), 15–38.

13. Angioni, A., Barra, A., Cereti, E., Barile, D., Coïsson, J. D., Arlorio, M., Dessi, S., Coroneo, V. & Cabras, P. (2004). Chemical composition, plant genetic differences, antimicrobial and antifungal activity investigation of the essential oil of *Rosmarinus officinalis* L. *J Agric Food Chem* **52**(11), 3530–3535.

14. del Baño, M. J., Lorente, J., Castillo, J., Benavente-García, O., del Río, J. A., Ortuño, A., Quirin, K. W. & Gerard, D. (2003). Phenolic diterpenes, flavones, and rosmarinic acid distribution during the development of leaves, flowers, stems, and roots of *Rosmarinus officinalis*. Antioxidant activity. *J Agric Food Chem* **51**(15), 4247–4253.

15. Frankel, E., Huang, S., Aescherbach, R. & Prior, E. (1996). Antioxidant activity of a rosemary extract and its constituents, carnosic acid, carnosol, and rosmarinic acid, in bilk oil and oil-in-water emulsion. *J Agric Food Chem* **44**(1), 131–135.

16. Slamenova, D., Kuboskova, K., Horvathova, E. & Robichova, S. (2002 Mar 28). Rosemary-stimulated reduction of DNA strand breaks and FPG-sensitive sites in mammalian cells treated with H_2O_2 or visible light-excited Methylene Blue. *Cancer Lett* **177**(2), 145–153.

17. Offord, E. A., Macé, K., Ruffieux, C., Malnoë, A. & Pfeifer, A. M. (1995). Rosemary components inhibit benzo[a]pyrene-induced genotoxicity in human bronchial cells. *Carcinogenesis* **16**(9), 2057–2062.

18. Singletary, K. W. & Rokusek, J. T. (1997). Tissue-specific enhancement of xenobiotic detoxification enzymes in mice by dietary rosemary extract. *Plant Foods Hum Nutr* **50**(1), 47–53.

19. Soyal, D., Jindal, A., Singh, I. & Goyal, P. K. (2007). Modulation of radiation-induced biochemical alterations in mice by rosemary (*Rosmarinus officinalis*) extract. *Phytomedicine* **14**(10), 701–705.

20. Sotelo-Félix, J. I., Martinez-Fong, D., Muriel, P., Santillán, R. L., Castillo, D. & Yahuaca, P. (2002). Evaluation of the effectiveness of *Rosmarinus officinalis* (Lamiaceae) in the alleviation of carbon tetrachloride-induced acute hepatotoxicity in the rat. *J Ethnopharmacol* **81**(2), 145–154.

21. Amagase, H., Sakamoto, K., Segal, E. R. & Milner, J. A. (1996). Dietary rosemary suppresses 7,12-dimethylbenz(a)anthracene binding to rat mammary cell DNA. *J Nutr* **126**(5), 1475–1480.

22. Singletary, K. W. & Nelshoppen, J. M. (1991). Inhibition of 7,12 dimethylbenz[a] anthracene (DMBA)-induced mammary tumorigenesis and of *in vivo* formation of mammary DMBA-DNA adducts by rosemary extract. *Cancer Lett* **60**(2), 169–175.

23. Alexandrov, K., Rojas, M. & Rolando, C. (2006). DNA damage by benzo(a)pyrene in human cells is increased by cigarette smoke and decreased by a filter containing rosemary extract, which lowers free radicals. *Cancer Res* **66**(24), 11938–11945.
24. Sancheti, G. & Goyal, P. K. (2006). Effect of *Rosmarinus officinalis* in modulating 7,12-dimethylbcnz(a)anthracene induced skin tumorigenesis in mice. *Phytother Res* **20**(11), 981–986.
25. Nolkemper, S., Reichling, J., Stintzing, F. C., Carle, R. & Schnitzler, P. (2006). Antiviral effect of aqueous extracts from species of the Lamiaceae family against *Herpes simplex* virus type 1 and type 2 *in vitro*. *Planta Med* **72**(15), 1378–1382.
26. Mahady, G. B., Pendland, S. L., Stoia, A., Hamill, F. A., Fabricant, D., Dietz, B. M. & Chadwick, L. R. (2005). *In vitro* susceptibility of *Helicobacter pylori* to botanical extracts used traditionally for the treatment of gastrointestinal disorders. *Phytother Res* **19**(11), 988–991.
27. Sharabani, H., Izumchenko, E., Wang, Q., Kreinin, R., Steiner, M., Barvish, Z., Kafka, M., Sharoni, Y., Levy, J., Uskokovic, M., Studzinski, G. P. & Danilenko, M. (2006). Cooperative antitumor effects of vitamin D3 derivatives and rosemary preparations in a mouse model of myeloid leukemia. *Int J Cancer* **118**(12), 3012–3021.
28. Yamamoto, J., Yamada, K., Naemura, A., Yamashita, T. & Arai, R. (2005). Testing various herbs for antithrombotic effect. *Nutrition* **21**(5), 580–587.
29. Scarpati, M. L. & Oriente, G. (1958). Isolamento e costituzione dell'acido rosmarinico (dal *rosmarinus off.*). *Ric Sci* **28**, 2329–2333.
30. Petersen, M. & Simmonds, M. S. (2003). Rosmarinic acid. *Phytochemistry* **62**(2), 121–125.
31. Al-Sereitia, M. R., Abu-Amerb, K. M. & Sena, P. (1999). Pharmacology of rosemary (*Rosmarinus officinalis* Linn.) and its therapeutic potentials. *Indian J Exper Biol* **37**, 124–131.
32. Baba, S., Osakabe, N., Natsume, M., Yasuda, A., Muto, Y., Hiyoshi, K., Takano, H., Yoshikawa, T. & Terao, J. (2005). Absorption, metabolism, degradation and urinary excretion of rosmarinic acid after intake of *Perilla frutescens* extract in humans. *Eur J Nutr* **44**(1), 1–9.
33. Nakazawa, T. & Ohsawa, K. (2000). Metabolites of orally administered *Perilla frutescens* extract in rats and humans. *Biol Pharm Bull* **23**(1), 122–127.
34. Osakabe, N., Yasuda, A., Natsume, M. & Yoshikawa, T. (2004). Rosmarinic acid inhibits epidermal inflammatory responses: Anticarcinogenic effect of *Perilla frutescens* extract in the murine two-stage skin model. *Carcinogenesis* **25**(4), 549–557.
35. Osakabe, N., Takano, H., Sanbongi, C., Yasuda, A., Yanagisawa, R., Inoue, K. & Yoshikawa, T. (2004). Anti-inflammatory and anti-allergic effect of rosmarinic acid (RA); inhibition of seasonal allergic rhinoconjunctivitis (SAR) and its mechanism. *Biofactors* **21**(1–4), 127–131.
36. Atsumi, T. & Tonosaki, K. (2007). Smelling lavender and rosemary increases free radical scavenging activity and decreases cortisol level in saliva. *Psychiatry Res* **150**(1), 89–96.
37. Huang, S. S. & Zheng, R. L. (2006). Rosmarinic acid inhibits angiogenesis and its mechanism of action *in vitro*. *Cancer Lett* **239**(2), 271–280.
38. Lee, J., Kim, Y. S. & Park, D. (2007). Rosmarinic acid induces melanogenesis through protein kinase A activation signaling. *Biochem Pharmacol* **74**(7), 960–968.

39. Kim, D. S., Kim, H. R., Woo, E. R., Hong, S. T., Chae, H. J. & Chae, S. W. (2005). Inhibitory effects of rosmarinic acid on adriamycin-induced apoptosis in H9c2 cardiac muscle cells by inhibiting reactive oxygen species and the activations of c-Jun N-terminal kinase and extracellular signal-regulated kinase. *Biochem Pharmacol* **70**(7), 1066–1078.

40. Kang, M. A., Yun, S. Y. & Won, J. (2003). Rosmarinic acid inhibits Ca^{2+}-dependent pathways of T-cell antigen receptor-mediated signaling by inhibiting the PLC-gamma 1 and Itk activity. *Blood* **101**(9), 3534–3542.

41. Chang, C. H., Chyau, C. C., Hsieh, C. L., Wu, Y. Y., Ker, Y. B., Tsen, H. Y. & Peng, R. Y. (2008). Relevance of phenolic diterpene constituents to antioxidant activity of supercritical CO(2) extract from the leaves of rosemary. *Nat Prod Res* **22**(1), 76–90.

42. Pérez-Fons, L., Aranda, F. J., Guillén, J., Villalaín, J. & Micol, V. (2006). Rosemary (*Rosmarinus officinalis*) diterpenes affect lipid polymorphism and fluidity in phospholipid membranes. *Arch Biochem Biophys* **453**(2), 224–236.

43. Munné-Bosch, S. & Alegre, L. (2001). Subcellular compartmentation of the diterpene carnosic acid and its derivatives in the leaves of rosemary. *Plant Physiol* **125**(2), 1094–1102.

44. Singletary, K., MacDonald, C. & Wallig, M. (1996). Inhibition by rosemary and carnosol of 7,12-dimethylbenz[a]anthracene (DMBA)-induced rat mammary tumorigenesis and *in vivo* DMBA-DNA adduct formation. *Cancer Lett* **104**(1), 43–48.

45. Huang, M. T., Ho, C. T., Wang, Z. Y., Ferraro, T., Lou, Y. R., Stauber, K., Ma, W., Georgiadis, C., Laskin, J. D. & Conney, A. H. (1994). Inhibition of skin tumorigenesis by rosemary and its constituents carnosol and ursolic acid. *Cancer Res* **54**(3), 701–708.

46. Huang, S. C., Ho, C. T., Lin-Shiau, S. Y. & Lin, J. K. (2005). Carnosol inhibits the invasion of B16/F10 mouse melanoma cells by suppressing metalloproteinase-9 through down-regulating nuclear factor-kappa B an c-Jun. *Biochem Pharmacol* **69**(2), 221–232.

47. Visanji, J. M., Thompson, D. G. & Padfield, P. J. (2006). Induction of G2/M phase cell cycle arrest by carnosol and carnosic acid is associated with alteration of cyclin A and cyclin B1 levels. *Cancer Lett* **237**(1), 130–136.

48. Costa, S., Utan, A., Speroni, E., Cervellati, R., Piva, G., Prandini, A. & Guerra, M. C. (2007). Carnosic acid from rosemary extracts: A potential chemoprotective agent against aflatoxin B1. *An in vitro study. J Appl Toxicol* **27**(2), 152–159.

49. Lee, J. J., Jin, Y. R., Lee, J. H., Yu, J. Y., Han, X. H., Oh, K. W., Hong, J. T., Kim, T. J. & Yun, Y. P. (2007). Antiplatelet activity of carnosic acid, a phenolic diterpene from *Rosmarinus officinalis*. *Planta Med* **73**(2), 121–127.

50. Rau, O., Wurglics, M., Paulke, A., Zitzkowski, J., Meindl, N., Bock, A., Dingermann, T., Abdel-Tawab, M. & Schubert-Zsilavecz, M. (2006). Carnosic acid and carnosol, phenolic diterpene compounds of the labiate herbs rosemary and sage, are activators of the human peroxisome proliferator-activated receptor gamma. *Planta Med* **72**(10), 881–887.

51. González-Mahave, I., Lobesa, T., Del Pozo, M. D., Blasco, A. & Venturini, M. (2006). Rosemary contact dermatitis and cross-reactivity with other labiate plants. *Contact Dermatitis* **54**(4), 210–212.

52. Nusier, M. K., Bataineh, H. N. & Daradkah, H. M. (2007). Adverse effects of rosemary (*Rosmarinus officinalis* L.) on reproductive function in adult male rats. *Exp Biol Med (Maywood)* **232**(6), 809–813.

53. Debersac, P., Heydel, J. M., Amiot, M. J., Goudonnet, H., Artur, Y., Suschetet, M. & Siess, M. H. (2001). Induction of cytochrome P450 and/or detoxication enzymes by various extracts of rosemary: Description of specific patterns. *Food Chem Toxicol* **39**(9), 907–918.

54. Peng, C. H., Su, J. D., Chyau, C. C., Sung, T. Y., Ho, S. S., Peng, C. C. & Peng, R. Y. (2007). Supercritical fluid extracts of rosemary leaves exhibit potent anti-inflammation and anti-tumor effects. *Biosci Biotechnol Biochem* **71**(9), 2223–2232.

55. Keokamnerd, T., Acton, J. C., Han, I. Y. & Dawson, P. L. (2008). Effect of commercial rosemary oleoresin preparations on ground chicken thigh meat quality packaged in a high-oxygen atmosphere. *Poult Sci* **87**(1), 170–179.

56. Bentayeb, K., Rubio, C., Batlle, R. & Nerín, C. (2007). Direct determination of carnosic acid in a new active packaging based on natural extract of rosemary. *Anal Bioanal Chem* **389**(6), 1989–1996.

57. Minich, D. M., Bland, J. S., Katke, J., Darland, G., Hall, A., Lerman, R. H., Lamb, J., Carroll, B. & Tripp, M. (2007). Clinical safety and efficacy of NG440: A novel combination of rho iso-alpha acids from hops, rosemary, and oleanolic acid for inflammatory conditions. *Can J Physiol Pharmacol* **85**(9), 872–883.

Licorice

58. Shin, B. C. & Lee, M. S. (2007). Effects of aromatherapy acupressure on hemiplegic shoulder pain and motor power in stroke patients: A pilot study. *J Altern Complement Med* **13**(2), 247–251.

59. Fiore, C., Eisenhut, M., Ragazzi, E., Zanchin, G. & Armanini, D. (2005). A history of the therapeutic use of liquorice in Europe. *J Ethnopharmacol* **99**(3), 317–324.

60. Hemphill, I. (2006). *The Spice and Herb Bible*, (2nd ed.) Robert Rose Inc, Toronto, Ontario, Canada.

61. Isbrucker, R. A. & Burdock, G. A. (2006). Risk and safety assessment on the consumption of Licorice root (*Glycyrrhiza* sp.), its extract and powder as a food ingredient, with emphasis on the pharmacology and toxicology of glycyrrhizin. *Regul Toxicol Pharmacol* **46**(3), 167–192.

62. Whorwood, C. B., Sheppard, M. C. & Stewart, P. M. (1993). Licorice inhibits 11 beta-hydroxysteroid dehydrogenase messenger ribonucleic acid levels and potentiates glucocorticoid hormone action. *Endocrinology* **132**(6), 2287–2292.

63. Sigurjónsdóttir, H. A., Franzson, L., Manhem, K., Ragnarsson, J., Sigurdsson, G. & Wallerstedt, S. (2001). Liquorice-induced rise in blood pressure: A linear dose-response relationship. *J Hum Hypertens* **15**(8), 549–552.

64. de Klerk, G. J., Nieuwenhuis, M. G. & Beutler, J. J. (1997). Hypokalaemia and hypertension associated with use of liquorice flavoured chewing gum. *BMJ* **314**(7082), 731–732.

65. Blumenthal, M. (2000). *The Complete German Commission E Monographs – Therapeutic Guide to Herbal Medicines*, Integrative Medicine Communications, Newton, MA.

66. Chevallier, A. (1996). *The Encyclopedia of Medicinal Plants*, DK Publishing Inc, New York, NY.

67. Saeedi, M., Morteza-Semnani, K. & Ghoreishi, M. R. (2003). The treatment of atopic dermatitis with licorice gel. *J Dermatol Treat* **14**(3), 153–157.
68. Chin, Y. W., Jung, H. A., Liu, Y., Su, B. N., Castoro, J. A., Keller, W. J., Pereira, M. A. & Kinghorn, A. D. (2007). Anti-oxidant constituents of the roots and stolons of licorice (*Glycyrrhiza glabra*). *J Agric Food Chem* **55**(12), 4691–4697.

Chamomile

69. Baumann, L. S. (2007). Less-known botanical cosmeceuticals. *Dermatol Ther* **20**(5), 330–342.
70. O'Hara, M., Kiefer, D., Farrell, K. & Kemper, K. (1998). A review of 12 commonly used medicinal herbs. *Arch Fam Med* **7**(6), 523–536.
71. Mann, C. & Staba, E. J. (1986). The chemistry, pharmacology, and commercial formulations of Chamomile. *In* Herbs, Spices, and Medicinal Plants: Recent Advances in Botany, Horticulture, and Pharmacology (L. E. Craker & J. E. Simon, Eds.), Vol. 1, pp. 235–280, Oryx Press, Phoenix.
72. McKay, D. L. & Blumberg, J. B. (2006). A review of the bioactivity and potential health benefits of chamomile tea (*Matricaria recutita* L.). *Phytother Res.* **20**(7), 519–530.
73. Kotov, A. G., Khvorost, P. P. & Komissarenko, N. F. (1991). Coumarins of Matricaria recutita. *Chem Nat Compd* **27**, 753.
74. Patel, D., Shukla, S. & Gupta, S. (2007). Apigenin and cancer chemoprevention: Progress, potential and promise (review). *Int J Oncol* **30**(1), 233–245.
75. Dragland, S., Senoo, H., Wake, K., Holte, K. & Blomhoff, R. (2003). Several culinary and medicinal herbs are important sources of dietary antioxidants. *J Nutr* **133**(5), 1286–1290.
76. Nakamura, H., Moriya, K., Oda, S., Yano, E. & Kakuta, H. (2002). Changes in the parameters of autonomic nervous system and emotion spectrum calculated from encephalogram after drinking chamomile tea. *[Japanese]. Aroma Res* **3**, 251–255.
77. Gould, L., Reddy, C. V. & Gomprecht, R. F. (1973). Cardiac effects of chamomile tea. *J Clin Pharmacol* **13**(11), 475–479.
78. de la Motte, S., Böse-O'Reilly, S., Heinisch, M. & Harrison, F. (1997). Double-blind comparison of an apple pectin-chamomile extract preparation with placebo in children with diarrhea [German]. *Arzneimittelforschung* **47**(11), 1247–1249.
79. Maiche, A. G., Gröhn, P. & Mäki-Hokkonen, H. (1991). Effect of chamomile cream and almond ointment on acute radiation skin reaction. *Acta Oncol* **30**(3), 395–396.
80. Glowania, H. J., Raulin, C. & Swoboda, M. (1987). Effect of chamomile on wound healing: A clinical double-blind study. *Z Hautkr* **62**(17), 1262, 1267–1271.
81. Hartman, D. & Coetzee, J. C. (2002). Two US practitioners' experience of using essential oils for wound care. *J Wound Care* **11**, 317–320.
82. Kyokong, O., Charuluxananan, S., Muangmingsuk, V., Rodanant, O., Subornsug, K. & Punyasang, W. (2002). Efficacy of chamomile-extract spray for prevention of post-operative sore throat. *J Med Assoc Thai* **85**(Suppl 1), S180–S185.
83. Subiza, J., Subiza, J. L., Hinojosa, M., Garcia, R., Jerez, M., Valdivieso, R. & Subiza, E. (1989). Anaphylactic reaction after the ingestion of chamomile tea: A study of cross-reactivity with other composite pollens. *J Allergy Clin Immunol* **84**(3), 353–358.

84. Reider, N., Sepp, N., Fritsch, P., Weinlich, G. & Jensen-Jarolim, E. (2000). Anaphylaxis to camomile: Clinical features and allergen cross-reactivity. *Clin Exp Allergy* **30**(10), 1436–1443.
85. Paulsen, E. (2002). Contact sensitization from Compositae-containing herbal remedies and cosmetics. *Contact Dermatitis* **47**(4), 189–198.
86. Nowack, R. & Nowak, B. (2005). Herbal teas interfere with cyclosporin levels in renal transplant patients. *Nephrol Dial Transplant* **20**(11), 2554–2556.
87. Heck, A. M., DeWitt, B. A. & Lukes, A. L. (2000). Potential interactions between alternative therapies and warfarin. *Am J Health Syst Pharm* **57**, 1221–1227.

Olive Oil

88. Waterman, E. & Lockwood, B. (2007). Active components and clinical applications of olive oil. *Altern Med Rev* **12**(4), 331–342.
89. Tuck, K. L. & Hayball, P. J. (2002). Major phenolic compounds in olive oil: Metabolism and health effects. *J Nutr Biochem* **13**(11), 636–644.
90. Trichopoulou, A. & Dilis, V. (2007). Olive oil and longevity. *Mol Nutr Food Res* **51**(10), 1275–1278.
91. Alarcón de la Lastra, C., Barranco, M. D., Motilva, V. & Herrerías, J. M. (2001). Mediterranean diet and health: Biological importance of olive oil. *Curr Pharm Des* **7**(10), 933–950.
92. Velasco, J. & Dobarganes, C. (2002). Oxidative stability of virgin olive oil. *Eur J Lipid Sci Technol* **104**, 661–676.
93. Carrasco-Pancorbo, A., Cerretani, L., Bendini, A., Segura-Carretero, A., Lercker, G. & Fernández-Gutiérrez, A. (2007). Evaluation of the influence of thermal oxidation on the phenolic composition and on the antioxidant activity of extra-virgin olive oils. *J Agric Food Chem* **55**(12), 4771–4780.
94. Visioli, F., Poli, A. & Gall, C. (2002). Antioxidant and other biological activities of phenols from olives and olive oil. *Med Res Rev* **22**(1), 65–75.
95. Gutiérrez-Rosales, F., Ríos, J. J. & Gómez-Rey, M. L. (2003). Main polyphenols in the bitter taste of virgin olive oil. Structural confirmation by on-line high-performance liquid chromatography electrospray ionization mass spectrometry. *J Agric Food Chem* **51**(20), 6021–6025.
96. Visioli, F., Bellomo, G., Montedoro, G. & Galli, C. (1995). Low density lipoprotein oxidation is inhibited *in vitro* by olive oil constituents. *Atherosclerosis* **117**(1), 25–32.
97. Bartsch, H., Nair, J. & Owen, R. W. (2002). Exocyclic DNA adducts as oxidative stress markers in colon carcinogenesis: Potential role of lipid peroxidation, dietary fat and antioxidants. *Biol Chem* **383**(6), 915–921.
98. Escrich, E., Moral, R., Grau, L., Costa, I. & Solanas, M. (Oct 2007). Molecular mechanisms of the effects of olive oil and other dietary lipids on cancer. *Mol Nutr Food Res* **51**(10), 1279–1292.
99. Keys, A., Menotti, A., Karvonen, M. J., Aravanis, C., Blackburn, H., Buzina, R., Djordjevic, B. S., Dontas, A. S., Fidanza, F., Keys, M. H. *et al.* (1986). The diet and 15-year death rate in the seven countries study. *Am J Epidemiol* **124**(6), 903–915.
100. Covas, M. I. (2007). Olive oil and the cardiovascular system. *Pharmacol Res* **55**(3), 175–186.

101. Psaltopoulou, T., Naska, A., Orfanos, P., Trichopoulos, D., Mountokalakis, T., Trichopoulou, A., Olive oil, the Mediterranean diet, and arterial blood pressure: The Greek European Prospective Investigation into Cancer and Nutrition (EPIC) study. *Am J Clin Nutr.* 2004 Oct; 80(4): 1012-8. Erratum in: *Am J Clin Nutr* 2005, **81**(5), 1181.

102. Trevisan, M., Krogh, V., Freudenheim, J., Blake, A., Muti, P., Panico, S., Farinaro, E., Mancini, M., Menotti, A. & Ricci G. Consumption of olive oil, butter, and vegetable oils and coronary heart disease risk factors. The Research Group ATS-RF2 of the Italian National Research Council. JAMA. 1990; 263(5): 688–692. Erratum in: *JAMA* 1990, **263**(13), 1768.

103. Alonso, A. & Martínez-González, M. A. (2004). Olive oil consumption and reduced incidence of hypertension: The SUN study. *Lipids* **39**(12), 1233–1238.

104. Alonso, A., Ruiz-Gutierrez, V. & Martínez-González, M. A. (2006). Monounsaturated fatty acids, olive oil and blood pressure: Epidemiological, clinical and experimental evidence. *Public Health Nutr* **9**(2), 251–257.

105. Ferrara, L. A., Raimondi, A. S., d'Episcopo, L., Guida, L., Dello Russo, A. & Marotta, T. (2000). Olive oil and reduced need for antihypertensive medications. *Arch Intern Med* **160**(6), 837–842.

106. Lopez-Miranda, J., Delgado-Lista, J., Perez-Martinez, P., Jimenez-Gómez, Y., Fuentes, F., Ruano, J. & Marin, C. (2007). Olive oil and the haemostatic system. *Mol Nutr Food Res* **51**(10), 1249–1259.

107. Ruano, J., López-Miranda, J., de la Torre, R., Delgado-Lista, J., Fernández, J., Caballero, J., Covas, M. I., Jiménez, Y., Pérez-Martínez, P., Marín, C., Fuentes, F. & Pérez-Jiménez, F. (2007). Intake of phenol-rich virgin olive oil improves the postprandial prothrombotic profile in hypercholesterolemic patients. *Am J Clin Nutr* **86**(2), 341–346.

108. Oubiña, P., Sánchez-Muniz, F. J., Ródenas, S. & Cuesta, C. (2001). Eicosanoid production, thrombogenic ratio, and serum and LDL peroxides in normo- and hypercholesterolaemic post-menopausal women consuming two oleic acid-rich diets with different content of minor components. *Br J Nutr* **85**(1), 41–47.

109. Visioli, F., Caruso, D., Grande, S., Bosisio, R., Villa, M., Galli, G., Sirtori, C. & Galli, C. Virgin. (2005). Olive Oil Study (VOLOS): Vasoprotective potential of extra virgin olive oil in mildly dyslipidemic patients. *Eur J Nutr* **44**(2), 121–127.

110. Bogani, P., Galli, C., Villa, M. & Visioli, F. (2007). Postprandial anti-inflammatory and antioxidant effects of extra virgin olive oil. *Atherosclerosis* **190**(1), 181–186.

111. Hargrove, R. L., Etherton, T. D., Pearson, T. A., Harrison, E. H. & Kris-Etherton, P. M. (2001). Low fat and high monounsaturated fat diets decrease human low density lipoprotein oxidative susceptibility *in vitro*. *J Nutr* **131**(6), 1758–1763.

112. Wiseman, S. A., Mathot, J. N., de Fouw, N. J. & Tijburg, L. B. (1996). Dietary non-tocopherol antioxidants present in extra virgin olive oil increase the resistance of low density lipoproteins to oxidation in rabbits. *Atherosclerosis* **120**(1–2), 15–23.

113. Machowetz, A., Poulsen, H. E., Gruendel, S., Weimann, A., Fitó, M., Marrugat, J., de la Torre, R., Salonen, J. T., Nyyssönen, K., Mursu, J., Nascetti, S., Gaddi, A., Kiesewetter, H., Bäumler, H., Selmi, H., Kaikkonen, J., Zunft, H. J., Covas, M. I. & Koebnick, C. (2007). Effect of olive oils on biomarkers of oxidative DNA stress in Northern and Southern Europeans. *FASEB J* **21**(1), 45–52.

114. Hodge, A. M., English, D. R., McCredie, M. R., Severi, G., Boyle, P., Hopper, J. L. & Giles, G. G. (2004). Foods, nutrients and prostate cancer. *Cancer Causes Control* **15**, 11–20.

115. Trichopoulou, A., Katsouyanni, K., Stuver, S., Tzala, L., Gnardellis, C., Rimm, E. & Trichopoulos, D. (1995). Consumption of olive oil and specific food groups in relation to breast cancer risk in Greece. *J Natl Cancer Inst* **87**, 110–116.

116. Braga, C., La Vecchia, C., Franceschi, S., Negri, E., Parpinel, M., Recarli, A., Giocosa, A. & Trichopoulos, D. (1998). Olive oil, other seasoning fats, and the risk of colorectal carcinoma. *Cancer* **82**, 448–453.

117. Franceschi, S., Favero, A., Conti, E., Talamini, R., Volpe, R., Negri, E., Barzan, L. & La Vecchia, C. (1999). Food groups, oils and butter, and cancer of the oral cavity and pharynx. *Br J Cancer* **80**, 614–620.

118. Escrich, E., Moral, R., Grau, L., Costa, I. & Solanas, M. (2007). Molecular mechanisms of the effects of olive oil and other dietary lipids on cancer. *Mol Nutr Food Res.* **51**(10), 1279–1292.

119. Llor, X., Pons, E., Roca, A., Alvarez, M., Mañé, J., Fernández-Bañares, F. & Gassull, M. A. (2003). The effects of fish oil, olive oil, oleic acid and linoleic acid on colorectal neoplastic processes. *Clin Nutr* **22**(1), 71–79.

120. Brunelleschi, S., Bardelli, C., Amoruso, A., Gunella, G., Ieri, F., Romani, A., Malorni, W. & Franconi, F. (2007). Minor polar compounds extra-virgin olive oil extract (MPC-OOE) inhibits NF-kappaB translocation in human monocyte/macrophages. *Pharmacol Res* **56**(6), 542–549.

121. Menendez, J. A., Vazquez-Martin, A., Colomer, R., Brunet, J., Carrasco-Pancorbo, A., Garcia-Villalba, R., Fernandez-Gutierrez, A. & Segura-Carretero, A. (2007). Olive oil's bitter principle reverses acquired autoresistance to trastuzumab (Herceptin) in HER2-overexpressing breast cancer cells. *BMC Cancer* **7**, 80.

122. Hashim, Y. Z., Rowland, I. R., McGlynn, H., Servili, M., Selvaggini, R., Taticchi, A., Esposto, S., Montedoro, G., Kaisalo, L., Wähälä, K. & Gill, C. I. (2008). Inhibitory effects of olive oil phenolics on invasion in human colon adenocarcinoma cells *in vitro*. *Int J Cancer* **122**(3), 495–500.

123. Fabiani, R., Rosignoli, P., De Bartolomeo, A., Fuccelli, R. & Morozzi, G. (2008). Inhibition of cell cycle progression by hydroxytyrosol is associated with upregulation of cyclin-dependent protein kinase inhibitors p21(WAF1/Cip1) and p27(Kip1) and with induction of differentiation in HL60 cells. *J Nutr* **138**(1), 42–48.

124. Fini, L., Hotchkiss, E., Fogliano, V., Graziani, G., Romano, M., De Vol, F. B., Qin, H., Selgrad, M., Boland, C. R. & Ricciardiello, L. (2007). Chemopreventive properties of pinoresinol-rich olive oil involve a selective activation of the ATM-p53 cascade in colon cancer cell lines. *Carcinogenesis*, [Epub ahead of print].

125. Garg, A. (1998). High-monounsaturated-fat diets for patients with diabetes mellitus: A meta-analysis. *Am J Clin Nutr* **67**(3 Suppl), 577S–582S.

126. Paniagua, J. A., de la Sacristana, A. G., Sánchez, E., Romero, I., Vidal-Puig, A., Berral, F. J., Escribano, A., Moyano, M. J., Peréz-Martinez, P., López-Miranda, J. & Pérez-Jiménez, F. (2007). A MUFA-rich diet improves postprandial glucose, lipid and GLP-1 responses in insulin-resistant subjects. *J Am Coll Nutr* **26**(5), 434–444.

127. Perona, J. S., Vögler, O., Sánchez-Domínguez, J. M., Montero, E., Escribá, P. V. & Ruiz-Gutierrez, V. (2007). Consumption of virgin olive oil influences membrane

lipid composition and regulates intracellular signaling in elderly adults with type 2 diabetes mellitus. *J Gerontol A Biol Sci Med Sci* **62**(3), 256–263.

128. Medina, E., de Castro, A., Romero, C. & Brenes, M. (2006). Comparison of the concentration of phenolic compounds in olive oils and other plant oils: Correlation with antimicrobial activity. *J Agric Food Chem* **54**, 4954–4961.

129. Bisignano, G., Tomaino, A., Lo Cascio, R., Crisafi, G., Uccella, N. & Saija, A. (1999). On the *in-vitro* antimicrobial activity of oleuropein and hydroxytyrosol. *J Pharm Pharmacol* **51**(8), 971–974.

130. Romero, C., Medina, E., Vargas, J., Brenes, M. & De Castro, A. (2007). *In vitro* activity of olive oil polyphenols against *Helicobacter pylori*. *J Agric Food Chem* **55**(3), 680–686.

131. Budiyanto, A., Ahmed, N. U., Wu, A., Bito, T., Nikaido, O., Osawa, T., Ueda, M. & Ichihashi, M. (2000). Protective effect of topically applied olive oil against photocarcinogenesis following UVB exposure of mice. *Carcinogenesis* **21**(11), 2085–2090.

132. Al-Waili, N. S. (2004). An alternative treatment for pityriasis versicolor, tinea cruris, tinea corporis and tinea faciei with topical application of honey, olive oil and beeswax mixture: An open pilot study. *Complement Ther Med* **12**(1), 45–47.

133. Pérez-Jiménez, F., Ruano, J., Perez-Martinez, P., Lopez-Segura, F. & Lopez-Miranda, J. (2007). The influence of olive oil on human health: Not a question of fat alone. *Mol Nutr Food Res* **20**, 1199–1208.

Chapter 27

Quercetin: A Potential Complementary and Alternative Cancer Therapy

Thilakavathy Thangasamy, Sivanandane Sittadjody and Randy Burd

Department of Nutritional Sciences, University of Arizona, Tucson, AZ, USA

Abstract

The role of flavonoids in the diet is of great interest and the biological activity of these polyphenolic compounds is of significant importance in understanding the health benefits derived from these compounds. Quercetin (3,5,7,3′,4′-pentahydroxyflavanone) is one of the most common flavonoids found in health foods or herbal products. It is believed to exert beneficial effects on human health based on its ability to act as a scavenger of free radicals and its potency to inhibit proliferation of transformed epithelial cells. However, high concentrations of quercetin have been reported to exert pro-oxidant and pro-apoptotic effects. Intake of dietary quercetin through food sources and supplementation results in little or no free circulating quercetin, rather it is found almost exclusively as glycoside conjugates. Therefore, the knowledge of achievable blood/tissue concentration of quercetin, the form of quercetin and cell-specific characteristics is of great importance because these factors may dictate different mechanisms of action and influence cell response. The current chapter discusses quercetin absorption, achievable blood concentration, its role as an antioxidant/pro-oxidant and its effect on cancer.

Keywords: *Quercetin, cancer, flavonoid, therapy, toxicity, blood levels, mechanisms*

INTRODUCTION

Flavonoids are plant polyphenolic compounds present in the daily diet and contribute to the flavor and color of fruit and vegetables. The six major subclasses of flavonoids include the flavones, flavonols, flavanones, catechins or flavanols, anthocyanidins and isoflavones. They have been proposed to exert beneficial effects in a multitude of disease states including cancer, cardiovascular disease and neurodegenerative disorders [1]. The daily intake of flavonoids calculated on the basis of the aglycones was estimated to range from approximately 3 mg to 70 mg in different countries, but this may be exceeded based on the particular diet [2]. The flavonoid quercetin is one of the most studied flavonols and is ubiquitously present in fruits and vegetables and its daily intake is calculated to range between 6 mg/day and 31 mg/day [3].

Quercetin is best known as an antioxidant, but at high concentrations also exhibits pro-oxidant activity. Quercetin has additional bio-modifying properties such as induction or inhibition of apoptosis, anti-inflammatory effects, cell cycle arrest and anti-proliferative effects. These effects appear to be concentration specific as well and are most commonly studied in cell culture systems. Quercetin is almost found exclusively as glycoside conjugates in the blood. Therefore, the achievable blood/tissue concentration of quercetin, the form of quercetin and cell-specific characteristics is of great importance because these factors may dictate different mechanisms of action and influence cell response.

The exploration of quercetin as a potential drug of the future is rapidly increasing, especially as an anti-cancer agent. Quercetin exhibits chemo-preventive action in animal models [4], and is known to inhibit the proliferation of colorectal, breast, gastric, ovarian and lymphoid cancer cell lines [5,6]. In addition to its antioxidant activity, the protective effects of quercetin have also been attributed to the inhibition of key signaling enzymes like protein kinase C, tyrosine kinase and phosphoinositide 3-kinase (PI-3 kinase) involved in the regulation of cell proliferation, angiogenesis, inhibition of DNA damage and apoptosis [7]. However, its cellular concentration plays a vital role in determining its biological action which may differ with different cell lines.

The goal of this chapter is to explore the concentration specific effects of quercetin as an anti-cancer agent. The effects of quercetin on cancer cells as well as the forms and concentrations of quercetin that are biologically available through diet will be explored. The absorption and bioavailability of quercetin and its conjugates are of significant importance due to the fact that little free quercetin is available in the blood after dietary intake or supplementation as a result of rapid glycosylation and methylation. Quercetin metabolism and absorption also represent major areas of interest in studies utilizing the dietary intake of quercetin because the cellular concentration of quercetin that is achievable plays a vital role in its biological activity.

ABSORPTION OF QUERCETIN

In plants and plant-derived foods, quercetin is found to be present mainly as glycosides. The hydrolysis of flavonoid glycosides can occur in the oral cavity and in the small intestine by glucosidase and/or lactase phloridizin hydrolase [8] and after this hydrolysis the aglycones formed are efficiently absorbed although the bioavailability may be extremely low due to extensive pre-systemic metabolism [9]. The absorption of quercetin occurs mainly in the small intestine and the sugar moiety is a major determining factor in the intestinal absorption. Pharmacological doses are mostly absorbed in the same amount as dietary concentrations. In most of the animal studies and human trials, quercetin aglycone results in absorption of approximately 20%. Studies carried out by Graf *et al.* [10] in rats indicate that 6% of dietary quercetin is absorbed from the gastro-intestinal (GI) tract. The stomach, small and large intestines appear to absorb and actively metabolize quercetin because the tissues contain both free quercetin as well as a complex and differing metabolite profile depending on the region of the GI tract [11].

Of the various forms of quercetin glycosides (rhamnosides, glucosides, etc.) hydrolysis occurs in the oral cavity (~60%) [12]. The absorption of quercetin glucosides is thought to occur through the interactions of quercetin with epithelial brush border membrane transporters such as sodium-dependant glucose transporter-1 (SGLT-1) followed by deglycosylation. It is further metabolized by conjugation to glucuronides and/or sulfates or methyl conjugates prior reaching to systemic circulation [13, 14].

The transport of quercetin and its glucosides like quercetin 4'-glucoside, quercetin 3,4'-diglucoside depends on the position and nature of glucosidic moiety [15]. The same authors further demonstrated that quercetin 4'-glucoside is transported by SGLT-1 across the apical membrane of enterocytes and its absorption is limited by a multidrug resistance associated protein (MRP2) mediated efflux across the apical membrane as well as by an unknown transporter on the basolateral membrane [16]. Exposure of the intestinal epithelium to high concentration of flavonoids also suggests that these compounds can have an important role in prevention of colon cancer by its role in the epithelial cells [17]. Quercetin metabolites may partly be responsible for the pharmacological activity of the parent flavonols and its elimination is found to be slow, with half-lives varying from 11 hours to 28 hours [18]. Studies on intestinal metabolism [19, 20] and *in vivo* bioavailability reports [21] suggest that quercetin is metabolized to the extent that very less or no free quercetin aglycone is present in the circulation. Quercetin conjugates have also been reported to retain the properties of parent molecule such as antioxidation [22] and to inhibit xanthine oxidase and lipoxygenase [23].

QUERCETIN DOSAGE AND ACHIEVABLE BLOOD CONCENTRATION

Quercetin is used in many countries as a vasoprotectant and as an ingredient in numerous multivitamin preparations and herbal remedies. It is sold as a dietary supplement with a recommended dose of 1200–1500 mg/day (400–500 mg, 3 times a day) [24]. Dihal *et al.* [25] reported that ingestion of 500 mg quercetin supplement would lead to an increase of approximately 40 times the physiological colon concentration (2–3 mM). However, there are no scientific reports regarding human safety in this concentration range. In humans receiving

TABLE 27.1 The Quercetin Concentration Achieved after Administration in Rats and Humans

Doses	Quercetin concentration	References
In Humans		
100 mg single dose	0.8 μM (serum)	[29]
100 mg single dose intravenous	12 μM (serum)	[86]
1 g/day for 28 days	0.10–1.5 μM (plasma)	[87]
8 mg, 20 mg, 50 mg orally	0.14, 0.22, 0.29 μM (plasma)	[26]
200 mg rutin (quercetin glycoside) orally	0.49 μM at 5 hours (plasma)	[88]
200–500 mg/day	1 μM and 5 μM aglycone (serum)	[89]
1–2 g (amount proposed by supplement makers)	10–50 μM (plasma)	[59]
In Rats		
Single meal, 0.2%	50 μM of quercetin metabolites (plasma)	[31]
0.25% for 21 days	61.2 ± 45 μM (plasma)	[90]
0.2% for 3 weeks	133 μM (sulfated and glucoronidated) (serum)	[76]
2 mg/day for 4 weeks	~6.054 μM (serum)	[44]
20 mg/day for 4 weeks	~45.13 μM (serum)	[44]

quercetin or rutin, the plasma concentration of the quercetin aglycone reaches 29 nM, 5 hours after ingestion [26] and a nearly similar concentration (25 nM) has been reported by Soleas *et al.* [27]. The plasma half-life of quercetin in humans ranges between 17 hours and 28 hours. Table 27.1 shows the quercetin concentration achieved in humans and rats.

Earlier investigations by Freireich *et al.* [28] compared blood levels and toxicity of quercetin in different species. The studies revealed the quercetin dose used in rats by in terms of body surface area was $40.6 \, mg/m^2$ (6.25 mg/kg), which was approximately 4.5% of the dose given to humans in this study ($945 \, mg/m^2$). The plasma level (14 μM) achieved in rats 5 minutes after quercetin administration was approximately 5% of that observed in humans immediately after quercetin administration, which was approximately 280 μM [29, 30]. Rats fed quercetin 0.5%, 0.25% and 0.125% for 10 days reported a plasma concentration of 118 ± 8 μM, 79 ± 7 μM and 45 ± 6 μM respectively [31]. In general, quercetin is considered safe, but at high doses, it has been suggested to possess mutagenic and carcinogenic properties, and there were indications of toxicity in humans. Table 27.2 illustrates the effects of quercetin administration in humans and animals.

TABLE 27.2 The Toxicity of Quercetin Administration in Humans and Animals

Quercetin administration	Side effects	References
Intravenous 100 mg in humans	None, well tolerated	[71]
Intravenous 1400 mg/m² once weekly for 3 weeks in humans	Renal toxicity in two of ten patients	[71]
Albino Norwegian rats 0.1% quercetin in diet treated for 406 days (grain-based diet)	80% developed intestinal tumors and 20% developed bladder tumors	[91]
1% Quercetin in diet (400 mg/kg) for 410 days in rats	No increase in gross pathology, no risk of cancer	[92]
F344 rats supplemented with dietary quercetin supplemented (2%)	Reduction in aberrant crypt foci (ACF) induced by azoxymethane (AOM) in the colon	[93]
10% Quercetin in diet for 850 days in rats (commercial diet)	No tumor incidence	[94]
Wistar rats fed 25 mg/kg body weight quercetin weekly once for 4 weeks	Significant reduction in tumor volume	[95]
Rats were fed quercetin at 1 g/kg after treatment with 1,2-dimethylhydrazine to induce aberrant crypt foci	Significant reduction in the number of aberrant crypts and larger aberrant crypt foci in colon	[96]
Mice bearing abdominal tumors given daily intraperitoneal injection of quercetin (doses 20, 200, 400 and 800 mg/kg)	Significant inhibition of tumor growth	[97]
10% Quercetin in diet to golden hamsters for 735 days	No tumor incidence	[98]

ANTIOXIDANT AND PRO-OXIDANT ACTIVITY OF QUERCETIN

Compounds that enhance defense mechanisms by inhibiting cellular damage inflicted by reactive oxygen species (ROS) may play an important role in disease prevention. The ROS are formed *in vivo* during normal aerobic metabolism and can cause damage to DNA, proteins and lipids, when there is an imbalance in the natural antioxidant defense systems. The chemical structure of quercetin makes them capable of stabilizing free electrons obtained from free radicals such as ROS [32]. In particular, the catechol moiety of quercetin with two hydroxyl groups can exert a powerful free radical scavenging action mainly due to its electron donating nature [33]. The catechol group is also directly related to the chelating action of quercetin as demonstrated by numerous studies in which quercetin inhibits lipid peroxidation by its free radical scavenging action. Quercetin at a concentration of 0.2 –1 mM has been shown to scavenge super oxide anion, singlet oxygen and lipid peroxyl radicals [34] as well as inhibit Cu-catalyzed oxidation and cytotoxicity of low density lipoprotein (LDL) *in vitro* [35]. A 0.5 μM of quercetin decreases the malondialdehyde or MDA production in LDL samples in serum of healthy persons [36]. Higher doses of quercetin (10–100 μM) also diminished MDA concentration [3]. Pretreatment for 2 or 20 hours with all doses of quercetin (0.1–10 μM) prevented the decrease of reduced glutathione (GSH) and the increase of MDA initiated in the presence of tert-butyl hydroperoxide in HepG2 cells [37]. ROS generation induced by tert-butyl hydroperoxide was significantly reduced when cells were pretreated for 2 or 20 hours with 10 μM and for 20 hours with 5 μM of quercetin in the same study. Studies in the same cell line later revealed increased lipid peroxidation at a concentration of 80 μM for 72 hours [38].

Cellular studies indicate that quercetin can exert both antioxidant and prooxidant effects depending upon its concentration (Fig. 27.1). And it is suggested that cellular oxidative balance and GSH content play a vital role in these effects. GSH is the main nonenzymatic antioxidant defense within the

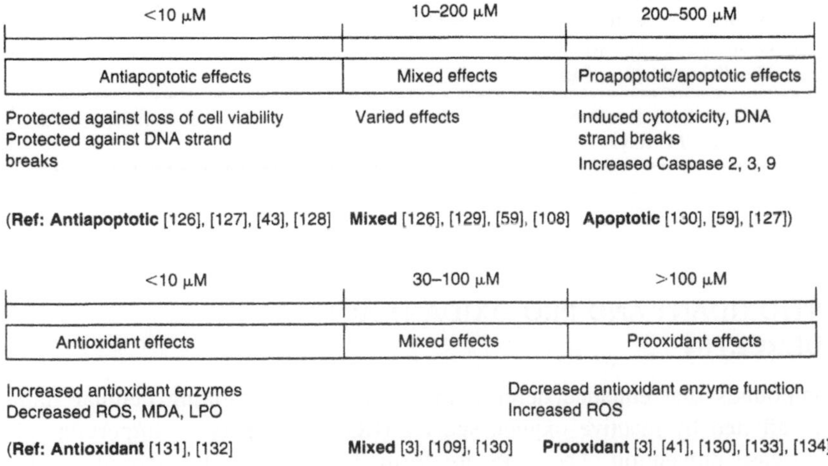

<10 μM	10–200 μM	200–500 μM
Antiapoptotic effects	Mixed effects	Proapoptotic/apoptotic effects
Protected against loss of cell viability Protected against DNA strand breaks	Varied effects	Induced cytotoxicity, DNA strand breaks Increased Caspase 2, 3, 9

(Ref: Antiapoptotic [126], [127], [43], [128]   **Mixed** [126], [129], [59], [108]   **Apoptotic** [130], [59], [127])

<10 μM	30–100 μM	>100 μM
Antioxidant effects	Mixed effects	Prooxidant effects
Increased antioxidant enzymes Decreased ROS, MDA, LPO		Decreased antioxidant enzyme function Increased ROS

(Ref: Antioxidant [131], [132]   **Mixed** [3], [109], [130]   **Prooxidant** [3], [41], [130], [133], [134])

FIGURE 27.1   Dual effect of quercetin in cells.

cell, bio-reducing different peroxides, hydroperoxides and radicals (alkyl, alkoxyl, peroxyl, etc.) [39]. Glutathione is also known to stimulate quercetin-related damage of DNA [40]. Spencer *et al.* [41] illustrated that quercetin concentrations upto $10\,\mu M$ rendered protection against fibroblast damage induced by oxidative stress and this effect was replaced by cytotoxicity following pre-treatment with $30\,\mu M$ quercetin. Quercetin treatment to rat hepatoma cells $(5-100\,\mu M)$ decreased the activities of enzymatic antioxidants like manganese superoxide dismutase, glutathione peroxidase and copper zinc superoxide dismutase mRNA expression levels by 30–40% [3, 42]. *In vitro* pre-treatment of human lymphocytes with quercetin (low concentrations $1-10\,\mu M$) was also reported to be very effective in preventing oxidative DNA damage in a concentration-dependant manner [43].

In animals, quercetin treatment 2 or $20\,mg/day$ for 4 weeks to male Sprague-Dawley rats significantly decreased the concentration of glutathione both in vitamin E deprived rats as well as in undeprived rats [44]. Similar investigations carried out by the same group later revealed that treatment of quercetin $(20\,mg/day)$ or vehicle alone for 6 weeks in rats, significantly increased the serum and liver alpha-tocopherol concentrations. Conversely, the treatment decreased glutathione concentration and glutathione reductase activity significantly confirming the pro-oxidant role of quercetin [45].

Cellular defense can also be regulated by genes with antioxidant responsive elements/electrophile responsive elements (ARE/EpRE) in their promoters. The antioxidant nature of quercetin has been attributed to its ability to chelate transition metal ions, such as Fe^{2+} and Cu^{2+}, catalyze electron transport and scavenge free radicals. Quercetin increases expression of the rate limiting enzyme γ-glutamylcysteine synthetase (GCS) in the synthesis of the most important endogenous cellular antioxidant, GSH which is required for numerous cellular functions and provides bio-reducing equivalents for many cellular reactions. NAD(P)H:quinone oxidoreductase 1 (NQO1) is a flavoprotein known to catalyze metabolic detoxification of quinones and protect cells from futile redox cycling, oxidative stress and neoplasia. Quercetin activates the promoter of NQO1 through ARE/EpRE-dependent mechanisms [46]. Investigation of the effect of quercetin on expression and enzymatic activity of NQO1 in the MCF-7 human breast carcinoma cell line revealed that treatment of these cells for 24 hours with $15\,\mu M$ quercetin results in a twofold increase in NQO1 protein levels and enzyme activity, and a three to fourfold increase in NQO1 mRNA expression [46]. Similar upregulation of NQO1 protein levels after $25\,\mu M$ quercetin treatment for 24 hours were also observed by our group [47]. The increase in NQO1 transcription in response to quercetin suggests that dietary plant polyphenols can stimulate transcription of phase II detoxifying systems, potentially through an ARE-dependent mechanism [46].

Recent studies illustrate NQO1 mediated protection against quercetin toxicity, in incubations in the presence of $1\,mM$ vitamin C in Chinese Hamster

Ovary (CHO) cells [48]. But Boots *et al.* [49] indicated that NQO1 offers no protection against quercetin. The overall reports based on the relationship between NQO1 and quercetin has been quite conflicting so far. However, Asher *et al.* [50] provided evidence that NQO1 stabilizes p53 and that reducing the NQO1 level by small interfering RNA decreases the level of p53. In our studies, cells that overexpressed tyrosinase and were exposed to quercetin, died by apoptosis due to conjugate formation and the stabilization of p53 by NQO1, as NQO1 can stabilize p53 via a redox mechanism involving oxidation of NAD(P)H [51]. It has also been suggested that a protein–protein interaction may be responsible for the stabilization of p53 by NQO1 [52]. Therefore, induction of NQO1 may result in detoxification and the stabilization of p53, thereby preventing cancer. While in other cells the induction of NQO1, by high levels of quercetin, may affect the metabolism of quercetin and produce pro-oxidant species. The subsequent stabilization of p53 may result in cell death of tumor cells or induce cell cycle arrest or aiding cancer treatment.

MOLECULAR ACTIONS OF QUERCETIN

Cell Cycle, DNA Damage and Apoptosis

The relationship between nutrition and cancers has been well illustrated in several epidemiological studies. Quercetin has various characteristics that makes it as a potential anti-cancer compound. These functions include cell cycle regulation, interaction with type II estrogen binding sites, reversal of multidrug resistance and induction of tumor cell apoptosis. Inactivation of Akt-1 protein, alterations in Bcl-2 family of proteins and phosphorylation of ERK are reported to be associated with quercetin-related apoptosis [53]. The inhibitory activity of quercetin is associated with its ability to compete with the binding of ATP to the nucleotide binding site on the kinases. Binding of quercetin to PI-3 kinase has been studied on the atomic level through crystallization of the kinase in the quercetin bound state. These studies reveal that quercetin and related kinase inhibitors bind in the ATP-binding pocket of the kinase [54]. The anti-cancer activity has also been related to the ability of quercetin to promote gap junctional communication between isolated cells stimulated by tumor promoters [55]. Park *et al.* [56] hypothesized that the anti-tumor effects of quercetin are mediated by its ability to down-regulate the β-catenin/Tcf signaling.

A number of investigations demonstrate the molecular actions of quercetin but for the purpose of this chapter we focus only on the role of quercetin pertaining to tumor growth. The protein p53 is a cellular gatekeeper for the cell growth and division and it can regulate cell cycle arrest, apoptosis, and DNA repair in a variety of cells. The p53 downstream effectors include p21, which participates in cell cycle arrest and Bax which triggers apoptosis [57]. Kuo *et al.* [58] observed that quercetin increased the levels of total p53, phospho-p53 (serine 15), and p21 proteins in A549 lung carcinoma cells. Quercetin is also known to regulate AP-1, which regulates the expression of genes associated with cell growth and cellular stress and induce DNA ladder formation between $100\,\mu M$ and $500\,\mu M$ concentrations. Incubation with $250\,\mu M$ quercetin for 24 hours in rat H4IIE cells increased caspase-2, caspase-3 and caspase-9 activity by 100–500% [59]. However in the same cell lines quercetin protected against H_2O_2-induced cytotoxicity, DNA strand breaks and apoptosis at a concentration of $10\,\mu M$, and this effect was attributed to the antioxidant activity of the polyphenol.

Intravenous administration of quercetin at a dosage of $60–1700\,mg/m^2$ to cancer patients in advanced stages led to inhibition of lymphocyte tyrosine kinase [30]. After exposure to $50\,\mu M$ quercetin, cell proliferation decreased to 51.3% of control, and further decrease in the percentage of cells in the G1 phase coincided with an increase in the percentage of cells in the sub-G1 phase. Studies with breast cancer cells [60, 61] show that micromolar concentrations of quercetin inhibits cell proliferation, thus acting as a cytotoxic agent. In other studies 10 pM [62] or 10 nM quercetin [63] have been demonstrated to reduce cell proliferation. However there are also reports which show that 1–10 nM quercetin stimulates the proliferation of breast cancer cells via an ER-mediated mechanism [60]. A biphasic effect of quercetin was observed on cell proliferation in HCT-116 and HT-29 colon carcinoma cell lines and mammary adenocarcinoma (MCF-7) cell lines after 24 hours of exposure. Inhibition of cell proliferation in HCT-116 and HT-29 was observed at 30 and $80\,\mu M$ while the viability of MCF-7 cells was unchanged at concentrations up to $100\,\mu M$ [64]. In a human squamous SCC-25 carcinoma cell line, growth stimulation was observed after 72 hours of exposure at concentrations of 1 and $10\,\mu M$, and growth inhibition with $100\,\mu M$ quercetin further illustrating its dual effect [65]. Fig. 27.1 illustrates the apoptotic and anti-apoptotic role of Quercetin.

Quercetin-mediated apoptosis is suggested to result from the induction of stress proteins, disruption of microtubules and mitochondrial release of cytochrome c, and activation of caspases [66, 67]. Quercetin-induced apoptosis of murine melanoma B16-BL6 cells was related to its injurious effects on mitochondria by decreasing the expression of Bcl-2 and increasing the activity of caspase-3 [68]. Pretreatment of HeLa cells to quercetin sensitizes to cisplatin-induced apoptosis and it was related to induction of caspase-3 activity and inhibition of both heat shock proteins (Hsp72) and multidrug resistance proteins (MRP) levels [69]. It could be therefore suggested from the available literature that low dose quercetin decreased apoptosis and necrosis occurring to some extent in the cultures, while higher concentrations increased both apoptosis and necrosis. Table 27.3 illustrates the molecular actions of Quercetin in certain tumor cell lines.

QUERCETIN AND CANCER TREATMENT

Several studies postulate the anti-tumorogenic effect of quercetin in cancer therapy. Quercetin dose-dependently suppressed PC-3 tumor growth both

TABLE 27.3 The molecular actions of quercetin in certain tumor cell lines

Cell lines	Dosage of Quercetin	Molecular action	References
Colon cancer cells	5 μM	Down-regulates the expression of CDC6, CDK4 and cyclin D1, cell proliferation and arrests cell cycle	[99]
Human colon cancer cells	10 μM	Inhibits expression of p21 ras oncogene	[100]
Human lung cancer cell line (NCI-H209)	10 μM (glucuronides)	DNA laddering	[101]
Murine osteoblastic cells (MC3T3-E1)	10 μM	TNF-α-mediated cytotoxicity	[102]
Human leukemia cells (U937)	20 μM	Caspase-mediated induction of apoptosis	[103]
Human chronic myeloid (K562)	25 μM	Cytotoxicity	[104]
Human hepatoma cells (HepG2)	25–50 μM	G1 phase arrest	[105]
HepG2 cells	25–75 μM	Increased expression of active caspase 3 and 9 levels	[106]
Colon cancer cell (HT-29)	25–100 μM	Markedly lowered phosphorylated and total levels of Akt	[107]
Human myelogenous leukemia (K562)	20–100 μM	Protective effect against H_2O_2-induced DNA damage	[108]
Human colon cells (SW480)	50 μM	β-Catenin/Tcf transcriptional activity	[56]
Human non-small lung cancer cells (A549)	50–200 μM	Concentration-dependent cytotoxicity	[109]
Human gastric cancer cells (HGC-27)	70 μM	Arrests G-1 phase of cell cycle, Reduction of cell growth	[110]
HeLa cells	100 μM	Inhibits cell proliferation and cell cycle progression	[111]
Human breast cancer cell MDA-MB468	248 μM	Down-regulates mutant p53	[112]

in vitro and *in vivo* [70]. Concentration up to 12 μM in serum was achieved in humans with single intravenous doses with no side effects [71], whereas up to 400 μM in serum showed minor toxicity [30]. A phase I clinical study carried out by Ferry *et al.* [30] showed that quercetin can be safely administered by intravenous bolus at a dose injection. The patients received a dosage of 945 mg/m^2 at 3-or 6-week intervals for the phase I clinical trials. From these studies, it was suggested a bolus dose of 1400 mg/m^2 be used for phase II trials. The plasma levels achieved inhibited lymphocyte tyrosine kinase activity and showed evidence of antitumor activity.

Dietary administration of quercetin (2 or 5%) to Sprague-Dawley rats reduced the incidence of mammary tumor induction to carcinogens 7,12, dimethyl benzanthracene or *N*-nitrosomethyl urea [72]. *In vivo* studies show that mice inoculated with ascites tumor cells and then treated intraperitoneally daily with either quercetin 40 mg/kg had a 20% increase in life span or its glycoside 160 mg/kg rutin had a 50% increase in life span [73]. Inhibition of metastatic growth of B16M-F10 cells in the liver (73%) was observed in mice after intravenous administration of pterostilbene and quercetin (20 mg/kg/day). This antimetastatic role has been correlated to the combined effect of quercetin and pterostilbene associated inhibition of Bcl-2 expression which sensitizes these cells to vascular endothelium-induced cytotoxicity [74]. However, Femia *et al.* [75] demonstrated that none of the diets supplemented with variable quercetin-glycoside content demonstrated a potential chemopreventive effect on azoxymethane-induced Aberrant Crypt Foci, preneoplastic lesions in the colon of rats.

In vitro quercetin has a wide range of inhibitory effects [76] and specific properties of quercetin are being explored as an adjuvant to therapy. For example, studies carried out by Debes *et al.* [77] in Ewing's tumor cell lines suggest that quercetin potentially may be useful in cancer therapy as a thermosensitizer by increasing the cell killing effect of hyperthermia and chemotherapy because of its ability to suppress heat shock protein expression.

Recently, cyclooxygenase (COX) enzymes, especially COX-2, have been implicated in the early changes associated with carcinogenesis in a number of tissues studied most extensively. A noteworthy fact is the ability of quercetin to interfere with COX by inhibiting COX-2 promoter activity [78], COX-2 protein expression [79] and COX enzyme activity. The IC$_{50}$ for COX enzyme inhibition of quercetin has been reported to be approximately 10 μM in HCA-7 cells [80]. We further demonstrated that quercetin can be used to selectively target cells that overexpress tyrosinase, such as in DB-1 melanoma cell lines [47]. Sensitization of these cell lines to apoptosis was observed at 25 μM, but 75 μM resulted in significant toxicity.

QUERCETIN METABOLITES AS BIOMARKERS

Determination of the relationship between dietary intake and cancer risk depends on the characterization of quercetin intake. The development and use

TABLE 27.4 Levels of Quercetin and its Metabolites in Human Plasma

Diet	Quercetin equivalent	Plasma (total level)	References
Onions	50 mg	0.83 µM	[18, 113]
Onions	186 mg	2.18 µM	[114]
129 g onion/day	13 mg	0.0727 µM	[115]
150 g fried onions	71.7 mg	0.65 µM	[116]
160 g onions	100 mg	7.6 µM	[117]
200 g fried onions	57 mg	0.67 µM	[118]
220 g onions/day	114 mg	1.48 ± 0.39 µM	[119]
225 g fried onions	56.49 mg	0.82 µM	[113]
260–360 g onions/day	67.32 mg	~0.69 µM	[120]
333 g fried onions	64.2 mg	0.648 µM	[116]
500 g fried onions	150 mg aglycone	1 µM	[121]
Quercetin aglycone	8, 20, 50 mg	0.14, 0.22, 0.29 µM	[26]
Quercetin 3-glucoside	151 mg	5–6 µM	[122]
Quercetin 4'-glucoside	150 mg	3.5 µM	[123]
Quercetin 4'-glucoside	154 mg	4.5–5.2 µM	[122]
Pure quercetin 3 rutinoside	100 mg	0.3 µM	[29]
Pure rutin	190 mg	0.18 µM	[123]
Rutin supplement	500 mg	0.13–0.73 µM	[124]
Quercetin 3-O rutinoside	200 mg	1.1 µM	[125]

of biomarkers for quercetin intake may provide a basis for the objective classification of this exposure. Most biomarker approaches refer to measurements of the original compound or its metabolite in blood and urine. After intake of a quercetin rich diet, quercetin metabolites accumulate in the circulation at a concentration of 10^{-7} to 10^{-5} M glucosides [22]. Moon *et al.* [81] isolated and identified a quercetin metabolite, quercetin 3–O-β-D-glucuronide (Q3GA), in rat plasma after oral administration of quercetin aglycone. Their studies also demonstrated that this metabolite possesses a considerable free radical scavenging activity because of its catechol group. Wittig et al. [82] reported 5' quercetin glucuronides in human plasma whereas Mullen et al. [14] identified 18 metabolites including O-methylated products, in addition to glucuronide and/or sulfate conjugates, from rat plasma after oral ingestion of Q4G. Table 27.4 illustrates the levels of quercetin metabolites in human plasma.

Absorbed phenols may be metabolized, stored or excreted through different routes and therefore the urinary content of phenols does not reflect absolute absorptive efficiency or can be served as an efficient biomarker. However Young et al. [83] stated that urinary excretion reflects the absorption and, therefore can serve as a better marker of bioavailability than dietary intake. Later studies by Kim et al. [84] portrayed urinary quercetin and kaempferol as biomarkers of dietary phenol absorption.

Fasting plasma quercetin concentrations seem to be promising biomarkers as they reflect dietary intake on the day before sampling as well as they serve as a measure for the usual dietary intake for a week. In healthy women on a 7–day diet protocol, the mean intake of quercetin was found to be 17.89 ± 9.5 mg/day, in fasting plasma samples collected at the end of the protocol period it was found to be 22.9 ± 16.6 nmol/l [85]. The flavonoid content in fasting plasma samples seems to be a suitable biomarker of short-term intake and a possible biomarker of the medium-term intake. The ability to detect and quantitate reliable marker of quercetin intake and bioavailability will lead to a better understanding of how diet and supplementation can influence quercetin concentration and modes of action.

CONCLUSION

Quercetin is a dietary polyphenolic compound with potentially beneficial effects on health. Most research has focused on the antioxidant properties of quercetin, its effects on several enzyme systems, and effects on biological pathways involved in carcinogenesis, inflammation and cardiovascular diseases. Upon absorption in the small intestine, quercetin is metabolized immediately by enzymes in the epithelial cells and further metabolized by the liver. Even if the bioavailability of quercetin is now relatively well documented, data is still lacking on the association of this flavonoid in the diet with respective to absorption and metabolism. As there is increasing evidence that there is little to no free quercetin in the plasma, the effects of the glucoconjugates and not free quercetin must be further investigated. Most of the studies presented focus on the aglycone form of quercetin, so the effects of the conjugates are still unkown, although, free quercetin may be readily absorbed and not detectable. Therefore, especially in the intestinal epithelial cells where there is evidence of deglycosylation, studying the effect of free quercetin may be of greater value.

Understanding the mechanism of action of quercetin and the determination of its free, and conjugated forms of quercetin in plasma and urine prior to or after supplementation seems to be an important aspect as its various biological actions seem to be dose-dependant in many of these studies we have cited in this chapter. The effects of quercetin concentration are varied with low doses ($0-10\,\mu M$) resulting in chemoprevention, mid ranges ($10-200\,\mu M$) resulting in mixed effects, and higher concentration ($>200\,\mu M$) in pro-oxidant or potential direct therapeutic properties. From the studies presented, these lower concentrations appear to be achievable by diet, while the therapeutic concentrations might require supplementation or intravenous administration and result in little or no side effects.

REFERENCES

1. Williams, R. J., Spencer, J. P. & Rice-Evans, C. (2004). Flavonoids: Antioxidants or signalling molecules? *Free Radic Biol Med* **36**, 838–849.
2. Graefe, E. U., Derendorf, H. & Veit, M. (1999). Pharmacokinetics and bioavailability of the flavonol quercetin in humans. *Int J Clin Pharmacol Ther* **37**, 219–233.
3. Alia, M., Mateos, R., Ramos, S., Lecumberri, E., Bravo, L. & Goya, L. (2006). Influence of quercetin and rutin on growth and antioxidant defense system of a human hepatoma cell line (HepG2). *Eur J Nutr* **45**, 19–28.
4. Elangovan, V., Sekar, N. & Govindasamy, S. (1994). Chemopreventive potential of dietary bioflavonoids against 20-methylcholanthrene-induced tumorigenesis. *Cancer Lett* **87**, 107–113.
5. De, A. W., Jr., Mueller-Dieckmann, H. J., Schulze-Gahmen, U., Worland, P. J., Sausville, E. & Kim, S. H. (1996). Structural basis for specificity and potency of a flavonoid inhibitor of human CDK2, a cell cycle kinase. *Proc Natl Acad Sci USA* **93**, 2735–2740.
6. Larocca, L. M., Teofili, L., Maggiano, N., Piantelli, M., Ranelletti, F. O. & Leone, G. (1996). Quercetin and the growth of leukemic progenitors. *Leuk Lymphoma* **23**, 49–53.
7. Agullo, G., Gamet-Payrastre, L., Manenti, S., Viala, C., Remesy, C., Chap, H. & Payrastre, B. (1997). Relationship between flavonoid structure and inhibition of phosphatidylinositol 3-kinase: A comparison with tyrosine kinase and protein kinase C inhibition. *Biochem Pharmacol* **53**, 1649–1657.
8. Day, A. J., Canada, F. J., Diaz, J. C., Kroon, P. A., Mclauchlan, R., Faulds, C. B., Plumb, G. W., Morgan, M. R. & Williamson, G. (2000). Dietary flavonoid and isoflavone glycosides are hydrolysed by the lactase site of lactase phlorizin hydrolase. *FEBS Lett* **468**, 166–170.
9. Walle, T., Walle, U. K. & Halushka, P. V. (2001). Carbon dioxide is the major metabolite of quercetin in humans. *J Nutr* **131**, 2648–2652.
10. Graf, B. A., Mullen, W., Caldwell, S. T., Hartley, R. C., Duthie, G. G., Lean, M. E., Crozier, A. & Edwards, C. A. (2005). Disposition and metabolism of [2–14C]quercetin-4'-glucoside in rats. *Drug Metab Dispos* **33**, 1036–1043.
11. Graf, B. A., Ameho, C., Dolnikowski, G. G., Milbury, P. E., Chen, C. Y. & Blumberg, J. B. (2006). Rat gastrointestinal tissues metabolize quercetin. *J Nutr* **136**, 39–44.

12. Walle, T., Browning, A. M., Steed, L. L., Reed, S. G. & Walle, U. K. (2005). Flavonoid glucosides are hydrolyzed and thus activated in the oral cavity in humans. *J Nutr* **135**, 48–52.

13. Day, A. J. & Williamson, G. (2001). Biomarkers for exposure to dietary flavonoids: A review of the current evidence for identification of quercetin glycosides in plasma. *Br J Nutr* **86**(Suppl 1), S105–S110.

14. Mullen, W., Graf, B. A., Caldwell, S. T., Hartley, R. C., Duthie, G. G., Edwards, C. A., Lean, M. E. & Crozier, A. (2002). Determination of flavonol metabolites in plasma and tissues of rats by HPLC-radiocounting and tandem mass spectrometry following oral ingestion of [2–(14)C]quercetin-4 -glucoside. *J Agric Food Chem* **50**, 6902–6909.

15. Walgren, R. A., Walle, U. K. & Walle, T. (1998). Transport of quercetin and its glucosides across human intestinal epithelial Caco-2 cells. *Biochem Pharmacol* **55**, 1721–1727.

16. Walgren, R. A., Lin, J. T., Kinne, R. K. & Walle, T. (2000). Cellular uptake of dietary flavonoid quercetin 4 -beta-glucoside by sodium-dependent glucose transporter SGLT1. *J Pharmacol Exp Ther* **294**, 837–843.

17. Salucci, M., Stivala, L. A., Maiani, G., Bugianesi, R. & Vannini, V. (2002). Flavonoids uptake and their effect on cell cycle of human colon adenocarcinoma cells (Caco2). *Br J Cancer* **86**, 1645–1651.

18. Manach, C., Williamson, G., Morand, C., Scalbert, A. & Remesy, C. (2005). Bioavailability and bioefficacy of polyphenols in humans. I. Review of 97 bioavailability studies. *Am J Clin Nutr* **81**, 230S–242S.

19. Shimoi, K., Okada, H., Furugori, M., Goda, T., Takase, S., Suzuki, M., Hara, Y., Yamamoto, H. & Kinae, N. (1998). Intestinal absorption of luteolin and luteolin 7-*O*-beta-glucoside in rats and humans. *FEBS Lett* **438**, 220–224.

20. Spencer, J. P., Chowrimootoo, G., Choudhury, R., Debnam, E. S., Srai, S. K. & Rice-Evans, C. (1999). The small intestine can both absorb and glucuronidate luminal flavonoids. *FEBS Lett* **458**, 224–230.

21. Scalbert, A. & Williamson, G. (2000). Dietary intake and bioavailability of polyphenols. *J Nutr* **130**, 2073S–2085S.

22. Manach, C., Morand, C., Crespy, V., Demigne, C., Texier, O., Regerat, F. & Remesy, C. (1998). Quercetin is recovered in human plasma as conjugated derivatives which retain antioxidant properties. *FEBS Lett* **426**, 331–336.

23. Day, A. J., Bao, Y., Morgan, M. R. & Williamson, G. (2000). Conjugation position of quercetin glucuronides and effect on biological activity. *Free Radic Biol Med* **29**, 1234–1243.

24. Volate, S. R., Davenport, D. M., Muga, S. J. & Wargovich, M. J. (2005). Modulation of aberrant crypt foci and apoptosis by dietary herbal supplements (quercetin, curcumin, silymarin, ginseng and rutin). *Carcinogenesis* **26**, 1450–1456.

25. Dihal, A. A., Woutersen, R. A., Ommen, B. V., Rietjens, I. M. & Stierum, R. H. (2006). Modulatory effects of quercetin on proliferation and differentiation of the human colorectal cell line Caco-2. *Cancer Lett* **238**, 248–259.

26. Erlund, I., Kosonen, T., Alfthan, G., Mäenpää, J., Perttunen, K., Kenraali, J., Parantainen, J. & Aro, A. (2000). Pharmacokinetics of quercetin from quercetin aglycone and rutin in healthy volunteers. *Eur J Clin Pharmacol* **56**, 545–553.

27. Soleas, G. J., Yan, J. & Goldberg, D. M. (2001). Measurement of trans-resveratrol, (+)-catechin, and quercetin in rat and human blood and urine by gas chromatography with mass selective detection. *Methods Enzymol* **335**, 130–145.

28. Freireich, E. J., Gehan, E. A., Rall, D. P., Schmidt, L. H. & Skipper, H. E. (1966). Quantitative comparison of toxicity of anticancer agents in mouse, rat, hamster, dog, monkey, and man. *Cancer Chemother Rep* **50**, 219–244.

29. Hollman, P. C., van Trijp, J. M., Buysman, M. N., van der Gaag, M. S., Mengelers, M. J., de Vries, J. H. & Katan, M. B. (1997). Relative bioavailability of the antioxidant flavonoid quercetin from various foods in man. *FEBS Lett* **418**, 152–156.

30. Ferry, D. R., Smith, A., Malkhandi, J., Fyfe, D. W., deTakats, P. G., Anderson, D., Baker, J. & Kerr, D. J. (1996). Phase I clinical trial of the flavonoid quercetin: Pharmacokinetics and evidence for *in vivo* tyrosine kinase inhibition. *Clin Cancer Res* **2**, 659–668.

31. Manach, C., Morand, C., Texier, O., Favier, M. L., Agullo, G., Demigne, C., Regerat, F. & Remesy, C. (1995). Quercetin metabolites in plasma of rats fed diets containing rutin or quercetin. *J Nutr* **125**, 1911–1922.

32. Pietta, P. G. (2000). Flavonoids as antioxidants. *J Nat Prod* **63**, 1035–1042.

33. Murota, K. & Terao, J. (2003). Antioxidative flavonoid quercetin: Implication of its intestinal absorption and metabolism. *Arch Biochem Biophys* **417**, 12–17.

34. Robak, J. & Gryglewski, R. J. (1988). Flavonoids are scavengers of superoxide anions. *Biochem Pharmacol* **37**, 837–841.

35. Negre-Salvayre, A. & Salvayre, R. (1992). Quercetin prevents the cytotoxicity of oxidized LDL on lymphoid cell lines. *Free Radic Biol Med* **12**, 101–106.

36. Filipe, P., Haigle, J., Silva, J. N., Freitas, J., Fernandes, A., Maziere, J. C., Maziere, C., Santus, R. & Morliere, P. (2004). Anti- and pro-oxidant effects of quercetin in copper-induced low density lipoprotein oxidation. Quercetin as an effective antioxidant against pro-oxidant effects of urate. *Eur J Biochem* **271**, 1991–1999.

37. Alía, M., Ramos, S., Mateos, R., Granado-Serrano, A. B., Bravo, L. & Goya, L. (2006). Quercetin protects human hepatoma HepG2 against oxidative stress induced by tert-butyl hydroperoxide. *Toxicol Appl Pharmacol* **212**, 110–118.

38. Chang, Y. F., Chi, C. W. & Wang, J. J. (2006). Reactive oxygen species production is involved in quercetin-induced apoptosis in human hepatoma cells. *Nutr Cancer* **55**, 209.

39. Ferraresi, R., Troiano, L., Roat, E., Lugli, E., Nemes, E., Nasi, M., Pinti, M., Fernandez, M. I., Cooper, E. L. & Cossarizza, A. (2005). Essential requirement of reduced glutathione (GSH) for the anti-oxidant effect of the flavonoid quercetin. *Free Radic Res* **39**, 1249–1258.

40. Formica, J. V. & Regelson, W. (1995). Review of the biology of Quercetin and related bioflavonoids. *Food Chem Toxicol* **33**, 1061–1080.

41. Spencer, J. P., Kuhnle, G. G., Williams, R. J. & Rice-Evans, C. (2003). Intracellular metabolism and bioactivity of quercetin and its *in vivo* metabolites. *Biochem J* **372**, 173–181.

42. Rohrdanz, E., Bittner, A., Tran-Thi, Q. H. & Kahl, R. (2003). The effect of quercetin on the mRNA expression of different antioxidant enzymes in hepatoma cells. *Arch Toxicol* **77**, 506–510.

43. Wilms, L. C., Hollman, P. C., Boots, A. W. & Kleinjans, J. C. (2005). Protection by quercetin and quercetin-rich fruit juice against induction of oxidative DNA damage and formation of BPDE-DNA adducts in human lymphocytes. *Mutat Res* **582**, 155–162.

44. Choi, E. J., Chee, K. M. & Lee, B. H. (2003). Anti- and prooxidant effects of chronic quercetin administration in rats. *Eur J Pharmacol* **482**, 281–285.

45. Choi, E. J., Lee, B. H., Lee, K. & Chee, K. M. (2005). Long-term combined administration of quercetin and daidzein inhibits quercetin-induced suppression of glutathione antioxidant defenses. *Food Chem Toxicol* **43**, 793–798.

46. Valerio, L. G., Jr., Kepa, J. K., Pickwell, G. V. & Quattrochi, L. C. (2001). Induction of human NAD(P)H:quinone oxidoreductase (NQO1) gene expression by the flavonol quercetin. *Toxicol Lett* **119**, 49–57.

47. Thangasamy, T., Sittadjody, S., Lanza-Jacoby, S., Wachsberger, P., Limesand, K. & Burd, R. (2007). Quercetin selectively inhibits bioreduction and enhances apoptosis in melanoma cells that overexpress tyrosinase. *Nutr Cancer* **59**, 1–11.

48. Gliszczynska-Swiglo, A., van der Woude, H., de Haan, L., Tyrakowska, B., Aarts, J. M. & Rietjens, I. M. (2003). The role of quinone reductase (NQO1) and quinone chemistry in quercetin cytotoxicity. *Toxicol In Vitro* **17**, 423–431.

49. Boots, A. W., Bast, A. & Haenen, G. R. (2005). No role of DT-diaphorase (NQO1) in the protection against oxidized quercetin. *FEBS Lett* **579**, 677–682.

50. Asher, G., Lotem, J., Kama, R., Sachs, L. & Shaul, Y. (2002). NQO1 stabilizes p53 through a distinct pathway. *Proc Natl Acad Sci USA* **99**, 3099–3104.

51. Asher, G., Lotem, J., Cohen, B., Sachs, L. & Shaul, Y. (2001). Regulation of p53 stability and p53-dependent apoptosis by NADH quinone oxidoreductase 1. *Proc Natl Acad Sci USA* **98**, 1188–1193.

52. Anwar, A., Dehn, D., Siegel, D., Kepa, J. K., Tang, L. J., Pietenpol, J. A. & Ross, D. (2003). Interaction of human NAD(P)H:quinone oxidoreductase 1 (NQO1) with the tumor suppressor protein p53 in cells and cell-free systems. *J Biol Chem* **278**, 10368–10373.

53. Nguyen, T. T., Tran, E., Nguyen, T. H., Do, P. T., Huynh, T. H. & Huynh, H. (2004). The role of activated MEK-ERK pathway in quercetin-induced growth inhibition and apoptosis in A549 lung cancer cells. *Carcinogenesis* **25**, 647–659.

54. Walker, E. H., Pacold, M. E., Perisic, O., Stephens, L., Hawkins, P. T., Wymann, M. P. & Williams, R. L. (2000). Structural determinants of phosphoinositide 3-kinase inhibition by wortmannin, LY294002, quercetin, myricetin, and staurosporine. *Mol Cell* **6**, 909–919.

55. Warngard, L., Flodstrom, S., Ljungquist, S. & Ahlborg, U. G. (1987). Interaction between quercetin, TPA and DDT in the V79 metabolic cooperation assay. *Carcinogenesis* **8**, 1201–1205.

56. Park, C. H., Chang, J. Y., Hahm, E. R., Park, S., Kim, H. K. & Yang, C. H. (2005). Quercetin, a potent inhibitor against beta-catenin/Tcf signaling in SW480 colon cancer cells. *Biochem Biophys Res Commun* **328**, 227–234.

57. Levine, A. J. (1997). p53, the cellular gatekeeper for growth and division. *Cell* **88**, 323–331.

58. Kuo, P. C., Liu, H. F. & Chao, J. I. (2004). Survivin and p53 modulate quercetin-induced cell growth inhibition and apoptosis in human lung carcinoma cells. *J Biol Chem* **279**, 55875–55885.

59. Watjen, W., Michels, G., Steffan, B., Niering, P., Chovolou, Y., Kampkotter, A., Tran-Thi, Q. H., Proksch, P. & Kahl, R. (2005). Low concentrations of flavonoids are protective in rat H4IIE cells whereas high concentrations cause DNA damage and apoptosis. *J Nutr* **135**, 525–531.

60. Balabhadrapathruni, S., Thomas, T. J., Yurkow, E. J., Amenta, P. S. & Thomas, T. (2000). Effects of genistein and structurally related phytoestrogens on cell cycle kinetics and apoptosis in MDA-MB-468 human breast cancer cells. *Oncol Rep* **7**, 3–12.

61. Maggiolini, M., Bonofiglio, D., Marsico, S., Panno, M. L., Cenni, B., Picard, D. & Ando, S. (2001). Estrogen receptor alpha mediates the proliferative but not the cytotoxic dose-dependent effects of two major phytoestrogens on human breast cancer cells. *Mol. Pharmacol* **60**, 595–602.

62. Damianaki, A., Bakogeorgou, E., Kampa, M., Notas, G., Hatzoglou, A., Panagiotou, S., Gemetzi, C., Kouroumalis, E., Martin, P. M. & Castanas, E. (2000). Potent inhibitory action of red wine polyphenols on human breast cancer cells. *J Cell Biochem* **78**, 429–441.

63. Han, D. H., Denison, M. S., Tachibana, H. & Yamada, K. (2002). Relationship between estrogen receptor-binding and estrogenic activities of environmental estrogens and suppression by flavonoids. *Biosci Biotechnol Biochem* **66**, 1479–1487.

64. van der, W. H., Gliszczynska-Swiglo, A., Struijs, K., Smeets, A., Alink, G. M. & Rietjens, I. M. (2003). Biphasic modulation of cell proliferation by quercetin at concentrations physiologically relevant in humans. *Cancer Lett* **200**, 41–47.

65. Elattar, T. M. & Virji, A. S. (2000). The inhibitory effect of curcumin, genistein, quercetin and cisplatin on the growth of oral cancer cells *in vitro*. *Anticancer Res*. **20**, 1733–1738.

66. Ong, C. S., Tran, E., Nguyen, T. T., Ong, C. K., Lee, S. K., Lee, J. J., Ng, C. P., Leong, C. & Huynh, H. (2004). Quercetin-induced growth inhibition and cell death in nasopharyngeal carcinoma cells are associated with increase in Bad and hypophosphorylated retinoblastoma expressions. *Oncol Rep* **11**, 727–733.

67. Gupta, K. & Panda, D. (2002). Perturbation of microtubule polymerization by quercetin through tubulin binding: A novel mechanism of its antiproliferative activity. *Biochemistry* **41**, 13029–13038.

68. Zhang, X. M., Chen, J., Xia, Y. G. & Xu, Q. (2005). Apoptosis of murine melanoma B16-BL6 cells induced by quercetin targeting mitochondria, inhibiting expression of PKC-alpha and translocating PKC-delta. *Cancer Chemother Pharmacol* **55**, 251–262.

69. Jakubowicz-Gil, J., Paduch, R., Piersiak, T., Glowniak, K., Gawron, A. & Kandefer-Szerszen, M. (2005). The effect of quercetin on pro-apoptotic activity of cisplatin in HeLa cells. *Biochem Pharmacol* **69**, 1343–1350.

70. Asea, A., Ara, G., Teicher, B. A., Stevenson, M. A. & Calderwood, S. K. (2001). Effects of the flavonoid drug quercetin on the response of human prostate tumours to hyperthermia *in vitro* and *in vivo*. *Int J Hyperthermia* **17**, 347–356.

71. Gugler, R., Leschik, M. & Dengler, H. J. (1975). Disposition of quercetin in man after single oral and intravenous doses. *Eur J Clin Pharmacol* **9**, 229–234.

72. Verma, A. K., Johnson, J. A., Gould, M. N. & Tanner, M. A. (1988). Inhibition of 7,12-dimethylbenz(a)anthracene- and *N*-nitrosomethylurea-induced rat mammary cancer by dietary flavonol quercetin. *Cancer Res* **48**, 5754–5758.

73. Molnar, J., Beladi, I., Domonkos, K., Foldeak, S., Boda, K. & Veckenstedt, A. (1981). Antitumor activity of flavonoids on NK/Ly ascites tumor cells. *Neoplasma* **28**, 11–18.

74. Ferrer, P., Asensi, M., Segarra, R., Ortega, A., Benlloch, M., Obrador, E., Varea, M. T., Asensio, G., Jorda, L. & Estrela, J. M. (2005). Association between pterostilbene and quercetin inhibits metastatic activity of B16 melanoma. *Neoplasia* **7**, 37–47.

75. Femia, A. P., Caderni, G., Ianni, M., Salvadori, M., Schijlen, E., Collins, G., Bovy, A. & Dolara, P. (2003). Effect of diets fortified with tomatoes or onions

with variable quercetin-glycoside content on azoxymethane-induced aberrant crypt foci in the colon of rats. *Eur J Nutr* **42**, 346–352.

76. Lamson, D. W. & Brignall, M. S. (2000). Antioxidants and cancer, part 3: Quercetin. *Altern Med Rev* **5**, 196–208.

77. Debes, A., Oerding, M., Willers, R., Gobel, U. & Wessalowski, R. (2003). Sensitization of human Ewing's tumor cells to chemotherapy and heat treatment by the bioflavonoid quercetin. *Anticancer Res* **23**, 3359–3366.

78. Mutoh, M., Takahashi, M., Fukuda, K., Komatsu, H., Enya, T., Matsushima-Hibiya, Y., Mutoh, H., Sugimura, T. & Wakabayashi, K. (2000). Suppression by flavonoids of cyclooxygenase-2 promoter-dependent transcriptional activity in colon cancer cells: Structure-activity relationship. *Jpn J Cancer Res* **91**, 686–691.

79. Raso, G. M., Meli, R., Di, C. G., Pacilio, M. & Di, C. R. (2001). Inhibition of inducible nitric oxide synthase and cyclooxygenase-2 expression by flavonoids in macrophage J774A.1. *Life Sci* **68**, 921–931.

80. Jones, D. J., Lamb, J. H., Verschoyle, R. D., Howells, L. M., Butterworth, M., Lim, C. K., Ferry, D., Farmer, P. B. & Gescher, A. J. (2004). Characterisation of metabolites of the putative cancer chemopreventive agent quercetin and their effect on cyclo-oxygenase activity. *Br J Cancer* **91**, 1213–1219.

81. Moon, J. H., Tsushida, T., Nakahara, K. & Terao, J. (2001). Identification of quercetin 3-*O*-beta-D-glucuronide as an antioxidative metabolite in rat plasma after oral administration of quercetin. *Free Radic Biol Med* **30**, 1274–1285.

82. Wittig, J., Herderich, M., Graefe, E. U. & Veit, M. (2001). Identification of quercetin glucuronides in human plasma by high-performance liquid chromatography-tandem mass spectrometry. *J Chromatogr B Biomed Sci Appl* **753**, 237–243.

83. Young, J. F., Nielsen, S. E., Haraldsdottir, J., Daneshvar, B., Lauridsen, S. T., Knuthsen, P., Crozier, A., Sandstrom, B. & Dragsted, L. O. (1999). Effect of fruit juice intake on urinary quercetin excretion and biomarkers of antioxidative status. *Am J Clin Nutr* **69**, 87–94.

84. Kim, H. Y., Kim, O. H. & Sung, M. K. (2003). Effects of phenol-depleted and phenol-rich diets on blood markers of oxidative stress, and urinary excretion of quercetin and kaempferol in healthy volunteers. *J Am Coll Nutr* **22**, 217–223.

85. Radtke, J., Linseisen, J. & Wolfram, G. (2002). Fasting plasma concentrations of selected flavonoids as markers of their ordinary dietary intake. *Eur J Nutr* **41**, 203–209.

86. Morand, C., Crespy, V., Manach, C., Besson, C., Demigne, C. & Remesy, C. (1998). Plasma metabolites of quercetin and their antioxidant properties. *Am J Physiol* **275**, R212–R219.

87. Conquer, J. A., Maiani, G., Azzini, E., Raguzzini, A. & Holub, B. J. (1998). Supplementation with quercetin markedly increases plasma quercetin concentration without effect on selected risk factors for heart disease in healthy subjects. *J Nutr* **128**, 593–597.

88. Ishii, K., Furuta, T. & Kasuya, Y. (2003). High-performance liquid chromatographic determination of quercetin in human plasma and urine utilizing solid-phase extraction and ultraviolet detection. *J Chromatogr B Analyt Technol Biomed Life Sci* **794**, 49–56.

89. Okamoto, T. (2005). Safety of quercetin for clinical application (Review). *Int J Mol Med* **16**, 275–278.

90. Silberberg, M., Morand, C., Manach, C., Scalbert, A. & Remesy, C. (2005). Co-administration of quercetin and catechin in rats alters their absorption but not their metabolism. *Life Sci* **77**, 3156–3167.

91. Pamukcu, A. M., Yalciner, S., Hatcher, J. F. & Bryan, G. T. (1980). Quercetin, a rat intestinal and bladder carcinogen present in bracken fern (*Pteridium aquilinum*). *Cancer Res* **40**, 3468–3472.

92. Ambrose, A. M., Robbins, D. J. & Deeds, F. (1952). Comparative toxicities of quercetin and quercitrin. *J Am Pharm Assoc* **41**, 119–122.

93. Matsukawa, Y., Nishino, H., Okuyama, Y., Matsui, T., Matsumoto, T., Matsumura, S., Shimizu, Y., Sowa, Y. & Sakai, T. (1997). Effects of quercetin and/or restraint stress on formation of aberrant crypt foci induced by azoxymethane in rat colons. *Oncology* **54**, 118–121.

94. Hirono, I., Ueno, I., Hosaka, S., Takanashi, H., Matsushima, T., Sugimura, T. & Natori, S. (1981). Carcinogenicity examination of quercetin and rutin in ACI rats. *Cancer Lett* **13**, 15–21.

95. Sankarasharma, D., Ganapathy, V. & Shyamaladevi, C. S. (2006). Suppression of tumor growth and invasion in 9,10 dimethyl benz(*a*) anthracene induced mammary carcinoma by the plant bioflavonoid quercetin. *Chem Biol Interact* **162**, 106–113.

96. Gee, J. M., Hara, H. & Johnson, I. T. (2002). Suppression of intestinal crypt cell proliferation and aberrant crypt foci by dietary quercetin in rats. *Nutr Cancer* **43**, 193–201.

97. Castillo, M. H., Perkins, E., Campbell, J. H., Doerr, R., Hassett, J. M., Kandaswami, C. & Middleton, E., Jr. (1989). The effects of the bioflavonoid quercetin on squamous cell carcinoma of head and neck origin. *Am J Surg* **158**, 351–355.

98. Morino, K., Matsukara, N., Kawachi, T., Ohgaki, H., Sugimura, T. & Hirono, I. (1982). Carcinogenicity test of quercetin and rutin in golden hamsters by oral administration. *Carcinogenesis* **3**, 93–97.

99. van Erk, M. J., Roepman, P., van der Lende, T. R., Stierum, R. H., Aarts, J. M., van Bladeren, P. J. & van Ommen, B. (2005). Integrated assessment by multiple gene expression analysis of quercetin bioactivity on anticancer-related mechanisms in colon cancer cells *in vitro*. *Eur J Nutr* **44**, 143–156.

100. Ranelletti, F. O., Maggiano, N., Serra, F. G., Ricci, R., Larocca, L. M., Lanza, P., Scambia, G., Fattorossi, A., Capelli, A. & Piantelli, M. (2000). Quercetin inhibits p21-RAS expression in human colon cancer cell lines and in primary colorectal tumors. *Int J Cancer* **85**, 438–445.

101. Yang, J. H., Hsia, T. C., Kuo, H. M., Lee Chao, P. D., Chou, C. C., Wei, Y. H. & Chung, J. G. (2006). Inhibition of lung cancer cell growth by quercetin glucuronides via G2/M arrest and induction of apoptosis. *Drug Metab Dispos* **34**, 296–304.

102. Son, Yo., Kook, S. H., Choi, K. C., Jang, Y. S., Jeon, Y. M., Lee, K. Y., Kim, J., Chung, M. S., Chung, G. H. & Lee, J. C. (2006). Quercetin, a bioflavonoid, accelerates TNF-alpha-induced growth inhibition and apoptosis in MC3T3-E1 osteoblastic cells. *Eur J Pharmacol* **529**, 24–32.

103. Lee, T. J., Kim, O. H., Kim, Y. H., Lim, J. H., Kim, S., Park, J. W. & Kwon, T. K. (2006). Quercetin arrests G2/M phase and induces caspase-dependent cell death in U937 cells. *Cancer Lett* **240**, 234–242.

104. Brisdelli, F., Coccia, C., Cinque, B., Cifone, M. G. & Bozzi, A. (2007). Induction of apoptosis by quercetin: Different response of human chronic myeloid (K562) and acute lymphoblastic (HSB-2) leukemia cells. *Mol Cell Biochem* **296**, 137–149.

105. Mu, C., Jia, P., Yan, Z., Liu, X., Li, X. & Liu, H. (2007). Quercetin induces cell cycle G1 arrest through elevating Cdk inhibitors p21 and p27 in human hepatoma cell line (HepG2). *Methods Find Exp Clin Pharmacol* **29**, 179–183.

106. Granado-Serrano, A. B., Martín, M. A., Bravo, L., Goya, L. & Ramos, S. (2006). Quercetin induces apoptosis via caspase activation, regulation of Bcl-2, and inhibition of PI-3-kinase/Akt and ERK pathways in a human hepatoma cell line (HepG2). *J Nutr* **136**, 2715–2721.

107. Kim, W. K., Bang, M. H., Kim, E. S., Kang, N. E., Jung, K. C., Cho, H. J. & Park, J. H. (2005). Quercetin decreases the expression of ErbB2 and ErbB3 proteins in HT-29 human colon cancer cells. *J Nutr Biochem* **16**, 155–162.

108. Horvathova, K., Novotny, L., Tothova, D. & Vachalkova, A. (2004). Determination of free radical scavenging activity of quercetin, rutin, luteolin and apigenin in H2O2-treated human ML cells K562. *Neoplasma* **51**, 395–399.

109. Robaszkiewicz, A., Balcerczyk, A. & Bartosz, G. (2007). Antioxidative and prooxidative effects of quercetin on A549 cells. *Cell Biol Int* **31**, 1245–1250.

110. Yoshida, M., Sakai, T., Hosokawa, N., Marui, N., Matsumoto, K., Fujioka, A., Nishino, H. & Aoike, A. (1990). The effect of quercetin on cell cycle progression and growth of human gastric cancer cells. *FEBS Lett* **260**, 10–13.

111. Triantafyllou, A., Liakos, P., Tsakalof, A., Chachami, G., Paraskeva, E., Molyvdas, P. A., Georgatsou, E., Simos, G. & Bonanou, S. (2007). The flavonoid quercetin induces hypoxia-inducible factor-1alpha (HIF-1alpha) and inhibits cell proliferation by depleting intracellular iron. *Free Radic Res* **41**, 342–356.

112. Avila, M. A., Velasco, J. A., Cansado, J. & Notario, V. (1994). Quercetin mediates the down-regulation of mutant p53 in the human breast cancer cell line MDA-MB468. *Cancer Res* **54**, 2424–2428.

113. McAnlis, G. T., McEneny, J., Pearce, J. & Young, I. S. (1999). Absorption and antioxidant effects of quercetin from onions, in man. *Eur J Clin Nutr* **53**, 92–96.

114. Aziz, A. A., Edwards, C. A., Lean, M. E. & Crozier, A. (1998). Absorption and excretion of conjugated flavonols, including quercetin-4'-*O*-beta-glucoside and isorhamnetin-4'-*O*-beta-glucoside by human volunteers after the consumption of onions. *Free Radic Res* **29**, 257–269.

115. de Vries, J. H., Hollman, P. C., Meyboom, S., Buysman, M. N., Zock, P. L., van Staveren, W. A. & Katan, M. B. (1998). Plasma concentrations and urinary excretion of the antioxidant flavonols quercetin and kaempferol as biomarkers for dietary intake. *Am J Clin Nutr* **68**, 60–65.

116. Hollman, P. C., vd, G. M., Mengelers, M. J., van Trijp, J. M., de Vries, J. H. & Katan, M. B. (1996). Absorption and disposition kinetics of the dietary antioxidant quercetin in man. *Free Radic Biol Med* **21**, 703–707.

117. Graefe, E. U., Wittig, J., Mueller, S., Riethling, A. K., Uehleke, B., Drewelow, B., Pforte, H., Jacobasch, G., Derendorf, H. & Veit, M. (2001). Pharmacokinetics and bioavailability of quercetin glycosides in humans. *J Clin Pharmacol* **41**, 492–499.

118. Dávalos, A., Castilla, P., Gómez-Cordovés, C. & Bartolomé, B. (2006). Quercetin is bioavailable from a single ingestion of grape juice. *Int J Food Sci Nutr* **57**, 391–398.

119. Janssen, K., Mensink, R. P., Cox, F. J., Harryvan, J. L., Hovenier, R., Hollman, P. C. & Katan, M. B. (1998). Effects of the flavonoids quercetin and apigenin on hemostasis in healthy volunteers: Results from an *in vitro* and a dietary supplement study. *Am J Clin Nutr* **67**, 255–262.

120. Moon, J. H., Nakata, R., Oshima, S., Inakuma, T. & Terao, J. (2000). Accumulation of quercetin conjugates in blood plasma after the short-term ingestion of onion by women. *Am J Physiol Regul Integr Comp Physiol* **279**, R461–R467.

121. Murota, K., Hotta, A., Ido, H., Kawai, Y., Moon, J. H., Sekido, K., Hayashi, H., Inakuma, T. & Terao, J. (2007). Antioxidant capacity of albumin-bound quercetin metabolites after onion consumption in humans. *J Med Invest* **54**, 370–374.

122. Olthof, M. R., Hollman, P. C., Vree, T. B. & Katan, M. B. (2000). Bioavailabilities of quercetin-3-glucoside and quercetin-4'-glucoside do not differ in humans. *J Nutr* **130**, 1200–1203.

123. Hollman, P. C. & Katan, M. B. (1999). Health effects and bioavailability of dietary flavonols. *Free Radic Res* **31**(Suppl), S75–S80.

124. Boyle, S. P., Dobson, V. L., Duthie, S. J., Hinselwood, D. C., Kyle, J. A. & Collins, A. R. (2000). Bioavailability and efficiency of rutin as an antioxidant: A human supplementation study. *Eur J Clin Nutr* **54**, 774–782.

125. Graefe, E. U., Wittig, J., Mueller, S., Riethling, A. K., Uehleke, B., Drewelow, B., Pforte, H., Jacobasch, G., Derendorf, H. & Veit, M. (2001). Pharmacokinetics and bioavailability of quercetin glycosides in humans. *J Clin Pharmacol* **41**, 492–499.

126. Liu, G. A. & Zheng, R. L. (2002). Protection against damaged DNA in the single cell by polyphenols. *Pharmazie* **57**, 852–854.

127. Saito, A., Sugisawa, A., Umegaki, K. & Sunagawa, H. (2004). Protective effects of quercetin and its metabolites on H_2O_2-induced chromosomal damage to WIL2-NS cells. *Biosci Biotechnol Biochem* **68**, 271–276.

128. Spencer, J. P., Rice-Evans, C. & Williams, R. J. (2003). Modulation of pro-survival Akt/protein kinase B and ERK1/2 signaling cascades by quercetin and its *in vivo* metabolites underlie their action on neuronal viability. *J Biol Chem* **278**, 34783–34793.

129. Shen, S. C., Chen, Y. C., Hsu, F. L. & Lee, W. R. (2003). Differential apoptosis-inducing effect of quercetin and its glycosides in human promyeloleukemic HL-60 cells by alternative activation of the caspase 3 cascade. *J Cell Biochem* **89**, 1044–1055.

130. Yen, G. C., Duh, P. D., Tsai, H. L. & Huang, S. L. (2003). Pro-oxidative properties of flavonoids in human lymphocytes. *Biosci Biotechnol Biochem* **67**, 1215–1222.

131. Makris, D. P. & Rossiter, J. T. (2001). Comparison of quercetin and a non-orthohydroxy flavonol as antioxidants by competing *in vitro* oxidation reactions. *J Agric Food Chem* **49**, 3370–3377.

132. Rao, Y. K., Geethangili, M., Fang, S. H. & Tzeng, Y. M. (2007). Antioxidant and cytotoxic activities of naturally occurring phenolic and related compounds: A comparative study. *Food Chem Toxicol* **45**, 1770–1776.

133. Awad, H. M., Boersma, M. G., Vervoort, J. & Rietjens, I. M. (2000). Peroxidase-catalyzed formation of quercetin quinone methide-glutathione adducts. *Arch Biochem Biophys* **378**, 224–233.

134. Metodiewa, D., Jaiswal, A. K., Cenas, N., Dickancaite, E. & Segura-Aguilar, J. (1999). Quercetin may act as a cytotoxic prooxidant after its metabolic activation to semiquinone and quinoidal product. *Free Radic Biol Med* **26**, 107–116.

Index

(−)-epigallocatechin-3-gallate (EGCG), 377, 378, 380, 381, 382, 385
2-E-caffeoylfukiic acid, *see* Fukinolic acid
2-cyano-3,12-dioxooleana-1,9-dien-28-oic acid (CDDO), 215
3-hydroxy-3-methylglutaryl-coenzyme A (HMG-CoA) reductase, 118–19
5-hydroxytryptophan (5-HTP), 70–1
6-alpha-hydroxyadoxoside, 306
6-beta-7-beta-epoxy-8-epi-splendoside, 306
7,12-dimethylbenz[a]anthracene (DMBA), 166, 167
8-hydroxy-2-deoxyguanosine (8-OH-dG), 453
8-isoprostane F_{2a}, 424
9,19-cycloartane triterpenes, 204
17β-estradiol (E2), 169
25-acetylcimigenol xylopyranoside (ACCX), 206
β-carotene, 344
β-fibrillogenesis, 463
γ-glutamylcysteine synthetase (GCS), 361

A

Acetic acid, 434
Achilles tendinopathies, 34
Actaea racemosa, see Black cohosh
Actein, 196
Activator protein-1 (AP-1), 356, 455, 477, 491, 571
Adenosine A_1 receptors, 405
Adenosine A_{2A} receptors, 405
Adriamycin, 204
Advanced sleep phase disorder (ASPD), 60
   melatonin supplementation for, 69
Agathosma betulina, 185
Agency for Research Health and quality (AHRC), 36
Aglycones, 201, 373
Albumen, *see* Egg white
Alles zutraut, 137
Alzheimer's disease (AD), 97, 98
   caffeine effects on, 409–10

donepezil, 107, 108
   EGb 761, efficacy of, 106–7
   therapeutic applications for, 99
Alzheimer's disease assessment scale-cognitive subscale (ADAS-Cog), 106
Androgen excess/hirsutism, botanical treatments for, 322–3
Androgen receptor (AR), 456
Anemarrhena asphodeloides, 262
Angelica sinensis, 234, 257
Angiotensin-converting enzyme (ACE), 435
Anovulation, botanical treatments for, 319–23
Anthocyanidin, 419
Anthocyanins, 352–3, 356, 447, 461
Anthroposophic medicine and homeopathy:
   for epilepsy treatment:
      arnica, 88
      Belladonna and Hyoscyamus, 87–8
      Bufo Rana, 88
      Viscum album, 87
Anti-diol-epoxide, 167
Antiepilepsirine (AES), 86
Anti-inflammation and noni, 305–6
Antioxidants:
   flavonoids, 376–80
   in fruits and vegetables, 419–20
   melatonin, 452
   quercetin, 567–70
Anti-tumorigenic phytochemical compounds:
   and chemoprotection, in berries:
      in vitro evidence, 355–9
      in vivo evidence, 360–3
      theories, 353–5
Apigenin, 68, 138
Arbutin, 184
Arctostaphylos uva-ursi, 184
Arnica, 88
Aromatase, 456
Artepillin C (ARC), 531
Arthritis treatment:
   botanical and marine oils for, 1–11
Aryl hydrocarbon receptor (AHR), 214, 456

585

Printed and bound by CPI Group (UK) Ltd, Croydon, CR0 4YY

03/10/2024

01040416-0013